10/2003

Cutaneous Manifestations of Rheumatic Diseases

Second Edition

Cutaneous Manifestations of Rheumatic Diseases

Second Edition

Editors

Richard D. Sontheimer, M.D.
John S. Strauss Endowed Chair in Dermatology
Head, Department of Dermatology
University of Iowa College of Medicine
Chief of Dermatology Service
University of Iowa Hospitals and Clinics
Iowa City, Iowa

Thomas T. Provost, M.D.
Johns Hopkins Distinguished Service Professor
Noxell Professor and Chairman (Emeritus)
Department of Dermatology
Johns Hopkins Medical Institutions
Baltimore, Maryland

LIPPINCOTT WILLIAMS & WILKINS
A **Wolters Kluwer** Company
Philadelphia • Baltimore • New York • London
Buenos Aires • Hong Kong • Sydney • Tokyo

Acquisitions Editor: Danette Somers
Developmental Editor: Denise Martin
Project Editor: Sheila Higgins
Manufacturing Manager: Benjamin Rivera
Cover Designer: Karen Quigley
Compositor: Lippincott Williams & Wilkins Desktop Division
Printer: Maple Press

530 Walnut Street
Philadelphia, PA 19106 USA
LWW.com

Printed in the USA

Library of Congress Cataloging-in-Publication Data

Cutaneous manifestations of rheumatic diseases / editors, Richard D. Sontheimer, Thomas T. Provost—2nd ed.
p. ; cm.
Includes bibliographical references and index.
ISBN 0-7817-3478-9
1. Cutaneous manifestations of general diseases. 2. Rheumatism—Complications. 3. Connective tissues—Diseases—Complications. I. Sontheimer, Richard D. II. Provost, Thomas T.
[DNLM: 1. Skin Manifestations. 2. Rheumatic Diseases. WR 143 C989 2003]
RL100.C88 2003
616.5—dc21

2003052175

10 9 8 7 6 5 4 3 2 1

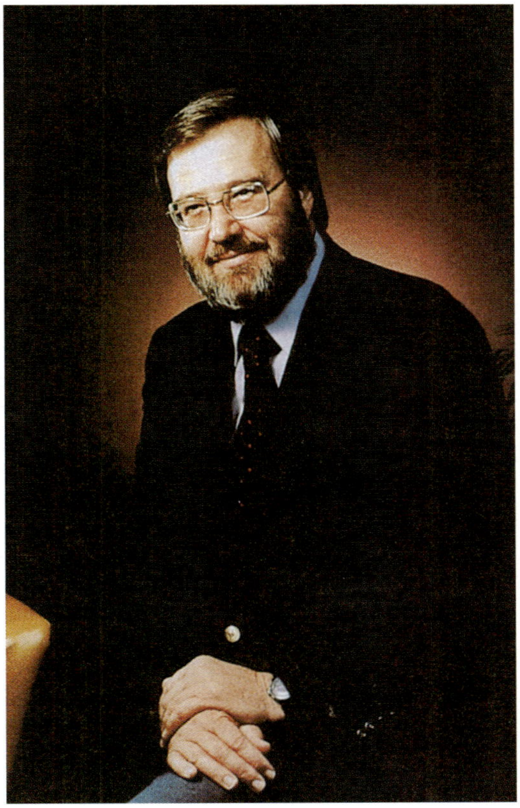

James N. Gilliam, M.D.
November 30, 1936–June 8, 1984

The idea for this book was originally conceived by Dr. James N. Gilliam who was serving as the Chairman of the Dermatology Department at the University of Texas Southwestern Medical Center at the time of his tragic and untimely death in 1984. Jim Gilliam was utterly fascinated by the plethora of ways that the skin can be affected by rheumatic disorders and how such cutaneous changes can be used to reflect the nature of the underlying systemic disease processes. On a number of occasions, he mentioned the need for a monograph that dealt with this subject specifically and in depth. As a memorial to our dear friend, mentor, and colleague, the editors and other contributors to this project have attempted to bring his idea to fruition.

Other thoughts concerning the measure of this warm-hearted physician-scholar and the impact that his brief but distinguished career had on the specialties of dermatology and rheumatology have been presented elsewhere (Bergstresser PR. In memoriam. *J Invest Dermatol* 1984;83:241; Sontheimer RD. Festschrift to Professor James N. Gilliam. *Clin Dermatol* 1988;6:1–2; and Norris DA, Bergstresser PR, Sontheimer RD. Dedication. *J Invest Dermatol* 1993;100:1S).

Contents

Contributing Authors

Jeffrey P. Callen, M.D.
Chief, Division of Dermatology
Professor of Medicine
Department of Dermatology
Univeristy of Louisville School of Medicine
Louisville, Kentucky

Benjamin F. Chong, B.A.
Department of Dermatology
Brigham & Women's Hospital
Boston, Massachusetts

M. Kari Connolly, M.D.
Associate Professor of Dermatology and Medicine
Department of Dermatology
University of California San Francisco
San Francisco, California

Melissa I. Costner, M.D.
Assistant Professor
Department of Dermatology
University of Texas Southwestern Medical Center
Dallas, Texas

Rebecca L. Euwer, M.D.
Clinical Associate Professor
Department of Dermatology
University of Texas Southwestern Medical Center
Dermatologist
Department of Internal Medicine
Robert H. Dedman Hospital
Dallas, Texas

Vincent Falanga, M.D.
Chairman
Department of Dermatology and Skin Surgery
Roger Williams Medical Center
Providence, Rhode Island

Steven R. Flint, B.D.S., M.B., Ph.D.
Senior Lecturer
School of Dental Science
Trinity College
Consultant
Department of Oral Medicine
Dublin Dental Hospital
Dublin, Ireland

Andrew G. Franks, Jr., M.D., F.A.C.P.
Clinical Professor
Department of Dermatology
New York University School of Medicine
Chief
Connective Tissue Disease Section
New York University Medical Center
New York, New York

Adam S. Greenberg, M.D.
Private Practice
Venice, Florida

Carlin B. Hollar, M.D.
Resident
Department of Dermatology
Wake Forest University School of Medicine
Winston-Salem, North Carolina

Joseph L. Jorizzo, M.D.
Professor and Chair
Department of Dermatology
North Carolina Baptist Hospital
Winston-Salem, North Carolina

Smeena Khan-Sabir, M.D.
Clinical Instructor
Department of Dermatology
Baylor University
Garland, Texas

Thomas S. Kupper, M.D.
Thomas B. Fitzpatrick Professor
Department of Dermatology
Harvard Medical School
Chairman
Department of Dermatology
Brigham & Women's Hospital
Boston, Massachusetts

Lela A. Lee, M.D.
Professor
Department of Dermatology and Medicine
University of Colorado School of Medicine
Chief, Dermatology Service
Denver Health Medical Center
Denver, Colorado

Daniel Mimouni, M.D.
Instructor
Department of Dermatology
Sackler Faculty of Medicine
Tel Aviv University
Tel Aviv, Israel
Rabin Medical Center
Petah Tiqva, Israel

Samuel L. Moschella, M.D.
Clinical Professor (Emeritus)
Department of Dermatology
Harvard Medical School
Cambridge, Massachusetts
Senior Consultant
Department of Dermatology
Lahey Clinic Foundation
Burlington, Massachusetts

Carlos H. Nousari, M.D.
Co-Director
Division of Dermatoimmunology
Assistant Professor
Department of Dermatology and Medicine
Johns Hopkins Hospital
Baltimore, Maryland

Warren W. Piette, M.D.
Professor and Vice-Chair
Department of Dermatology
University of Iowa
Roy J. and Lucille A. Carver College of Medicine
Iowa City, Iowa

Thomas T. Provost, M.D.
Johns Hopkins Distinguished Service Professor
Noxell Professor and Chairman (Emeritus)
Department of Dermatology
Johns Hopkins Medical Institutions
Baltimore, Maryland

Adrienne Rencic, M.D., Ph.D.
Clinical Instructor
Department of Dermatology
University of Maryland
Attending Dermatologist
Department of Internal Medicine
Mercy Medical Center
Baltimore, Maryland

Richard D. Sontheimer, M.D.
John S. Strauss Endowed Chair in Dermatology
Head, Department of Dermatology
University of Iowa College of Medicine
Chief of Dermatology Service
University of Iowa Hospitals and Clinics
Iowa City, Iowa

Denny L. Tuffanelli, M.D.
University of California
at San Francisco
San Francisco, Caifornia

Rosemarie Watson, M.D.
Lecturer
Department of Medicine
Trinity College
Consultant Dermatologist
Department of Dermatology
St. James Hospital
Dublin, Ireland

Victoria P. Werth, M.D.
Associate Professor
Department of Dermatology
University of Pennsylvania
Chief
Department of Dermatology
Philadelaphia VA Hospital
Philadelphia, Pennsylvania

William L. Weston, M.D.
Professor and Chairman (Emeritus)
Department of Dermatology
University of Colorado
School of Medicine
Denver, Colorado

Foreword

This second edition of *Cutaneous Manifestations of Rheumatic Diseases* is a book that will be valuable and interesting for all physicians caring for patients with rheumatic diseases.

Written entirely by dermatologists, this book describes in detail the skin findings in a broad range of diseases—from vasculitis to systemic rheumatic diseases to a host of diseases pairing polyarthritis with skin disease. Although there is a clear emphasis on the description of the cutaneous findings, there is a thorough analysis of the underlying pathogenic mechanisms that are most often immunologic. In addition to the emphasis on pathogenesis, all of the chapters contain sections on differential diagnosis, relationship of the skin disease to the systemic aspects of the disease, prognosis, and therapy.

The first chapter describes the innate and acquired immune systems in detail. Basically, all elements of these aspects of host defense are well developed in the skin where the organism meets the environment and, in most instances, disposes of the invading microbes. In a symmetry of literary structure, the final chapter spells out the details of immunosuppressive therapies and how they are applied to the management of the diseases described in this book. Although these drugs are useful in almost all of the diseases in this book, clearly the therapy of infectious disease affecting the skin and joints requires specific antibiotics appropriate for each particular infectious agent.

The heart of the book is composed of chapters on lupus erythematosus, dermatomyositis, systemic sclerosis, localized cutaneous sclerosis, Sjögren syndrome, rheumatoid and psoriatic arthritis, and primary systemic vasculitis. There are two chapters on assorted miscellaneous diseases that also affect the skin, and there is a concise chapter on rheumatic and cutaneous disease in children.

Although it is a daunting task to read this book in its entirety, physicians will be delighted to use this book as a reference when evaluating patients afflicted with these disorders. The quality and clarity of all these chapters is remarkable and will not only make the book useful, but will also provide intellectual pleasure to the reader.

Clearly, this is a group of physicians who in the tradition of the late Dr. James Gilliam are skilled at both the analysis of the skin pathology and a thorough understanding of the systemic rheumatic diseases existing in the patients described in this book. Those who use this book will be rewarded with new and deeper insights into the relationship of the skin diseases to the systemic rheumatic diseases that they accompany.

Morris Reichlin, M.D.
Oklahoma City, Oklahoma

Preface

During the past four decades, many dermatologists have spent considerable time studying the cutaneous manifestations of the autoimmune connective tissue (rheumatic) diseases. A good deal of knowledge has been amassed from these studies. Clinical manifestations, new cutaneous features, and pathophysiologic mechanisms have been elucidated.

Among this group was a cadre of physicians, trained in dermatology in the 1960s, who decided to devote a major part of their efforts to the study of the cutaneous manifestations of rheumatic diseases. Several individuals had extensive training in internal medicine. A number of individuals, but not all, sought training in basic immunology laboratories to carry out their studies. In addition, successful long-term collaborations with rheumatologists and immunologists were established. These collaborations contributed greatly to the data amassed. A special note of thanks must be given to immunologists Morris Ziff, Thomas Tomasi, Henry Claman, Morris Reichlin, Robert Good, Frank Austen, and others who opened their laboratories to dermatologists desiring specialized training. It is our hope that this book will serve to stimulate a future generation of dermatologists to pursue similar career paths and to devote their energy to the further advancement of this fascinating field.

The original concept of this book was to provide a comprehensive summary of information pertaining to the cutaneous manifestations of the disorders that concurrently affect the skin and musculoskeletal system. We believed that this might be best accomplished by having a group of dermatologists with significant personal experience in managing such diseases combine the elements of a color atlas with systematic, comprehensive discussions of these various disorders, focusing especially on the cutaneous manifestations and how the skin changes correlate with the underlying disease processes.

The Arthritis Foundation's *Primer on the Rheumatic Diseases (9th edition)* was used to compile the list of disorders covered in this book. Unfortunately, certain compromises were necessary to address all of these disorders. Publication constraints did not allow all aspects of each of these clinical disorders to be covered with equal depth. Space was just not available for comprehensive discussions of all topics such as pathology and etiology/pathogenesis. Perhaps this will become more feasible in the future.

Richard D. Sontheimer, M.D.
Thomas T. Provost, M.D.

Acknowledgments

The editors would like to acknowledge those in the Sontheimer clan (Liz, Kristin, CJ, Erin, Pat, John, and Buck) and the Provost clan (Carol, Chip, Christie, and Tommie) whose unceasing support over the years has been absolutely vital in providing the emotional foundation from which efforts such as this evolve. In addition, Dr. Sontheimer would like to thank his former chairman, Dr. Paul R. Bergstresser, for selflessly preserving and fostering an academic environment conducive to the completion of scholarly pursuits, such as the first edition of this book, in an era of ever-increasing financial constraints. There is an increasing threat that the growing financial constraints within U.S. academic healthcare centers might inhibit or eliminate such clinical scholarship endeavors in the future.

Several corporate sponsors contributed the financial support that made possible the liberal use of color illustrations in the first edition of this book that were vital to its success. These sponsors include Hoffmann La Roche Inc., Owen/Galderma, and Curatek Pharmaceuticals. Their patronage continues to be greatly appreciated.

Cutaneous Manifestations of Rheumatic Diseases

Second Edition

CHAPTER 1

The Cutaneous Immune System

A Skin-based Perspective on Immunology

Benjamin F. Chong and Thomas S. Kupper

As the interface that separates us from the outside environment, the skin is constantly exposed to potential pathogens. Skin has developed a series of defense mechanisms utilizing various elements to effectively combat infection. A well-developed host defense apparatus is essential to meeting the daunting challenge of fighting a vast array of microbes. The secret to the versatility of the host defense lies in the complex and synergistic interaction between two immune pathways: innate immunity and acquired immunity. Innate immunity, the more evolutionarily ancient of the two, provides a potent but limited defense against pathogens, whereas acquired immunity generates a plethora of antigen-specific responses that can expand and change over the course of the host's lifetime.

INNATE IMMUNITY

Innate immunity is a phylogenetically ancient defense mechanism; elements of innate immunity are shared by both vertebrates and invertebrates. Similar effector molecules and signaling pathways can be found in a wide range of animal and insect species (1). Because its function is to efficiently protect against a wide range of pathogens, innate immunity acts as the first line of defense, in part by enabling the recruitment of various leukocytes to sites of injury. All leukocytes share a common pathway in reaching areas of inflammation via a multistep process (discussed later).

Innate immunity provides immediate protection against invasion by pathogens. This happens in part through the receptor-mediated recognition of commonly shared constituents of pathogens, referred to as "pathogen-associated molecular patterns" (PAMPs). For example, lipopolysaccharides (LPSs), which are integral components of all gram-negative bacteria, can be easily detected by cell-surface receptors on leukocytes, such as macrophages and neutrophils (2). These pattern-recognition receptors (PRRs), which have evolved to bind to PAMPs, are often found on the cell surface, allowing them to initially bind to pathogens (3). Toll-like receptors (TLRs), which are human homologs of the *Drosophila* Toll protein, are examples of PRRs with ligands that include PAMPs (2); for example, TLR2 is the PRR that binds to LPS (Table 1.1). Binding through TLRs activates intracellular signaling pathways via induction of AP-1, nuclear factor κB (NF-κB), and mitogen-activated protein kinase transcription factors, which ultimately induces the expression of cytokines, chemokines, and adhesion molecules that recruit leukocytes to sites of inflammation (2).

In addition to PRRs and PAMPs, innate immunity also relies on secreted effector molecules, including complement proteins, acute-phase proteins, and antimicrobial peptides. Complement proteins, present in the plasma and on cell surfaces, contribute to the elimination of bacteria by recognizing and binding to carbohydrate residues expressed by these microbes. There are three pathways through which complement is activated: the classic, alternative, and lectin pathways. Whereas the alternative pathway proceeds spontaneously on the surface of bacteria, the lectin pathway requires the activation of complement by mannose-binding protein. A complex of mannose-binding protein and other proteins attaches to epitopes such as mannose or *N*-acetylglucosamine on the bacterial surface (5). After complement binds to these microorganisms, phagocytic cells expressing complement receptors bind and internalize these pathogens. Activated complement proteins can also directly lyse pathogens via a membrane attack complex (MAC) forming pores on their surface (6). If microorganisms evade these complement-mediated mechanisms, host cells can release cytokines that induce production of acute-phase proteins by the liver. Some of these, like C-reactive protein, bind to the surface of microbes, aiding in both the activation of complement and phagocytosis (7). See Walport (8) for a review of the alternative and mannose-binding lectin complement pathways.

One of the oldest features of innate immunity is the production of antimicrobial peptides by epithelial cells and leukocytes. Small antimicrobial peptides bind to the surface of bacteria, fungi, and viruses, and form pores, leading to cell injury and death. Two types of antimicrobial peptides, β-defensins and cathelicidins, have been located on mammalian skin as products of keratinocytes (9,10). In addition to their antimicrobial activity on epithelial tissue, β-defensins and cathelicidins can also act as chemokines for T cells and neutrophils, respectively (11,12). Their expression in the skin is either constitutive, such as the case for human β-defensin 1 (HBD-1), or inducible on

TABLE 1.1. Toll-Like Receptors

Toll-like Receptor	Ligands	Comments
TLR2	Peptidoglycan, bacterial lipoproteins, LPS from *Prophyromonas gingivitis* and *Leptospira interrogans,* phenol soluble factor from *Staphylococcus epidermidis,* glycosy phosphatidylinositol lipid from *Trypanosoma cruzi,* and zymosan from yeast cell walls	TLR2 recognizes ligands through heterodimer formation with TLR1 or TLR6.
TLR4	LPS on gram-negative bacteria, liptocheic acid, heat shock protein hsp60, fusion protein of respiratory syncytial virus	TLR4 also requires LPS-binding protein CD14, and MD-2 to recognize LPS. TLR4 is the first characterized mammalian TLR.
TLR5	Flagellin (bacteria flagella)	TLR5 recognizes the hydrophobic portion of flagellin.
TLR7	Imiquimod, R-848 (resiquimod) loxoribine, bropirimine	TLR7 recognizes Imiquimod (Aldara) which is used to treat malignant skin lesions.
TLR9	Unmethylated CpG motifs on bacterial DNA	Most mammals have methylated DNA, whereas bacteria do not. TLR9 may work intracellularly to bind to its ligand.

LPS, lipopolysaccharide; TLR, toll-like receptor.
From Janeway CA Jr, Medzhitov R. Innate immune recognition. *Annu Rev Immunol* 2002;20:197, and Akira S, Hemmi H. Recognition of pathogen-associated molecular patterns by TLR family. *Immunol Lett* 2003;85:85.

inflammatory stimuli (i.e., human β-defensin 2 [HBD-2] and LL-37 cathelicidin) (8,9). Low levels of HBD-2 and LL-37 cathelicidin may be responsible for the higher incidence of *Staphylococcus aureus* skin infections in patients with atopic dermatitis (12).

The skin is a major site where innate immunity mediates defense for the host. Although the stratum corneum of the epidermis provides a physical barrier separating the environment from the internal body, its disruption via trauma or microbial invasion results in the up-regulation of inflammatory mediators and antimicrobial peptides. Cytokines are soluble factors released by multiple cell types that bind to specific receptors on target cells and induce gene expression. Cells resident to the skin produce multiple cytokines, including so-called primary cytokines: interleukin-1 α (IL-1α), IL-1β, and tumor necrosis factor-α (TNF-α). These potent cytokines signal through receptors that share intracellular signaling pathways with the TLRs; indeed, the cytoplasmic domains of the TLRs and the type I IL-1R (IL-1 receptor) are homologous (13). Through activation of NFκB, AP-1, and mitogen-activated protein kinase pathways, these cytokines can induce expression of endothelial adhesion molecules, secondary cytokines, and chemokines that recruit leukocytes to the site of primary cytokine release (2). In the epidermis, both keratinocytes and Langerhans cells are capable of producing primary cytokines, and keratinocytes store preformed IL-1α, which can be released on disruption (14). In the dermis, mast cells store TNF-α for release, and resident dendritic cells (DCs) can release primary cytokines on stimulation (15). Other cytokines important in cutaneous inflammation are produced by T cells recruited to skin. Release of unique cytokines like interferon-γ (IFN-γ), IL-4, and IL-14, as well as primary cytokines like TNF-α and TNF-β, induces inflammation through additional pathways.

Chemokines are a subset of cytokines that are integral to the recruitment of leukocytes. Nearly every cell in the body can produce chemokines, which bind to specific G protein–coupled receptors on target cells. At last count, there were 45 chemokines and 19 chemokine receptors (16). In general, chemokines have two functions. The first is to activate leukocytes that are rolling along the surface of endothelial cells in postcapillary venules (described later). On activation, such leukocytes mobilize their integrins to bind firmly to ligands on the endothelium, resulting in firm adhesion and extravasation into tissue. Different chemokines target different subsets of leukocytes via unique chemokine receptors. Some chemokines are produced constitutively and mediate physiologic trafficking of cell into tissues (i.e., lymph nodes), whereas most others are induced by primary cytokines or T cell–derived cytokines (17). The other major function of chemokines is to form chemotactic gradients, attracting leukocytes that have already extravasated through tissue to the site of inflammation (described later).

Cells in the skin that produce chemokines and cytokines include keratinocytes, fibroblasts, and DCs. Activated keratinocytes produce several chemokines, including IL-8/CXCL1, GRO-α/CXCL2, IP-10/CXCL10, Mig/CXCL9, I-TAC/CXCL11, and CTACK/CCL27 (Table 1.2). Similarly, fibroblasts produce a similar assortment of chemokines, including RANTES/CCL5 and eotaxin/CCL11 (18) (Table 1.2). Langerhans cells produce a different set of chemokines including MIP-1α /CCL3 (19) and MDC/CCL22 (20) (Table 1.2). Certain chemokines are highly specific for certain target cells: For example, CXCL1 is specific for neutrophils, and CCL27 is specific for skin-homing T cells. Other chemokines chemoattract multiple cell types; for example, CCL5 binds to its various receptors (CCR1, -3, -5) on T cells, monocytes, eosinophils, and DCs (Table 1.2).

Despite their many differences, both innate and acquired immunity share a common set of pathways in the recruitment of leukocytes to sites of inflammation via the aid of adhesion molecules and their receptors. This process contains a series of steps that include (a) rolling and tethering of leukocytes along postcapillary venule endothelium, (b) activation of integrins on leukocytes, (c) firm adhesion of leukocytes on endothelium, and (d) extravasation of leukocytes. In the skin, inflammatory stimuli trigger a complex sequence of events that draws leukocytes to areas of damage. For example, microbial invasion results in the release of cytokines such as IL-1 and TNF-α, which bind to their receptors and initiate the NF-κB pathway, increasing the expression of adhesion molecules (i.e., E-selectin) and chemokines in the postcapillary venule endothelium. Skin-homing leukocytes carry unique markers that help them reach their destination. One of them is CLA (cutaneous lymphocyte-associated antigen), whose attachment to E-selectin initiates the tethering (binding under physiologic flow) and rolling of leukocytes along the vessel wall. This decrease in velocity increases the chance for further binding between chemokines present on the endothelium and chemokine receptors on leukocytes, resulting in a conformational shape change of leukocyte integrins (i.e., LFA-1 [lymphocyte function-associated antigen-1]) that facilitate their binding to their ligands (i.e., ICAM-1 [intercellular adhesion molecule-1]). The binding of activated inte-

TABLE 1.2. Chemokines Involved in Directing Leukocytes to Skin

Chemokine	Receptor	Origin of Expression in Skin	Constitutive or Inducible	Function
CC Chemokines				
MCP-1 (CCL2)	CCR2	Keratinocytes, endothelial cells	Constitutive, inducible	Integrin activation and extravasation of monocytes, chemotaxis of lymphocytes and monocytes
MIP-1α (CCL3)	CCR1,5	Langerhans cells	Inducible	Chemotaxis of eosinophils, monocytes, lymphocytes
RANTES (CCL5)	CCR1,3,5	Keratinocytes, endothelial cells, dermal fibroblasts	Inducible	Integrin activation of eosinophils, chemotaxis of eosinophils, monocytes, and lymphocytes
MCP-3 (CCL7)	CCR1,2,3	Dermal fibroblasts	Inducible	Integrin activation of eosinophils, chemotaxis of eosinophils and lymphocytes
MCP-2 (CCL8)	CCR3	—	Inducible	Chemotaxis of eosinophils and lymphocytes
Eotaxin (CCL11)	CCR3	Dermal fibroblasts, keratinocytes	Inducible	Chemotaxis of eosinophils
MCP-4 (CCL13)	CCR2,3	Dermal fibroblasts	Inducible	Chemotaxis of eosinophils and monocytes
TARC (CCL17)	CCR4	Keratinocytes, endothelial cells, dendritic cells	Constitutive, inducible	Integrin activation of lymphocytes (i.e., T_H2 cells)
LARC (MIP-3α, CCL20)	CCR6	Keratinocytes, endothelial cells, dendritic cells, dermal fibroblasts	Constitutive, inducible	Integrin activation and chemotaxis of lymphocytes
MDC (CCL22)	CCR4	Dermal dendritic cells, mature Langerhans cells, keratinocytes	Constitutive, inducible	Chemotaxis of lymphocytes (i.e., T_H2 cells)
Eotaxin-2 (CCL24)	CCR3	Dermal fibroblasts	Inducible	Chemotaxis of eosinophils
CTACK (CCL27)	CCR10	Keratinocytes	Constitutive, inducible	Chemotaxis of lymphocytes
CXC Chemokines				
GRO-α (CXCL1)	CXCR2	Keratinocytes, endothelial cells	Inducible	Integrin activation and chemotaxis of neutrophils
ENA-78 (CXCL5)	CXCR2	—	Inducible	Chemotaxis of neutrophils
IL-8 (CXCL8)	CXCR1,2	Keratinocytes, endothelial cells	Inducible	Integrin activation and chemotaxis of neutrophils
Mig (CXCL9)	CXCR3	Keratinocytes, endothelial cells	Inducible	Chemotaxis of lymphocytes (i.e., T_H1 cells)
IP-10 (CXCL10)	CXCR3	Keratinocytes, endothelial cells	Inducible	Chemotaxis of lymphocytes (i.e., T_H1 cells)
I-TAC (CXCL11)	CXCR3	Keratinocytes	Inducible	Chemotaxis of lymphocytes (i.e., T_H1 cells)
Fractalkine (CX_3CL1)	CX_3CR1	Endothelial cells, dermal APCs	Constitutive, inducible	Extravasation and chemotaxis of lymphocytes

APCs, antigen-presenting cells.
From Olson TS, Ley K. Chemokines and chemokine receptors in leukocyte trafficking. *Am J Physiol Regul Integr Comp Physiol* 2002;283:R7, with permission.

grins to endothelial adhesion molecules allows leukocytes to firmly adhere and flatten against the endothelium in preparation for extravasation into the skin. After passing between endothelial cells to enter the skin, the leukocytes follow a chemotactic gradient established by chemokines directing them to sites of injury (21–23) (Fig. 1.1). It is important to recall that both neutrophils (of the innate immune system) and T cells (of the acquired immune system) use this multistep pathway, albeit with cell-specific variations on the theme.

Innate immunity is powerful and can be mobilized rapidly. It is the sole form of immunity used by invertebrates. Its repertoire, however, is limited, and microorganisms can evolve to evade its weapons. Another weakness of innate immunity is its lack of memory. That is, the innate immune system responds to each attack by a pathogen in the same fashion and with the same kinetics. In contrast, the acquired immune system (discussed later) does have the features that are consistent with memory. Clonally expanded (memory) T and B cells respond to subsequent challenges by pathogens differently—qualitatively and quantitatively—than their response to the initial encounter. Finally, it is important to appreciate that innate immunity and acquired immunity work together synergistically and are codependent. A successful immune response uses elements of both systems.

ACQUIRED IMMUNITY

Although innate immunity can effectively combat common microbial infections, it is limited in its reliance on recognition of common surface patterns in pathogens. Acquired immunity, which is exclusive to vertebrates, can provide a stronger line of defense by recognizing a nearly unlimited range of pathogens through its highly specific antigen recognition capabilities. This capacity is mediated through antigen receptors, which are derived from complex genes that genetically recombine their germline DNA to form novel cell-specific coding sequences. In B cells, these are known as antibodies or immunoglobulins, whereas in T cells, they are known generically as T cell receptors. The precise pattern of gene recombination, and thus the specific sequence of the T cell or B cell receptor protein, is unique to each naïve lymphocyte. Different subgroups of specific regions of antigen-receptor genes, known as V (variable), D

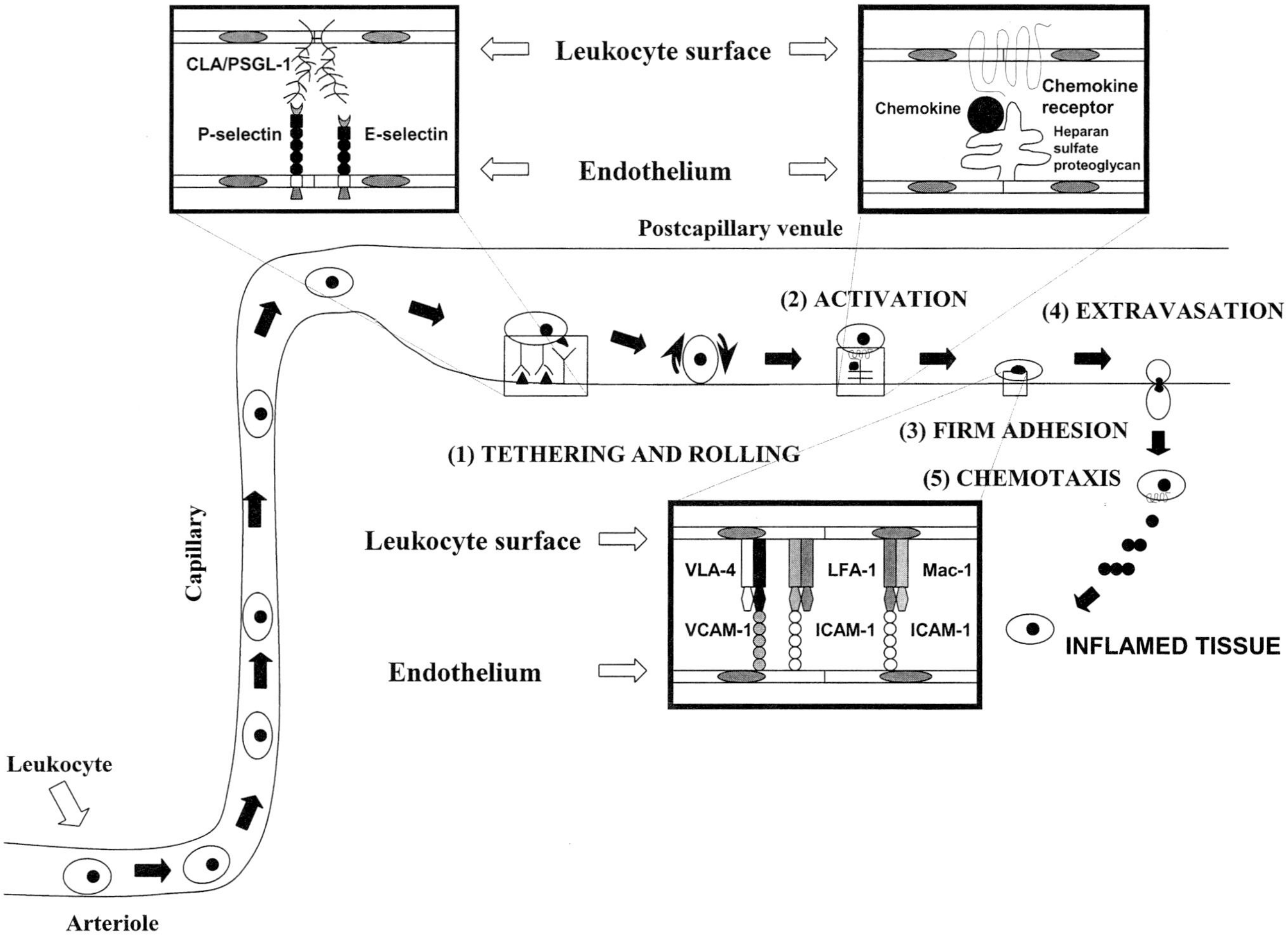

Figure 1.1. After traveling through arterioles and capillaries, leukocytes arrive at postcapillary venules and undergo a series of steps to target inflamed skin. First, they roll and tether on endothelium (*1*), displaying P- and E-selectin ligands, CLA/PSGL-1 (From Fuhlbrigge RC, Kupper TS. Molecular mechanisms of allergic skin responses. *Allergic skin disease: a multidisciplinary approach*. Leung DYM, Greaves MW, eds.New York: Marcel Dekker Inc., 2000:37, with permission). The lectin domain of selectins binds to carbohydrate epitopes, specifically sialyl Lewis X. Leukocytes then undergo activation of integrins (*2*) expressed on their surface via the interaction between chemokines and their respective 7-transmembrane–spanning receptors. Heparan sulfate proteoglycans bind chemokines to the endothelium, immobilizing them for presentation to leukocytes. Integrin activation increases the avidity of integrins (VLA-4, LFA-1, Mac-1) to endothelial adhesion molecules (VCAM-1, ICAM-1), which are members of the immunoglobulin superfamily (From Luster AD. Chemokines - chemotactic chemokines that mediate inflammation. *N Engl J Med* 1998;338:436, with permission). This interaction causes the firm arrest of leukocytes on endothelium (*3*), which is immediately followed by extravasation of the leukocyte from the blood vessel (*4*). Leukocytes are guided to sites of inflammation by tracking a gradient set by chemokines. This process of chemotaxis (*5*) is aided by glycosaminoglycans in the extracellular matrix that bind chemokines for presentation. CLA, cutaneous lymphocyte antigen; PSGL-1, P-selectin glycoprotein ligand-1; PNAd, peripheral node addressin; VLA-4, very late antigen-4; LFA-1, lymphocyte function antigen-1; ICAM-1, intercellular adhesion molecule-1; VCAM-1, vascular cell adhesion molecule-1.

(diversity), J (joining), and C (constant), join together with some intentional imprecision, which introduces a tremendous amount of sequence variability. This creates a multitude of genetic sequences that encode receptors that are collectively capable of recognizing a vast number of antigens on pathogenic organisms. Lymphocytes that recognize their antigen through their antigen receptor expand clonally, and these clonal progeny differentiate into effector and memory cells. This process is called clonal expansion, which provides the foundation for a targeted immune response to an infection. After proliferation and a successful immune response, many of the clonally expanded cells undergo apoptosis, but a significant number survive and remain with the host for years or decades. These remaining cells provide immunologic memory by inducing a faster, more robust, and often tissue-specific response upon a subsequent encounter with the same antigen. However, whereas innate immunity recognizes PAMPs, antigen receptors recognize peptides (T cells) or shapes of proteins (B cells), and these can include sequences or shapes that are similar or even identical to those of host proteins. Self-reactive T cells are typically deleted during thymic development or actively suppressed in the periphery, but dysfunction or failure of these processes can lead to autoimmune disease. T cell and B cell receptors are discussed later.

B CELLS AND ANTIBODIES

B-lymphocytes, or B cells, are formed from lymphoid progenitor cells that undergo maturation in the bone marrow. On the surface of B cells are B cell antigen receptors, known as immunoglobulins or antibodies. Antibodies are Y-shaped dimers consisting of two heavy and two light chains, each encoded by a uniquely recombined immunoglobulin gene. The heavy chain includes the so-called Fc region, which determines antibody isotype. Naïve B cells that have not seen antigen before express IgM, but after antigen recognition, B cells switch their isotype as well as proliferate. Most frequently, this involves switching to one of the IgG isotypes, but IgE, IgD, and IgA isotypes can also be expressed. Each isotype-specific Fc region is capable of binding to a specific Fc receptor on different classes of leukocytes; this Fc receptor binding can mediate a variety of different responses. The other end of the antibody contains the Fab, or variable region, which binds to antigen. During B cell development, gene segments, each responsible for part of the variable region, rearrange to form the extensive gamut of antibody specificities. This antigen binding part of the antibody, to which both heavy and light chains contribute, contains the most variable sequence, which is unique to every naïve B cell. Unlike T cell receptors, antibodies bind with high affinity to antigens by recognizing their tertiary structure or their three-dimensional conformation. Although antibodies are present on the cell surface of the B cell, they are most abundant in the circulation, where they also bind to antigens with high affinity.

Antibodies mediate the so-called humoral response of acquired immunity, which effectively fights pathogens in extracellular compartments. They can aggregate along the surface of microbes, allowing phagocytes to engulf the microorganism in a process called opsonization. They can also directly bind to pathogens or toxins and inhibit their toxic effects. Certain antibodies can activate complement via the classic pathway, leading to formations of the MAC on the pathogen cell surface. Complexes of antibodies bound to antigen, which are then carried by erythrocytes, are typically cleared by macrophages and other phagocytes in the liver and spleen (6). Small immune complexes that are not successfully removed can injure small blood vessels and contribute to vasculitis (23), systemic lupus erythematosus (25,26), rheumatoid arthritis (27,28), and other rheumatologic diseases. See Walport (7) for a review on the classic pathway and Janeway et al. (6) for a review of B cells and antibodies.

T CELLS AND T-CELL RECEPTORS

T cells are the captains of cellular immunity and play central roles in inflammatory skin disease, including those with rheumatologic components. T cells are derived from bone marrow–derived progenitors that mature in the thymus (Fig. 1.2). This maturation involves recombination of T cell receptor gene expression of a heterodimeric T cell receptor on the cell surface. Genes for T cell receptors rearrange in a process similar to antibodies on B cells, known as V(D)J-recombination (29), and produce a variety of receptors, each of which differs in primary sequence. Intrathymic maturation includes an editing process, and most T cells are destroyed *in situ*, either because they have too much affinity for self-proteins or because they have no affinity for MHC (major histocompatibility complex) molecules. The surviving T cells exit thymus and enter blood, where they are classified as naïve T cells. Naïve T cells, which by definition have not yet encountered their specific antigen, characteristically express the RA isoform of CD45, and circulate between the blood and secondary lymphoid organs, such as lymph nodes. Naïve T cells are drawn to T cell–rich areas of lymph nodes, which are also frequented by DCs that have come from tissue. If the T cell recognizes the antigen for which its T cell receptor is specific, it proliferates by clonal expansion and differentiates into either an effector T cell or memory T cell (discussed later) (30) (Fig. 1.2).

T cell receptors are heterodimeric proteins composed of either α/β (the majority) or γ/δ chains. Whereas antibodies identify the three-dimensional conformation of proteins, T cell receptors recognize peptides bound to a groove of MHC molecules, which are glycoproteins on the surface of antigen-presenting cells (APCs). T cell receptors are specific for peptides in the context of MHC molecules, not peptides free in solution. The sheer magnitude of T cell receptor sequences, which number in the billions, means that there are likely to be several T cells that can recognize at least some peptides derived from any pathogen protein. Although this greatly increases the breadth of responsiveness to potential pathogens, it also creates a logistic challenge for the T cell. A T cell must both find the peptide for which its antigen receptor is specific and interact with the APC over the tiny distance between MHC molecules and T cell receptors needed for a stable interaction: 1 nm, or 1⁄800 of the T cell diameter (31). This would never happen if T cells and APCs were distributed randomly throughout the body. Secondary lymphoid tissue help solve this problem by permitting APCs, including DCs, to colocalize in a compact and unique site: the lymph node. Peripheral lymph nodes (PLNs) are strategic microenvironments where antigen-presenting DCs, loaded with environmental antigens, and naïve lymphocytes meet to initiate immune responses.

To understand how T cells become activated by antigen, it is vital to understand how antigens are processed and presented to T cells by APCs.

ANTIGEN PROCESSING

Extracellular pathogens are internalized by APCs, such as immature DCs, into an endosome. Immature DCs use receptor-mediated endocytosis to efficiently capture antigens (32,33). The endosome merges with lysosomes, and pathogen proteins are cleaved into peptides. At the same time, a vesicle with a MHC class II molecule (HLA-DR, -DQ, -DP) merges with the acidified endosome. This event results in the release of the invariant chain, which blocks the peptide-binding groove of the MHC class II molecule. Peptides from the pathogen can now bind to the MHC class II molecule with the help of another molecule, HLA-DM (34). The vesicle is transported to the cell surface, and the MHC molecule, now loaded with peptide, is available for recognition by $CD8^+$ T cells.

The pathway described above is useful for extracellular pathogens, but would not be an effective way of recognizing intracellular bacteria or viruses. The class I MHC pathway meets this challenge by allowing cytoplasmic peptides to be sampled on the cell surface by $CD8^+$ T cells. Normally, the proteosome complex acts not unlike a cellular garbage disposal, digesting both non-self and self-cytoplasmic proteins into peptides. Transporter associated with antigen processing (TAP) shuttle these peptides from the cytosol to the lumen of the endoplasmic reticulum, where they bind to a partially folded MHC class I molecule (HLA-A, -B, -C). Peptide binding completes the folding of the MHC class I molecule. A vesicle

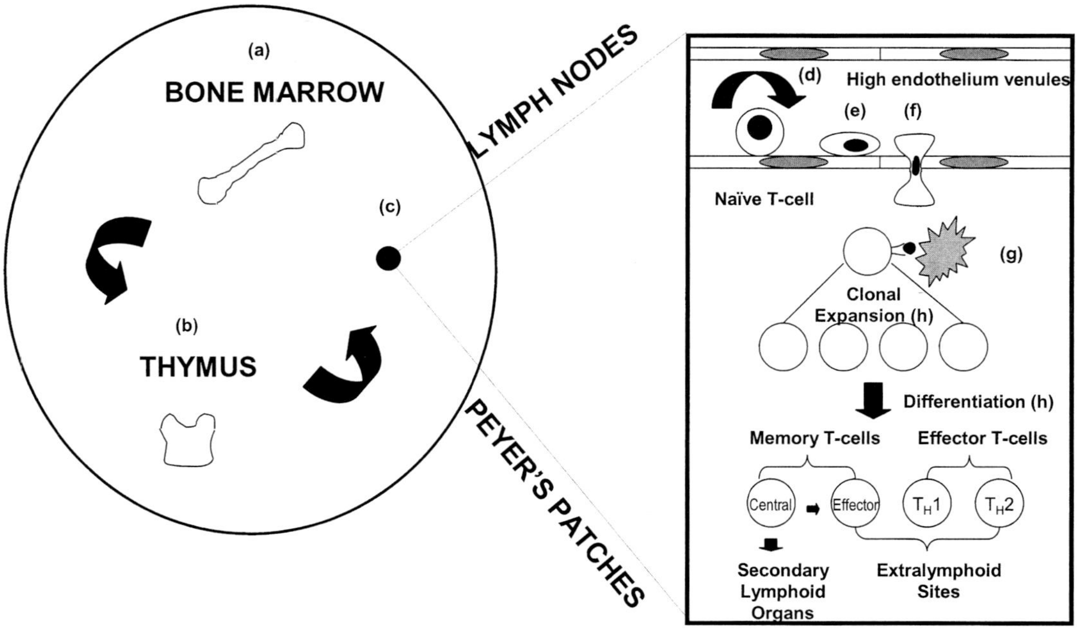

Figure 1.2. The life of a T cell originates in the bone marrow (*a*), where progenitor cells are created. They then migrate to the thymus (*b*) to develop, and are sent out to the bloodstream as naïve T cells. To maximize their chances of finding the correct antigen, they travel to secondary lymphoid organs (*c*), such as lymph nodes and Peyer patches in the small intestine. In the high endothelium venules, these T cells tether and roll (*d*), firmly adhere (*e*), and extravasate (*f*) into the lymphoid organ via the interaction of adhesion molecules expressed on both T cells and high endothelium venules. Naïve T cells will subsequently sample a variety of antigens on antigen-presenting cells, which have been internalized, processed, and presented at the surface. When T cells find their appropriate antigen, the signals for activation include the proper interactions between T cell receptors and the major histocompatibility antigen complex as well as co-stimulatory molecules on T cells and antigen-presenting cells. Activation of the T cell results in clonal expansion of the T cell (*g*) with the production of interleukin-2, and subsequent differentiation (*h*) into either memory or effector T cells. Memory T cells can be divided into central memory T cells, which, like naïve T cells, home to secondary lymphoid organs to search for antigen, and effector memory T cells, which originate from central memory T cells and travel to extralymphoid sites. Central memory T cells differ from effector memory T cells by their unique expression of L-selectin, CCR7, and lymphocyte function antigen-1. Effector T cells, which act in extralymphoid sites, differentiate into T_H1 and T_H2 cells. If the antigen-presenting cell produces interleukin-12, the formation of T_H1 cells occurs. T_H1 cells produce interferon-γ, which activates macrophages. If IL-4 is manufactured by the antigen-presenting cell, T_H2 cells are generated and become responsible for humoral immunity.

containing peptide-loaded class I MHC molecules buds off of the endoplasmic reticulum and travels to the plasma membrane, where it can be recognized by $CD8^+$ T cells (35). See Jensen (35) for a review on both antigen-processing pathways.

Although $CD4^+$ T cell/MHC class II pathways survey the extracellular milieu (think of the Central Intelligence Agency [CIA]), and $CD8^+$ T cell/MHC class I pathways survey the intracellular milieu (conversely, think of the Federal Bureau of Investigation [FBI]), the two pathways described above are not always mutually exclusive. The phenomenon of "cross-priming" occurs when exogenous peptides are presented by MHC class I molecules and endogenous peptides by MHC class II molecules. Thus, $CD8^+$ T cells have the opportunity to be activated by exogenous proteins, whereas endogenous proteins can be presented to $CD4^+$ T cells. For example, with the ability to process both endogenous and exogenous peptides and arrange them with MHC class I molecules, DCs have the ability to "cross-prime" T cells (36).

COLOCALIZATION OF NAÏVE T CELLS AND DENDRITIC CELLS FOR SUCCESSFUL ANTIGEN PRESENTATION

Once antigen is processed and delivered to the surface of the APC in the context of MHC molecules, it is ready to be presented to T cells. Lymph nodes, which drain environmental interfaces such as the skin via afferent lymphatics, concentrate DCs derived from a large surface area to a single site. Naïve T cells extravasate into lymph nodes from the blood with the help of adhesion molecules and chemokines on the endothelium of postcapillary venules and chemokine receptors and selectins on the T cells. This mechanism is a specific variation of the multistep leukocyte-trafficking model with the same steps involved: tethering/rolling, chemokine-mediated integrin activation, firm adhesion, and extravasation (Fig. 1.3). L-selectin, expressed on naïve T cells, binds to PNAd (peripheral node addressin) in lymph node postcapillary venules, resulting in

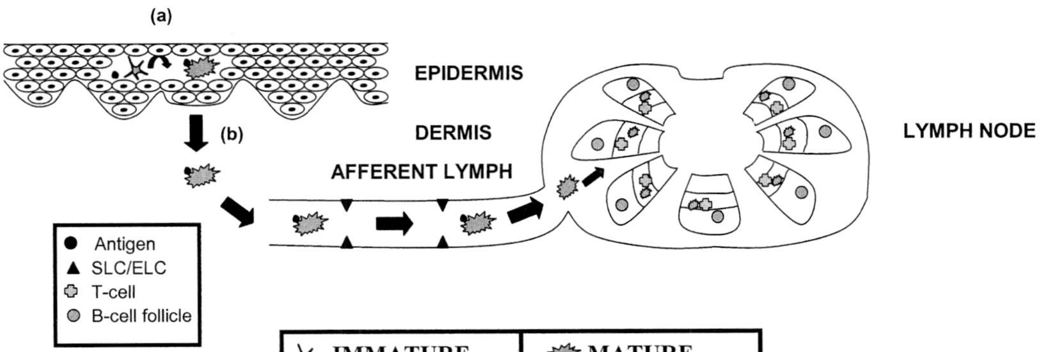

	IMMATURE DENDRITIC CELL	MATURE DENDRITIC CELL
FUNCTION	**Internalize antigen (via phagocytosis, macropinocytosis, endocytosis), antigen processing**	**Stimulate T-cells with antigen presentation, enhance survival of CD4+ T-cells**
FcR LEVEL	↑	↓
MHC LEVEL	↓	↑
CO-STIMULATORY MOLECULE LEVEL	↓	↑
MOBILITY	**Restricted to peripheral tissue**	**Travel to lymph nodes via afferent lymph and chemokines SLC and ELC**

Figure 1.3. Dendritic cells (DCs) initially reside in peripheral tissues such as skin. In their immature stage, they mimic their distant relatives, phagocytes, and internalize antigen by a variety of processes such as receptor-mediated endocytosis via high levels of Fc receptor. During this phase, immature DCs contain low levels of major histocompatibility complex and co-stimulatory molecules on their surface. Once antigen enters the DC, it becomes processed for later presentation. Although antigen internalization serves as a maturation signal (*a*) for DCs, other stimuli include lipopolysaccharide, tumor necrosis factor α, and interleukin-1. However, interleukin-10 and ceramide can prevent maturation. Maturation induces DCs to prepare for T cell activation through a number of processes. Levels of major histocompatibility and co-stimulatory molecules are up-regulated for antigen presentation and T cell stimulation, respectively, whereas the number of Fc receptor is reduced, decreasing their antigen internalization capabilities. Mature DCs migrate to lymph nodes via afferent lymphatics (*b*) where they can present their antigens to T cells. Their trafficking to T cell zones in lymph nodes is mediated by the secondary lymphoid tissue chemokine/CCL21 and EBV-induced molecule 1 ligand chemokine/CCL19 and their receptor, CCR7, which is up-regulated on the DC's surface during maturation.

tethering (i.e., binding under flow) of T cells and their rolling in the direction of flow. PNAd belongs to the family of addressins and is constitutively expressed in so-called high-endothelial venules (HEVs) in lymph nodes (30). The chemokine SLC (secondary lymphoid tissue chemokine)/CCL21, which is constitutively present on high-endothelium venules of lymph nodes and lymphatic endothelium (37), activates the naïve T cell via its receptor CCR7, allowing the integrin LFA-1 on T cells to change conformation and bind with high affinity to ICAM-1 (38), which is also constitutively expressed on the lymph node venular endothelium luminal surface. These interactions result in the firm arrest and extravasation of naïve T cells into the lymph nodes. Thus, naïve T cells are specifically plucked from the circulation into lymph nodes, leaving the rest of the leukocytes in the bloodstream. Once they have traversed the venule, naïve T cells are attracted to the paracortex of the lymph node, where they mix with DCs collected from the surrounding environment. T cells and DCs collide randomly, and if the T cell receptor does not recognize its peptide antigen bound to MHC, T cells travel to the medulla of the lymph node and exit via efferent lymphatics to the blood. Little is known about the mechanism and regulation of T cell exiting the lymph node (31).

DCs change as they migrate from environmental interfaces to the lymph node (Fig. 1.3). When stimulated via injury or infection, epidermal Langerhans cells break their adhesion to keratinocytes, cross the basement membrane into the dermis, and move into afferent lymphatics, a process facilitated by the chemotactic properties of SLC/6Ckine (39,40) and MIP-3β (macrophage inducible protein-3β)/ELC (EBV-induced molecule 1 ligand chemokine)/CCL19 produced in the lymph node

(39,41). These chemokines are ligands for the chemokine receptor, CCR7, whose expression is up-regulated on the surface of activated Langerhans cells (41). Together, they direct DCs to lymph node T cell zones. Moreover, the levels of other chemokine receptors produced in response to inflammation (i.e., CCR1, CCR5) are decreased (42,43). By the time it reaches the lymph node, the Langerhans cell has become a mature DC, capable of activating a naïve T cell. Unlike its immature precursor, a mature DC has elevated levels of MHC molecules, has lost the capacity to internalize pathogens, and expresses high levels of co-stimulatory molecules (Fig. 1.3). The role of these last molecules is described later.

T cells require more than just recognition via the T cell receptor of the appropriate peptide–MHC complex, the so-called first signal. A second signal is required; in fact, the absence of this second signal can result in the lack of T cell responsiveness called anergy (45). Second signals are delivered by so-called co-stimulatory molecules, which are up-regulated on the surface of DCs during their maturation process. The dominant co-stimulatory pathway involves the interaction of B7 molecules and CD28. DCs express CD80 (or B7.1) and CD86 (or B7.2). They subsequently bind to CD28, which is constitutively expressed on naïve T cells, promoting clonal expansion and survival of naïve T cells and IL-2 production (46). Other co-stimulatory molecules can initiate T cell activation but do not sustain T cell proliferation and survival as well as CD28, possibly because of lower IL-2 production (47). One such molecule is ICOS (inducible costimulator), which attaches to LICOS (Ligand ICOS) (B7-H2) on APCs (48). Found only on activated T cells, ICOS increases T cell expression of CD40 ligand (CD40L), another co-stimulatory molecule (46). CD40L's interaction with CD40 on DCs helps sustain T cell activation by increasing B7 molecule expression on APCs (7). Members of the TNF receptor family have been implicated as co-stimulatory molecules on T cells, including 4-1BB, which maintains T cell activation in the face of decreasing levels of CD28 (49), and OX40, which promotes cytokine secretion and proliferation of effector T cells (46). However, co-stimulatory pathways can also be used to inhibit T cell activation. For example, CTLA-4 (cytotoxic T-lymphocyte antigen-4), a CD28-related protein expressed on T cell surfaces, binds to B7 molecules on APCs and down-regulates the activation signal to T cells (50). CTLA-4 may be one means of turning off immune responses and maintaining tolerance to self-antigens; its absence may facilitate autoimmunity.

DENDRITIC CELL MATURATION

Originally derived from bone marrow, DCs are potent APCs in that small numbers of DCs presenting are only needed for vigorous T cell activation *in vivo* and *in vitro* (36). The incipient stages of a DC's life are spent in peripheral tissues, such as the skin. These immature DCs are phagocytic cells that can capture microbes via phagocytosis (50) and macropinocytosis, a process in which DCs brings in extracellular fluid to sample for antigens (31). They can also internalize microbes bound by antibody through Fc-mediated endocytosis (32). However, they express low levels of MHC and co-stimulatory molecules, making them incapable of activating naïve T cells (6). Once antigen is internalized, immature DCs concentrate their efforts from antigen capture to antigen processing and production of MHC–peptide complexes, which can accumulate in large amounts and stabilize at the cell surface (35) (Fig. 1.3).

Maturation of a DC results in the ability to stimulate T cells. The signals for a DC to undergo maturation can come from a variety of sources, including antigen internalization, LPS activation of TLR2 (52), and cytokines such as IL-1, granulocyte-macrophage colony-stimulating factor, and TNF-α (36). These are all features of innate immunity. However, IL-10 (53) and ceramide (54) can both inhibit DC maturation, thus indirectly inhibiting T cell activation. Once DCs receive the appropriate signals to mature, their cell-surface expression changes dramatically. The number of MHC complexes increases, co-stimulatory molecules are up-regulated, and cytokines such as IL-12 and IL-23 are up-regulated (55). Maturation signals also induce mature DCs to leave peripheral tissues and migrate to lymphoid tissues, such as lymph nodes, via afferent lymphatics. They can subsequently present their MHC–peptide complexes to T cells. Other functions of mature DCs include attracting T cells via chemokines (56) and prolonging the survival of mature $CD4^+$ T cells (57) (Fig. 1.3).

DCs are heterogeneous from other perspectives as well. Lymphoid and myeloid DCs have been described, and each derives from different progenitors. Their functions are distinct and incompletely understood, but lymphoid DCs appear to mediate tolerance in naïve T cells, and myeloid DCs stimulate T cell activation (59). Myeloid DCs can also help direct differentiation of effector T cells (see below) by promoting T helper cell type 1 (T_H1) T cell differentiation. IFN-γ serves as a potent factor that induces the formation of such DCs, which subsequently produce IL-12 and favor a T_H1 response (60). Factors such as prostaglandin E_2 (PGE_2) (61) and histamine (62) promote the polarization of effector T cells to T_H2 and decrease the amount of IL-12 generated (60).

T CELL ACTIVATION AND DIFFERENTIATION

The result from the binding of naïve T cells and their receptors to mature DCs carrying the appropriate MHC–peptide complexes and co-stimulatory molecules is T cell activation. This event leads not only in the clonal expansion of T cells but also to their transformation into effector cells. Features of the lymph node microenvironment where the T cell is first activated can influence its subsequent effector functions.

Activated T cells gain the ability to replicate and differentiate through their own production of IL-2 and expression of a high-affinity IL-2 receptor. After several rounds of division, T cells can differentiate into effector T cells, depending on their lineage: $CD8^+$ cells can become cytolytic T cells, and $CD4^+$ cells can become T_H1 or T_H2 cells, depending on the panel of cytokines they produce (described later). Effector T cells acquire the capacity to migrate to peripheral extralymphoid tissues and can be further activated by antigen at these sites (Fig. 1.2).

The classification of T cells based on their cytokine profile into T_H1 and T_H2 cells, first proposed in 1986, has stood the test of time. T_H1 T cells, also known as inflammatory T cells, produce IFN-γ, TNF, and GM-CSF (62). Differentiation of an activated proliferating T cell into a T_H1 cell is facilitated by cytokines, such as IL-12 and IL-23 (63). Typically, microbes induce T_H1 cells to initiate the cell-mediated immunity response in which macrophages are activated by IFN-γ to mediate phagocytosis of pathogens. IFN-γ works cooperatively with other cytokines. For example, IFN-γ and IL-2 can induce $CD8^+$ T cells to become cytotoxic T cells (64). Together with TNF-α, IFN-γ can stimulate production of nitric oxide, which has antimicrobial properties (65). IFN-γ also aids in T_H1 self-propagation by increasing IL-12 production by APCs (66) and inhibiting the function of T_H2 cells (67). T_H1 cells have characteristic chemokine receptors such as CCR5 and CXCR3, which aid in the trafficking of T_H1 cells to sites of inflammation (68).

If IL-4 is present during T cell activation, T_H2 cells are generated. The newly differentiated T_H2 cell produces type II cytokines (IL-4, IL-5, IL-10, IL-13) (62,64). These cytokines mediate isotype switching of B cell immunoglobulins from IgM to IgE and IgG_1 (IL-4, IL-13), eosinophil growth and activation (IL-5), mast cell activation (IL-4) and inhibition of DC maturation and function. This last property also serves to inhibit generation of T_H1 cells by inhibiting DC IL-12 production (69). Allergens and parasitic infections can induce production of IL-4, which can induce B cells to generate allergen- and parasite-specific IgE antibodies (70,71). IL-4 participates in the recruitment of eosinophils by up-regulating levels of adhesion molecules (i.e., VCAM-1 (vascular cell adhesion molecule-1)) (72) and chemokines specific for eosinophils on vascular endothelium (73). Eosinophils are further affected by IL-5, which acts as a prominent eosinophil growth and activation factor (74). T_H2 cells express the chemokine receptor CCR3, whose ligand is eotaxin/CCL11 (75), and thus T_H2 cells, eosinophils (76), and basophils (77) are recruited together by this chemokine. T_H2 cells may also possess the chemokine receptor CCR4 (68).

The classification of T cells based on cytokine profile has expanded to regulatory T cells. Contrary to helper T cells, regulatory T cells inhibit the activation of T cells on reexposure of antigen, preventing destructive immune responses. A subset called T_H3 cells primarily secretes the inhibitory cytokine TGF-β (transforming growth factor-β) and is thought to mediate the phenomenon of oral tolerance, the suppression of immune responses to antigens entering the body via the oral route (78). T_R1 cells, formed from naïve T cell precursors under the presence of IL-10 and IFN-α, synthesize both IL-10 and TGF-β, which down-regulate T cell–mediated responses (79). It has also been postulated that $CD4^+$ $CD25^+$ T cells, which constitutively produce IL-10 and TGF-β and express the regulatory co-stimulatory molecule, CTLA-4 (80), can prevent autoimmune diseases through their regulatory functions (81,82).

IMMUNOLOGIC MEMORY

Immunologic memory is the major distinction between innate and acquired immunity. Memory is based partly on clonal expansion and persistence of T cells. Memory T cells originate from the surviving clonally expanded T cells at the end of an immune response (83,84). Recently, memory T cells have been divided into two categories, based on their homing properties: central memory T cells and effector memory T cells. This model is still evolving (85).

Central memory T cells retain the capacity to enter secondary lymphoid organs and maintain expression of L-selectin, CCR7, and LFA-1. They enter PLNs using the same mechanism as naïve T cells. They can be readily activated by DCs due to a low activation threshold and the up-regulation of CD40L. In theory, these cells can differentiate into effector memory cells on subsequent encounter with antigen (85) (Fig. 1.2). In contrast, effector memory cells lack expression of either L-selectin or CCR7 and are thus excluded from lymph nodes. They do express higher levels of β_2 and β_1 integrins, other chemokine receptors specific for inflammatory chemokines, and specialized homing molecules that all direct them to different tissues (85). Both T_H1 and T_H2 cells belong to the effector memory T cell subset, and activation of effector memory cells in tissue by antigen leads to cytokine release. Both classes of memory cell are antigen-specific, and each patrols a different anatomic compartment.

T CELL HOMING TO SKIN AND OTHER TISSUES

Recently, another element of T cell memory has been recognized. It appears that T cells can remember not only the identity of their antigen, but also where it was last encountered. Specifically, naïve T cells encountering antigens in skin-draining lymph nodes will differentiate into effector T cells that express cell-surface markers that target them to skin (21). The mechanism by which this occurs is unclear, but it appears that the milieu where naïve T cells is activated can control the expression of certain homing molecules on T cells (86). Whether DCs in skin-draining nodes have unique features that mediate this differentiation, or whether factors in afferent lymph play a role, is unknown at present and is the subject of intense investigation.

T cells activated by antigen in skin-draining lymph nodes will proliferate and begin to express CLA (Table 1.3). Defined by the monoclonal antibody HECA-452 (87), CLA is produced by a unique glycosylation of P-selectin glycoprotein 1 (PSGL-1) via the activity of the α(1,3) fucosyltransferase Fuc-TVII (88). CLA^+ T cells contribute about 10% to 15% of all total peripheral blood T cells (89), or about 35% to 40% of CD45RO (i.e., effector/memory) T cells. CLA^+ T cells are not restricted with regard to other phenotypic features, can produce type I and II cytokines, and can be either $CD4^+$ or $CD8^+$ (90). The CLA glycoform of PSGL-1 is also present on neutrophils, monocytes, and DCs (91). The tethering and rolling of CLA to its principal ligand, E-selectin (92), is required in preparation for T cell extravasation to inflamed skin (93). Although CLA has been well documented as a homing molecule for $CD8^+$ T cells, CLA has been recently established as having the same role for virus-specific $CD8^+$ memory T cells (94). E-selectin is an important adhesion molecule whose expression is up-regulated by cytokines such as IL-1 (95) and whose presence is key to the development of inflammatory reactions in the skin. It binds sialyl-Lewis X epitopes expressed on CLA from skin-homing T cells.

CCR4, which serves as a receptor for the chemokines TARC (thymus- and activation-related chemokine)/CCL17 and MDC (macrophage-derived chemokine)/CCL22, is strongly expressed in CLA^+ T cells, but found in very low levels on T cells that home to other tissues (96) (Table 1.3). CLA^+ $CCR4^+$ T cells accumulate at high levels in the skin of patients with cutaneous T cell lymphoma (97). CCR10 is another chemokine receptor expressed on a subset of CLA^+ $CCR4^+$ skin-homing T cells (98). It binds to the chemokine CTACL (cutaneous T cell atracting chemokine)/CCL27, which appears to be uniquely expressed by keratinocytes, and this results in the recruitment of a subset of skin-homing T cells to epidermis (99,100).

Skin is not the only epithelial interface with the environment to have its own dedicated populations of memory T cells. Gut-homing memory T cells express a set of homing receptors different from those of skin-homing lymphocytes. These gut-specific lymphocytes contain high levels of $\alpha_4\beta_7$ integrin, which allow them to efficiently interact with MAdCAM-1 (mucosal addressin cell adhesion molecule-1)on postcapillary venules in lamina propria (101). Their expression of $\alpha_4\beta_7$ integrin is greater than that on naïve T cells, allowing them to roll in endothelium of both lamina propria venules and high endothelium venules in Peyer patches (102). DCs have been postulated to play a role in the homing of gut-specific lymphocytes by up-regulating their expression of $\alpha_4\beta_7$ integrin (103) (thymus-expressed

TABLE 1.3. Markers Designating T Cells for Skin and Gut

Adhesion Molecule	Ligand	Function in T-Cell Homing	Evidence for Specificity
Skin			
CLA	E-selectin	Tethering/rolling	T cells expressing CLA have increased homing potential to skin[a,b] with very few traversing to extracutaneous inflammatory sites,[c] CLA⁺ T cells were congregated in cutaneous delayed-type hypersensitivity lesions,[d] patch stage mycosis fungoides,[c] milk-induced eczema.[e] E-selectin is not as skin-specific as CLA; its expression has been found up-regulated in various cutaneous and extracutaneous inflammatory sites (93).[f]
CCR4	TARC (CCL17)	Integrin activation	Most skin-homing CLA⁺ T cells express CCR4, helping them respond better to TARC/CCL17 in preparation for firm adhesion than gut-homing T cells, which contain small amounts of CCR4. In addition, immunohistochemical studies showed TARC reactivity in venules of inflamed skin but not in the lamina propria of the GI tract (96). TARC has been found up-regulated in cutaneous inflammatory lesions of psoriatic,[g] atopic dermatitis,[h,i] and cutaneous T cell lymphoma skin (97).
CCR6	LARC (CCL20)	Integrin activation, chemotaxis	CLA⁺ T cells highly express CCR6, and these cells have been located near LARC/CCL20–expressing keratinocytes in the skin of psoriasis[j] and patients with atopic dermatitis.[k] However, CCR6 is not totally specific to CLA⁺ T cells, for its presence has been located on other T cell subsets such as those containing $\alpha_4\beta_7$ integrin.[l]
CCR10	CTACK (CCL27)	Chemotaxis, integrin activation	CTACK/CCL27, the only skin-specific chemokine known, preferentially recruits CLA⁺ T cells to the skin via chemotaxis (99). The presence of CCR10 in T cells is highly associated with expression of CLA,[m] and CCR4, but not with $\alpha_4\beta_7$ integrin (98). Inhibition of both CCR10 and CCR4 significantly decreases cutaneous T cell trafficking to the skin.[m] Immunohistochemical stainings have demonstrated increased CCL27 and CCR10 expression in the skin of patients with atopic dermatitis, allergic contact dermatitis, and psoriasis (111).
Gut			
$\alpha_4\beta_7$ Integrin	MAdCAM-1	Firm adhesion	Gut-homing lymphocytes express $\alpha_4\beta_7$ integrin, which directs them to the MAdCAM-1-expressing venules in the GI tract, such as those in Peyer patches and lamina propria (101). Specific antibodies against the $\alpha_4\beta_7$ integrin have decreased lymphocyte homing to mucosal areas[n] and helped resolve colonic colitis in murine models.[o]
$\alpha_E\beta_7$ Integrin	E-cadherin	Adhesion to epithelial cells	$\alpha_E\beta_7$ integrin can draw lymphocytes to the epithelium by attaching them to epithelial cells expressing E-cadherin.[p] However, $\alpha_E\beta_7$ integrin is not exclusive to intraepithelial lymphocytes in the gut (106), for they have been also located in synovial lymphocytes in patients with rheumatoid arthritis,[q] and skin-homing lymphocytes in cutaneous T cell lymphoma patients.[r]
CCR9	TECK (CCL25)	Firm adhesion, extravasation	CCR9⁺ lymphocytes are specifically drawn to the small intestine, where TECK/CCL25 is primarily found. Expression of CCR9 and CCL25 in the small intestine is substantially larger than other sites, including the rest of the digestive tract.[s] CCL25 preferentially attracts gut-homing lymphocytes amongst other T cells.[t]
Secondary Lymphoid Organs			
CCR7	SLC (CCL21)	Integrin activation	The binding of SLC/CCL21 to CCR7 on naïve lymphocytes and central memory T cells results in firm adhesion on high endothelial venules in lymph nodes and Peyer's patches, where SLC is abundantly expressed (37). Mice lacking the capacity to produce SLC demonstrate fewer T cells congregating in lymph nodes.[u] When flooded with CCR7 ligands, T cells are unable to firmly adhere on HEVs *in vitro*.[v] In addition, in the absence of CCR7 or its ligands, firm adhesion of T cells to the high endothelium venules of Peyer patches is not visualized.[w]

L-selectin	PNAd	Tethering/Rolling	The expression of L-selectin on naïve and central memory T cells allows for their specific interaction with PNAd, permitting them to roll and tether on high endothelial venules of secondary lymphoid organs[x]. Monoclonal antibodies against L-selectin and PNAd have decreased rolling of T cells in HEVs[x] as well as lymphocyte homing to lymph nodes[y].

GI, gastrointestinal.

[a]From Picker LJ, Martin RJ, Trumble A, et al. Differential expression of lymphocyte homing receptors by human memory/effector T cells in pulmonary versus cutaneous immune effector sites. *Eur J Immunol* 1994;24:1269, with permission.

[b]From Pitzalis C, Cauli A, Pipitone N, et al. Cutaneous lymphocyte antigen-positive T lymphocytes preferentially migrate to the skin but not to the joint in psoriatic arthritis. *Arthritis Rheum* 1996;39:137, with permission.

[c]From Picker LJ, Michie SA, Rott LS, et al. A unique phenotype of skin-associated lymphocytes in humans: preferential expression of the HECA-452 epitope by benign and malignant T cells at cutaneous sites. *Am J Pathol* 1990;136:1053, with permission.

[d]From Picker LJ, Treer JR, Ferguson-Darnell B, et al. Control of lymphocyte recirculation in man. II. Differential regulation of the cutaneous lymphocyte-associated antigen, a tissue-selective homing receptor for skin-homing T cells. *J Immunol* 1993;150:1122, with permission.

[e]From Abernathy-Carver KJ, Sampson HA, et al. Milk-induced eczema is associated with the expansion of T cells expressing cutaneous lymphocyte antigen. *J Clin Invest* 1995;95:913, with permission.

[f]From Koch AE, Burrows JC, Haines GK, et al. Immunolocalization of endothelial and leukocyte adhesion molecules in human rheumatoid and osteoarthritis synovial tissues. *Lab Invest* 1991;64:313, with permission.

[g]From Rottman JB, Smith TL, Ganley KG, et al. Potential role of the chemokine receptors CXCR3, CCR4, and the integrin $\alpha_E\beta_7$ in the pathogenesis of psoriasis vulgaris. *Lab Invest* 2001;81:335, with permission.

[h]From Vestergaard C, Bang K, Gesser B, et al. A T_H2 chemokine, TARC, produced by keratinocytes may recruit CLA^+CCR4^+ lymphocytes into lesional atopic dermatitis skin. *J Invest Dermatol* 2000;115:640, with permission.

[i]From Kakinuma T, Nakamura K, Wakugawa M, et al. Thymus and activation-regulated chemokine in atopic dermatitis: serum thymus and activation-regulated chemokine level is closely related with disease activity. *J Allergy Clin Immunol* 2001;107:535, with permission.

[j]From Homey B, Dieu-Nosjean M, Wiesenborn A, et al. Up-regulation of macrophage inflammatory protein-3α/CCL20 and CC chemokine receptor 6 in psoriasis. *J Immunol* 2000;164:6621, with permission.

[k]From Nakayama T, Fujisawa R, Yamada H, et al. Inducible expression of a CC chemokine liver- and activation-regulated chemokine (LARC)/macrophage inflammatory protein (MIP)-3α/CCL20 by epidermal keratinocytes and its role in atopic dermatitis. *Int Immunol* 2001;13:95, with permission.

[l]From Liao F, Rabin RL, Smith CS, et al. CC-chemokine receptor 6 is expressed on diverse memory subsets of T cells and determines responsiveness to macrophage inflammatory protein-3α. *J Immunol* 1999;162:186, with permission.

[m]From Reiss Y, Proudfoot AE, Power CA, et al. CC chemokine receptor (CCR4) and the CCR10 ligand cutaneous T cell-attracting chemokine (CTACK) in lymphocyte trafficking to inflamed skin. *J Exp Med* 2001;194:1541, with permission.

[n]From Hamann A, Andrew DP, Jablonski-Westrich D, et al. Role of α_4-integrins in lymphocyte homing to mucosal tissues *in vivo*. *J Immunol* 1994;152:3282, with permission.

[o]From Hesterberg PE, Winsor-Hines D, Briskin MJ, et al. Rapid resolution of chronic colitis in the cotton-top tamarin with an antibody to a gut-homing integrin $\alpha_4\beta_7$. *Gastroenterology* 1996;111:1373, with permission.

[p]From Cepek KL, Shaw SK, Parker CM, et al. Adhesion between epithelial cells and T lymphocytes mediated by E-cadherin and the $\alpha_E\beta_7$ integrin. *Nature* 1994;372:190, with permission.

[q]From Trollmo C, Nilsson IM, Sollerman C, et al. Expression of the mucosal lymphocyte integrin $\alpha_E\beta_7$ and its ligand E-cadherin in the synovium of patient with rheumatoid arthritis. *Scan J Immunol* 1996;44:293, with permission.

[r]From Dietz SB, Whitaker-Menezes D, Lessin SR. The role of the $\alpha_E\beta_7$ integrin (CD103) and E-cadherin in epidermotropism in cutaneous T cell lymphoma. *J Cutan Pathol* 1996;23:312, with permission.

[s]From Kunkel EJ, Campbell JJ, Haraldsen G, et al. Lymphocyte CC chemokine receptor 9 and epithelial thymus-expressed chemokine (TECK) expression distinguish the small intestinal immune compartment: epithelial expression of tissue-specific chemokines as an organizing principle in regional immunity. *J Exp Med* 2000;192:761, with permission.

[t]From Zabel BA, Agace WW, Campbell JJ, et al. Human G protein-coupled receptor GPR-9-6/CC chemokine receptor 9 is selectively expressed on intestinal homing T lymphocytes, mucosal lymphocytes, and thymocytes and is required for thymus-expressed chemokine-mediated chemotaxis. *J Exp Med* 1999;190:1241, with permission.

[u]From Gunn MD, Kyuwa S, Tam C, et al. Mice lacking expression of secondary lymphoid organ chemokine have defects in lymphocyte homing and dendritic cell localization. *J Exp Med* 1999;189:451, with permission.

[v]From Campbell JJ, Butcher EC. Chemokines in tissue-specific and microenvironment-specific lymphocyte homing. *Curr Opin Immunol* 2000;12:336, with permission.

[w]From Warnock RA, Campbell JJ, Dork ME, et al. The role of chemokines in the microenvironmental control of T versus B cell arrest in Peyer's patch high endothelial venules. *J Exp Med* 2000;191:77, with permission.

[x]From Von Andrian UH. Intravital microscopy of the peripheral lymph node microcirculation in mice. *Microcirculation* 1996;3:287, with permission.

[y]From Berg EL, Robinson MK, Warnock RA, et al. The human peripheral lymph node vascular addressin is a ligand for LECAM-1, the peripheral lymph node homing receptor. *J Cell Biol* 1991;114:343, with permission.

chemokine)/CCL25. T cells trafficking to small intestine preferentially express the chemokine receptor CCR9, whose ligands include TECK (104). A small group of gut-homing T cells also display the integrin $\alpha_E\beta_7$ at significant levels, allowing them to congregate at the basement membrane near gut epithelium and bind to E-cadherin on epithelial cells (105,106) (Table 1.3).

IMMUNOSURVEILLANCE: MECHANISMS AND PROPERTIES

Although the concept of immunosurveillance is not new, its mechanistic basis has been elusive. Several studies have shown spontaneous rolling of leukocytes in cutaneous venules in noninflamed skin via interactions with endothelial selectins (107–109). Whereas lymphocytes and monocytes were found to roll on dermal postcapillary venules in a rat model, granulocytes were the predominant leukocyte involved, suggesting the importance of innate immunity in maintaining a constant cutaneous defense system. The ability of E-selectin–blocking antibodies to diminish leukocyte rolling fractions in this same model demonstrated the importance of E-selectin in rolling (109). Moreover, immunohistochemical studies have demonstrated the constitutive presence of E-selectin in noninflamed skin (95,107). P-selectin may also be involved in this rolling (107), as it has also been shown to be constitutively expressed (110). The presence of spontaneous rolling suggests that leukocytes in general, and skin-homing T cells in particular, can be quickly drawn to sites of inflammation. In addition, other factors downstream in the multi-step inflammation model that would be crucial in recruiting leukocytes have been shown to be constitutively expressed in normal skin. Immunohistochemical stainings have demonstrated the presence of TARC in dermal venules (96) and CTACK in epidermal keratinocytes (99) and superficial dermal vessels (111) in noninflamed human skin. Furthermore, ICAM-1 has been located on endothelial cells in normal skin (112–114).

Innate immunosurveillance is easy to understand and is ubiquitous. Production of defensins and complement proteins can directly kill microorganisms, and release of primary cytokines and chemokines by epidermal and dermal cells via injury or infection is an efficient way of recruiting leukocytes to specific areas of skin. Innate immunosurveillance depends broadly on the recognition of patterns or PAMPs, as described before. Leukocytes that do not bear antigen receptors circulate through microvessels in skin and can tether and roll on constitutively expressed selectins. These cells are poised to exit vessels at the first hint of injury and its attendant molecular signals. Innate immunosurveillance is highly efficient, but its scope is limited.

Primary acquired immunosurveillance takes advantage of the vast repertoire of antigen receptors available to the T cell population at large. It is facilitated by the co-localization of DCs derived from environmental interfaces and naïve T cells in lymph nodes that drain epithelial tissues. Langerhans cells internalize pathogen fragments, digest proteins into peptides, and express them on class II (and by cross-priming class I) cell-surface molecules, which are expressed in abundance as these cells differentiate into mature DCs. By the time the former Langerhans cell arrives in the lymph node, it is a mature DC, which expresses co-stimulatory molecules like CD80 and CD86, but cannot internalize further extracellular material. It is into this microenvironment that naïve T cells (and central memory cells) are shuttled with impressive precision. Naïve T cells are plucked out of the circulation by their expression of L-selectin, CCR7, and LFA-1, and the constitutive expression of their ligands PNAd, CCL21, and ICAM-1 on lymph node venules. In this fashion, the external environment is surveyed at a distance in these specialized immunologic microenvironments. DCs and their contents from large surface areas of skin can be localized to a single site and exposed to large numbers of naïve T cells. If there is recognition between a T cell receptor and a DC MHC molecule presenting a peptide, the T cell becomes activated and proliferates vigorously. It also differentiates, and in skin-draining lymph nodes, these newly minted effector memory cells express CLA, CCR4 (and sometimes CCR10), and high levels of LFA-1. Some of these cells become effector cells and express either type 1 or type 2 cytokines, and others become central memory cells, retaining the ability to enter lymph nodes.

Secondary acquired immunosurveillance has two components. In the first, central memory cells enter lymph nodes just as naïve T cells do, and look for antigen presented by DCs. Another form of immunosurveillance is performed by effector memory cells, which survive for long periods of time and maintain expression of CLA, CCR4, and LFA-1. It is likely that these cells can exit vessels in uninflamed skin by tethering and rolling on E-selectin, undergoing activation via CCR4 ligands, and firmly adhering and extravasating through LFA-1/ICAM-1 interactions. It appears likely that E-selectin, CCL17, and ICAM-1 are all expressed at low levels in postcapillary venules of skin (and can be up-regulated on traumatic injury). In this fashion, memory T cells continuously migrate out of vessels into skin, looking for their cognate antigen within the dermis and epidermis. If they see it, they become activated within skin, releasing cytokines. These cytokines, whether T_H1 or T_H2, will induce endothelial adhesion molecule expression and chemokine production, recruiting additional leukocytes and amplifying the inflammatory response.

Immunologically mediated skin diseases are typically driven by recognition of antigen by T cells that are persistent or dysfunctional. For example, in allergic contact dermatitis, vigorous T cell–mediated immunity is used against innocuous environmental chemicals. In atopic dermatitis, exaggerated T_H2 reactions occur to similarly innocuous proteins, leading to T_H2 cytokine–mediated skin disease. In psoriasis, it may be that an autoantigen in the epidermis is the target of a vigorous T cell response (90). Whether these T cells are dysfunctional in their capacity to be turned off or whether additional features of psoriasis are an exaggerated hyperplastic response of epidermis to T cell activation is currently unknown. There may be other T cell–mediated skin diseases, some of which feature vasculitis, that are likely to be catalyzed by antigens that are currently obscure. The delivery of antigen-specific effector memory T cells to skin, however, is a process that we are beginning to understand. This process is highly adaptive and appears to be essential to survival. It is striking that 35% to 40% of memory T cells (judged by CD45RO) expression are CLA^+. If expression of CLA on a memory effector T cell is an indication that the naïve-to-memory transition occurred in a skin-draining lymph node, it would appear that 35% to 40% of immune responses made by the average individual occur to agents encountered through our cutaneous interface with the environment.

REFERENCES

1. Hoffmann JA, Kafatos FC, Janeway CA Jr, et al. Phylogenetic perspectives in innate immunity. *Science* 1999;284:1313.
2. Medzhitov R. Toll-like receptors and innate immunity. *Nat Rev Immunol* 2001; 1:135.
3. Medzhitov R, Janeway CA Jr. Innate immunity: impact on the adaptive immune response. *Curr Opin Immunol* 1997;9:4.

4. Matsushita M. The lectin pathway of the complement system. *Microbiol Immunol* 1996;40:887.
5. Song W, Sarrias MR, Lambris JD. Complement and innate immunity. *Immunopharmacology* 2000;49:187.
6. Janeway CA Jr, Travers P, Walport M, et al. *Immunobiology: the immune system in health and disease,* 5th ed. New York: Garland Publishing, 2001:78–80, 368–369, 304–305, 307.
7. Walport MJ. Complement: first of two parts. *N Engl J Med* 2001;344:1058.
8. Harder J, Bartels J, Christophers E, et al. A peptide antibiotic from human skin. *Nature* 1997;387:861.
9. Frohm M, Agerberth B, Ahangari G, et al. The expression of the gene coding for the antibacterial peptide LL-37 is induced in human keratinocytes during inflammatory disorders. *J Biol Chem* 1997;272:15258.
10. Zasloff M. Antimicrobial peptides in health and disease. *N Engl J Med* 2002; 347:1199.
11. Yang D, Chen Q, Schmidt AP, et al. LL-37, the neutrophil granule- and epithelial cell-derived cathelicidin, utilizes formyl peptide receptor-like 1 (FPRL1) as a receptor to chemoattract human peripheral blood neutrophils, monocytes, and T cells. *J Exp Med* 2000;192:1069.
12. Ong PY, Ohtake T, Brandt C, et al. Endogenous antimicrobial peptides and skin infections in atopic dermatitis. *N Engl J Med* 2002;347:1151.
13. Janeway CA Jr, Medzhitov R. Innate immune recognition. *Annu Rev Immunol* 2002;20:197.
14. Lee RT, Briggs WH, Cheng GC, et al. Mechanical deformation promotes secretion of IL-1α and IL-1 receptor antagonist. *J Immunol* 1997;159:5084.
15. Fuhlbrigge RC, Kuper TS. Molecular mechanisms of allergic skin responses. Allergic skin disease: a multidisciplinary approach. Leung DYM, Greaves MW, eds. New York: Marcel Dekker Inc., 2000:32-33.
16. Olson TS, Ley K. Chemokines and chemokine receptors in leukocyte trafficking. *Am J Physiol Regul Integr Comp Physiol* 2002;283:R7.
17. Mantovani A. The chemokine system: redundancy for robust outputs. *Immunol Today* 1999;20:254.
18. Homey B, Zlotnik A. Chemokines in allergy. *Curr Opin Immunol* 1999;11:626.
19. Matsue H, Cruz PD Jr, Bergstresser PR, et al. Langerhans cells are the major source of mRNA for IL-1β and MIP-1α among unstimulated mouse epidermal cells. *J Invest Dermatol* 1992;99:537.
20. Hwang ST. Mechanisms of T cell homing to skin. *Adv Dermatol* 2001;17:211.
21. Butcher EC, Picker LJ. Lymphocyte homing and homeostasis. *Science* 1996; 272:60.
22. Springer TA. Traffic signals for lymphocyte recirculation and leukocyte emigration: the multistep paradigm. *Cell* 1994;76:301.
23. Butcher EC. Leukocyte-endothelial cell recognition: three (or more) steps to specificity and diversity. *Cell* 1991;67:1033.
24. Csernok E, Gross WL. Primary vasculitides and vasculitis confined to skin: clinical features and new pathogenic aspects. *Arch Dermatol Res* 2000;292:427.
25. Wener MH, Mannik M, Schwartz MM, et al. Relationship between renal pathology and the size of circulating immune complexes in patients with systemic lupus erythematosus. *Medicine* 1987;66:85.
26. Steinberg AD, Gourley MF, Klinman DM, et al. NIH conference. Systemic lupus erythematosus. *Ann Intern Med* 1991;115:548.
27. Edwards JCW, Cambridge G. Rheumatoid arthritis: the predictable effect of small immune complexes in which antibody is also antigen. *Br J Rheumatol* 1998;37:126.
28. Smith JB, Haynes M. Rheumatoid arthritis–a molecular understanding. *Ann Intern Med* 2002;136:908.
29. Agrawal A, Eastman QM, Schatz DG. Implications of transposition mediated by V(D)J-recombination proteins RAG1 and RAG2 for origins of antigen-specific immunity. *Nature* 1998;394:744.
30. Von Andrian UH, MacKay CR. T cell function and migration: two sides of the same coin. *N Engl J Med* 2000;343:1020.
31. Westermann J, Ehlers E, Exton MS, et al. Migration of naïve, effector, and memory T cells: implications for the regulation of immune responses. *Immunol Rev* 2001;184:20.
32. Sallusto F, Cella M, Danieli C, et al. Dendritic cells use macropinocytosis and the mannose receptor to concentrate macromolecules in the major histocompatibility complex class II compartment: downregulation by cytokines and bacterial products. *J Exp Med* 1995;182:389.
33. Harkiss GD, Hopkins J, McConnell I. Uptake of antigen by afferent lymph dendritic cells mediated by antibody. *Eur J Immunol* 1990;20:2367.
34. Jensen PE, Weber DA, Thayer WP, et al. HLA-DM and the MHC class II antigen presentation pathway. *Immunol Res* 1999;20:195.
35. Jensen PE. Mechanisms of antigen presentation. *Clin Chem Lab Med* 1999;37: 179.
36. Banchereau J, Steinman RM. Dendritic cells and the control of immunity. *Nature* 1998;392:245.
37. Gunn MD, Tangemann K, Tam C, et al. A chemokine expressed in lymphoid high endothelial venules promotes the adhesion and chemotaxis of naïve T-lymphocytes. *Proc Natl Acad Sci U S A* 1998;95:258.
38. Baggiolini M, Loetscher P. Chemokines in inflammation and immunity. *Immunol Today* 2000;21:418.
39. Kellermann S, Hudak S, Oldham ER, et al. The CC chemokine receptor-7 ligands 6Ckine and macrophage inflammatory protein-3β are potent chemoattractants for *in vitro*- and *in vivo*-derived dendritic cells. *J Immunol* 1999;162: 3859.
40. Saeki H, Moore AM, Brown MJ, et al. Cutting edge: secondary lymphoid-tissue chemokine (SLC) and CC chemokine receptor 7 (CCR7) participate in the emigration pathway of mature dendritic cells from the skin to regional lymph nodes. *J Immunol* 1999;162:2472.
41. Ngo VN, Tang HL, Cyster JG. Epstein-Barr virus-induced molecule 1 ligand chemokine is expressed by dendritic cells in lymphoid tissues and strongly attracts naïve T cells and activated B cells. *J Exp Med* 1998;188:181.
42. Campbell JJ, Bowman EP, Murphy K, et al. 6-C-kine (SLC), a lymphocyte adhesion-triggering chemokine expressed by high endothelium, is an agonist for the MIP-3β receptor CCR7. *J Exp Med* 1998;141:1053.
43. Cyster JG. Chemokines and the homing of dendritic cells to the T cell areas of lymphoid organs. *J Exp Med* 1999;189:447.
44. Sallusto F, Schaerli P, Loetscher P, et al. Rapid and coordinated switch in chemokine receptor expression during dendritic cell maturation. *Eur J Immunol* 1998;28:2760.
45. Lenschow DJ, Walunas TL, Bluestone JA. CD28/B7 system of T cell costimulation. *Annu Rev Immunol* 1996;14:233.
46. Watts TH, DeBenedette MA. T cell co-stimulatory molecules other than CD28. *Curr Opin Immunol* 1999;11:286.
47. Yashiro Y, Tai X, Toyo-oka K, et al. A fundamental difference in the capacity to induce proliferation of naïve T cells between CD28 and other co-stimulatory molecules. *Eur J Immunol* 1998;28:926.
48. Wang S, Zhu G, Chapoval AI, et al. Co-stimulation of T cells by B7-H2, a B7-like molecule that binds ICOS. *Blood* 2000;96:2808.
49. Kim Y, Kim SH, Mantel P, et al. Human 4-1BB regulates CD28 co-stimulation to promote T_H 1 cell responses. *Eur J Immunol* 1998;28:881.
50. Krummel MF, Allison JP. CD28 and CTLA-4 have opposing effects on the response of T cells to stimulation. *J Exp Med* 1995;182:459.
51. Inaba K, Inaba M, Naito M, et al. Dendritic cell progenitors phagocytose particulates, including bacillus Calmette-Guerin organisms, and sensitize mice to mycobacterial antigens in vivo. *J Exp Med* 1993;178:479.
52. Hertz CJ, Kiertscher SM, Godowski PJ, et al. Microbial lipopeptides stimulate dendritic cell maturation via Toll-like receptor 2. *J Immunol* 2001;166:2444.
53. Beissert S, Hosoi J, Grabbe S, et al. IL-10 inhibits tumor antigen presentation by epidermal antigen-presenting cells. *J Immunol* 1995;154:1280.
54. Sallusto F, Nicolò C, De Maria R, et al. Ceramide inhibits antigen uptake and presentation by dendritic cells. *J Exp Med* 1996;184:2411.
55. Pulendran B, Palucka K, Banchereau J. Sensing pathogens and tuning immune responses. *Science* 2001;293:253.
56. Adema GJ, Hartgers F, Verstraten R, et al. A dendritic-cell-derived C-C chemokine that preferentially attracts naïve T cells. *Nature* 1997;387:713.
57. Brocker T. Survival of mature CD4 T lymphocytes is dependent on major histocompatibility complex class II-expressing dendritic cells. *J Exp Med* 1997;186:1223.
58. Fazekas de St Groth B. The evolution of self-tolerance: a new cell arises to meet the challenge of self-reactivity. *Immunol Today* 1998;19:448.
59. Kalinski P, Hilkens CMU, Wierenga EA, et al. T cell priming by type-1 and type-2 polarized dendritic cells: the concept of a third signal. *Immunol Today* 1999;20:561.
60. Kalinski P, Schuitemaker JH, Hilkens CM, et al. Prostaglandin E2 induces the final maturation of IL-12-deficient $CD1a^+CD83^+$ dendritic cells: the levels of IL-12 are determined during the final dendritic cell maturation and resistant to further modulation. *J Immunol* 1998;161:2804.
61. Caron G, Delneste Y, Roelandts E, et al. Histamine polarizes human dendritic cells into T_H 2 cell-promoting effector dendritic cells. *J Immunol* 2001;167: 3682.
62. Mosmann TR, Coffman RL. T_H 1 and T_H 2 cells: different patterns of lymphokine secretion lead to different functional properties. *Annu Rev Immunol* 1989;7:145.
63. Oppmann B, Lesley R, Blom B, et al. Novel p19 protein engages IL-12p40 to form a cytokine, IL-23, with biological activities similar as well as distinct from IL-12. *Immunity* 2000;13:715.
64. Abbas AK, Murphy KM, Sher A. Functional diversity of helper T lymphocytes. *Nature* 1996;383:787.
65. Munoz-Fernandez MA, Fernandez MA, Fresno M. Synergism between tumor necrosis factor-α and interferon-γ on macrophage activation for the killing of intracellular *Trypansoma cruzi* through a nitric oxide-dependent mechanism. *Eur J Immunol* 1992;22:301.
66. Trinchieri G. Interleukin-12: a proinflammatory cytokine with immunoregulatory functions that bridge innate resistance and antigen-specific adaptive immunity. *Annu Rev Immunol* 1995;13:251.
67. Fitch FW, McKisic MD, Lancki DW, et al. Differential regulation of murine T lymphocyte subsets. *Annu Rev Immunol* 1993;11:29.
68. Bonecchi R, Bianchi G, Bordignon PP, et al. Differential expression of chemokine receptors and chemotactic responsiveness of type 1 T helper cells (T_H 1s) and T_H 2s. *J Exp Med* 1998;187:129.
69. Ria F, Penna G, Adorini L. T_H 1 cells induce and T_H 2 inhibit antigen-dependent IL-12 secretion by dendritic cells. *Eur J Immunol* 1998;28:2003.
70. O'Hehir RE, Bal V, Quint D, et al. An *in vitro* model of allergen-dependent IgE synthesis by human B lymphocytes: comparison of the response of an atopic and a non-atopic individual to *Dermatophagoides* spp. (house dust mite). *Immunology* 1989;66:499.
71. King CL, Nutman TB. IgE and IgG subclass regulation by IL-4 and IFN-γ in human helminth infections. Assessment by B cell precursor frequencies. *J Immunol* 1993;151:458.
72. Schleimer RP, Sterbinsky SA, Kaiser J, et al. IL-4 induces adherence of human

eosinophils and basophils but not neutrophils to endothelium. Association with expression of VCAM-1. *J Immunol* 1992;148:1086.
73. Mochizuki M, Bartels J, Mallet AI, et al. IL-4 induces eotaxin: a possible mechanism of selective eosinophil recruitment in helminth infection and atopy. *J Immunol* 1998;160:60.
74. Sanderson CJ. Interleukin-5: an eosinophil growth and activation factor. *Dev Biol Stand* 1988;69:23.
75. Sallusto F, Mackay CR, Lanzavecchia A. Selective expression of the eotaxin receptor CCR3 by human T helper 2 cells. *Science* 1997;277:2005.
76. Ponath PD, Qin S, Ringler DJ, et al. Cloning of the human eosinophil chemoattractant, eotaxin. Expression, receptor binding, and functional properties suggest a mechanism for the selective recruitment of eosinophils. *J Clin Invest* 1996;97:604.
77. Yamada H, Hirai K, Miyamasu M, et al. Eotaxin is a potent chemotaxin for human basophils. *Biochem Biophys Res Commun* 1997;231:365.
78. Weiner HL. Induction and mechanism of action of transforming growth factor-β-secreting T_H3 regulatory cells. *Immunol Rev* 2001;182:207.
79. Roncarolo MG, Bacchetta R, Bordignon C, et al. Type 1 T regulatory cells. *Immunol Rev* 2001;182:68.
80. Papiernik M. Natural $CD8^+CD25^+$ regulatory T cells. Their role in the control of superantigen responses. *Immunol Rev* 2001;182:180.
81. Sakaguchi S, Sakaguchi N, Asano M, et al. Immunologic self-tolerance maintained by activated T cells expressing IL-2 receptor alpha-chains (CD25). Breakdown of a single mechanism of self-tolerance causes various autoimmune diseases. *J Immunol* 1995;155:1151.
82. Asano M, Toda M, Sakaguchi N, et al. Autoimmune disease as a consequence of developmental abnormality of a T cell subpopulation. *J Exp Med* 1996;184:387.
83. Ahmed R, Gray D. Immunological memory and protective immunity: understanding their relation. *Science* 1996;272:54.
84. Sprent J, Tough DF. T cell death and memory. *Science* 2001;293:245.
85. Sallusto F, Lenig D, Förster R, et al. Two subsets of memory T lymphocytes with distinct homing potentials and effector functions. *Nature* 1999;401:708.
86. Picker LJ, Treer JR, Ferguson-Darnell B, et al. Control of lymphocyte recirculation in man. I. Differential regulation of the peripheral lymph node homing receptor L-selectin on T cells during the virgin to memory cell transition. *J Immunol* 1993;150:1105.
87. Bos JD, de Boer OJ, Tibosch E, et al. Skin-homing T lymphocytes: detection of cutaneous lymphocyte associated antigen (CLA) by HECA-452 in normal human skin. *Arch Dermatol Res* 1993;285:179.
88. Fuhlbrigge, RC, Kieffer, JD, Armerding D, et al. Cutaneous lymphocyte antigen is a specialized form of PSGL-1 expressed on skin-homing T cells. *Nature* 1997;389:978.
89. Picker LJ, Terstappen LW, Rott LS, et al. Differential expression of homing-associated adhesion molecules by T cell subsets in man. *J Immunol* 1990;145:3247.
90. Robert C, Kupper TS. Inflammatory skin diseases, T cells, and immune surveillance. *N Engl J Med* 1999;341:1817.
91. Erdmann I, Scheidegger EP, Koch FK, et al. Fucosyltransferase VII-deficient mice with defective E-, P-, and L-selectin ligands show impaired $CD8^+$ and $CD8^+$ T cell migration into the skin, but normal extravasation into visceral organs. *J Immunol* 2002;168:2139.
92. Berg EL, Yoshino T, Rott LS, et al. The cutaneous lymphocyte antigen is a skin lymphocyte homing receptor for the vascular lectin endothelial cell-leukocyte adhesion molecule 1. *J Exp Med* 1991;174:1461.
93. Picker LJ, Kishimoto TK, Smith CW, et al. ELAM-1 is an adhesion molecule for skin-homing T cells. *Nature* 1991;349:796.
94. Koelle DM, Liu Z, McClurkan CM, et al. Expression of cutaneous lymphocyte-associated antigen by $CD8^+$ T cells specific for a skin-tropic virus. *J Clin Invest* 2002;110:537.
95. Groves RW, Ross E, Barker JNWN, et al. Effect of *in vivo* interleukin-1 on adhesion molecule expression in normal human skin. *J Invest Dermatol* 1992;98:384.
96. Campbell JJ, Haraldsen G, Pan J, et al. The chemokine receptor CCR4 in vascular recognition by cutaneous but not intestinal memory T cells. *Nature* 1999;400:776.
97. Ferenczi K, Fuhlbrigge RC, Pinkus J, et al. Increased CCR4 expression in cutaneous T cell lymphoma. *J Invest Dermatol* 2002;119:1405.
98. Hudak S, Hagen M, Liu Y, et al. Immune surveillance and effector functions of $CCR10^+$ skin homing T cells. *J Immunol* 2002;169:1189.
99. Morales J, Homey B, Vicari AP, et al. CTACK, a skin-associated chemokine that preferentially attracts skin-homing T cells. *Proc Natl Acad Sci U S A* 1999;96:14470.
100. Homey B, Wang W, Soto H, et al. The orphan chemokine receptor G protein-coupled receptor-2 (GPR-2, CCR10) binds the skin-associated chemokine CCL27 (CTACK/ALP/ILC). *J Immunol* 2000;164:3465.
101. Berlin C, Berg EL, Briskin MJ, et al. $\alpha_4\beta_7$ Integrin mediates lymphocyte binding to the mucosal vascular addressin MAdCAM-1. *Cell* 1993;74:185.
102. Berlin C, Bargatze RF, Campbell JJ, et al. α_4 integrins mediate lymphocyte attachment and rolling under physiologic flow. *Cell* 1995;80:413.
103. Stagg AJ, Kamm MA, Knight SC. Intestinal dendritic cells increase T cell expression of $\alpha_4\beta_7$ integrin. *Eur J Immunol* 2002;32:1445.
104. Wurbel MA, Philippe JM, Nguyen C, et al. The chemokine TECK is expressed by thymic and intestinal epithelial cells and attracts double- and single-positive thymocytes expressing the TECK receptor CCR9. *Eur J Immunol* 2000;30:262.
105. Cepek KL, Parker CM, Madara JL, et al. Integrin $\alpha^*_E\beta_7$ mediates adhesion of T lymphocytes to epithelial cells. *J Immunol* 1993;150:3459.
106. Agace WW, Higgins JMG, Sadasivan B, et al. T-lymphocyte-epithelial cell interactions: integrin α_E(CD103)β_7, LEEP-CAM and chemokines. *Curr Opin Cell Biol* 2000;12:563.
107. Weninger W, Ulfman LH, Cheng G, et al. Specialized contributions by α(1,3)-fucosyltransferase-IV and FucT-VII during leukocyte rolling in dermal microvessels. *Immunity* 2000;12:665.
108. Janssen GHGW, Tangelder GJ, Oude Egbrink MGA, et al. Spontaneous leukocyte rolling in venules in untraumatized skin of conscious and anesthestized animals. *Heart Circ Physiol* 1994;36:H1199.
109. Oude Egbrink MGA, Janssen GHGW, Ookawa K, et al. Especially polymorphonuclear leukocytes, but also monomorphonuclear leukocytes, roll spontaneously in venules of intact rat skin: involvement of E-selectin. *J Invest Dermatol* 2002;118:323.
110. Hickey MJ, Kanwar S, McCafferty DM, et al. Varying roles of E-selectin and P-selectin in different microvascular beds in response to antigen. *J Immunol* 1999;162:1137.
111. Homey B, Alenius H, Müller A, et al. CCL27-CCR10 interactions regulate T cell-mediated skin inflammation. *Nat Med* 2002;8:157.
112. Veale D, Rogers S, Fitzgerald O. 1995. Immunolocalization of adhesion molecules in psoriatic arthritis, psoriatic, and normal skin. *Br J Dermatol* 1995;132:32.
113. Menage H du P, Sattar NK, Haskard DO, et al. A study of the kinetics and pattern of E-selectin, VCAM-1, and ICAM-1 expression in chronic actinic dermatitis. *Br J Dermatol* 1996;134:262.
114. Sigurdsson V, de Vries IJ, Toonstra J, et al. Expression of VCAM-1, ICAM-1, E-selectin, and P-selectin on endothelium *in situ* in patients with erythroderma, mycosis fungoides, and atopic dermatitis. *J Cutan Pathol* 2000;27:436.

CHAPTER 2

Lupus Erythematosus

Melissa I. Costner, Richard D. Sontheimer, and Thomas T. Provost

Lupus erythematosus (LE) refers to a heterogeneous disease whose protean clinical features are united by aberrant autoimmune activation. Patients may have single organ involvement affecting only the skin, or may have systemic, multiorgan life-threatening disease. Indeed, the occurrence of disease along a spectrum is a key feature of many of the rheumatic illnesses discussed in this book. It is important for the scholar of rheumatic diseases of the skin to remain cognizant of this spectrum to (a) stratify risk for underlying visceral involvement, (b) workup and follow up patients for the development of underlying illness, and (c) allay patients' fears in regard to the development of internal illness when cutaneous symptoms are the only presentation of their disease process.

This chapter will emphasize the cutaneous features of LE. Because of space limitations, a detailed discussion about the systemic features of LE will not be possible. For those interested, there are several excellent texts that provide a thorough review (1–9). The classification of cutaneous LE is still somewhat controversial; therefore, the authors have chosen to use the Gilliam classification scheme for skin disease in LE (10–12) (Table 2.1). Following the introductory discussions of the history, definition/classification, and pathogenesis of systemic LE (SLE), the remainder of the chapter will be divided into two sections: LE-specific skin disease and LE-nonspecific skin disease.

HISTORICAL PERSPECTIVE

Because none of the authors claims to be serious students of the history of this disease, it would be presumptuous of us to attempt to improve on the work of a true scholar, John Talbott. In his review of the history of LE in the fourth edition of *Dubois' Lupus Erythematosus,* Talbott (13) points out that this disease was initially recognized by its cutaneous manifestations long before its systemic manifestations were known. In this section, we will attempt to highlight the people and events relating to the evolution of thought concerning the cutaneous manifestations of this disease process. For more information, see Talbott's excellent chapter (13), and the overview of this subject by one of the present authors, which has been derived, in part, from an abstraction of Talbott's work (14):

1851 Cazenave first used the term "lupus erythemateaux" in referring to Biett's earlier description of what appears to have been discoid LE (DLE) skin lesions (15). The term "lupus erythemateaux" helped to further distinguish this entity from cutaneous tuberculosis (lupus vulgaris), a cutaneous malady with which it had been earlier confused.

1875 Kaposi expanded Hebra's earlier description of what is now recognized as the systemic manifestations of LE, and used the "butterfly" simile, first used by Hebra, to describe the facial skin lesions of LE (16). He also commented on the relationship between DLE skin lesions and the systemic manifestations of this disease, noting that DLE can occasionally progress to systemic LE (SLE).

1880 Hutchinson (17), and later Osler at the turn of the 20th century (18), emphasized the multisystem nature of LE, and the patient-to-patient variation with which its cutaneous and systemic manifestations are expressed.

1894 Payne first treated DLE with the natural antimalarial, quinine (19).

1916 Freidberg's presentation of the heretical idea that the systemic manifestations of LE could occur in the absence of any type of skin lesion (20).

1925 Brocq's initial description of "symmetric erythema centrifugum" (21), probably representing the earliest description of what Gilliam later referred to as "subacute cutaneous LE" (SCLE) (10).

1934 O'Leary's introduction of the term "disseminated DLE" as part of his new classification scheme that included both its cutaneous and systemic manifestations (22). The term "disseminated" in his classification scheme was used somewhat ambiguously in referring both to a widespread distribution of LE skin lesions and the transition from disease limited to skin to the systemic illness that we now recognize as SLE. Thereafter, several forms of widespread LE-specific skin disease (i.e., generalized DLE and SCLE) were often lumped together under the designation "disseminated DLE" or "subacute disseminated LE," obscuring the clinical and laboratory correlates of each of these clinically distinctive types of cutaneous LE. As a result, when the large LE population studies were later presented in which the clinical features of patients with LE were correlated with the newly identified autoimmune serologic manifestations of the disease, the distinction between patients having generalized DLE and SCLE was often blurred.

1948 Hargrave's (23) description of the LE cell factor and Friou's (24) subsequent description of the antinuclear antibody assay in 1957 ushered in the era of serologic–clinical correlation in LE.

TABLE 2.1. Gilliam Classification of Lupus Erythematosus (LE)–Associated Skin Lesions

LE-specific skin lesions
Acute cutaneous LE
Localized
Generalized
Subacute cutaneous LE
Annular
Papulosquamous
Chronic cutaneous LE
"Classic" DLE
Localized
Generalized
Hypertrophic (verrucous) DLE
Lupus panniculitis (profundus)
Mucosal LE
Lupus tumidus
Chilblains lupus
DLE–lichen planus overlap
LE-nonspecific skin lesions
Cutaneous vascular disease
Vasculitis
Leukocytoclastic
Palpable purpura
Urticarial vasculitis
Periarteritis nodosa–like
Vasculopathy
Dego disease–like
Atrophy blanche-like
Periungual telangiectasia
Livedo reticularis
Thrombophlebitis
Raynaud phenomenon
Erythromelalgia (erythermalgia)
Alopecia (nonscarring)
"Lupus hair"
Telogen effluvium
Alopecia areata
Sclerodactyly
Rheumatoid nodules
Calcinosis cutis
LE-nonspecific bullous lesions
Epidermolysis bullosa acquisita–like bullous LE
Dermatitis herpetiformis–like bullous LE
Pemphigus erythematosus
Bullous pemphigoid
Porphyria cutanea tarda
Urticaria
Papulonodular mucinosis
Anetoderma/cutis laxa
Acanthosis nigricans (type B insulin resistance)
Erythema multiforme
Leg ulcers
Lichen planus

DLE, discoid LE; LE, lupus erythematosus.

1951 Introduction of the synthetic antimalarial, quinacrine (25), and corticosteroids (26) for the treatment of LE.

1963 Neville Rowell's description of erythema multiforme-like lesions occurring in patients with LE with autoantibodies to the Sjögren syndrome antigen Sj-T, which is now thought to represent the La(SS-B) specificity (27). Rowell's other work has contributed significantly to our current understanding of various aspects of cutaneous LE including chilblain lupus (lupus pernio) and classic DLE.

1963 Burnham and coworkers' identification of the "lupus band" (28).

1963 Edmund Dubois and Denny Tuffanelli present their landmark description of 520 consecutive patients with SLE, 29% of whom had DLE skin lesions (29). Dubois was among the first to use the "spectrum" analogy for LE, emphasizing that this illness represented a disease continuum extending from localized DLE at the more benign pole to fully expressed SLE at the more severely affected pole. He also emphasized that various transitional forms commonly occurred within this spectrum including the appearance of SLE in patients who had initially presented with DLE lesions alone, as well as the development of DLE lesions in patients with preexisting SLE. These concepts were emphasized in the first edition of his classic book (30), which is currently in its sixth edition (3). Dubois' spectrum concept profoundly influenced Jim Gilliam's thinking concerning the classification of cutaneous LE.

1969 Morris Reichlin and coworkers' description of anti-Ro(SS-A) antibodies (31), later to be identified as the serologic marker for SCLE and neonatal LE.

1975 James N. Gilliam extended Edmund Dubois' spectrum analogy, focusing especially on the relationships that exist between the various cutaneous and systemic manifestations of LE (32). He also stressed the value of the various forms of cutaneous LE as markers for subsetting LE (the exercise of identifying more homogeneous subgroups or phenotypes of patients with LE on the basis of the sharing of common clinical, pathologic, and laboratory features) that had become popular by the 1970s (11).

1976 Publication of a comprehensive monograph by Marian W. Ropes (1) detailing the experience gained from a large number of patients with SLE followed over several decades in the inpatient and outpatient settings at Massachusetts General Hospital. Careful observations concerning the mucocutaneous manifestations of this disease were reported.

1979 Gilliam and coworkers' characterization of the immunogenetically homogeneous LE subset marked by the presence of SCLE skin lesions (33–35). These were virtually the same group of patients being described concurrently by Thomas Provost and his colleagues under the designation of "ANA-negative SLE" (36,37). The concept of SCLE was originally introduced by Gilliam as a component of a new classification of cutaneous LE that emphasized the clinical differences that exist between different types of histopathologically specific LE skin lesions (10,11). Gilliam's earlier work at Stanford with the dermatopathologist, Alvin Cox, and later at University of Texas Southwestern with Robert Freeman greatly influenced his thinking in this area.

1981 Description by investigators led by William Weston and Thomas Provost of anti-Ro(SS-A) autoantibody as the serologic marker for neonatal LE (38,39). Also, the description by these and other investigators of the association of anti-Ro(SS-A) antibodies with a heterogeneous group of patients with lupus with prominent photosensitive skin disease (40–42).

1984 Original report by David Norris and colleagues that ultraviolet (UV) irradiation was capable of modulating the expression of Ro(SS-A) antigens by epidermal keratinocytes, thus offering a potential molecular explanation for the pathogenesis of anti-Ro(SS-A) antibody–associated forms of photosensitive cutaneous LE such as SCLE and neonatal LE (43).

The significance of Norris' work is just now becoming realized. This work has stimulated other investigators to explore programmed cell death (apoptosis) and how it may relate to the pathogenesis of systemic lupus erythematosus (44) (see pathogenesis later).

DEFINITION AND CLASSIFICATION

LE is the root designation for a heterogeneous autoimmune syndrome whose diverse features are linked by a common pathogenesis. It may affect only one organ (i.e., cutaneous LE) or many organ systems and is best thought of as occurring along a spectrum (44a,b). Because there is such variation in presentation, nomenclature can potentially be fraught with difficulty and confusion. In this section, we will attempt to clarify controversies in classification and subclassification of this complex disease.

Systemic lupus erythematosus (SLE) refers to the end of the spectrum occupied by multisystem disease in which constitutional symptoms and musculoskeletal and visceral organ inflammation usually predominate. The American College of Rheumatology (ACR) has formulated a set of revised clinical and laboratory criteria for the classification of SLE (Table 2.2). Patients who meet four of 11 criteria are classified as having SLE. It should be emphasized that the ACR criteria for classification of SLE were devised primarily to provide some degree of uniformity to the patient populations of clinical studies (45). This classification system is also commonly used by clinicians, to some degree erroneously, to establish a diagnosis of SLE in a given patient. Those experienced in evaluating patients with this disorder consider SLE a diagnosis arrived on following a history and physical examination supported by laboratory evaluation, including serologic testing.

The term "SLE" has been used in the past synonymously with the term "LE" to designate all patients with this autoimmune disease process (unfortunately, many physicians continue to use the term in this manner). However, in this sense the term "SLE" unfairly stigmatizes those patients with LE whose disease is expressed only in their skin throughout their entire disease course. The term "SLE" will be used in this discussion to refer only to the systemic manifestations of the fundamental underlying disease process, LE.

Cutaneous LE (CLE) will be used in an umbrella fashion in this chapter to refer to all skin lesions that have some form of association with LE. One should consider CLE as one of the potential end organ targets that might be the result of injury due to LE activity. CLE may be the only manifestation of the LE disease phenotype or may be one of several involved organs.

The term "discoid LE" (DLE) was often used generically in the past to designate the subgroup of patients with LE whose disease was expressed only in the skin. The use of the term "DLE" in this sense can create confusion because this same term is also commonly used to identify one morphologically distinct form (coined shaped) of LE-specific skin disease. In the following discussion the term "DLE" will be used in the latter, more restricted, sense to refer only to a certain morphologic form of cutaneous LE.

The clinical expression of skin involvement in LE is very common and extremely heterogeneous (Table 2.1). Because the type of skin involvement in LE can be reflective of the underly-

TABLE 2.2. The 1982 Revised Criteria for Classification of Systemic Lupus Erythematosus (SLE)

Criterion	Definition
1. Malar rash	Fixed erythema, flat or raised, over the malar eminences, tending to spare the nasolabial folds
2. Discoid rash	Erythematous raised patches with adherent keratotic scaling and follicular plugging; atrophic scarring may occur in older lesions
3. Photosensitivity	Skin rash as a result of unusual reaction to sunlight, by patient history or physician observation
4. Oral ulcers	Oral or nasopharyngeal ulceration, usually painless, observed by a physician
5. Arthritis	Nonerosive arthritis involving two or more peripheral joints, characterized by tenderness, swelling, or effusion
6. Serositis	a. Serositis—convincing history of pleuritic pain or rub heard by a physician or evidence of pleural effusion or b. Pericarditis—documented by electrocardiogram or rub or evidence of pericardial effusion
7. Renal disorder	a. Persistent proteinuria—0.5 g/day or greater than 3 if quantification not performed or b. Cellular casts—may be red cell, hemoglobin, granular, tubular, or mixed
8. Neurologic disorder	a. Seizures—in the absence of offending drugs or known metabolic derangement (e.g., uremia, ketoacidosis, or electrolyte imbalance) or b. Psychosis—in the absence of offending drugs or known metabolic derangement (e.g., uremia, ketoacidosis, or electrolyte imbalance)
9. Hematologic disorder	a. Hemolytic anemia with reticulocytosis or b. Leukopenia—leukocytes <4,000/μL on two or more occasions or c. Lymphopenia—lymphocytes <1,500/μL on two or more occasions or d. Thrombocytopenia—platelets <100,000/μL in the absence of offending drugs
10. Immunologic disorder	a. Anti-DNA—antibody to native DNA in abnormal titer or b. Anti-Sm—presence of antibody to Sm nuclear antigen or c. Positive finding of antiphospholipid antibodies based on (a) an abnormal serum level of IgG or IgM anticardiolipin antibodies, (b) a positive test result for lupus anticoagulant using a standard method, or (c) a false-positive serologic test for syphilis known to be positive for at least 6 months and confirmed by *Treponema pallidum* immobilization or fluorescent treponemal antibody absorption test
11. Antinuclear antibody	An abnormal titer of antinuclear antibody by immunofluorescence of an equivalent assay at any time and in the absence of drugs known to be associated with "drug-induced lupus" syndrome

The proposed classification is based on 11 criteria. For the purpose of identifying patients in clinical studies, a person shall be said to have systemic lupus erythematosus if any four or more of the 11 criteria are present, serially or simultaneously, during any interval of observation.
From Tan et al, (45), with permission.

ing pattern of SLE activity, it is important to have a common language when referring to LE skin lesions. Much attention has been paid to the issue of classifying LE from the dermatologic perspective in the past, and there continues to be considerable debate in this area (46–50). For the purposes of this discussion, we will use the classification system developed by Gilliam (10). That system divides the skin lesions that can be encountered in patients with LE into those that have the characteristic histologic changes of LE (i.e., *LE-specific skin disease*) and those that do not show these changes (i.e., *LE-nonspecific skin disease*) (10,11). The histologically characteristic skin lesions share the following elements of a lichenoid tissue reaction (51): hyperkeratosis; epidermal atrophy; vacuolar alteration of the epidermal basal cell layer; a mononuclear cell infiltrate focused at the dermal–epidermal junction, perivascular areas, and perifollicular areas; thickening of the epidermal basement membrane; melanin pigment incontinence, and dermal mucin deposition. There are three broad categories of LE-specific skin disease: *acute cutaneous LE* (ACLE), *subacute cutaneous LE* (SCLE), and *chronic cutaneous LE* (CCLE). LE-nonspecific skin lesions such as cutaneous vasculitis have clinicohistopathologic changes that are seen in conditions other than LE and are thus not specific for this disorder.

The classification and subclassification of CLE and its association with SLE can be seen as being analogous to LE activity in other organ systems (Fig. 2.1). Consider the hematologic system. Patients with autoimmune disorders of the blood and its precursors may have localized single organ (blood) involvement (i.e., idiopathic thrombocytopenic purpura [ITP], autoimmune hemolytic anemia), or their cytopenia(s) may be part of a multiorgan presentation of SLE. It is not uncommon to see overlap (i.e., both ITP and hemolytic anemia may occur in a patient with SLE).

The LE disease spectrum can be subdivided in a number of ways: clinically, serologically, or pathologically. Using this approach, various patterns (or subsets) of illness can be identified (i.e., some patients will share common patterns of clinical, immunologic, and pathologic abnormalities). One example is SCLE. Patients who present with SCLE skin lesions have a clinically and pathologically distinctive form of cutaneous LE, frequently produce anti-Ro(SS-A) autoantibodies, and share a common HLA phenotype (HLA B8 DR2 (DRB1*1501) DR3 (DRB1*0301). Similarly, patients with immune thrombocytopenia (with or without underlying SLE) have a clinically and pathologically distinctive form of thrombocytopenia. Patients frequently produce antiplatelet (anti–glycoprotein IIb/IIIa) antibodies and often share the major histocompatibility complex (MHC) class II allele HLA DRB1 DQB1 (52,53).

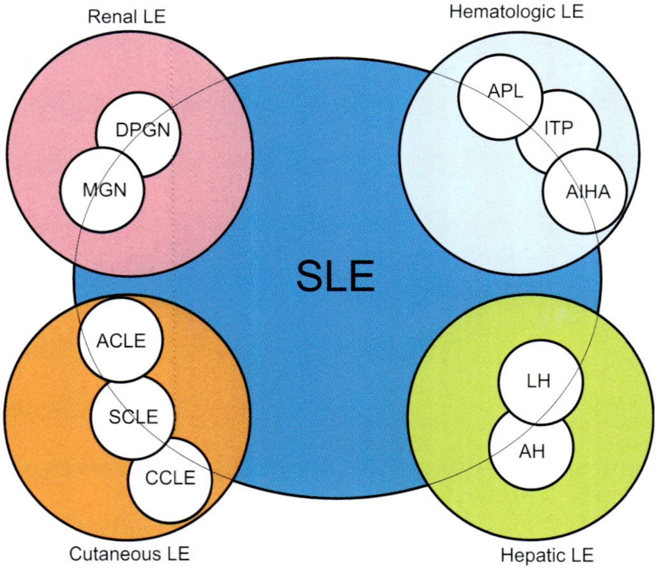

Figure 2.1. Spectrum of lupus erythematosus activity. The classification of cutaneous lupus erythematosus may be viewed as similar to other organ systems affected in systemic lupus erythematosus.

The authors believe that the Gilliam classification scheme best emphasizes that CLE is a heterogeneous subset of LE and that certain conclusions can be drawn about patients with specific clinicopathologic manifestations of CLE based on their subgrouping of CLE (i.e., risk for scarring from CLE, risk for underlying systemic illness, etc.) However, utilization of the Gilliam classification requires several points of clarification. First, it is important to note that the designations "acute, subacute, and chronic" concerning LE-specific skin disease, refer to the pace and severity of any associated SLE as well as how long individual lesions are present. For example, ACLE usually occurs in the setting of acutely flaring SLE, whereas CCLE often occurs in the absence of SLE or in the presence of mild smoldering SLE. SCLE occupies an intermediate position in this clinical spectrum.

"LE-specific skin disease" has been used synonymously with the term "LE-specific histology." In consideration of the term LE-specific histology, one must use caution. There are several examples of entities that are histologically similar to CLE, including dermatomyositis, medication hypersensitivity reactions with an interface pattern of inflammation, and some forms of polymorphic light eruption, among others (53a). "LE-specific histology" does not imply that the characteristic histologic changes seen in LE-specific skin disease may absolutely not be seen in any other cutaneous disease process, but rather merely attempts to subclassify cutaneous lesions in patients with SLE into two groups: those united by the lichenoid tissue reaction described before and those with other histologic findings.

With any arbitrary subdivision of a disease continuum such as LE, exceptions can occur. Overlap of different subsets of LE-specific skin disease is common. For example, patients may be difficult to subclassify because they have two or three subsets of LE-specific skin disease concomitantly (i.e., patients with predominately SCLE lesions can also develop scarring DLE or ACLE lesions at some point in their course). However, in most patients, one form of LE-specific skin involvement will predominate. In addition, some patients (especially black patients in our experience) have LE-specific skin disease that is clinically indeterminate. That is, the clinical appearance of these patients' skin lesions does not clearly conform to one of the conventional categories within the Gilliam classification scheme. Although clinically indeterminate, histologic sections from their skin biopsies will show many of the characteristic changes of LE-specific skin disease (Fig. 2.2).

It should also be remembered that patients with LE not infrequently develop unrelated common dermatologic disorders that are not the direct result of LE activity in the skin. In their study of 84 consecutive patients with SLE, Weinstein et al. (54) found that 42% had dermatoses attributable to SLE, whereas 69% had dermatoses that were not directly attributable to SLE. Some conditions (i.e., acne rosacea and tinea fasciae) can simulate the clinical appearance of different forms of cutaneous LE (55). Harm to patients can result when this principle is not kept in mind. Corticosteroid-induced acne vulgaris is an example of a skin condition that could occur in a patient with LE as a result of treatment of LE rather than the LE autoimmune process itself.

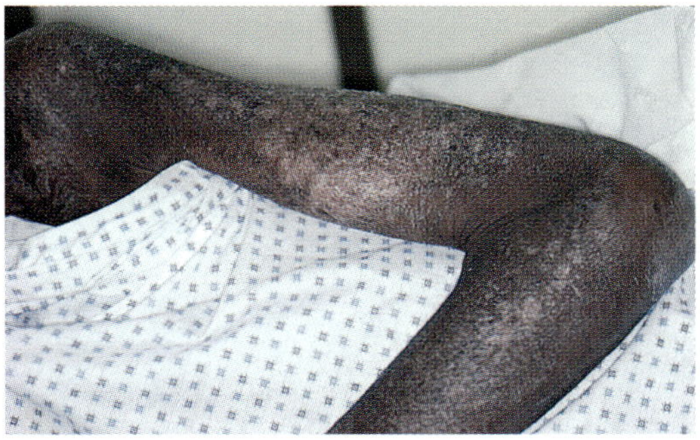

Figure 2.2. Clinically indeterminate LE–specific skin disease. Although the biopsy demonstrated clear changes of LE-specific skin disease, the clinical appearance in this middle-aged black man was not typical of ACLE, SLE, or DLE.

ETIOLOGIC FACTORS AND PATHOGENESIS OF SYSTEMIC LUPUS ERYTHEMATOSUS

Although much remains unknown about the cause of this complex syndrome, many recent insights have been gained (56). An attractive contemporary model of SLE pathogenesis describes four theoretic temporally sequential phases that are prerequisite for the clinical expression of this disease. These phases are the inheritance of susceptibility genes, induction of autoimmunity, expansion of autoimmune processes, and immunologic injury (Fig. 2.3).

The first phase is the *susceptibility phase* and refers to the genetic predisposition of the patient with SLE. The predisposition state likely also includes genes that promote a sustained autoimmune response following the initial activation or, in some way, lower the threshold for self-reactivity or determine the pattern and extent of end-organ injury (56). The important role of genetics in the development of SLE has been confirmed with many recent advances in the study of both murine and human lupus genetics. A familial prevalence of 10% to 12% has been estimated using surveys of patients with SLE who report lupus in first-degree relatives. There is a 10-fold difference in heritability of SLE between dizygotic and monozygotic twins (57). Linkage analyses performed in lupus-prone mice strains have identified more than 30 genes that may play a role in lupus susceptibility. Multiple crosses of these mice have shown localization to three chromosomes: 1, 4, and 7. The susceptibility locus on chromosome 1 appears to confer loss of B-cell tolerance to subnucleosomal antigens, whereas that on chromosome 4 is associated with B-cell hyperreactivity, including overproduction of IgM. The locus on chromosome 7 confers overproduction of IgG and mild glomerulonephritis (58). Studies with transgenic mice have pointed to pathways in which candidate genes may have altered expression, conferring susceptibility to SLE in humans. These include genes involved in apoptosis, antigen presentation, and lymphocyte activation (59). Genes associated with apoptosis have been particularly compelling candidates because it is well known that apoptosis exposes potential autoantigens that might have been previously hidden (60). This in turn might lead to loss of self-tolerance of these cryptic peptides and induction of autoimmunity (see second phase later) (61). A murine model of lupus erythematosus (MRL-lpr) has been shown to have defective apoptosis, pre-

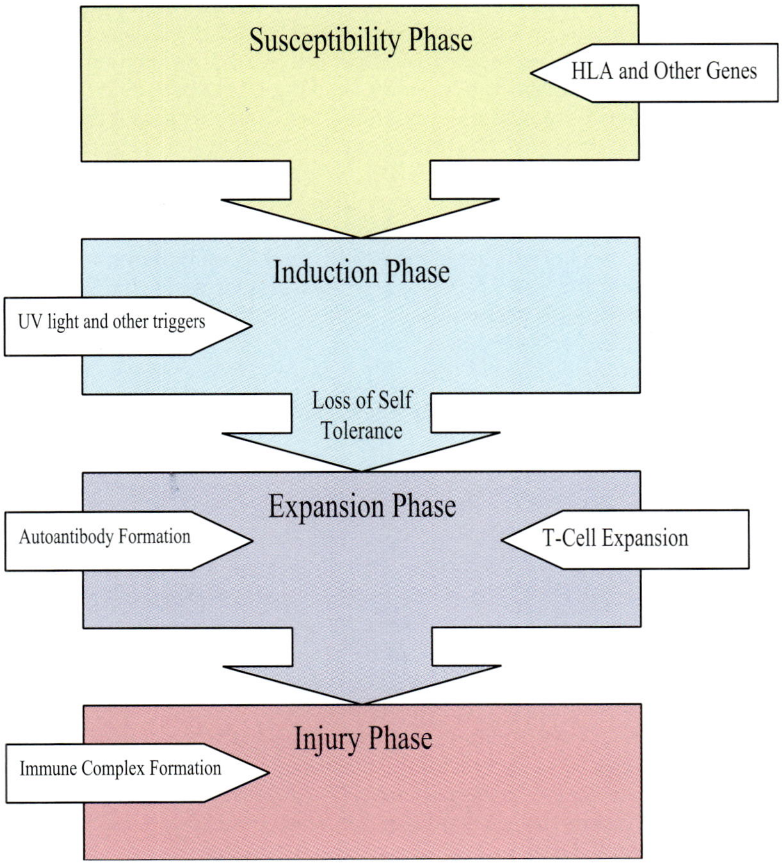

Figure 2.3. Pathogenesis of systemic lupus erythematosus. This model summarizes current theories regarding pathogenesis of systemic lupus erythematosus and lupus-specific skin disease.

sumably due to mutations or insertions into *Fas* or *gld* genes (62,63).

In human lupus, association studies comprise most of what we know about the genetics of SLE. Numerous case control studies have established associations of SLE with certain MHC class II alleles (DRB and DQA) (64). The association between CLE and inheritance of class II alleles is well known and is described in detail later. Additionally, there have been recent studies documenting polymorphisms in MHC class III genes, tumor necrosis factor-α (TNF-α), complement proteins C19, C2 and C4, and complement receptor 1 (65). Inherited complement deficiencies have been associated with SLE (65). Ninety-three percent of individuals identified who have complete congenital deficiency of C19 have developed SLE, often with photosensitive cutaneous LE (65a). Genes encoding complement proteins are compelling candidate genes for two reasons. Genetic studies involving New Zealand white mice have also pointed to a gene encoding complement receptors 1 and 2 as a strong candidate gene for conferring lupus susceptibility (66). Furthermore, complement is involved in the opsonization and clearing of potentially autoimmunogenetic cells (including apoptotic cells), suggesting that a defect in this "waste clearance" mechanism might lead to lupus-like illness (67). Recent evidence suggests that deficiency of mannose-binding lectin (MBL), an acute-phase reactant that is able to activate both the classic and alternative pathways of the complement cascade and opsonize bacteria, confirms a minor risk for the development of SLE (68,69). Several studies have shown the TNF-α allele to be an independent risk factor for susceptibility to SLE, and recent attention has focused on studying the TNF receptors I and II as potential candidate genes, because they are major regulators for apoptosis of mature T cells (70). A polymorphism in one of the genes encoding TNF-α has recently been associated with photosensitivity in patients with SCLE (70,71). In addition, a single nucleotide polymorphism in the C19A gene has recently been associated with the SCLE phenotype and low C19 serum levels (71a). Specifics regarding genetic susceptibility of LE-specific skin disease will be discussed further later.

The second phase of SLE pathogenesis, *the induction phase,* involves the initiation of autoimmunity characterized by the appearance of autoreactive T cells that exhibit the loss of self-tolerance. Potential mechanisms include aberrant expression of HLA-DR molecules, molecular mimicry induced by infection, failure of central thymic or peripheral tolerance mechanisms, and the presentation of cryptic peptides during apoptosis. There has been much recent data suggesting the role of apoptosis in the induction of self-tolerance. Apoptosis is characterized by chromatin condensation with a very characteristic fragmentation of DNA, producing a ladder effect on gel electrophoresis, as well as shrinkage of the cytoplasm with nuclear and cytoplasm bleb formation. Recent studies by Casciola-Rosen et al. (44) have demonstrated the compartmentalization of specific nucleosome constituents, including ribonuclear proteins, to the cytoplasmic cell surface blebs of keratinocytes undergoing UV light–induced apoptosis (72–75). UV light likely plays a large role in the second phase of LE pathogenesis, especially in the pathogenesis of LE-specific skin disease (see later). The tendency for patients with complement deficiencies to develop LE might be related to their inability to opsonize apoptotic cells resulting in defective initiation of self-tolerance (75a).

The third or *expansion phase* seems to involve progressive augmentation of the aberrant autoimmune clonal expression of B and T cells capable of autorecognition. Although SLE has been classically thought of as a disease characterized by overexpression of B cells and subsequent autoantibody production, there is compelling evidence for the central role of the T cell in the autoimmune response of SLE. Autoantigen-specific $CD4^+$, MHC class II–restricted, T-cell clones or lines have been identified in both murine models and humans with SLE. These autoreactive T cells are capable of providing the requisite "help" to B cells that produce pathogenic antibodies (56,70). The T-cell compartment in SLE is characterized by extensive, unexplained activation, and may be related to the decreased requirement for costimulatory signals necessary for normal activation of T cells. During the expansion phase, there are cognitive interactions of T and B cells that occur in germinal centers of lymphoid follicles. CD40 and CD40L play a crucial role in regulating this interaction, and monoclonal antibodies to CD40L are currently being studied as potential novel therapeutic targets in SLE (76). The cognate interaction between T and B cells leads to the production of higher affinity and titers of serologically detectable autoantibodies produced by a population of clonally expanded B cells. Despite their abundance, autoantibodies in SLE are directed against a limited number of nuclear and cytoplasmic antigens. Three major targets are the nucleosome (anti-DNA and antihistone antibodies), the spliceosome (anti-Sm and anti-RNP antibodies), and the Ro and La molecules (anti-Ro and anti-LA). Interestingly, these autoantibodies often arise in grouped sets probably because these targets are available to the immune system as intact rather than as individual particles. The aggregation of these autoantibodies and the source of the triggering autoantigens was a mystery until it was realized that most of the lupus target autoantigens are clustered in distinct structures at the surface of apoptotic cells. Once immune tolerance to the intact particles is broken down, the autoantibody response diversifies to the individual components via recognition of new epitopes within the intact complex. This phenomenon has been referred to as epitope spreading (44,70).

The last and perhaps clinically most relevant stage that heralds the onset of clinical disease is the *injury phase.* Much of this injury phase can be attributed to the action of autoantibodies and the immune complexes they form that may cause tissue damage by many means: direct cell death, complement activation and opsonization, or by blocking target molecule function. Passively transferred autoantibodies directed against the snNPs of the SS-A/Ro, SS-B/La group are thought to be directly pathogenic in neonatal LE (77). Thrombocytopenia in SLE and Coombs-positive anemia are likely due to uptake of antibody-coated cells by phagocyte Fc receptors (56). Injury patterns seen in vasculitis and nephritis in SLE are the result of immune complexes that are deposited within glomeruli or blood vessel walls, which subsequently bind to C1q and initiate injury via complement activation (75a).

Lupus Erythematosus–specific Skin Disease

EPIDEMIOLOGY

There are very few population-based data concerning the epidemiology of LE—cutaneous or systemic. Most studies are reported by rheumatologists or dermatologists working separately, and as a result, selection bias is often present in the data that are commonly reported. In most large clinical studies of selected patients with LE, the skin is second only to joints as the most frequently affected organ system, and skin disease is the second most common way that LE initially presents clinically (78–80). The same finding was documented in a population-based cohort of 80 patients (81). In some study populations, cutaneous disease has been the most common disease manifestation (82,83).

Together, all forms of cutaneous LE have a significant socioeconomic impact within the United States. It has been suggested that cutaneous LE is the third most common cause of industrial disability from dermatologic disease, with 45% of patients with CLE experiencing some degree of vocational handicap (84).

Acute Cutaneous Lupus Erythematosus

In most large clinical studies carried out by rheumatologists or internists, ACLE is reported under the designations "malar rash" or "butterfly rash" (i.e., presumably localized ACLE), and "rash," "maculopapular rash," or "photosensitive lupus dermatitis" (presumably generalized ACLE). In such studies, the skin lesions are usually not biopsied, and thus it is difficult to know whether they in fact represent LE-specific skin disease. Because dermatologists are not usually the primary managers of such patients because of the strong association between ACLE and systemic LE activity, few data concerning this form of LE-specific skin disease are available in the dermatologic literature. Because of its strong association with SLE, the epidemiology of ACLE might be expected to closely parallel that of unselected patients with SLE. The epidemiology of SLE has been comprehensively reviewed (81–83).

DEMOGRAPHICS

Malar rash or butterfly rash has been reported in 20% to 60% of large LE patient cohorts (54,78–80,82,83,85). Limited data suggest that the "maculopapular rash" of SLE is present in about 35% of patients with SLE (80). Malar rash is more common in women than in men (80,86). Because photosensitivity is seen more frequently in whites than blacks (81), one might infer that the same could be true for ACLE, and in fact, a recent study comparing features of SLE in different populations in central Australia showed that malar rash and photosensitivity are much more common in whites than in darkly skinned aboriginal patients (87). Malar rash has been suggested to be associated with a younger age of disease onset (80). A clinically nonspecific maculopapular rash resembling a drug eruption but which was believed to be related to SLE was present in 59% of the 81 patients studied by Wysenbeek et al. (85); however, because biopsy data were not presented it cannot be certain whether this "rash" was related to generalized ACLE.

GENETIC ASSOCIATIONS

ACLE lesions usually occur in the context of SLE, and as described above, genetic susceptibility is paramount to the development of SLE. It is curious however, that very few studies have been performed to determine whether ACLE has any specific MHC class II or other genetic associations. Rao et al. performed a linkage analysis of individual clinical components of SLE in 101 SLE-affected sibling pairs and found that "malar rash" was linked significantly to chromosome 7 (88). SLE has been associated with HLA B8 DR2 (DRB1*1501) DR3 (DRB1*0301) (88a,89). However these HLA associations may be more closely associated with the anti-Ro(SS-A) antibody responses (reviewed in [88],89), and recent studies indicate that the malar dermatitis is the most common cutaneous lesion in patients with anti-Ro(SS-A)–positive lupus (90).

ENVIRONMENTAL FACTORS

Exposure to natural or UV irradiation is a frequent precipitating factor for patients with SLE (91), especially those who produce anti-Ro(SS-A) autoantibodies (92,93). UV radiation induces lesions of ACLE and SCLE and to a lesser extent DLE (94). UV radiation can displace autoantigens such as Ro/SS-A and related autoantigens, La/SS-B and calreticulin, from their normal locations inside epidermal keratinocytes to the cell surface. Evidence suggests that UV-induced keratinocyte apoptosis is a major mechanism responsible for this aberrant pattern of cell surface autoantigen expression (44,95). Other potential mechanisms include UV alteration of cellular DNA and aberrant expression of HLA-DR. UV light may cause an exaggerated release of immune mediators such as interleukin-1 (IL-1), TNF-α, prostaglandin E, proteases, oxygen free radicals, and histamine in genetically predisposed individuals with LE, which might in turn lead to induction of self-tolerance (i.e., induction phase of LE pathogenesis) or might be directly involved in keratinocyte cytotoxicity (i.e., injury phase of LE pathogenesis).

Chemicals such as L-canavanine, present in alfalfa sprouts, can induce an SLE-like illness (96). Numerous drugs have been implicated in inducing various features of SLE (97), although the skin is generally spared in classic drug-induced SLE (i.e., hydralazine, isoniazid, and procainamide). There has been much speculation regarding the role of infectious agents, particularly viruses in the induction of SLE and cutaneous LE. Infections of all types have long been known to exacerbate SLE. Infection by α viruses such as Sindbis, rubella, and cytomegalovirus appears able to induce cell surface expression of Ro/SS-A and related autoantigens in cells undergoing virus-induced apoptosis. Seroconversion to Epstein–Barr virus among patients with SLE is nearly universal. Epstein–Barr virus infection is associated with overexpression of bcl2 and the inability of lupus T cells to suppress growth of infected/activated B cells (98).

Subacute Cutaneous Lupus Erythematosus

DEMOGRAPHICS

Patients with SCLE comprised 9% of the total LE patient population examined by Sontheimer et al. (33). Others have found SCLE lesions in 7% to 27% of their populations of patients with LE (54,80,85,99–103). SCLE is primarily a disease of white females of all ages. Seventy percent of the original cohort of patients with SCLE were female and 85% were white (33). The mean age of this group of patients was 43.3 years with a range of 17 to 67 years. Others have reported similar racial and sex demographic data (80,99–106).

GENETIC ASSOCIATIONS

Most studies have found that at least half of patients with SCLE have the HLA-DR3 phenotype (34,99,105,107,108), although some groups have found a lower frequency of HLA-DR3 (104, 109). HLA-DR3 is normally found in only 25% of the U.S. white population (110). One group has suggested that the HLA-DR3 phenotype is most strongly associated with the annular form of SCLE (111) and that annular SCLE lesions denote the most immunogenetically homogeneous subgroup of patients with SCLE (111). HLA-DR2 has also been associated with SCLE (112). Patients with SCLE with overlapping features of SCLE and Sjögren syndrome (SSj) are more likely to have the HLA B8 DR2 (DRB1*1501) DR3 (DRB1*0301) extended haplotype (113) and these phenotypes have also been shown to be statistically increased in anti-Ro(SS-A) antibody–positive neonatal lupus erythematosus (NLE) mothers and patients with SSj/LE overlap (114). It has been suggested that the HLA-DR antigen associations of SCLE relate more to the anti-Ro(SS-A) antibody response in these patients than to the SCLE skin lesions (112). Patients with the extended haplotype produce very high levels of Ro(SS-A) autoantibodies (115,116). High Ro(SS-A) antibody titers have also been associated in individuals with HLA-DQw1/DQw2 (116).

IL-1 receptor antagonist and TNF-α gene polymorphisms have been implicated as genetic factors in SCLE. Werth et al. (71) found a substantial increase in the prevalence of a promoter polymorphism of TNF-α-308A in patients with SCLE. Additionally, they found that there was a striking synergy between UVB and added IL-1α (a photo-induced cytokine) in the induction of transcription of the TNF-α-308A promoter (71). This suggests that this polymorphism may directly contribute to the photosensitivity of patients with SCLE.

Homozygous deficiency of various complement components including C1 (especially C1q), C2, C3, C4, and C5 (40,42, 117–120), as well as C1 esterase inhibitor (121,122), has been reported in association with SCLE and DLE. As previously noted, a specific C19A gene single nucleotide polymorphism has been associated with SCLE and low C19 blood levels (71a).

ENVIRONMENTAL FACTORS

Earlier studies (123) and the more recent data (108,124,125) have indicated that most patients with SCLE are highly sensitive to UV irradiation (see before). Exposure to certain drugs and other treatment modalities including hydrochlorothiazide (123, 126–130), procainamide (131), D-penicillamine (123), sulfonylureas (123), oxprenolol (132), griseofulvin (133), piroxicam (134), naproxen (135), spironolactone (136), UVB (137), PUVA (138), terbinafine (139–143), diltiazem (144) and the antiangiogenesis tetracycline-derived drug COL-3 (145) have been associated with the development of SCLE, or an acute phototoxic widespread dermatitis, or both.

Chronic Cutaneous Lupus Erythematosus

No reliable population-based data exist pertaining to the true prevalence or incidence of classic DLE (the most common form of chronic cutaneous LE) presenting in the absence of systemic LE activity. Such patients tend to be underrepresented in studies reported by rheumatologists and internists and overrepresented by those reported by dermatologists. In addition, the epidemiologic data available that pertains to DLE are difficult to interpret. Studies before 1970 did not stratify patients according to the ACR's classification criteria for SLE. In addition, these workers did not have access to the various laboratory parameters that gauge the presence and degree of activity of systemic autoimmunity. In addition, before 1979, investigators did not distinguish between DLE and SCLE, usually lumping these two varieties of cutaneous LE together under the generic designations of "DLE" or "disseminated DLE." Thus, it can be difficult to gain an accurate view of the prevalence or incidence of DLE from the data presented in studies before that time.

DEMOGRAPHICS

On the basis of data from the available studies, the following points can be made concerning the epidemiology of DLE, as distinguished from SCLE. DLE skin lesions are present in 15% to 30% of variously selected study populations of SLE (29,80,82, 83,146). Approximately 5% to 10% of SLE populations have DLE skin lesions as their presenting disease manifestation (29). For every patient affected primarily with DLE, seven will be affected primarily by SLE (79). The most common age of onset of DLE is between 20 and 40 years in both males and females (32,147–152). DLE lesions, however, can appear in infancy as well as the elderly. The female-to-male ratio for DLE has been reported to be between 3:2 and 3:1 (29,147–156), which is much lower than the ratio of females to males (9:1) with SLE. Any race can be affected, although most of the classic studies have found DLE to be more frequent in whites (32,147,149,150,157). Our collective experience indicates that blacks generally have a much more cosmetically severe form of DLE with increased scarring and postinflammatory hypo- and hyperpigmentation. Some earlier studies suggested that blacks were relatively protected from DLE; however, Hochberg et al. (82) have presented data that argue that DLE might actually be more prevalent in blacks (82).

GENETIC ASSOCIATIONS

Knop et al. (158) found significant increases of HLA-B7, B8, Cw7, DR2, DR3, and DQW1, and a significant decrease in HLA-A2 in a large group of German patients with DLE. The combinations of HLA-Cw7, DR3, DQW1, and HLA-B7, Cw7, DR3 conferred the maximum relative risk (7.4) for DLE. Fischer et al. (159) have reported a significant association with HLA-DQA1*0102 conferring a relative risk of 4.7. No associations were found with the HLA-DPB1 locus.

ENVIRONMENTAL FACTORS

Skin lesions are precipitated or aggravated by UV irradiation, especially UVB, in approximately half the patients with DLE. Drug-induced DLE lesions are extremely rare. We have observed several patients whose previously refractory DLE lesions improved spontaneously in a dramatic fashion following the cessation of cigarette smoking. Other investigators have recently confirmed this finding (160,161). Nonspecific injury to the skin can precipitate the development of DLE activity within the areas of trauma (the Köebner phenomenon).

Recent studies suggest that exposure to cold damp weather may induce pernio lesions in some anti-Ro(SS-A) antibody–positive patients (see discussion on chilblain lupus).

CUTANEOUS MANIFESTATIONS

Acute Cutaneous Lupus Erythematosus

ACLE can present in either a localized or generalized distribution. Localized ACLE (the classic "butterfly rash" or "malar rash" of SLE) is the most common pattern. Localized ACLE is

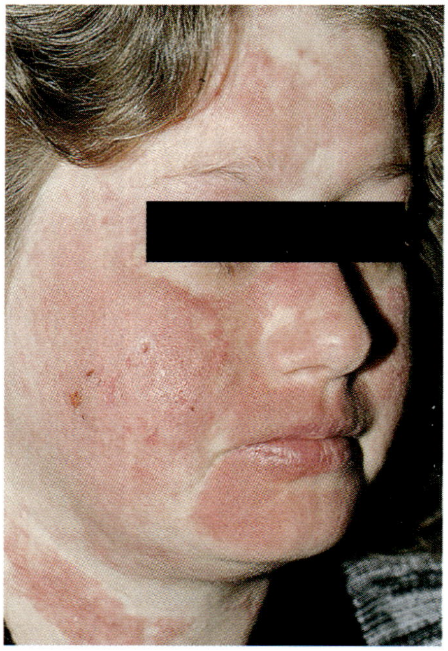

Figure 2.4. Localized acute cutaneous lupus erythematosus (ACLE). ACLE confined to the face and neck is classified under the Gilliam scheme as localized ACLE. The most typical presentation as seen in this case is that of a confluent erythema that can be associated with some degree of induration due to edema formation. As the inflammation subsides, postinflammatory hyper- or hypopigmentation can remain; however, atrophic dermal scarring is not seen.

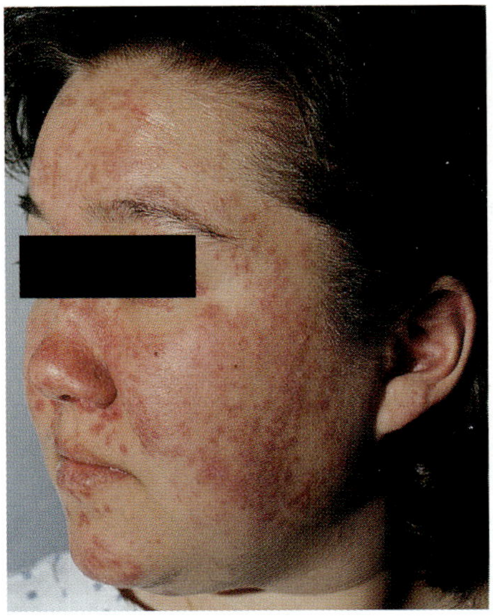

Figure 2.5. Macular/papular acute cutaneous lupus erythematosus (ACLE). Acute cutaneous lupus erythematosus less commonly presents as a macular and/or papular erythema as demonstrated in this young woman who ultimately died from systemic lupus erythematosus.

typically characterized by confluent symmetric erythema and edema centered over the malar eminences (unilateral involvement with ACLE has been described (1) (Fig. 2.4). Inflammation extending over the bridge of the nose completes the body of the classic butterfly. However, the nasolabial folds are typically spared. The forehead and V-area of the neck can be similarly involved. Facial swelling may be severe in some patients with ACLE (1,162). Occasionally, ACLE begins on the face as small, discrete macular, or papular lesions, or both, that later become confluent and hyperkeratotic (163) (Fig. 2.5).

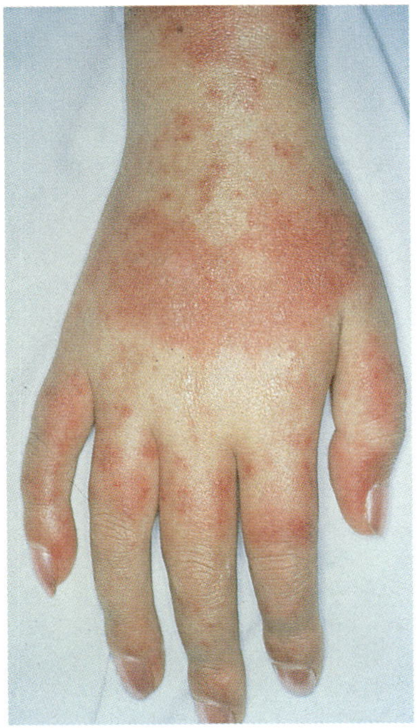

Figure 2.6. Generalized acute cutaneous lupus erythematosus (ACLE). ACLE present both above and below the neck is classified as generalized ACLE. Note the macular erythema over the extensor aspect of the wrists that becomes confluent over the dorsal aspect of the hand and interphalangeal areas.

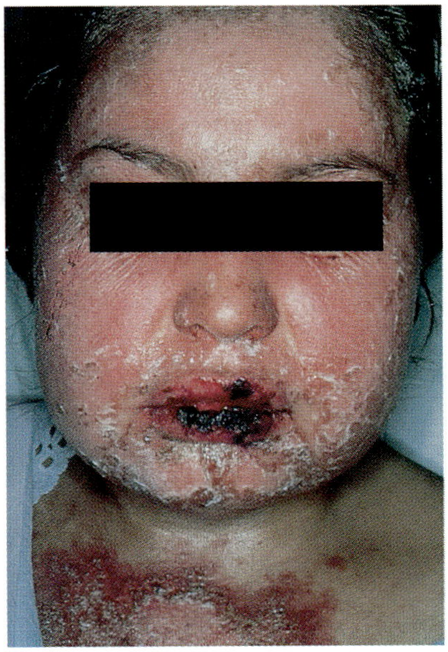

Figure 2.7. Acute cutaneous lupus erythematosus (ACLE) simulating the appearance of toxic epidermal necrolysis. Note the hemorrhagic crusting of the lips and the erosions over the V-area of the neck and upper chest. These skin changes developed during an acute flare of this patient's systemic lupus erythematosus (SLE) that followed her decision to abruptly discontinue all of her medications. Therefore, there was no possibility that her toxic epidermal necrolysis–like skin changes were the result of a drug hypersensitivity reaction.

Generalized ACLE, a less common variety, presents as a more widespread morbilliform or exanthematous eruption (Fig. 2.6). This presentation has been referred to as the "maculopapular rash" or "photosensitive lupus dermatitis."

Some patients experience an extremely acute form of ACLE that can simulate toxic epidermal necrolysis (Fig. 2.7). This form of bullous LE results from dissolution of the epidermal basal cell layer due to intense lichenoid inflammation (164). Su and Alegre (165) present a framework for considering how this form of bullous LE skin change relates to the other clinical patterns of bullous cutaneous injury that can be seen in patients with LE. The other bullous skin lesions that occur in LE are discussed separately later and listed in Table 2.3.

ACLE is very photosensitive and can be transient, lasting only several days or weeks. Occasionally lesions will wax and wane over a period of several hours. Some patients will experience more prolonged disease activity. Postinflammatory pigmentary change is most prominent in patients with LE with

TABLE 2.3. Bullous Skin Lesions That Can Be Seen in Patients with Lupus Erythematosus (LE)

LE-specific ("classic" bullous LE)
Toxic epidermal necrolysis–like ACLE and SCLE
Vesiculobullous annular SCLE
Bullous DLE
LE-nonspecific
"Bullous SLE"
Dermatitis herpetiformis–like cutaneous LE
Epidermolysis bullosa acquisita-like cutaneous LE
Bullous disorders anecdotally reported to occur in patients with LE
Bullous pemphigoid
Pemphigus erythematosus
Porphyria cutanea tarda

ACLE, acute cutaneous LE; DLE, discoid LE; LE, lupus erythematosus; SCLE, subacute cutaneous LE.

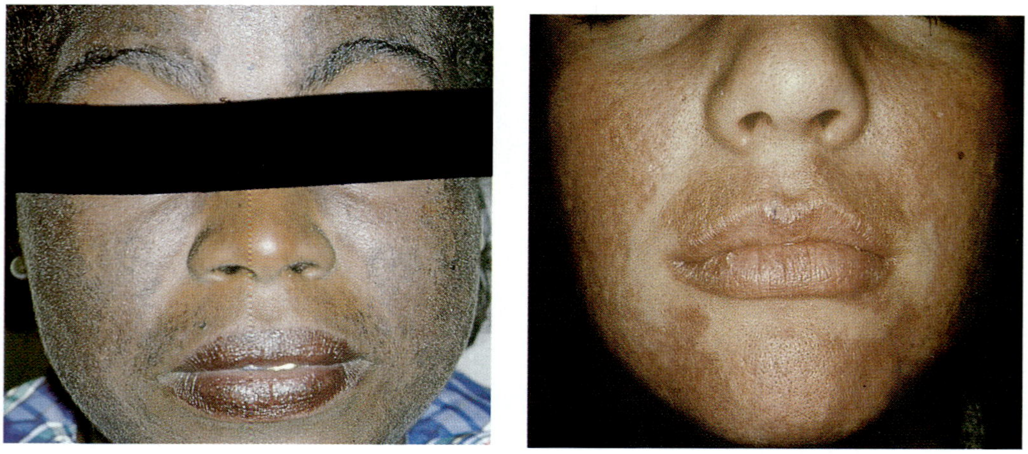

A B

Figure 2.8. Hyperpigmented acute cutaneous lupus erythematosus (ACLE). **A:** Hyperpigmentation can often soon follow the onset of ACLE inflammation in darkly pigmented individuals. This rather stoic patient's only presenting complaint was darkening of the skin of her face. However, her evaluation revealed the presence of active systemic lupus erythematosus (SLE) including renal involvement. Soon after starting prednisone and hydroxychloroquine, she developed an acute abdominal crisis resulting in an unrevealing exploratory laparotomy. The source of her abdominal pain was subsequently realized to have been due to antimalarial-induced acute hepatotoxicity in the setting of clinically silent porphyria cutanea tarda. **B:** Anti-Ro (SS-A) woman who developed postinflammatory hyperpigmentation on the face in areas of previous ACLE.

darkly pigmented skin (Fig. 2.8). ACLE lesions do not result in scarring. Patients with localized ACLE will occasionally have SCLE lesions elsewhere on their bodies, although the simultaneous occurrence of ACLE and active DLE is very unusual.

Superficial ulceration of the oral or nasal mucosa is a frequent accompaniment of ACLE (Fig. 2.9). Such lesions can be the source of extreme discomfort in some individuals, and produce virtually no pain in others. The posterior areas of the hard palate are most commonly affected, however, the labial, gingival, buccal, and lingual mucosa may also be involved. In the early stages of such lesions, the pathology is usually nonspecific; however, changes similar to DLE can be seen at biopsy of more established lesions.

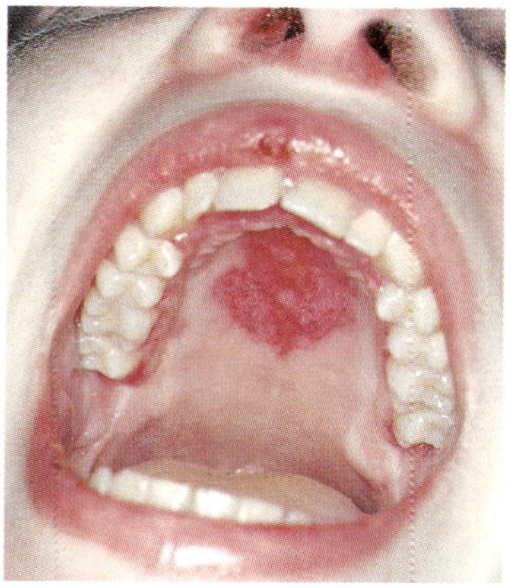

Figure 2.9. Oral mucosal ulceration in systemic lupus erythematosus (SLE). As seen in this case, superficial ulcers often occur in the junctional area of the hard and soft palates; however, ulceration of the gingival, buccal, and lingual mucosa can also occur. In the early stages of such lesions, the histopathology is often nonspecific. Although difficult to see in this photograph, this young woman with active systemic lupus erythematosus (SLE), including nephritis, also had ulceration of the nasal mucosa. Oral and nasal mucosal ulceration in this setting can be associated with severe pain or can be painless.

Subacute Cutaneous Lupus Erythematosus

SCLE was first discussed as a distinct disease entity by Gilliam (10) in 1977, with expanded discussion in 1981 (11). SCLE skin lesions have been referred to in the past under a number of other designations including symmetric erythema centrifugum, disseminated DLE, autoimmune annular erythema, subacute disseminated LE, superficial disseminated LE, psoriasiform LE, pityriasiform LE, and maculopapular photosensitive LE (33). The entity "lupus erythematosus gyratum repens" is now also considered synonymous with annular SCLE (166). The original cohort of patients with SCLE presented in 1979 (33), and the others that have followed, indicate that SCLE is a distinct subset of cutaneous LE having characteristic clinical, serologic, and genetic features (34,35,99,101,104–109,113,124,125,163,167–174).

SCLE consists of nonscarring papulosquamous or annular skin lesions that have a LE-specific histopathology (175) and occur in a characteristic photo-distribution (33). Approximately 85% of patients with SCLE report photosensitivity (99,104, 123,169–171), although some ethnic groups such as the Japanese and Chinese appear to be much less so (106,176). Approximately 70% of patients with SCLE are anti-Ro(SS-A) antibody–positive (35). Female patients with SCLE have a higher frequency of anti-Ro(SS-A) antibody positivity (114). The strong relationship between SCLE and anti-Ro(SS-A) antibodies is depicted in Table 2.4 (113,114). A number of anti-Ro(SS-A)–positive patients with SCLE "burn through window glass," indicating that long-wave, low-energy UV light is capable of activating their skin disease. The frequency of photosensitivity in anti-Ro antibody-positive lupus patients is striking. Approximately 80% of anti-Ro(SS-A) antibody–positive patients described under the rubric of antinuclear antibody (ANA)–negative LE were photosensitive (37). Furthermore, a more recent study examining anti-Ro antibody–positive patients by a group of rheumatologists has detected a 90% frequency of photosensitivity (93). Although circulating autoantibodies to the Ro(SS-A) ribonucleoprotein particle support this diagnosis (35), their presence is not required to make a diagnosis of SCLE according to its original definition (33).

TABLE 2.4. Comparison of Serologic Findings in Patients with Subacute Cutaneous Lupus Erythematosus (SCLE) and Systemic Lupus Erythematosus (SLE)

Antibody	Subacute Cutaneous Lupus Erythematosus (%) ($N = 32$)	Systemic Lupus Erythematosus (%) ($N = 150$)	p Value
Anti-Ro(SS-A)	59	32	<0.05
Anti-La(SS-B)	12	12	NS
Anti-dsDNA	0	28	<0.005
Anti-ssDNA	10	89	<0.005
Anti-U_1RNP	9	34	<0.05
Anti-Sm	0	17	<0.05
Anticardiolipin	10	63	<0.005

From Watson RM, et al. Subacute cutaneous lupus erythematosus—immunogenic associations. *J Autoimmun* 1991;4:73; Hochberg MC, et al. Systemic lupus erythematosus: a review of clinicolaboratory features and immunogenetic markers in 150 patients with emphasis on demographic subsets. *Medicine* 1985;64:285–295; and Provost TT, Watson RM. Anti-Ro(SSA), HLA-DR3 positive females: the interrelationship between some ANA negative, SS, SCLE, NLE mothers and SS/LE overlap female patients. *J Invest Dermatol* 1993;100:145, with permission.

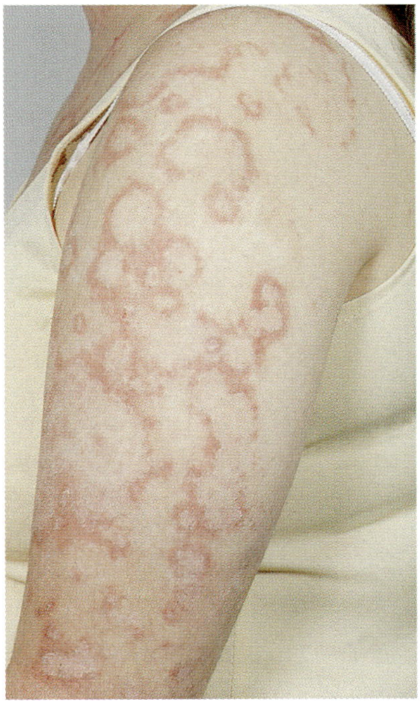

Figure 2.11. Annular subacute cutaneous lupus erythematosus (SCLE). Note the polycyclic array resulting from the confluence of the individual annular lesions. This young woman ultimately died from complications of chronic active hepatitis.

SCLE lesions present initially as erythematous macules or papules that evolve into scaly, papulosquamous or annular/polycyclic plaques. Approximately 50% of patients have predominately papulosquamous or psoriasiform lesions (Fig. 2.10), whereas the other half has the annular/polycyclic form (Fig. 2.11). A few patients may develop both types of lesions. Some researchers have observed a predominance of papulosquamous lesions (101,104,109), whereas others have noted an abundance of the annular/polycyclic form (99,106,111). The central areas of annular SCLE lesions typically become hypopigmented (Fig. 2.12). SCLE lesions characteristically occur in sun-exposed areas (i.e., upper back, shoulders, extensor aspects of the arms, V-area of the neck, and less commonly, on the face) (Fig. 2.13).

Infrequently, SCLE lesions present initially with an appearance of erythema multiforme (177,178) (Fig. 2.14). Such cases can simulate the appearance of Rowell syndrome (erythema multiforme–like lesions occurring in patients with SLE in the presence of La(SS-B) autoantibodies) (27). In addition, lesions similar to erythema annulare centrifugum can be seen (Fig. 2.15). As a result of hyperacute basal cell layer injury, on rare

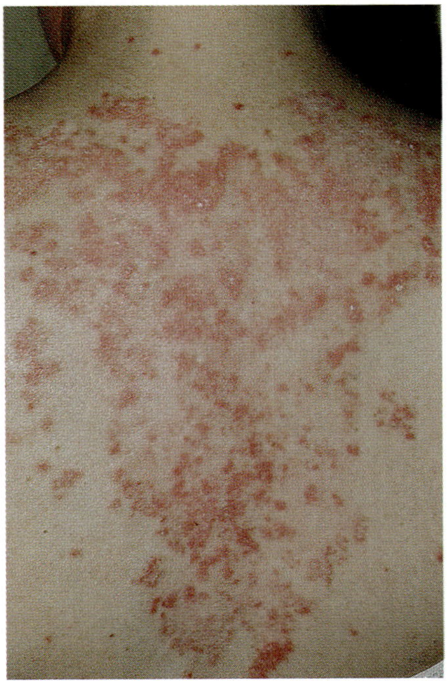

Figure 2.10. Papulosquamous subacute cutaneous lupus erythematosus (SCLE) on the mid- and upper back of a patient having no extracutaneous manifestations of systemic lupus erythematosus (SLE). Note the superficial scale and the tendency for the individual lesions to merge into a retiform pattern.

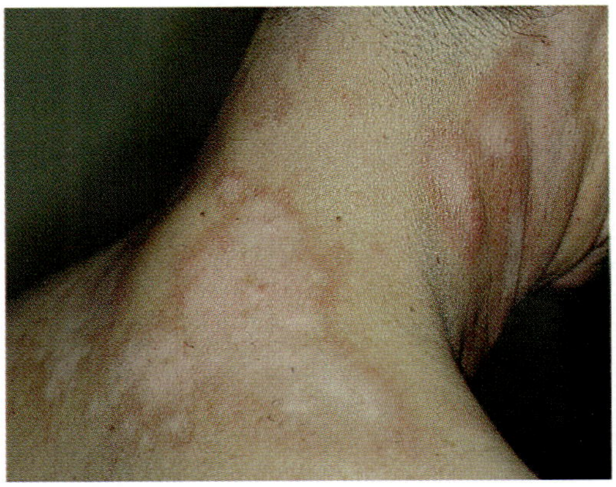

Figure 2.12. Annular subacute cutaneous lupus erythematosus (SCLE) with central hypopigmentation. As opposed to other types of annular skin lesions, the central portions of annular SCLE lesions characteristically display hypopigmentation in areas where the inflammation has subsided, reflecting the pigment compartment injury pattern that is commonly seen on biopsy. Although not visible in this photograph, telangiectasia can also frequently be observed in the inactive central areas of annular SCLE lesions.

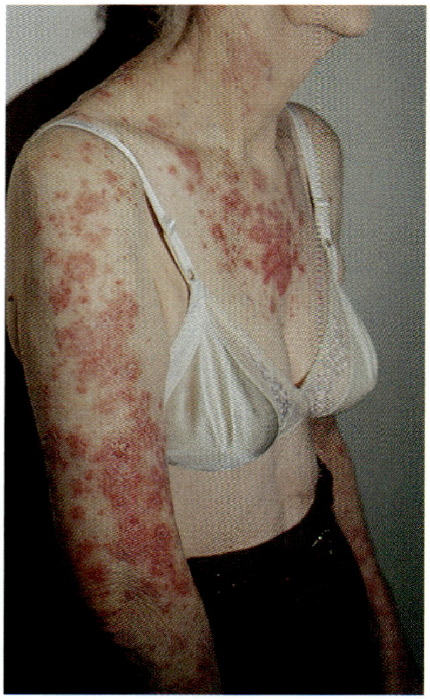

Figure 2.13. Characteristic photodistribution of subacute cutaneous lupus erythematosus (SCLE). Curiously, the face of this patient with hydrochlorothiazide-induced SCLE was not affected. In the experience of one of the authors (R.D.S.), sparing of the face in patients with SCLE has been the rule rather than the exception.

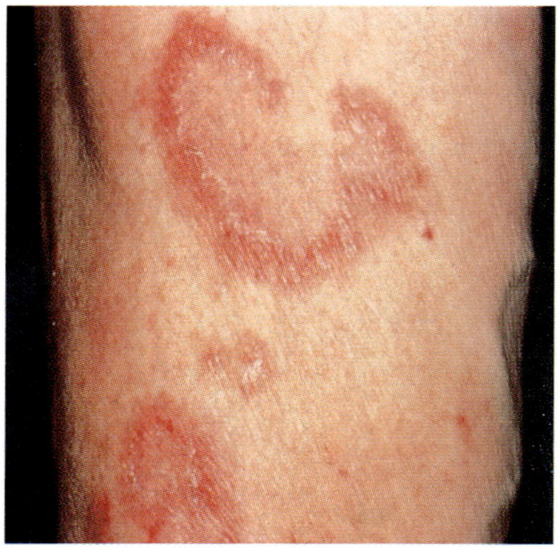

Figure 2.15. An arcuate lesion of biopsy-confirmed subacute cutaneous lupus erythematosus (SCLE) simulating the appearance of erythema annulare centrifugum. Although the fine scale at the trailing edge of the actively inflamed border is characteristic of erythema annulare centrifugum, it can also be seen in arcuate and annular lesions of subacute cutaneous lupus erythematosus (SCLE).

occasions, the active edge of annular SCLE lesions undergoes a vesicular change that breaks down to produce a striking crusted appearance (177–181) (Fig. 2.16). On at least one occasion, such lesions have progressed to mimic toxic epidermal necrolysis (182). One patient with SCLE was reported to initially present with exfoliative erythroderma (183), whereas another presented with a curious acral distribution of annular lesions (184). Pityriasiform (123,171,185) (Fig. 2.17) and exanthematous (177) variants of SCLE have been reported anecdotally on rare occasions. In addition, a follicular erythematous lesion is occasionally seen in patients with SCLE.

Lesions typically heal without scarring but can leave long-lasting and occasionally permanent vitiligo-like leukoderma and telangiectasias (Fig. 2.18). In one case, annular SCLE lesions

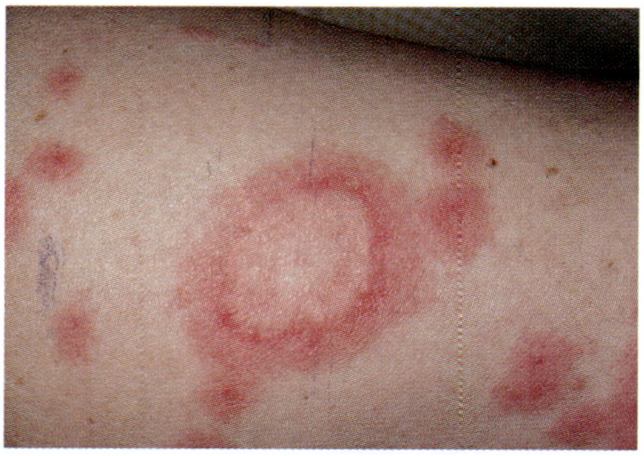

Figure 2.14. Annular subacute cutaneous lupus erythematosus (SCLE) presenting with an appearance highly similar to that of erythema multiforme. Note the targetoid appearance of the small primary lesions surrounding the more established annular subacute cutaneous lupus erythematosus (SCLE) lesion in the center of the photograph.

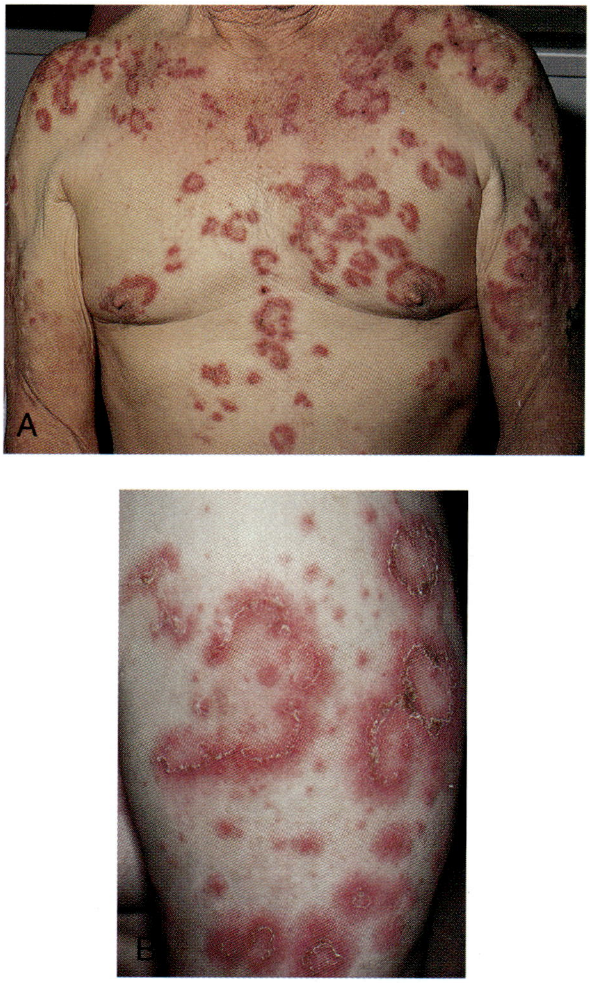

Figure 2.16. Vesiculobullous annular subacute cutaneous lupus erythematosus (SCLE). On rare occasions, the active advancing border of annular SCLE lesions undergoes a vesiculobullous change due to extensive liquefactive degeneration of the epidermal basal cell layer **(A).** As these vesicular elements break down, crusts can form (this is more evident in the closer view shown in **B**). Such eroded areas can at times become secondarily infected with gram-positive bacteria. Intact pustules can occasionally be seen intermixed with vesicles at the border of annular SCLE lesions such as this.

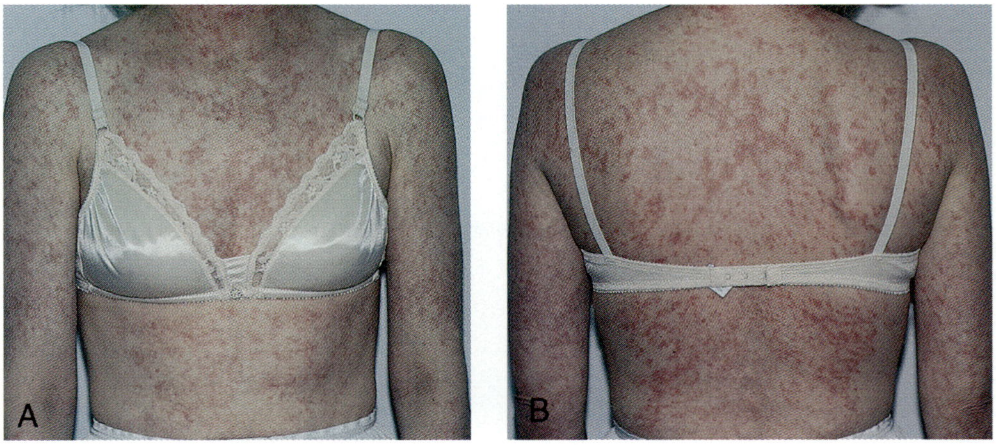

Figure 2.17. Pityriasiform subacute cutaneous lupus erythematosus (SCLE). This anti-Ro(SS-A) antibody–positive patient had a generalized eruption of focal, minimally scaling, nonscarring lesions demonstrating lupus erythematosus–specific skin disease at biopsy **(A,B)**.

were reported over time to progress to plaques of morphea (186).

Patients with SCLE lesions may also develop ACLE (Fig. 2.19) or classic DLE (Fig. 2.20). Localized facial ACLE lesions have been seen in 20% of the patients with SCLE examined by one of the authors (R.D.S.). Other investigators have reported ACLE lesions in 7% to 100% of patients with SCLE (101,106, 169,177). One of the authors (T.T.P.) has examined the frequency of ACLE, SCLE, and CCLE lesions in 50 anti-Ro(SS-A) antibody–positive patients with SLE. Fifty-eight percent had ACLE, 20% had SCLE, and 20% had CCLE (90). ACLE skin lesions tend to be more transient than SCLE and heal with less pigmentary change. They tend to be more edematous and less scaly than SCLE lesions. ACLE more commonly affects the malar areas of the face. The experience of the authors and others (125) suggests that SCLE affects the face much less often.

Various reports have noted that 0% to 29% of patients with SCLE manifest DLE lesions sometime during their clinical course (33,90,101,104,106,169,187) (Fig. 2.20). Nineteen percent of the original cohort of patients with SCLE had classic DLE lesions (33). DLE lesions can predate the onset of SCLE lesions. DLE lesions in patients with SCLE are usually confined to the head and neck but may be more widely distributed. DLE lesions in this setting are generally associated with a greater degree of hyper- and hypopigmentation, may display atrophic dermal scarring, and are more characteristically associated with follicular plugging and adherent scale. DLE lesions are characteristically indurated, whereas those of SCLE are not (125).

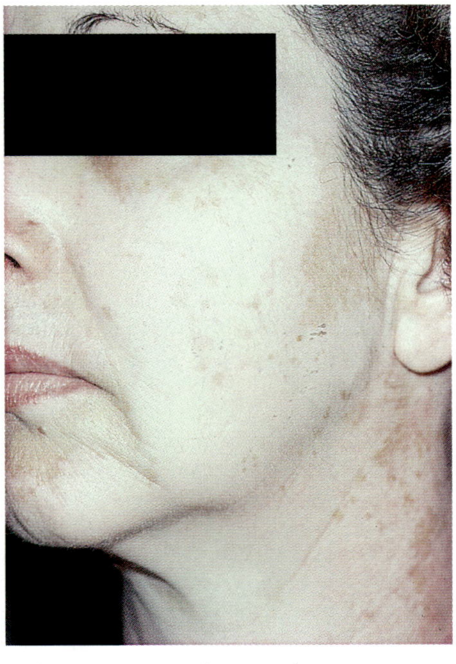

Figure 2.18. Subacute cutaneous lupus erythematosus (SCLE) of the neck and face resolving with permanent vitiligo-like depigmentation.

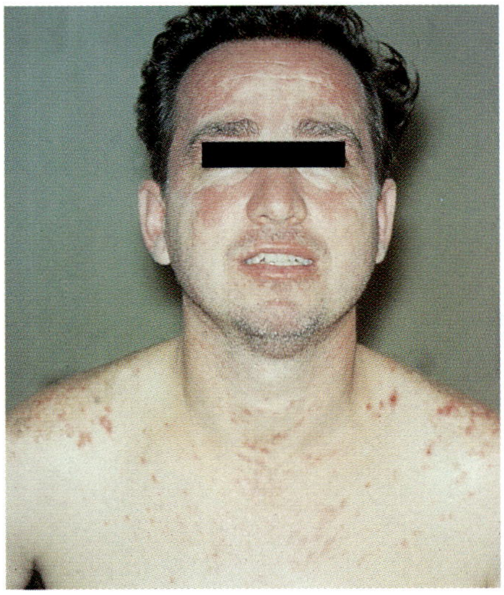

Figure 2.19. Facial acute cutaneous lupus erythematosus (ACLE) occurring in a patient with subacute cutaneous lupus erythematosus (SCLE). This man had experienced uncomplicated papulosquamous SCLE for several years before developing confluent malar erythema at a point in his illness where he experienced clear evidence of extracutaneous systemic lupus erythematosus (SLE) activity, including nephritis. It has been the experience of one of the authors (R.D.S.) that the superimposition of ACLE on SCLE is a worrisome prognostic sign with respect to the risk for developing extracutaneous manifestations of systemic lupus erythematosus (SLE).

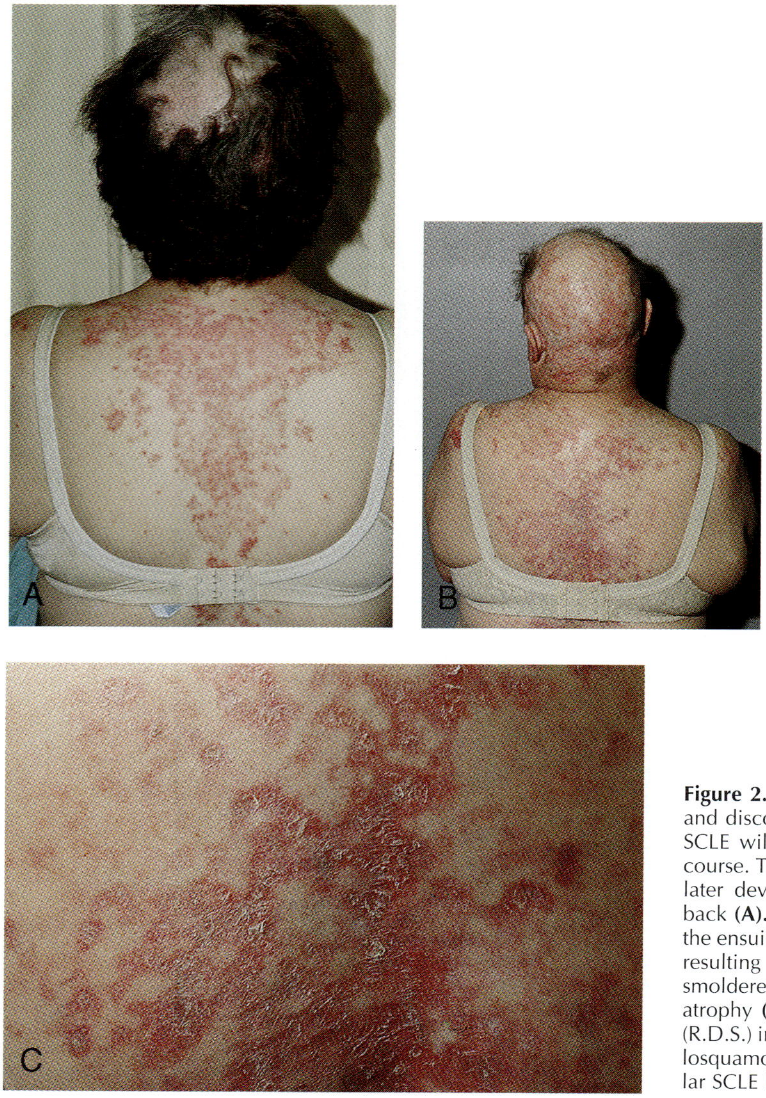

Figure 2.20. Coexistence of subacute cutaneous lupus erythematosus (SCLE) and discoid lupus erythematosus (DLE). Approximately 20% of patients with SCLE will develop classic scarring DLE skin lesions at some point in their course. This patient presented initially with DLE of her scalp and several years later developed typical nonscarring papulosquamous SCLE lesions on her back **(A).** Her cutaneous disease was extremely resistant to therapy and over the ensuing 5 years she experienced progression of her DLE scalp involvement resulting in extensive scarring alopecia **(B).** The SCLE activity on her back smoldered throughout this period, resulting in the development of superficial atrophy **(C).** This is one of two such cases observed by one of the authors (R.D.S.) in which dermal atrophy has developed within long-smoldering papulosquamous SCLE lesions. Such a progression has not been observed in annular SCLE lesions.

A number of other skin lesions that are not histopathologically specific for LE can be found in patients with SCLE (123). The most frequently encountered of these include alopecia, painless mucous membrane lesions, livedo reticularis, periungual telangiectasias, vasculitis, and Raynaud phenomenon (33,90,101,104,168,169,177,188). Cutaneous vasculitis (palpable and nonpalpable purpura) of the lower extremities is a frequent finding in anti-Ro(SS-A)–positive patients with SCLE described under the rubric of SSj/LE overlap syndrome (107,189). Cutaneous sclerosis and calcinosis may be seen rarely in patients with SCLE. Multiple HPV-11-associated squamous cell carcinomas of the skin were noted in one patient with SCLE (190).

Chronic Cutaneous Lupus Erythematosus

CLASSIC DISCOID LUPUS ERYTHEMATOSUS

The most common form of chronic cutaneous LE is classic DLE (hereafter, the unqualified term "DLE" will be used to refer to this form of DLE lesion). DLE lesions of this type begin as flat or slightly elevated, well-demarcated, red-purple macules or papules with a scaly surface. Early DLE lesions most commonly evolve into larger, coin-shaped ("discoid") erythematous plaques covered by a prominent, adherent scale that extends into dilated hair follicles (Fig. 2.21). These discoid plaques can enlarge and merge to form even larger, confluent, disfiguring plaques (Fig. 2.22).

Involvement of hair follicles is a prominent clinical feature of DLE lesions (Fig. 2.23). Scales accumulate in dilated follicular openings, which soon become devoid of hair. When the adherent scale is peeled back from more advanced lesions, follicle-sized keratotic spikes similar in appearance to carpet tacks can be seen to project from the undersurface of the scale (the "carpet tack sign"). Follicular DLE involvement is especially prominent in the conchae of the ear (Fig. 2.24).

Erythema and hyperpigmentation are present during the initial phase of DLE lesions. The lesions slowly expand with active inflammation and hyperpigmentation at the periphery leaving depressed central scarring, telangiectasia, and depigmentation. The central atrophic scarring is highly characteristic (Figs. 2.21 and 2.22). Pigment changes alone do not constitute scarring when referring to cutaneous LE lesions. In some ethnic groups, such as Indians from the Asian subcontinent, the DLE histopathology can present clinically as isolated areas of macular hyperpigmentation (191).

Typical DLE lesions occur most often on the face, scalp, ears, V-area of the neck, and extensor aspects of the arms. Any area

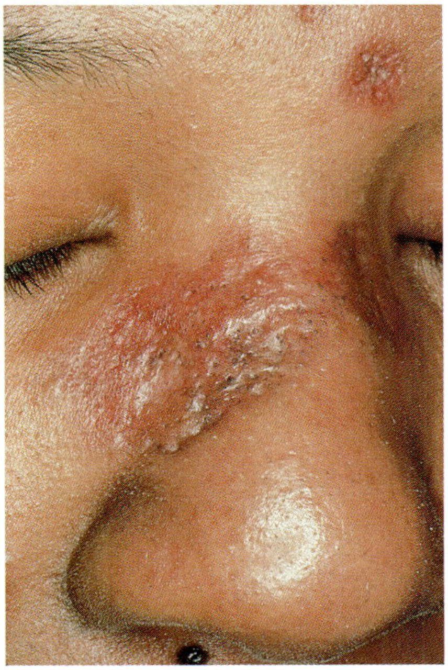

Figure 2.21. Classic discoid lupus erythematosus (DLE) lesion. Note the erythema (indicating disease activity), keratin-plugged follicles, and dermal atrophy. This is a relatively early lesion that lacks the typical adherent scale that usually accompanies more established lesions.

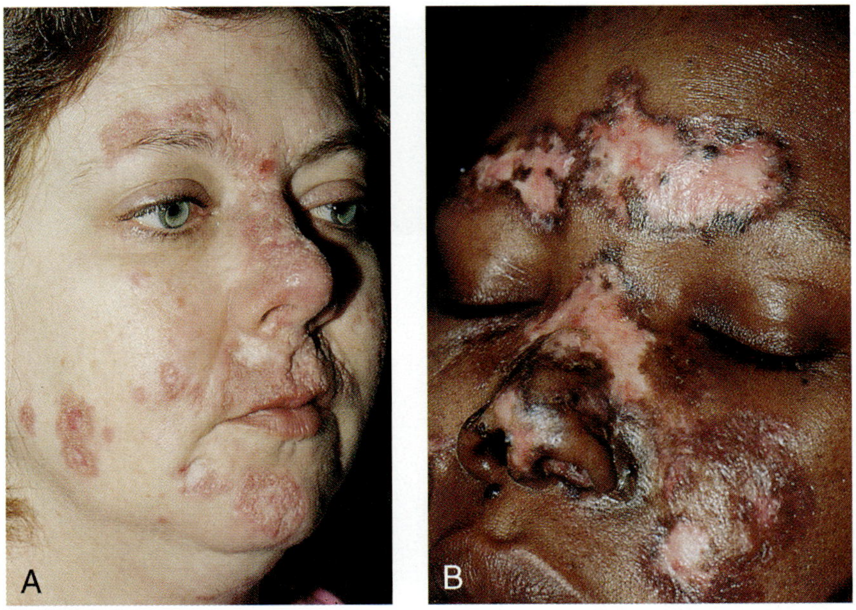

Figure 2.22. More extensive examples of therapeutically refractory facial (DLE) lesions that produce large areas of disfigurement on confluence **(A,B).** The characteristic pattern of hyperpigmentation at the active border and hypopigmentation at the inactive center is especially evident in black patients as shown in **B.** Facial involvement of this sort can produce extreme psychosocial disability. The proper application of corrective camouflage cosmetics can be of great psychologic benefit to such patients.

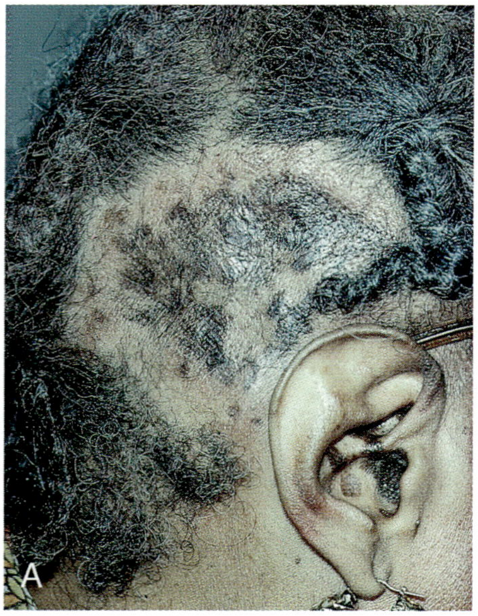

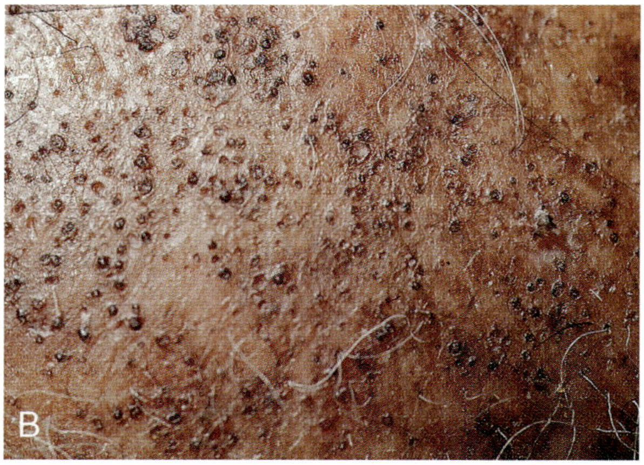

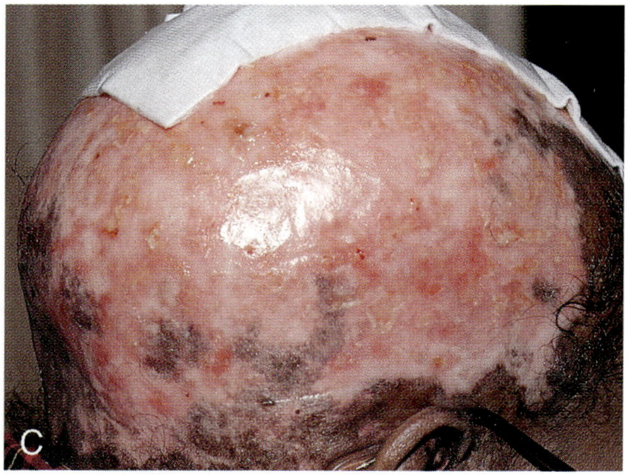

Figure 2.23. Discoid lupus erythematosus (DLE) of the scalp. The DLE scalp lesion shown in **A** is a relatively early one. At this stage, the alopecia might to some degree be reversible with effective treatment. **B:** A close-up view of the pattern of keratin-plugged follicles that can be observed in such lesions. **C:** A patient in whom the DLE disease process has progressed to the point of total, irreversible scarring alopecia. The areas of crusting represent a superimposed secondary bacterial infection.

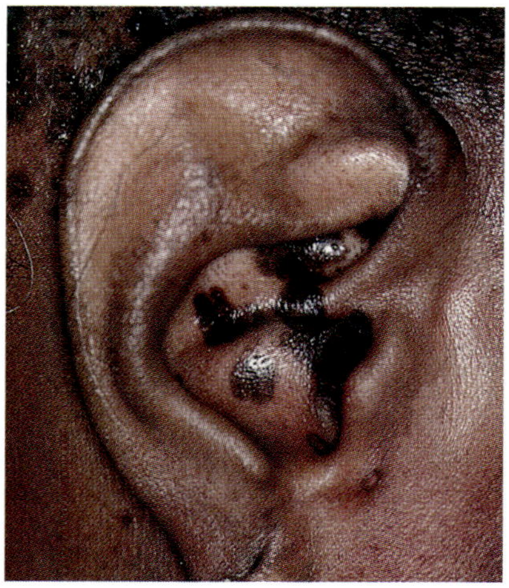

Figure 2.24. Discoid lupus erythematosus (DLE) involvement of the ear. Note the patulous, keratin-plugged follicles within areas of hyperpigmentation in the concha. This pattern of clinical involvement is highly specific for discoid lupus erythematosus (DLE). This is a close-up view of the ear of the patient shown in **A** of Fig. 2.23.

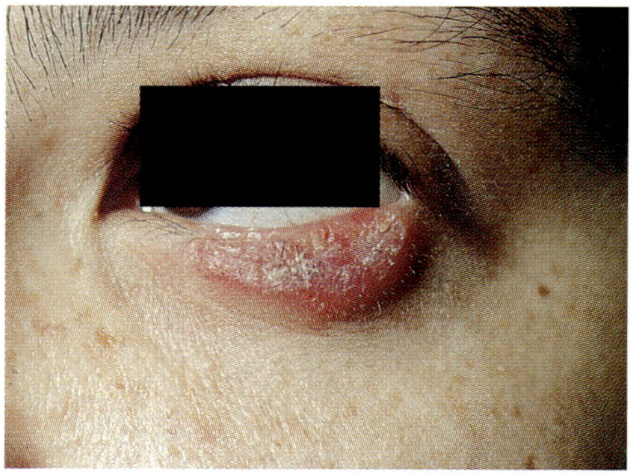

Figure 2.25. Discoid lupus erythematosus (DLE) of the lower eyelid resulting in loss of the eyelashes.

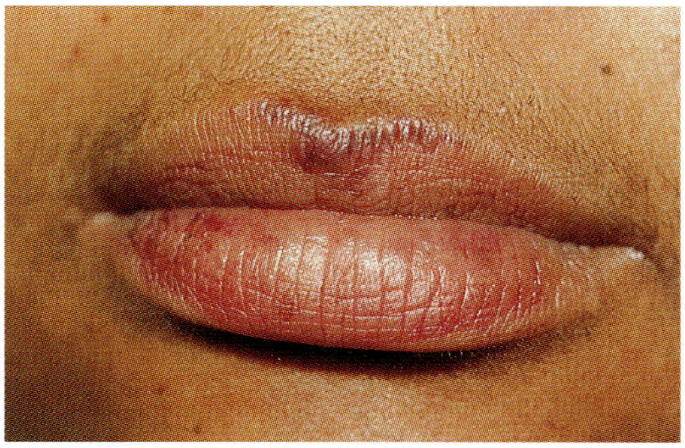

Figure 2.26. Discoid lupus erythematosus (DLE) of the vermillion border of the upper lip. Although the lower lip is more exposed to sunlight, for some curious reason the upper lip is more often affected with lupus erythematosus–specific skin disease (LE).

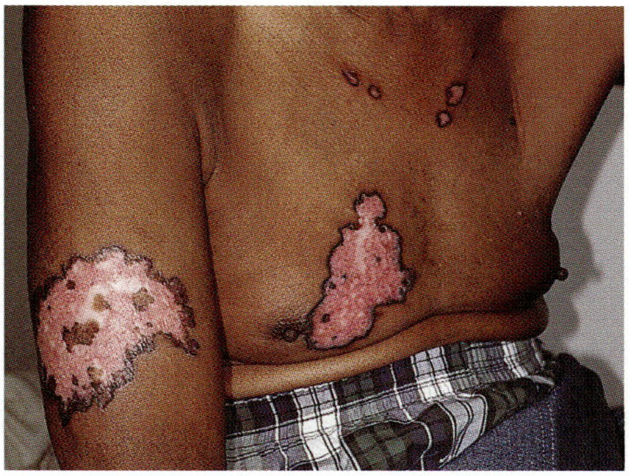

Figure 2.28. Generalized Discoid lupus erythematosus (DLE). There is a somewhat higher risk for developing SLE in patients with generalized DLE compared with those with localized DLE (i.e., head and neck involvement only).

of the face can be affected, including the eyebrows, eyelids (Fig. 2.25), nose, and lips (Fig. 2.26). Linear DLE facial lesions following Blashko lines have been described (192). A symmetric, butterfly-shaped DLE plaque will occasionally be found over the malar areas and bridge of the nose. Such DLE lesions are not to be confused with the more transient, edematous erythema reactions that occur over the same distribution in ACLE lesions. As with ACLE, DLE usually spares the nasolabial folds. Perioral DLE lesions can occur and often resolve with a striking acneiform pattern of pitted scarring (Fig. 2.27). DLE often involves the external ear, especially the concha. The earliest lesions in this area present as dilated, hyperpigmented follicles (Fig. 2.24).

Scalp involvement occurs in 60% of patients with DLE, and is the only area involved in approximately 10% (149) (Fig. 2.23). Irreversible scarring alopecia resulting from permanent follicular destruction occurred in 34% of patients in one recent series (193). The irreversible, scarring alopecia that occurs as the result of persistent DLE activity in a localized area differs from the more widespread, reversible, nonscarring alopecia that patients with SLE often develop during periods of systemic disease activity. DLE lesions that occur only on the head or neck are referred to as "localized DLE." DLE lesions occurring both above and below the neck are referred to as "generalized DLE." The presence of DLE lesions solely below the neck is extremely uncommon. DLE lesions occurring below the neck are most commonly found on the extensor aspects of the arms, forearms, and hands (Fig. 2.28), although DLE lesions can occur at virtually any site on the body, including completely sun-protected sites such as the inguinal folds (Fig. 2.29). Painful erosive palmar-plantar DLE involvement can predominate in some cases producing significant disability and presenting an especially

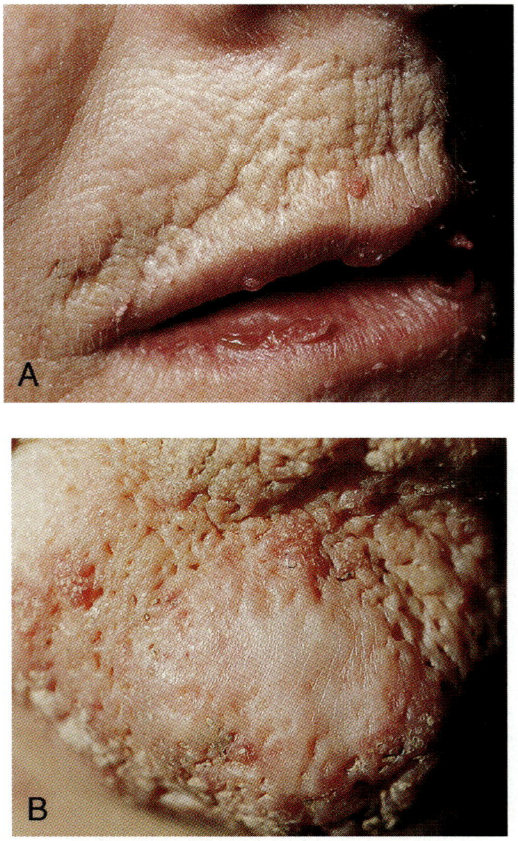

Figure 2.27. Perioral pitted scarring resulting from prior discoid lupus erythematosus (DLE) involvement **(A).** This pattern of scarring over the chin of a different patient was improved by dermabrasion as shown in **B** (note the smoother surface and improved appearance of the central part of the photograph that was treated as a test area). This patient was on antimalarial treatment at the time of the dermabrasion to minimize the chance for köebnerization.

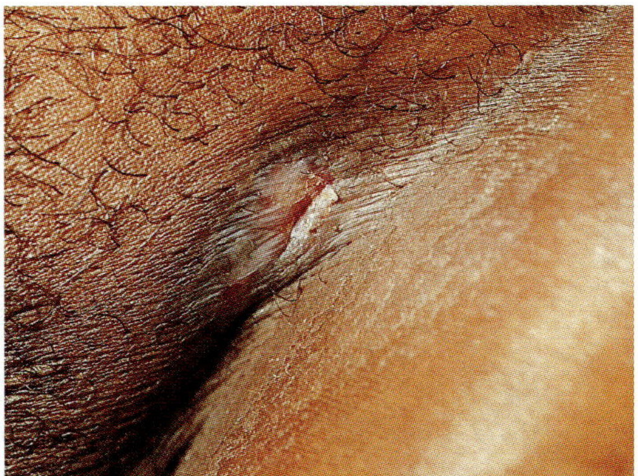

Figure 2.29. Biopsy-confirmed discoid lupus erythematosus (DLE) lesion of the inguinal fold.

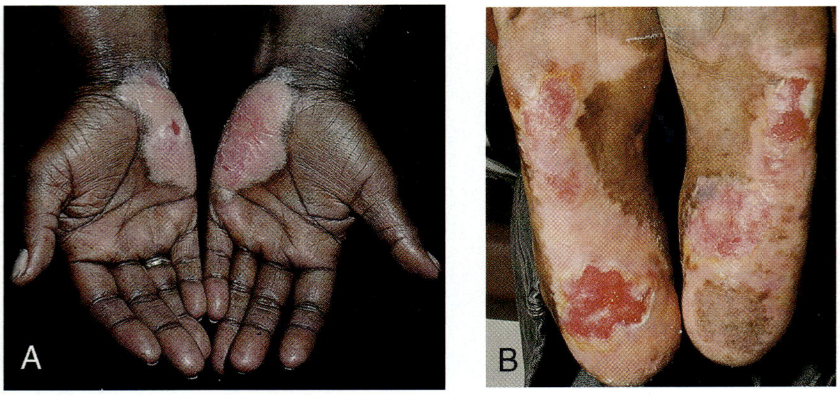

Figure 2.30. Palmar–plantar discoid lupus erythematosus (DLE). DLE involvement of the palms of the hands **(A)** and soles of the feet **(B)** can present a very difficult management problem. Erosions that can develop in such areas can cause extreme pain and result in occupational disability **(B).**

difficult management problem (194,195) (Fig. 2.30). Occasionally, DLE lesions can remain as small, discrete, follicle-based papules having a diameter of 1 cm or less. Such "follicular DLE" lesions are often seen around the elbow(Fig. 2.31), but can occur elsewhere as well. These lesions may also be more common in Chinese and other Asian patients (196).

The appearance of DLE lesions or other forms of LE skin disease in unusual locations may be evidence that these lesions can follow in the wake of any form of trauma to the skin (the Köebner or isomorphic response) (Fig. 2.32). Rowell and Goodfield (7) reported that in their Leeds series, DLE lesions were initiated by trauma in 11%, sunburn in 5%, infection in 3%, and exposure to cold in 2%. Lodin (197) has noted a frequency of the emergence of DLE lesions with trauma to be 2.2%. DLE lesions have been noted to occur following exposure to x-ray, diathermy, and chemical burns, and have arisen in scars associated with herpes zoster. Discoid lupus (DLE) lesions reportedly occurred in the scars of smallpox vaccination (197).

DLE lesions can be precipitated by sunlight exposure; however, this occurs less frequently than with ACLE and SCLE. It is predominately UVB that aggravates DLE lesions, although increasing evidence suggests that the longer UVA wavelengths can also be deleterious in some patients with LE (198–201). However, in as many as 50% of patients sun exposure does not appear to be related to the cause of their DLE lesions. DLE lesions in the hair-bearing scalp, external auditory canal, or perineal areas are examples where this form of cutaneous LE may not be related to light exposure.

DLE can also localize to the nail unit (14,202). Focal lesions of DLE occurring over the nailfold can produce nail plate dystrophy (Fig. 2.33). The nail unit can be impacted by other forms of cutaneous LE as well as SLE, producing nailfold erythema and telangiectasia, red lunulae, clubbing, paronychia, pitting, leukonychia striata, and onycholysis (14).

HYPERTROPHIC DISCOID LUPUS ERYTHEMATOSUS

Hypertrophic DLE (hyperkeratotic DLE, verrucous DLE) is a rare variant of chronic cutaneous LE in which the hyperkeratosis that is normally present in classic DLE lesions is greatly exaggerated (Fig. 2.34). These lesions can occur at any site where classic DLE lesions develop, although the extensor aspects of the arms, the upper back, and the face are the areas

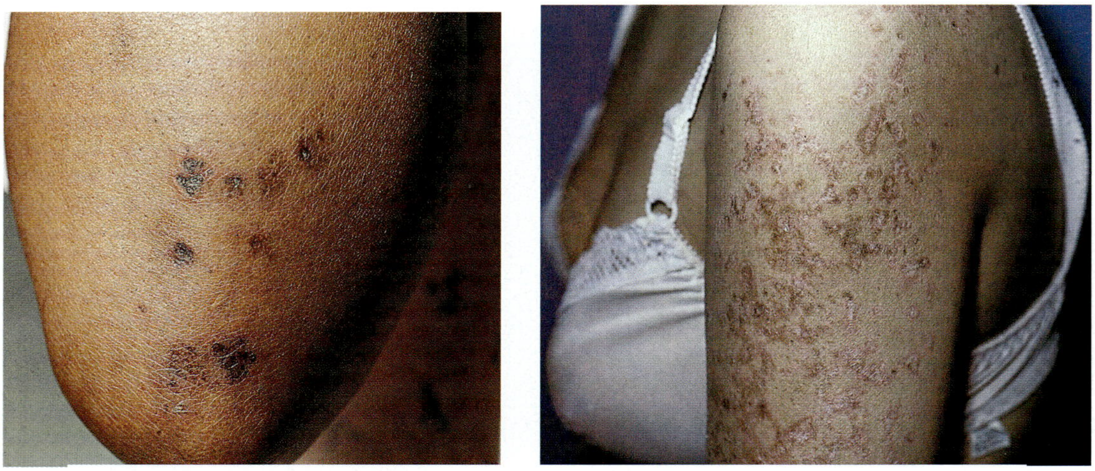

A B

Figure 2.31. Discoid lupus erythematosus (DLE) presenting as discrete follicular lesions. **A:** Follicular DLE lesions around the elbow, the most common site for this pattern of involvement. **B:** Follicular inflammatory DLE lesions on the upper arm of a Chinese American anti- Ro (SS-A) antibody–positive patient with systemic lupus erythematosus (SLE).

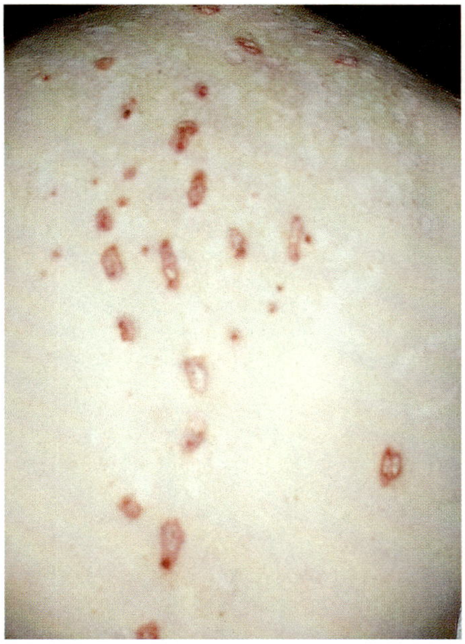

Figure 2.32. Köebnerized discoid lupus erythematosus (DLE). Discoid lupus erythematosus (DLE) lesions occurring in areas of neurotic excoriation. Note the linear shape of some of these lesions.

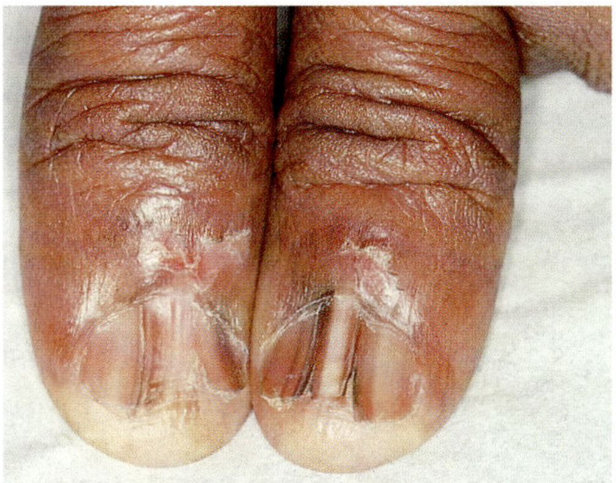

Figure 2.33. Symmetric discoid lupus erythematosus (DLE) lesions of the nailfold producing medial nail plate dystrophy. None of the other fingernails was affected.

most frequently affected. Overlapping features of hypertrophic LE and lichen planus have been described (203,204). Patients with hypertrophic DLE lesions often have classic DLE lesions elsewhere on their bodies. When it occurs in whites, hypertrophic DLE has been confused both clinically and histologically with squamous cell carcinoma (205).

The entity "lupus erythematosus hypertrophicus et profundus" that was originally described by Behçet in 1942 (206–208) appears to represent a very rare form of hypertrophic DLE affecting the face, associated with the additional features of violaceous (or dull red), indurated, rolled borders, and striking central, crateriform atrophy. The name of this entity is somewhat ambiguous because its pathology does not include a significant degree of LE profundus/LE panniculitis.

LUPUS ERYTHEMATOSUS PROFUNDUS/LUPUS ERYTHEMATOSUS PANNICULITIS

Historically referred to as Kaposi–Irgang disease (209), this unusual form of chronic cutaneous LE is characterized by inflammatory lesions in the lower dermis and subcutaneous tissue. This lesion occurs more commonly in women and approximately 1% to 3% of patients with SLE have this complication. Lupus panniculitis/profundus may occur in the absence of systemic disease (210). The lesions present as deep, firm nodules, 1 to 3 cm in diameter, often without overlying clinical change at the surface of the skin (211,212). On rare occasions, xanthomatous changes in the panniculitis lesions have been described (213). The overlying skin ultimately becomes attached to the firm, subcutaneous nodular lesions and is drawn inward to pro-

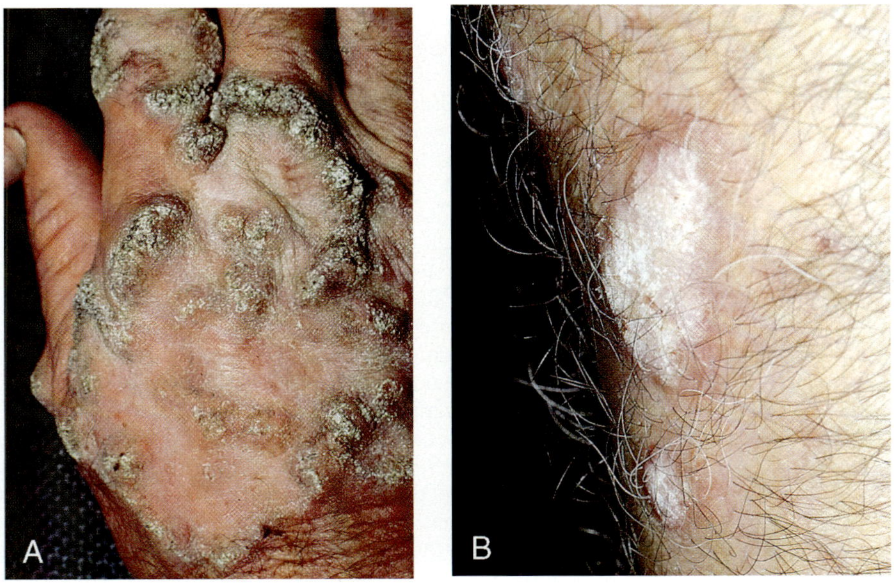

Figure 2.34. Two clinical patterns of hypertrophic (verrucous) discoid lupus erythematosus (DLE). **A:** Demonstration of a pattern where warty hyperkeratosis occurs at the active edge of an active DLE lesion. **B:** Illustration of a DLE lesion that is entirely covered by a thickened shield of hyperkeratosis, presenting a clinical appearance that could be mistaken for other common dermatoses such as keratoacanthoma, squamous cell carcinoma, or prurigo nodularis.

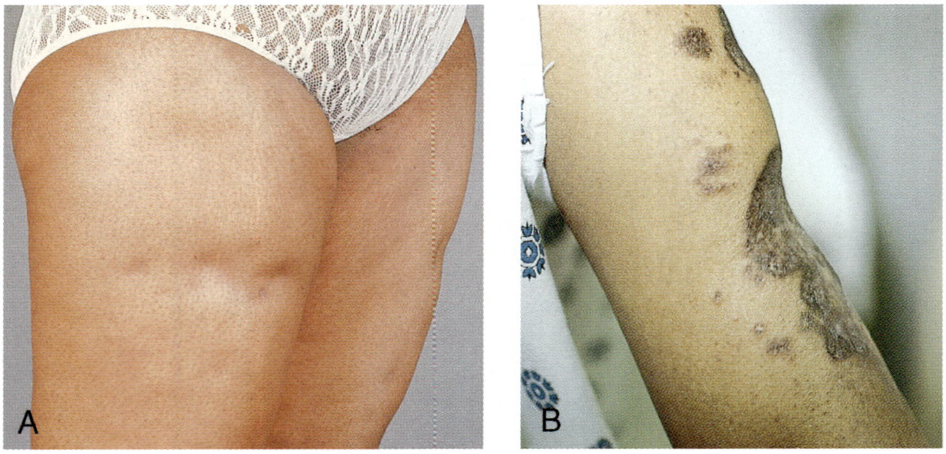

Figure 2.35. Lupus erythematosus (LE) panniculitis/profundus. An example of LE panniculitis without overlying discoid lupus erythematosus (DLE) is shown in **A.** The primary lesion is a firm subcutaneous nodule that is associated with saucerized areas of atrophy at the surface of the skin. The combination of LE panniculitis with overlying discoid lupus erythematosus (DLE) involvement **(B)** is referred to as LE profundus.

duce deep, saucerized depressions as the lesions mature (Fig. 2.35). The head, proximal upper arms, chest, buttocks, and thighs are the sites of predominant involvement. Reports also indicate the development of periorbital edema in some cases of facial lupus panniculitis (214,215). Confluent involvement of the face can simulate the appearance of lipoatrophy (Fig. 2.36). Linear involvement of the extremities has also been observed (216). Some of these lesions may have the appearance of morphea (217). Dystrophic calcification within older lesions of LE profundus is common and at times can be a prominent clinical feature of the disease requiring surgical excision. In addition, LE panniculitis may produce breast nodules ("lupus mastitis") that can mimic carcinoma, clinically and radiologically (217).

Approximately 70% of the patients with this type of chronic cutaneous LE also have typical DLE lesions, often overlying the panniculitis lesions (218). The term "lupus (LE) profundus" is used by some to designate those patients in whom classic DLE changes are superimposed on those of LE panniculitis.

MUCOSAL DISCOID LUPUS ERYTHEMATOSUS

It has long been recognized that mucosal membrane involvement can occur in patients with chronic cutaneous LE (219–222).

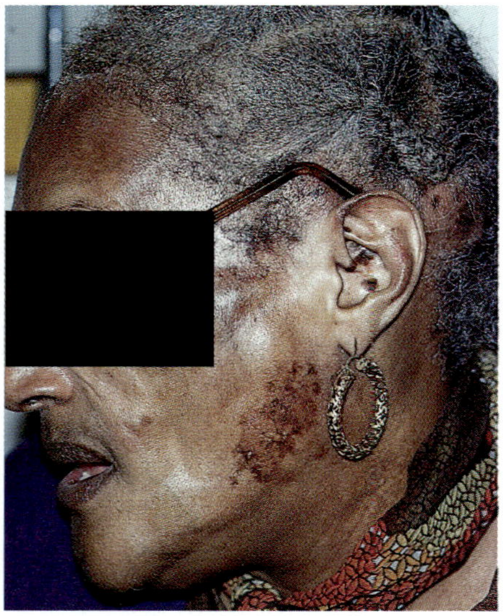

Figure 2.36. Lipoatrophy of the face resulting from lupus erythematosus (LE) profundus.

However, on unusual occasions, SLE may be heralded by the presence of oral mucosal lesions (220–227). Studies by Burge et al. (225) have confirmed that the prevalence of mucous membrane involvement in chronic cutaneous LE is about 25%. Although the oral mucosa is most frequently involved, nasal, conjunctival, and genital mucosal surfaces can also be affected.

Within the mouth, the buccal mucosal surfaces are most commonly involved, with the palate, alveolar processes, and tongue less frequently involved. Dentures may aggravate these lesions. Individual lesions begin as painless, erythematous patches, later maturing to a chronic plaque that can present an appearance quite similar to that of lichen planus (Fig. 2.37). The chronic buccal mucosal plaques have a sharply marginated, irregularly scalloped white border with radiating white striae and telangiectasia (225). The surfaces of these plaques overlying the palatal mucosa often have a well-defined meshwork of raised hyperkeratotic white strands that encircle zones of punctate erythema, which gives a "honeycomb" appearance (225). The centers of older lesions can become depressed and occasionally undergo painful ulceration. Well-defined chronic DLE plaques can also appear on the vermillion border of the lips (Fig. 2.26). At times DLE involvement of the lips can present as a diffuse cheilitis, especially on the more sun-exposed lower lip. Although lesions can appear on the tongue, they are quite rare (225).

Urman et al. (226) have extensively studied oral ulcerations in 47 of 182 patients with SLE (25%). These investigators have noted no significant correlation between the oral ulcerations and cutaneous manifestations. They did find, however, an increased frequency of these mucosal lesions with increased clinical activity of SLE. They found no detectable correlation between oral ulcerations and serologic parameters. The oral ulcerations histologically demonstrate features of DLE and not vasculitis.

Chronic oral mucosal DLE lesions can occasionally degenerate into squamous cell carcinoma (226), as can cutaneous DLE lesions. Any area of asymmetric nodular induration within a mucosal DLE lesion should be carefully evaluated for the possibility of malignant degeneration.

Discrete DLE plaques can also develop on the nasal, conjunctival, and genital mucosa (224). Nasal septum perforation is relatively rare and is more often associated with SLE than DLE (228–231). However, nasal mucosal involvement has recently been suggested to be relatively common in patients with LE in general (230). Conjunctival DLE lesions begin as small areas of nondescript inflammation most commonly affecting the palpebral conjunctivae or the margin of the eyelid. The lower lid is affected more often than the upper lid. As the early lesions

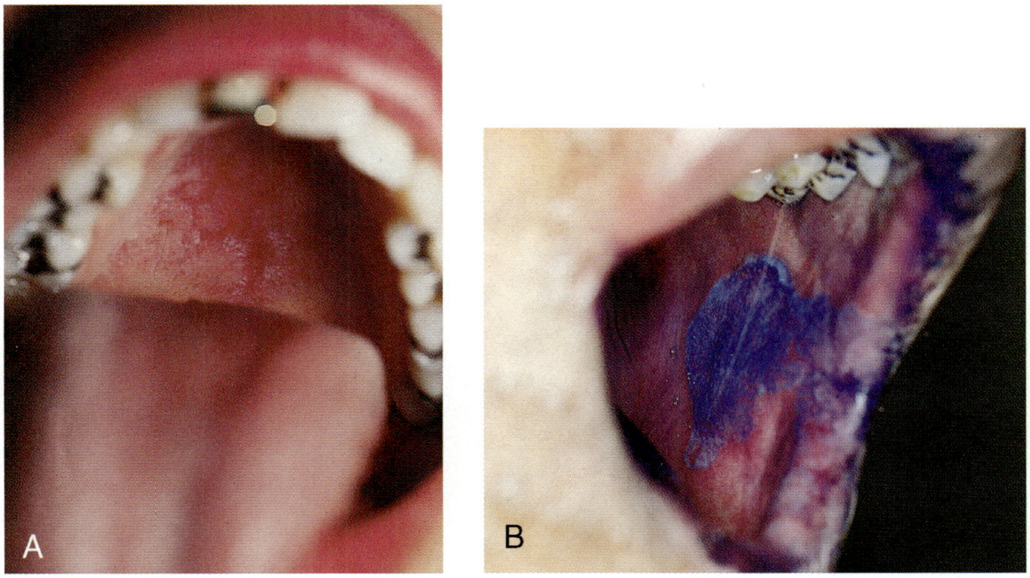

Figure 2.37. Discoid lupus erythematosus (DLE) of the oral mucosa. The typical appearance of a lesion on the hard palate is shown in **A.** Note the honeycomb appearance. These lesions show a typical lupus erythematosus (LE)–specific histopathology and are usually painless. The margins of a DLE lesion on the buccal mucosa of another patient are demarcated by staining with a toluidine blue mouthwash **(B).** The patient in **B** ultimately developed a squamous cell carcinoma within a different area of chronic DLE involvement on his buccal mucosa.

progress, scarring becomes more evident and can produce permanent loss of eyelashes and ectropion (Fig. 2.25). DLE involvement of the eyelid can produce considerable disability (232–234). It has recently been suggested that corneal stromal keratitis can also occur as a result of DLE ocular involvement (235). Although quite rare, anogenital mucosal DLE lesions have also been observed (224).

CHILBLAIN LUPUS

Some patients with LE develop red–purple patches and plaques on their toes, fingers, heels, calves, elbows, knees, and nose that are precipitated by cold, damp climates. Fissuring of the knuckles and heels is common, producing a good deal of discomfort. Such lesions are highly reminiscent of simple chilblain or pernio lesions (226–240). As these lesions evolve, however, they take on the typical appearance of DLE lesions, clinically and histopathologically. One could question whether such patients have simple pernio that in the predisposed individual produces a Köebner response that results in a DLE lesion. The terms "chilblain lupus" and "perniotic LE" have been used to describe such lesions (Fig. 2.38). Unfortunately, the term "lupus pernio" has also been used for such lesions, although this term is more properly used to designate a form of cutaneous sarcoidosis (241). Patients with chilblain lupus often have typical DLE lesions on the face and head (240).

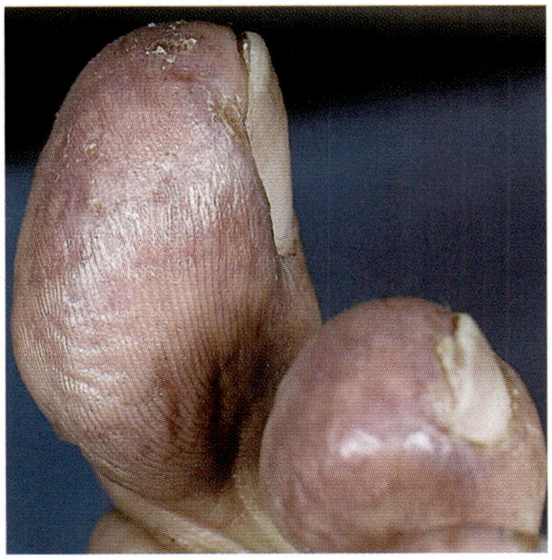

Figure 2.38. Chilblain lupus erythematosus (LE) (perniotic LE). Note the rather nondescript appearance of this early lesion. At this stage the pathology might be nonspecific; however, with time such lesions can present a typical discoid lupus erythematosus (DLE) histopathology.

Chilblain lupus is rare in the United States. Tuffanelli and Dubois (224) failed to detect these lesions among 520 patients with lupus. In marked contrast, Millard and Rowell (236) in Great Britain detected 17 cases of chilblain lupus erythematosus (LE) in a review of 150 patients (11.3%) with CLE. Four of these patients demonstrated erythema multiforme–like lesions. Three of these 17 patients subsequently developed features of SLE. Recent studies indicate in general that most cases of pernio are not related to LE (237). However, among chilblain LE, there appears to be an enrichment of anti-Ro(SS-A) antibodies (238,239). During a recent cold, damp winter, one of the authors noted that two patients with anti-Ro(SS-A)–positive LE developed pernio-like lesions. In a study of the relationship between chilblain and LE, Viguier et al. (237) suggested that persistence of lesions beyond the cold months, a positive ANA, or presence of one of the other ACR criteria for SLE at the time of diagnosis of chilblain lesions helps to distinguish chilblain LE from idiopathic chilblain.

LUPUS ERYTHEMATOSUS TUMIDUS

The accumulation of excessive dermal mucin early in the course of DLE skin lesions can result in the succulent, edematous, urticaria-appearing plaques of lupus erythematosus (LE) tumidus (LET) (Fig. 2.39). The characteristic epidermal histologic changes of DLE are often not as prominent in lupus erythematosus (LE) tumidus (LET) lesions. When this occurs, confusion often arises concerning the diagnosis. Recently, there

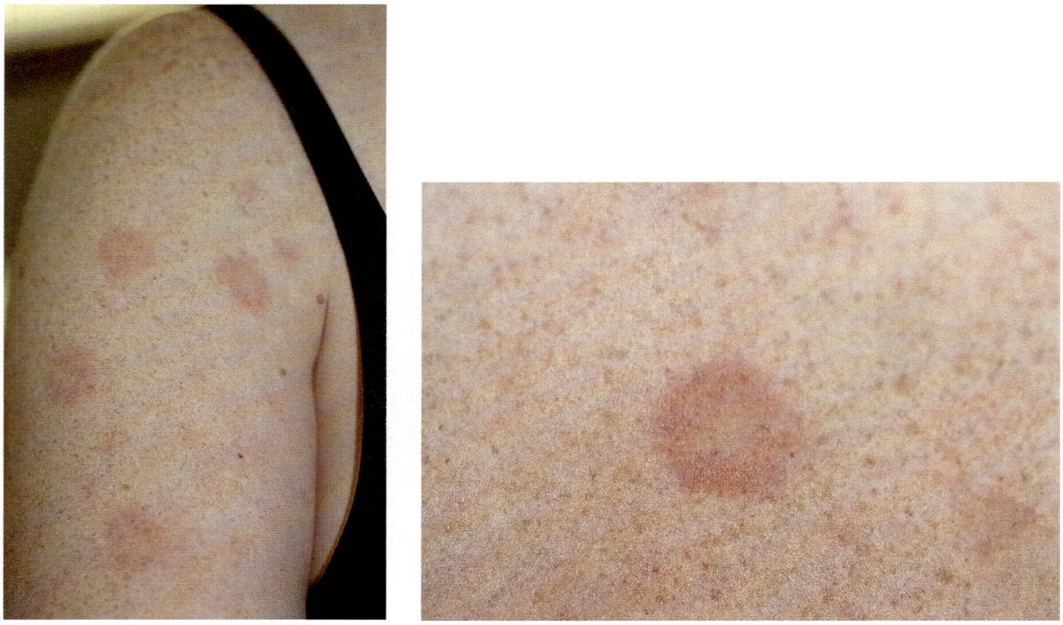

A B

Figure 2.39. Lupus (LE) tumidus. This form of chronic cutaneous lupus erythematosus (LE) , which is uncommon in the authors' experience, presents as succulent, elevated plaques occurring in a sun-exposed distribution. In the case shown in this photograph (which is not typical of all cases of lupus (LE) tumidus), there was a pattern of surface color change reminiscent of Wickham striae; however, the biopsy did not show changes of lichen planus nor were lupus erythematosus (LE)–specific skin disease changes clearly present at the dermal–epidermal junction. The predominant pathologic change was mononuclear cell infiltration around the superficial and deep dermal blood vessels. It is quite likely that lupus (LE) tumidus lesions and lesions described by others under different designations such as "urticarial plaque lupus erythematosus" represent the same disease process (Irwin M. Braverman, personal communication).

have been several reports of patients with this clinicopathologic presentation that have helped to alleviate some of this confusion and have led credence to the hypothesis that LET is a subtype of DLE. Ruiz and Sanchez reported four patients who had firm diagnoses of classic DLE or SLE in addition to red–violet plaques of LET on the upper body, in whom histology showed the dermal changes seen in LE-specific skin disease (242). Kuhn et al. (243) reported a cohort of 40 patients with similar clinical and histologic features. These patients were markedly photosensitive and had a very high response rate to antimalarial therapy. They had a very low incidence of SLE, further suggesting LET is a subset of DLE. It is interesting to note that unlike classic DLE, however, LET lesions tend to resolve completely in the absence of either scarring or atrophy (243).

Table 2.5 presents a comparison of the selected clinical and laboratory features of patients presenting with ACLE, SCLE, and classic DLE skin lesions.

BULLOUS SKIN LESIONS IN LUPUS ERYTHEMATOSUS

Confusion has always existed concerning the nosology and classification of the bullous skin changes that can occur in patients with LE, and there currently is no consensus in this area. Like nonbullous LE skin disease, the varieties of bullous skin lesions that can occur in patients with LE can be divided into those that do and those that do not have a LE-specific histopathology (Table 2.3). Bullae may develop in LE-specific skin lesions such as ACLE and SCLE as a direct extension of the vacuolar degeneration of the epidermal basal layer (165). Skin cleavage occurs as a result of dissolution of the basal cell layer, resulting in a subepidermal cleavage plane. In both ACLE (164) (Fig. 2.6) and SCLE (182), large areas of sheetlike cleavage occasionally develop, resulting in the clinical appearance of toxic epidermal necrolysis. Anti-Ro(SS-A) antibody–positive patients

TABLE 2.5. Comparison of Forms of Lupus Erythematosus (LE)–Specific Skin Disease

Disease Features	ACLE	SCLE	Classic DLE
Clinical features of skin lesions			
Induration	0	0	+++
Scarring	0	0	+++
Pigment changes	+	++	+++
Follicular plugging	0	0	+++
Hyperkeratosis	+	++	+++
Histopathology			
Thickened basement membrane	0	+	+++
Lichenoid infiltrate	+	++	+++
Periappendageal inflammation	0	+	+++
Lupus band			
Lesional	++	++	+++
Nonlesional	++	+	0
Antinuclear antibodies	+++	++	+
Ro(SS-A) antibodies			
By immunodiffusion	+	+++	0
By ELISA	++	+++	+
Anti–native DNA antibodies	+++	+	0
Hypocomplementemia	+++	+	+
Risk for developing SLE	+++	++	+

ACLE, acute cutaneous lupus erythematosus; DLE, discoid lupus erythematosus; ELISA, enzyme-linked immunosorbent assay; SCLE, subacute cutaneous lupus erythematosus; SLE, systemic lupus erythematosus; +++, strongly associated; ++, moderately associated; +, weakly associated; 0, negative, no association.

appear to be at increased risk for developing this complication following UV light exposure (137,243). Documentation of LE as the causal factor in this type of bullous skin change can be difficult because such patients are also frequently on systemic medication and toxic epidermal necrolysis most commonly develops as a result of drug hypersensitivity reaction. In some patients with SCLE, vesiculobullous changes develop at the active advancing edge of annular SCLE lesions (177,179,180, 182) (Fig. 2.15). Subepidermal bullous changes have also been reported to occur in DLE lesions; however, these changes appear to be extremely rare (244).

The term "bullous SLE" has classically been used to refer to an acquired autoimmune blistering disorder of the skin seen in the setting of patients with active SLE, in which histologic sections show a subepidermal blistering dermatitis with collections of neutrophils in dermal papillae. Such histologic findings mimic those of dermatitis herpetiformis and epidermolysis bullosa acquisita. Antibodies to type VII collagen are frequently isolated from patients' sera, but are not required for diagnosis (245). Direct immunofluorescence studies show multiple immunoreactants that exhibit a granular band at the dermal–epidermal junction. This type of bullous skin lesion in the patient with LE might more accurately be called *dermatitis herpetiformis-like blistering eruption of LE* or *epidermolysis bullosa acquisita–like blistering eruption of LE.* It is helpful to consider that patients with SLE may develop any of a number of autoantibodies to self antigens (double-stranded DNA [dsDNA], antiplatelet antibodies, and so on) and that type VII collagen antibodies may be part of the antibody spectrum in SLE in patients who develop this particular constellation of clinicoimmunopathologic findings (246). It is important to emphasize that although this blistering eruption resembles dermatitis herpetiformis (DH) or epidermolysis bullosa acquisita (EBA) very closely clinically and histologically, it should not be viewed merely as an overlap between SLE and DH or EBA because there are distinct immunopathologic and clinical differences, namely multiple immunoreactants at the dermal–epidermal junction and predilection for either extensor or flexural sites (247,248).

Relationship Between Cutaneous and Systemic Disease Features

Figure 2.40 illustrates the different relationships that exist between the three forms of LE-specific skin disease and the systemic autoimmune manifestations of LE.

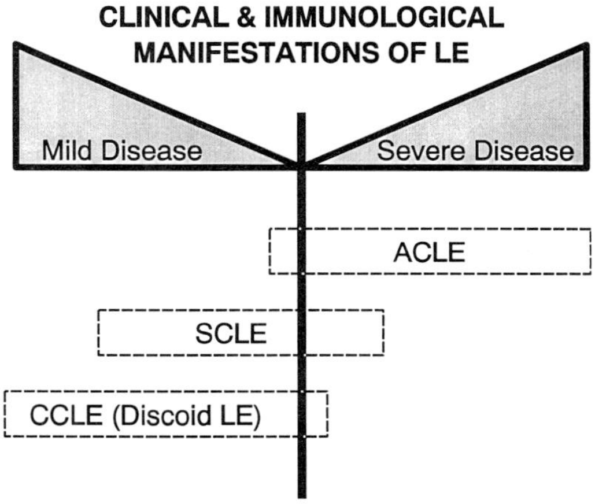

Figure 2.40. Relative risks for systemic lupus erythematosus (SLE) disease activity that are associated with the three major forms of lupus erythematosus (LE)–specific skin disease.

ACUTE CUTANEOUS LUPUS ERYTHEMATOSUS

Because the "malar rash" or "butterfly rash" is so common in patients with SLE, and because such lesions are considered to be a fundamental component of the clinical expression of SLE disease activity, few workers have directly examined the relationship that exists between ACLE and SLE disease activity. Ropes (1) noted that the "butterfly rash" of SLE often waxed and waned in parallel with underlying SLE disease activity. However, Ropes was unable to demonstrate a positive correlation with evidence of LE nephritis. Curiously, a significant negative correlation was noted with both psychosis and serum protein electrophoresis abnormalities. Vlachoyiannopoulos et al. (83) found that flaring of the "rash" of SLE frequently accompanies flares of SLE activity. Wysenbeek et al. (85) have also demonstrated that the generalized "nonspecific rash" of SLE (presumably generalized ACLE) correlated positively with lymphadenopathy, anti–native DNA antibody, low complement levels, and higher prednisone doses. However, these workers found no such correlation with renal disease, central nervous system disease, or SLE disease activity index.

It has always been our impression that either localized or generalized ACLE is associated with a high risk for aggressive SLE activity, including the risk for LE nephritis.

SUBACUTE CUTANEOUS LUPUS ERYTHEMATOSUS

Approximately half the patients with SCLE meet the ACR's revised criteria for the classification of SLE (45,123). However, it has been the experience of most observers that severe SLE (i.e., LE nephritis, central nervous system disease) develops in only 10% of patients with SCLE (123). Although most patients with SCLE who develop four or more SLE classification criteria tend to have a relatively mild disease course overall, there are reports of such patients who have had severe and sometimes fatal outcomes, usually from renal and central nervous system involvement (99,104,113,174,245). There is some indication that patients with the papulosquamous variety of SCLE might be at more risk for developing renal involvement (103,168,177,187).

Sontheimer et al. (177) identified five patients in a cohort of 47 individuals with SCLE that had evidence of lupus nephritis (169). All five of these patients had the papulosquamous type of SCLE, leukopenia, high-titer ANA (< 1:640), and anti-dsDNA antibodies. All five also developed ACLE lesions at some point during their disease courses, and all had been refractory to antimalarial treatment. Lymphocytopenia may also be a marker of underlying systemic disease in patients with either SCLE or DLE. Another report noted that patients with SCLE with renal disease were more likely to have the papulosquamous type of lesions (168). Men with papulosquamous SCLE may have higher risk for severe SLE (103).

SCLE can overlap with other autoimmune disorders. Some patients with SCLE will later manifest clear evidence of SSj, whereas some patients whose illness begins as SSj later have SCLE lesions. Patients with SS/LE overlap may have significant systemic features including central nervous system disease, pulmonary manifestations, and vasculitis (189). Of patients who present with SCLE skin lesions, 3-12% later develop Sjo–

gren syndrome (34,104,106,107). It is interesting to note in this regard that both SCLE and Sjogren syndrome have been associated with the same immunogenetic background—circulating Ro(SS-A) and La(SS-B) autoantibodies and the presence of the HLA-B8, DR3, DRW6, DQ2, and DRW52 extended haplotype (113,114).

A number of Japanese patients with SSj and Ro(SS-A) or La (SS-B) autoantibodies have been reported to have an annular erythema reaction that appears clinically similar to annular SCLE, although biopsies of the lesions have revealed histopathologic findings somewhat distinct from SCLE with a mucinous component (246–251). It is possible that genetic differences between Asians and whites could account for this difference in disease expression. For example, the HLA-DR3 allele is distinctly unusual in Japanese patients.

Roughly one third of patients with SCLE produce rheumatoid factor (33,123). It is not surprising, therefore, that on occasion, patients with patients have subsequently been noted to develop rheumatoid arthritis (RA) (252). In addition, patients presenting with RA can subsequently develop SCLE lesions. One group reported that of 12 patients with RA who produced Ro(SS-A) autoantibodies, two had SCLE skin lesions (253). An association between SCLE and antithyroid autoantibodies and Hashimoto thyroiditis has also been reported (254,255).

There have been case reports suggesting an occasional association between SCLE and malignancy (breast, lung, gastric, and uterus) (256–260). In some of these reports, the SCLE lesions have been suggested to represent a paraneoplastic manifestation of the underlying malignancy. Other disorders that have been anecdotally related to SCLE have been Sweet syndrome (261–263), porphyria cutanea tarda (264), gluten-sensitive enteropathy (265), and Crohn disease (266). The infrequency of these associated conditions militates against anything more than a casual association. However, it should be kept in mind that the usual dose of aminoquinoline antimalarial agents used in the management of SCLE (or DLE) can cause significant hepatotoxicity and exacerbate cutaneous features in patients who have subclinical porphyria cutanea tarda.

CHRONIC CUTANEOUS LUPUS ERYTHEMATOSUS

The relationship that exists between classic DLE and SLE has been the subject of debate throughout the 20th century. Daniel Wallace (157) has presented a comprehensive overview of this subject that systematically and thoughtfully addresses the following issues:

What is the risk for patients presenting with classic DLE subsequently developing SLE? Of patients presenting with classic DLE lesions, 5% to 10% will subsequently develop unequivocal evidence of SLE (29,147,150,155–157,266). Because of the failure in the past to distinguish DLE from SCLE lesions, the actual progression of DLE to SLE may occur less frequently. For example, one of the authors was only able to identify two of approximately 100 patients with DLE observed over a 10-year period who developed clinical and serologic evidence of SLE (T.T.P., unpublished observations). Considerable effort has been made to identify clinical or laboratory features that might correlate with such a pattern of disease progression. One clinical feature that can be useful in this regard is the extent and distribution of the DLE lesions. Patients with generalized DLE (i.e., lesions both above and below the neck) have a higher rate of immunologic abnormalities and risk for progressing to SLE compared with patients with localized DLE (147,149,155,156, 220,268). In addition, patients with generalized DLE are at higher risk for developing the more severe manifestations of SLE (147,155,156,269). In some instances, patients with SLE may develop DLE skin lesions late in the course of their disease when their SLE disease activity has fully remitted (270).

Other physical findings that should alert one to the possibility of underlying systemic disease are diffuse, nonscarring alopecia, generalized lymphadenopathy, periungual nailfold telangiectasia, Raynaud phenomenon, SCLE, and LE-nonspecific skin lesions such as vasculitis (149,266).

The following laboratory findings have been reported to be risk factors for the development of SLE in patients with DLE: unexplained anemia, marked leukopenia, false-positive tests for syphilis, persistently positive high-titer ANA, anti-single-stranded DNA antibody, hypergammaglobulinemia, an elevated erythrocyte sedimentation rate (especially of greater than 50 mm per hour), and immune deposits at the dermal–epidermal junction of nonlesional skin (i.e., a positive lupus band test) (147,155,156,266,271). Some research has also suggested that elevated soluble IL-2 receptor levels might also be a risk factor for SLE in patients with DLE (272).

What are the clinical implications of classic DLE lesions occurring in patients with SLE? Approximately one fourth of patients with SLE will develop DLE lesions at some point in the course of their disease. Some work has suggested that such patients tend to have less severe forms of SLE. Because life-threatening complications such as diffuse proliferative glomerulonephritis are uncommon in these patients, survival is greater when compared with patients with SLE without DLE lesions (266,273).

What are the risks for developing systemic disease associated with other forms of CCLE? Patients with hypertrophic DLE do not appear to have a greater risk for developing SLE than do patients with classic DLE lesions (274). Approximately 50% of the patients with LE profundus/panniculitis have a relatively mild form of SLE (208,210,211,218,275). The systemic features of patients with LE panniculitis/profundus tend to be less severe, and are similar to those in patients with SLE who have DLE skin lesions (208,211,218,275). Severe nephritis is an uncommon complication in patients with SLE with LE panniculitis. In one study, three (20%) of 15 patients presenting with chilblain LE later developed SLE (239); in another study, three of 17 patients developed SLE (235).

The risk for systemic disease activity in patients with LE with mucosal involvement is a function of the type of mucosal lesion that is present. Superficial, transient oral or nasal mucosal ulcerations having a relatively nonspecific histopathology are commonly seen in patients with active SLE (such mucosal lesions represent one of the 11 ACR's revised classification criteria for SLE). Chronic mucosal LE plaques, however, are seen most commonly in patients with LE who do not have life-threatening SLE. The more severe manifestations of SLE such as renal disease appear to be quite uncommon in patients with SLE who develop chronic mucosal plaques (224). Another study noted no significant correlation of oral ulcerations with cutaneous manifestations and serologic parameters (225).

Figure 2.41 illustrates the relative risks for systemic disease activity that are associated with the various clinical varieties of chronic cutaneous LE.

LUPUS BAND TEST

No discussion of the relationship between the cutaneous and systemic manifestations of LE would be complete without addressing the lupus band test. Using direct immunofluorescence microscopy, Burnham et al. (28) identified the presence of immunoglobulins and complement components along the der-

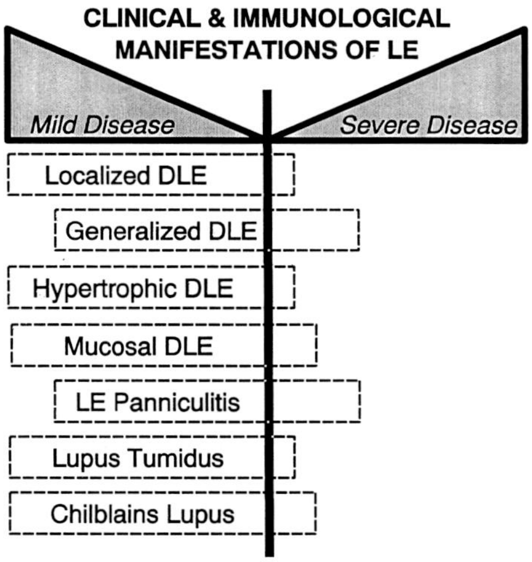

Figure 2.41. Relative risks for systemic lupus erythematosus (SLE) disease activity that are associated with the various clinical varieties of chronic cutaneous lupus erythematosus (LE).

mal–epidermal junction of LE lesional skin biopsies. This phenomenon, subsequently referred to as the "lupus band" (276), was initially believed to be quite specific for LE; however, subsequent work has documented that the lupus band can be found in other skin disorders (277).

Cormane (278) described similar findings in biopsies from clinically normal skin of patients with SLE in the complete absence of any signs of cutaneous inflammation. Because patients with DLE lacked this finding in their nonlesional skin, it was suggested that such results might have diagnostic specificity for SLE. The search for immunoreactant deposition in *nonlesional* skin of patients with LE has subsequently been referred to by many as the "lupus band test" (LBT).

Controversies concerning terminology have clouded this field from the beginning. Although some workers use the term "LBT" to refer to LE lesional as well as nonlesional immunopathologic findings (278), others reserve this designation for reference to the results of immunopathologic examination of nonlesional skin (279). Less confusion might exist in this area if the terms "lesional LBT" and "nonlesional LBT" were uniformly adopted by those working in this area.

The immunopathologic findings in nonlesional skin of patients with LE must be distinguished from those present in LE lesional skin biopsies. Issues related to immunopathologic findings in LE-specific skin lesions (i.e., the lesional LBT) will be discussed later in this chapter in the pathology/immunopathology section. The remainder of this discussion will be limited to the presence or absence of immunoreactants at the dermal–epidermal junction of nonlesional skin (i.e., the nonlesional LBT).

All three major immunoglobulin classes (IgG, IgM, and IgA), and a variety of complement components including constituents of the membrane attack complex, have been identified in these dermal–epidermal junction deposits (276). Studies have suggested that the presence of membrane attack complex in lesional skin is relatively sensitive and specific for LE (280). The immunoglobulin-staining pattern of immunoreactants in nonlesional LE skin under low power is generally described as granular. On high-power magnification, the pattern of fluorescence has been variously described as appearing homogeneous, stippled, fibrillar, shaggy, lumpy–bumpy, linear, or thready (details related to the appearance and significance of these various patterns have been reviewed) (281). Ultrastructurally, these immunoreactants are seen to be deposited on and below the lamina densa of the dermal–epidermal junction (282). The intensity of the staining and the number of immunoreactants present in these deposits can vary considerably (276,278). Most authorities require a continuous pattern of immunoreactant deposition along the dermal–epidermal junction for a positive nonlesional LBT. Numerous studies have suggested that a discontinuous or interrupted nonlesional LBT can be seen in a number of other disorders and thus is much less specific for SLE (276). In addition, the presence of IgM alone appears to be very nonspecific (276).

The diagnostic and prognostic significance of the nonlesional LBT has been the subject of much controversy over the past two decades. In-depth analyses of these issues are available elsewhere (276,278,281). The following summary can serve to acquaint the reader with the clinically relevant issues pertaining to the nonlesional LBT.

STANDARDIZATION

It is quite curious that a test such as this that has been used clinically for well over two decades has been so poorly standardized. Only recently have large numbers of clinically healthy individuals been studied to determine the incidence of a false-positive nonlesional LBT in both sun-exposed and nonexposed skin regions. Such studies have suggested that as many as 20% of healthy young adults have a positive LBT in sun-exposed nonlesional skin regions such as the lateral aspect of the neck, whereas virtually none are positive in sun-protected nonlesional sites such as the buttocks (282). Thus, considerable caution must be taken when interpreting the results of immunopathologic findings in lesional and nonlesional biopsies taken from fully sun-exposed skin sites (e.g., face, neck, extensor aspect of forearm and hand) or partially sun-exposed skin sites (flexor aspect of the forearm, deltoid region) with respect to the diagnosis of cutaneous or systemic LE.

Autofluorescence of dermal collagen and elastin fibers can give the appearance at low power of a positive nonlesional LBT (the "fibrillar pseudoband") (276). At higher power, the artifactual nature of this false-positive finding becomes apparent. A false-negative nonlesional LBT can occur when high levels of extravascular dermal IgG are present. This finding, which correlates with hypergammaglobulinemia, can obscure the distinct nature of the lupus band at the dermal–epidermal junction (284).

It is also important to understand that considerable anatomic regional variation exists with respect to the nonlesional LBT (284). It has been suggested that there is a cephalocaudal gradient in the frequency of a positive lesional LBT in DLE lesions, with lesions on the head more often positive than those on the trunk (278). There are indications that a similar phenomenon might exist with the LBT in nonlesional skin of NZB/W mice, a murine model of SLE (33). Firm data addressing this issue in human patients with LE have not been presented.

Diagnostic Specificity

Because the strongest clinical association of the nonlesional LBT has been with SLE, it is not surprising that patients with classic DLE without clinical or laboratory evidence of extracutaneous disease have been uniformly nonlesional LBT–negative (149). Only about 25% of the patients with SLE who have DLE lesions have a positive nonlesional LBT (149). Approximately 25% of the patients with SCLE (an LE subset that frequently has mild symptoms of SLE) are nonlesional LBT–positive in relatively sun-protected flexor forearm skin (33).

As noted earlier, the diagnostic specificity of the nonlesional LBT for SLE has become a point of controversy. Factoring in the profile of individual immunoreactants present in a positive nonlesional LBT has been suggested as one approach to enhancing the specificity of this test. Several studies have suggested that when three or more immunoreactants are present in the nonlesional LBT, the diagnostic specificity for SLE is very high (86,285). These observations, along with the fact that actinically damaged skin can yield a false-positive result (286), would suggest that a positive nonlesional LBT (confirmed under high-power observation to exclude the artifacts such as the fibrillar pseudoband) in fully sun-protected skin from the buttock or inner aspect of the upper arm that consists of three or more immunoglobulin or complement components, might have the greatest specificity for SLE. Under these conditions, a positive nonlesional LBT can serve as a very useful piece of diagnostic information in those difficult cases of SLE where the clinical and laboratory manifestations of this disorder are being expressed atypically.

Prognostic Significance

Although the nonlesional LBT was initially adopted because of its perceived diagnostic specificity for SLE, subsequent work suggested that it also correlated positively with a more aggressive course of systemic disease, including the development of lupus nephritis (287–294). The presence of IgG in the nonlesional LBT correlated with the presence of anti-dsDNA antibodies and was suggested to be more indicative of severe SLE than the presence of IgM alone (289,292). The idea that the nonlesional LBT had prognostic value also became a point of contention. However, a follow-up study has confirmed the predictive value of a positive nonlesional LBT (281). Whether the nonlesional LBT provides incremental value in prognosis assessment over more generally available and less-invasive tests such as circulating dsDNA antibody levels is not clear; however, there are those who continue to believe that this is the case (285). It is the authors' opinion that a properly interpreted nonlesional LBT has its greatest utility as an additional diagnostic maneuver in patients with atypical clinical and laboratory presentations of SLE.

Pathology and Immunopathology

ACUTE CUTANEOUS LUPUS ERYTHEMATOSUS

Histopathology

The histologic picture in ACLE is generally less impressive than that seen in SCLE and DLE lesions. The dermal cellular infiltrate is often relatively sparse. The most prominent changes are edema of the upper dermis and focal liquefactive degeneration of the epidermal basal cell layer. In the most severe forms of ACLE, epidermal necrosis may occur, producing a histopathologic pattern strongly resembling toxic epidermal necrolysis.

Immunopathology

Curiously, there are very few published data concerning direct immunofluorescence findings in ACLE. In one study, five (100%) of five skin biopsies from ACLE (i.e., "diffuse erythema") lesions were reported to be lesional LBT–positive (293). Recent work has indicated that the lesional LBT is positive in 60% of patient having the "malar rash" of SLE (294).

SUBACUTE CUTANEOUS LUPUS ERYTHEMATOSUS

Histopathology

Although the histopathology of SCLE is clearly that of LE-specific skin disease, it may be impossible to clearly differentiate SCLE from ACLE and DLE. Characteristically ACLE, SCLE, and DLE have variable degrees of hyperkeratosis, basal cell degeneration, dermal edema, and mononuclear cell infiltration around the dermal–epidermal junction extending into the dermis. In SCLE, there is focal basal cell injury and disorientation with liquefaction degeneration, sparse upper dermal mononuclear cell infiltrate that may partially obscure the dermal–epidermal junction, dermal edema, and rarely epidermal necrosis (175). The mononuclear infiltrate is usually limited to perivascular and adnexal structures in the upper third of the dermis, and the epidermis may be mildly atrophic. Vesicular changes can occur in SCLE lesions, particularly at the active border of annular SCLE lesions (99,179,180). It has been suggested that such patients more likely have HLA-DR3 alleles and have Ro(SS-A) autoantibodies (99).

SCLE lesions generally have less hyperkeratosis, follicular plugging, mononuclear cell infiltration of adnexal structures, and dermal melanophages compared with DLE lesions. Qualitative differences in the histopathology of SCLE versus DLE have been noted (102,125,175,295); however, not all agree on this point (296). Bangert et al. (175) were unable to differentiate papulosquamous from annular SCLE by blinded histopathologic examination.

Immunopathology

As in other LE-specific lesions, immune deposits can be frequently detected by immunofluorescence staining in SCLE skin lesions. The initial studies indicated that these deposits consist of immunoglobulin (IgM, IgG, or IgA) and complement components arranged in a granular bandlike pattern along the dermal–epidermal junction (33). Approximately 60% of SCLE lesions from the original cohort of patients with SCLE had such deposits compared with somewhat higher percentages for ACLE and DLE lesions. Others have found similar results in SCLE skin lesions (99), whereas some workers have found even greater frequencies (191). Thus, the presence of immune deposits at the dermal–epidermal junction can help confirm a diagnosis of SCLE, but its absence does not necessarily rule it out. These immune deposits are not specific for LE because similar deposits can be found in normal or sun-damaged skin (282), and in other non-LE dermatologic conditions (276).

Nonlesional deltoid and flexor forearm skin biopsies from the original group of patients with SCLE contained junctional immune deposits in 46% and 26%, respectively (33). The prognostic significance of such deposits has not yet been determined.

Nieboer et al. (172) have reported finding a "dustlike particle" pattern of IgG deposition deposited in and around the epidermal basal keratinocytes and subepidermal regions in 30% of SCLE lesional skin biopsies. This group suggested that this pattern of immunoglobulin deposition is specific for SCLE, although its presence did not correlate with the presence of circulating Ro(SS-A) autoantibodies. Others have noted this same immunofluorescence pattern in patients with SCLE (125,297). It is curious, however, that one of the authors (R.D.S.) as well as a number of other observers (54,191,285,298) have not been impressed by this pattern of immunofluorescence in SCLE lesional biopsies, suggesting that it might be somewhat technique-dependent. This dustlike pattern of IgG is similar to that found in human skin explants grafted onto nude mice that resulted from intravenous infusion of human Ro(SS-A) autoimmune sera (299). One of the authors has noted a similar pattern of IgG and IgM deposition in guinea pig skin following intradermal injections of human Ro(SS-A) autoimmune sera (R.D.S., personal/unpublished observation).

CHRONIC CUTANEOUS LUPUS ERYTHEMATOSUS

Classic Discoid Lupus Erythematosus

The epidermal basal cell layer is the principal site of injury in all three forms of LE-specific skin disease (175). In classic DLE, there is also prominent hyperkeratosis and follicular plugging. The spinous layer of the epidermis is generally not thickened and may be somewhat atrophic. Epidermal basal layer changes include loss of the normal organization and orientation of basal cells, edema with vacuole formation between and sometimes within basal cells (i.e., liquefaction or vacuolar degeneration), partial obliteration of the dermal–epidermal junction by a mononuclear cell infiltrate, thickening of the epidermal basement membrane, increased melanin pigment formation, and interruption of pigment transfer between melanocytes and keratinocytes leading to the accumulation of melanin by phagocytosis in dermal macrophages (pigment incontinence).

The dermal histopathologic changes are less specific. A mononuclear cell infiltrate composed mainly of T-lymphocytes and macrophages is present most predominately in the periappendageal and perivascular areas. Plasma cells are occasionally seen in the more chronic lesions, and dermal mucin deposition can at times be quite prominent. The chronically scarring DLE lesions more often have a denser inflammatory cell infiltrate that extends well into the deeper reticular dermis, or subcutis, or both. In contrast, ACLE and SCLE lesions contain a less dense inflammatory infiltrate that is confined to the upper dermis but still shows the distinctive pattern of injury along the dermal–epidermal junction (166). The periappendageal inflammation that is characteristic of DLE is less prominent in SCLE and ACLE.

Direct immunofluorescence examination of biopsy specimens taken from DLE lesions often reveals a thick continuous band of immunoreactants along the dermal–epidermal junction (276,278). This band also extends along the basement membrane of the hair follicle, a finding that is not often seen in those other disorders that have been reported to have similar dermal–epidermal junction immunoreactants deposited in a bandlike pattern. Multiple immunoglobulin classes (IgG, IgA, IgM) are usually present within this band and various complement components (C3, C4, Clq, properdin, factor B, and the membrane attack complex, C5b-C9) can present in many of these lesions (276,278,289).

Early reports suggested that more than 90% of DLE lesions had lesional immunoreactants at the dermal–epidermal junction (293); however, other studies have reported somewhat lower frequencies (276,278). The frequency with which immunoreactants are found in DLE lesions also appears to vary with the anatomic region from which the biopsy is taken. In one study, lesions on the head, neck, and arms were more often positive (80%) than those on the trunk (20%) (300). The frequency of bandlike immunoreactant deposition at the dermal–epidermal junction appears also to be a function of the age of the lesion being examined, with older lesions (> 3 months) being more often positive than younger ones (< 3 months) (301). Ultrastructural localization of immunoglobulin at the dermal–epidermal junction has confirmed that these proteins are deposited on the upper dermal collagen fibers and along the lamina densa of the epidermal basement membrane zone (302,303).

Hypertrophic Discoid Lupus Erythematosus

The histopathology and immunopathology is similar to that of classic DLE lesions except for a much greater degree of epidermal acanthosis and hyperkeratosis. Overlap between the histologic features of hypertrophic DLE and lichen planus has been described (203,204). Hypertrophic DLE has been mistaken for squamous cell carcinoma in some histologic sections because of pronounced acanthosis and squamatization of basal keratinocytes (247).

Lupus Erythematosus Profundus/Lupus Erythematosus Panniculitis

Absence of the characteristic epidermal and dermal changes of LE can make the histologic diagnosis sometimes challenging, and controversy has existed in the past as to the specificity of the histopathologic changes of LE panniculitis when overlying changes of DLE are not present at the dermal–epidermal junction. The histologic features are those of a lobular lymphocytic panniculitis: perivascular infiltration with lymphocytes, plasma cells, and histiocytes in the deep dermis and subcutaneous fat (including lymphoid nodule formation); vessel-wall thickening and invasion by mononuclear cells ("lymphocytic vasculitis"); absence of polymorphonuclear leukocytes. There is a characteristic hyaline fat necrosis and prominent fibrinoid degeneration of collagen; as well as mucinous degeneration and calcification in old established lesions (211,303,304). Immunoglobulin and complement deposits are usually found in blood vessel walls of the deep dermis and subcutis by direct immunofluorescence staining of biopsy specimens (218). Immunoglobulin deposits at the dermal–epidermal junction may or may not be present depending on the site biopsied, the presence or absence of accompanying SLE, and the presence or absence of overlying changes of DLE at the dermal–epidermal junction.

Mucosal Discoid Lupus Erythematosus

Except for the differences related to the absence of hair follicles and stratum corneum in mucous membranes, the microscopic changes are highly reminiscent of those seen in cutaneous DLE lesions (220,224).

Chilblain Lupus Erythematosus

Lesions of chilblain LE show interface dermatitis, with superficial and deep perivascular lymphocytic infiltration much like classic DLE. However, a lymphocytic vasculitis and fibrin within the lumina of dermal blood vessels are present in addition (247,305).

Lupus Erythematosus Tumidus

In LET, one sees the dermal changes of DLE, namely a variable perivascular mononuclear infiltrate with prominent mucin between collagen bundles, but the classic epidermal changes noted in other forms of LE-specific skin disease are not present (242,306).

Laboratory Manifestations

ACUTE CUTANEOUS LUPUS ERYTHEMATOSUS

Few data are available concerning specific laboratory associations of ACLE. Wysenbeek et al. (85) have recently reported that anti-

TABLE 2.6. Autoantibodies Encountered in Patients with Systemic Lupus Erythematosus (SLE)

	Autoantibody Frequency			
Antigen	**ID**	**SPA/RIA**	**Specificity**	**Clinical Association**
High disease specificity				
dsDNA	—	40%–60%	Native DNA	LE nephritis
Sm	25%	–	Ribonucleoprotein	–
rRNP	10%	–	Ribosomal P protein	CNS LE
PCNA	3%	–	Cyclin	
Low disease specificity				
ssDNA	—	60%–80%	Denatured DNA	Risk for SLE in DLE patients
C1q		60%	C1q	Active SLE with nephritis
Histones	—	50%–70%	Histones	Drug-induced SLE
U_1RNP	35%	–	Ribonucleoprotein	Overlap CTD (MCTD)
Ro(SS-A)	25%	50%	Ribonucleoprotein	SCLE, SSj neonatal LE
La(SS-B)	10%	—	Ribonucleoprotein	SSj, SCLE
Ku	10%	–	Transcription factor	Overlap CTD

CNS, central nervous system; CTD, connective tissue disease; DLE, discoid LE; ID, immunodiffusion; LE, lupus erythematosus; MCTD, mixed connective tissue disease; RIA, radioimmunoassay; SCLE, subacute cutaneous LE; SLE, systemic LE; SPA, solid-phase immunoassay (i.e., enzyme-linked immunosorbent assay); SSj, Sjögren syndrome.

dsDNA antibodies and low complement levels were more common in patients who had the nonspecific "rash" of SLE (presumably generalized ACLE). An overview of the autoantibodies that can be encountered in patients with LE is presented in Table 2.6.

SUBACUTE CUTANEOUS LUPUS ERYTHEMATOSUS

Autoantibodies

ANAs have been detected in 60% to 81% of patients with SCLE when human tissue substrate was used (33–35,104,106,171,177), but only in 49% to 55% of patients when mouse or rat substrates were used (97,101,168). Ro(SS-A) antibodies have been observed in frequencies ranging from 40% to 100% of patients by immunodiffusion techniques (123,307,308). Much higher percentages of patients are anti-Ro(SS-A)–positive by the more sensitive enzyme-linked immunosorbent assay (ELISA) (264,265). Some have recently suggested that anti-Ro(SS-A) precipitins are more often associated with patients with annular SCLE (111), although this has not been the experience of the authors. Most investigators report finding La(SS-B) antibodies by immunodiffusion in 12% to 42% of their patients with SCLE (99,104,105,168); however, two groups of investigators outside of the United States found that considerably higher percentages of their patients had these antibodies (106,167). A comparison of the frequency of laboratory abnormalities seen in SCLE to those seen in ACLE and DLE is presented in Table 2.5.

False-positive VDRL reactions, indicative of antiphospholipid antibodies, have been detected in anywhere from 7% to 33% of patients with SCLE (123). Anticardiolipin antibodies have been detected by ELISA in approximately 10% to 16% of patients (123,309) (Table 2.6). Recent studies indicate that the lupus anticoagulant is found in association with the DQ7 allele (310). In SCLE, as noted before, DQ1 and DQ2 alleles predominate. Rheumatoid factor has been present in approximately one third of patients with SCLE (123); however, relatively few patients with SCLE have developed RA (252). Sm, dsDNA, and U_1RNP antibodies have been reported to occur in approximately 10% of patients with SCLE (123) (Table 2.6). One report has found anti-U_1RNP antibodies in eight (53%) of 15 patients (311), although others have noted a much lower frequency (35,99,106,168). Antilymphocyte antibodies were found in 33% of patients in one study (35). Antithyroid antibodies have been reported in 18% (143) and 44% (214) of patients with SCLE. A comparison of the frequency of autoantibodies in patients with SCLE and classic DLE is presented in Table 2.5.

Other Laboratory Findings

Patients with SCLE, particularly those with systemic involvement, may have a number of laboratory abnormalities. Various studies have found the following: anemia, leukopenia, thrombocytopenia, an elevated erythrocyte sedimentation rate, hypergammaglobulinemia, proteinuria, hematuria, urine casts, elevated serum creatine and blood urea nitrogen levels, and depressed complement levels (123). Levels of complement components such as C2 or C4 can be depressed as a result of genetic deficiency (40,117,312). It may be difficult to determine if low C2 or C4 complement levels are due to an absence or defect in an individual's C2 or C4 genes, or are secondary to complement consumption resulting from systemic disease activity. Diagnosis is easier in an individual with complete C2 or C4 deficiency secondary to defects on both chromosomes because the total hemolytic complement activity will be zero.

CHRONIC CUTANEOUS LUPUS ERYTHEMATOSUS

Autoantibodies

Only a small percentage of patients with classic DLE who have no evidence of systemic disease by history or physical examination have detectable immunologic abnormalities (149,155). ANAs may be detected in low titer in as many as 30% to 40% of patients with DLE; however, less than 5% will have the higher ANA levels that are characteristically seen in severe SLE. Although antibodies to single-stranded DNA are not uncommon in DLE, antibodies to dsDNA are distinctly unusual (147,313,314). Precipitating antibodies to U_1RNP are sometimes found in patients whose disease course is dominated by DLE lesions; however, such patients usually have evidence of mild SLE or overlapping connective tissue disease (147). Ro(SS-A) precipitins can also occasionally be seen in patients with DLE (306,314). The presence of precipitating Sm and La(SS-B) antibodies are, however, distinctly unusual in patients with isolated DLE lesions (314). Fewer than 10% of patients with DLE have IgG anticardiolipin antibodies (315).

TABLE 2.7. Frequency of Anti-DNA and Anti-Ribonuclear Protein Antibodies in Systemic and Discoid Lupus Erythematosus (SLE) and (DLE)

	Anti DNA	U1RNP	Sm	Ro	La
SLE+	42%	36%	24%	24%	9%
DLE++	0%	10.5%	0%	24%	2.6%

++DLE, discoid lupus erythematosus 38 patients; RNP, ribonuclear protein; +SLE, systemic lupus erythematosus 150 patients.

ANAs are present in 70% to 75% of patients with LE profundus/panniculitis, but anti-dsDNA antibodies are uncommon (201,211,218).

One of us (T.T.P.) has addressed the frequencies of autoantibodies in patients with discoid lupus (DLE) by evaluating sera from 38 patients with DLE provided by Drs. Denny Tuffanelli and John Epstein. The results of this study and comparison with the serologies obtained in 150 untreated patients with SLE are presented in Table 2.7. (unpublished personal observation July, 2003).

Other Laboratory Abnormalities

A small percentage of patients with DLE will have biologic false-positive serologic tests for syphilis (VDRL), positive rheumatoid factor tests, slight depressions in serum complement levels, modest elevations in γ-globulin, and modest leukopenia. The significance of such findings will be discussed later.

Differential Diagnosis

ACUTE CUTANEOUS LUPUS ERYTHEMATOSUS

There are a number of dermatoses unrelated to LE that can produce a red face (14,55,316,317). Among those more commonly confused with ACLE are acne rosacea, dermatomyositis, and seborrheic dermatitis. Facial swelling may be severe in patients with ACLE and SLE, sometimes simulating the facial skin changes that are characteristic of dermatomyositis (1,162). The authors have detected a group of patients with photosensitive dermatomyositis sine myositis (amyopathic dermatomyositis) with facial and histologic features reminiscent of ACLE (see Chapter 3 for further discussion). Generalized ACLE can be confused with other causes of widespread exanthematous reactions such as drug hypersensitivity reactions as well as erythema multiforme.

SUBACUTE CUTANEOUS LUPUS ERYTHEMATOSUS

The cutaneous lesions of papulosquamous SCLE can be most closely mimicked by psoriasis (particularly photosensitive psoriasis). Occasionally, they can also be confused with pityriasis rubra pilaris (318) and crusted scabies (319). Seborrheic dermatitis, polymorphous light eruption, dermatophyte infections, nummular eczema, contact dermatitis, dermatomyositis, and cutaneous T-cell lymphoma/mycosis fungoides can also be confused with SCLE on occasion. Annular SCLE lesions are more apt to be misdiagnosed as granuloma annulare, erythema multiforme, or types of figurate erythemas such as erythema annulare centrifugum and erythema gyratum repens. The photo-distribution of SCLE lesions and the LE-specific histopathology are often crucial in helping the clinician differentiate SCLE from these other skin diseases. The central, inactive areas of annular SCLE tend to be hypopigmented, which distinguishes these lesions from other causes of annular erythema. The presence of circulating Ro(SS-A) autoantibodies can serve to support further a diagnosis of SCLE. It should be remembered that a number of different drugs can precipitate SCLE.

CHRONIC CUTANEOUS LUPUS ERYTHEMATOSUS

Classic Discoid Lupus Erythematosus

With respect to diagnosis, discoid-shaped skin lesions that have erythema and hyperpigmentation at their active borders, and depigmentation, telangiectasia, and atrophy at the centers are very unlikely to result from dermatologic disorders other than cutaneous LE. However, other dermatoses can produce persistent red plaques on the face that at times can be confused with DLE.

Polymorphous light eruption (PMLE), as the name implies, is an exclusively photo-triggered dermatosis that can be expressed in several clinical forms, including succulent red plaques that can occasionally mimic the earlier phases of evolving DLE lesions. PMLE lesions, however, clinically lack the keratinaceous follicular plugging, telangiectasia, and atrophy that are characteristic of DLE lesions. Histopathologically, PMLE lacks the prominent liquefaction degeneration of the epidermal basal cell layer and basement membrane thickening that is characteristic of DLE lesions. In the dermis, the lymphoid cell infiltrate is predominately perivascular in PMLE and does not involve the cutaneous appendages as in DLE. Immunoglobulins and complement components are not deposited at the dermal–epidermal junction in PMLE as in DLE. In addition, none of the clinical forms of PMLE have been associated with clinical or laboratory evidence of an underlying systemic disease process.

Granuloma faciale can also present as indolent, red–brown–to-purple facial plaques that can be very resistant to all forms of treatment. Although dilated patulous follicles are often present, hyperkeratosis and atrophy are not seen in this disorder. The epidermis is spared by the histopathologic process seen in granuloma faciale and the pattern of dermal inflammation is quite distinct from that seen in DLE lesions.

Sarcoidosis, Jessner benign lymphocytic infiltration of the skin, pseudolymphoma of Spiegler–Fendt (Spiegler–Fendt sarcoid), lymphocytoma cutis, angiolymphoid hyperplasia with eosinophilia, lymphoma cutis, lupus vulgaris (320), and tertiary syphilis (321) are other disorders that can clinically simulate some phases of DLE lesions and that may present diagnostic confusion. The histopathologies of these conditions are quite distinct from those of DLE and each is usually negative for immunoglobulin and complement components at the dermal–epidermal junction at direct immunofluorescence examination.

Hypertrophic Discoid Lupus Erythematosus

Uitto et al. (322) have pointed out that the verrucous, hyperkeratotic character of these lesions could be mistaken for keratoacanthoma, squamous cell carcinoma, prurigo nodularis, or hypertrophic lichen planus.

Lupus Erythematosus Profundus/Lupus Erythematosus Panniculitis

The differential diagnosis of patients with lupus panniculitis includes Weber–Christian panniculitis, factitial panniculitis, Talwin-induced panniculitis, pancreatic panniculitis, traumatic panniculitis, morphea profundus, eosinophilic fasciitis, sarcoidosis, subcutaneous granuloma annulare, and rheumatoid nodules. Deep excisional biopsy is often required to distinguish LE panniculitis from these other disorders, particularly when classic DLE lesions are not present.

Mucosal Discoid Lupus Erythematosus

With respect to differential diagnosis, oral lichen planus presents the closest clinical appearance to that of oral mucosal DLE.

Management

ACUTE CUTANEOUS LUPUS ERYTHEMATOSUS

ACLE lesions respond to the more aggressive regimens of systemic corticosteroids and other immunosuppressive agents (e.g., azathioprine, cyclophosphamide) that are often required to manage the more severe systemic manifestations of LE that frequently accompany this form of LE-specific skin disease. Increasing evidence suggests that drugs such as hydroxychloroquine can have a steroid-sparing effect on SLE (323). This is likely to be true for ACLE as well.

SUBACUTE CUTANEOUS LUPUS ERYTHEMATOSUS

The management of patients with SCLE should include evaluation to rule out underlying systemic disease at the time of diagnosis, then again at 6- to 12-month intervals, unless the patient develops symptoms that dictate an earlier reassessment (324). The initial evaluation should include a history, including a careful medication history to rule out drug-induced SCLE (see before), and a review of systems and physical examination to elicit symptoms and signs of underlying systemic disease (i.e., arthritis, serositis, central nervous system disease, renal disease). Initial laboratory evaluation should include, at the minimum, a complete blood count, platelet count, erythrocyte sedimentation rate, urinalysis, and blood chemistry profile. Additional determinations that can be of help include C3, C4, and CH_{50}, dsDNA, and Sm.

The initial management of all patients with SCLE should include education regarding protection from sun and artificial sources of UV light (323a) and the elimination of potentially provocative photosensitizing drugs such as hydrochlorothiazide, griseofulvin, and piroxicam. Also, calcium channel blockers and terbenifine should be eliminated. With regard to specific medical therapy, local measures should be maximized first and then systemic agents used if significant disease activity continues.

Sun Protection

Patients should be advised to avoid direct sun exposure, particularly during the midday hours and during the summer months when the UV component of sunlight is least attenuated by the atmosphere. Tightly woven clothing and hats should be worn with broad-spectrum sunscreens to achieve maximal shielding from sunlight. A clothing line offering maximized UV protection is currently being marketed (Ultra Sun Protective Clothing; Solumbra, Everett, WA). Patients should select broad-spectrum sunscreens that contain agents that block UVB with a sun protective factor (SPF) of 15 or greater. Preparations containing Parsol 1789 (avobenzone) and titanium dioxide provide the broadest degree of UVA protection (325), and such products may have benefit in patients with SCLE (326). Products should also be selected that are most resistant to being washed off by sweating or bathing. Sunscreens should be liberally applied at least 30 minutes before sun exposure and reapplied after bathing or appreciable perspiration. Several reviews addressing comparative sunscreen efficacy have been published (325,327). UV light–blocking films can be applied to home and automobile windows. Plastic shields can be placed over fluorescent light bulbs to block the small amount of UV irradiation that can leak from such sources (327).

Corrective camouflage cosmetics such as Dermablend (Dermablend Corrective Products, Chicago, IL) and Covermark offer the dual benefit of being highly effective physical sunscreens as well as aesthetically pleasing cosmetic masking agents for patients having psychological effects from therapeutically refractory, chronic, disfiguring skin disease as a result of cutaneous LE.

Local Corticosteroids

Initial treatment usually includes the use of a potent topical corticosteroid, such as clobetasol propionate 0.05% (Temovate; GlaxoSmithKline, Pittsburgh, PA; Olux, Connetics Co., Palo Alto, CA), betamethasone dipropionate in optimized vehicle 0.05% (Diprolene; Schering, Kenilworth, NJ), diflorasone diacetate 0.05% (Psorcon; Dermik, Berwyn, PA), or amcinonide 0.1% (Cyclocort; Fujisawa, Deerfield, IL). Twice-daily application of these products to lesional skin for 2 weeks followed by a 2-week rest period can minimize the risk for local complications such as steroid atrophy and telangiectasia. Cutaneous LE represents one the very few clinical situations where such potent topical fluorinated corticosteroids can be recommended for use on atrophy-prone areas such as the face, because the alternatives are unchecked, disfiguring skin disease or the potential for side effects from systemic therapy. Unfortunately, topical corticosteroids alone do not provide adequate improvement for most patients with SCLE. The lesions of most patients with SCLE are too numerous to be managed by intralesional corticosteroid injections and oral corticosteroids should be avoided as long as possible when treating this chronic cutaneous condition.

Antimalarials

Although a number of systemic medications have been reported to be of benefit to patients with SCLE, by far the most useful are the aminoquinoline antimalarial agents. The authors as well as others (328–330) have found that approximately 80% of patients with SCLE will respond to single-agent or combined antimalarial therapy. The three agents most frequently prescribed for patients with SCLE are hydroxychloroquine sulfate (Plaquenil-Sanofi Labs), chloroquine phosphate (Aralen-Sanofi Labs), and quinacrine (currently only available as a dihydrochloride salt which must be compounded into capsules). In general, hydroxychloroquine is best tolerated with the least side effects.

When using either hydroxychloroquine or chloroquine, ophthalmologic examination is required to minimize the risk for retinal toxicity (quinacrine has not been confirmed to be retinopathic). The most recent set of guidelines published by the American Academy of Ophthalmologists in April 2002 suggests the following approach (331a). The American Academy of Ophthalmology recommends that all individuals beginning treatment with either hydroxychloroquine or chloroquine have a complete baseline ophthalmologic exam within the first year. This should include examination of the retina through a dilated pupil and testing of central visual field sensitivity. *Low-risk patients* (those having normal eye exams who have received low daily doses of these drugs [i.e., hydroxychloroquine, ≤6.5 mg per kilogram per day or chloroquine, ≤3 mg per kilogram per day for less than 5 years] need no further ophthalmologic testing for the following 5 years. *High-risk patients* (those having used the drug for longer than 5 years; those taking larger daily doses; those having other risk factors [high body fat level, concomitant kidney, liver disease, or retinal disease, age ≥60 years]) should have ophthalmologic exams repeated annually. There does not appear to be an upper limit on the "safe" total lifetime dose of these drugs if these daily maximum dosing recommendations are not exceeded.

Periodic assessments of hematologic and hepatic function should be obtained during antimalarial therapy to identify the occasional patient who will have an idiosyncratic reaction. Quinacrine hydrochloride is more likely to induce hemolysis in glucose-6-phosphate dehydrogenase–deficient patients than is hydroxychloroquine or chloroquine. Neurotoxicity and muscular toxicity can occur but was much more of a problem in the past when higher daily doses of these drugs were used.

Antimalarial agents can induce a number of dermatologic changes. All can cause a blue–black pigmentation of the skin (particularly in the sun-exposed areas), palatal mucosa, nails, and pretibial surfaces. They can also rarely cause bleaching of lightly pigmented hair. Quinacrine frequently causes diffuse yellowing of the skin, sclera, and bodily secretions that is fully reversible on discontinuation of the drug. On very rare occasions, quinacrine produces a lichenoid drug reaction that can be the harbinger of severe bone marrow toxicity (332). Lichenoid drug reactions to antimalarials can at times simulate the appearance of SCLE or DLE (332a).

Therapy with hydroxychloroquine alone at 6 to 6.5 mg/kg (400 mg per day in an average-sized person) should be tried initially. Because hydroxychloroquine reaches steady-state levels in 6 to 8 weeks, if there is no significant improvement by 2-3 months, quinacrine 100 mg daily can be added to the hydroxychloroquine (332,333). If the response is inadequate after 4 to 6 weeks of hydroxychloroquine plus quinacrine, chloroquine 250 mg daily can be substituted for the hydroxychloroquine while continuing the quinacrine (an occasional patient with cutaneous LE will respond better to chloroquine than hydroxychloroquine). Once disease activity is controlled, the hydroxychloroquine can be decreased to 200 mg daily for maintenance. As noted previously, there is evidence that cigarette smoking interferes with efficacy of antimalarials in treating cutaneous disease possibly by interfering with antimalarial metabolism.

Dapsone

Dapsone (diaminodiphenylsulfone; Jacobus Pharmaceutical, Princeton, NJ) is best for treating the occasional patient who has DH-like or EBA-like vesiculobullous skin lesions of LE ("bullous SLE"). Within days, 100 mg per day of this drug can provide significant improvement. Higher doses will be required by some patients. Hematologic, renal, and hepatic toxicities can occur with this drug and thus frequent monitoring is required. The authors have had relatively little positive experience in treating patients with SCLE with this agent, although others have reported benefit within a few weeks after starting therapy in isolated cases (312,334,335).

Retinoids

The synthetic retinoids isotretinoin (Accutane; Roche Pharmaceuticals, Nutley, NJ) and acitretin (Soriatane; Roche Pharmaceuticals) at approximately 1 mg/kg per day have been shown to significantly improve SCLE lesions (336–340). These agents have also been advocated for hypertrophic DLE (340). The great potential for teratogenic effects with the retinoids makes it imperative that fertile females use contraceptive techniques according to guidelines set forth specifically for patients on retinoids. A common dose-related side effect is mucocutaneous dryness. It is advisable to have patients use sunscreens judiciously while being treated with these agents to minimize their tendency to aggravate photosensitivity. Drug-induced hepatitis and hypertriglyceridemia can occur with these agents and require periodic laboratory evaluation. Occasionally, these drugs can also induce bony changes consistent with the diffuse idiopathic skeletal hyperostosis (DISH) syndrome. Hair loss and peeling of the hands and feet are seen more often with acitretin.

Clofazimine

Crovoto (341) reported the successful use of clofazimine (Lamprene) in a patient with annular SCLE in 1981. He used a dose of 100 mg per day and noted clearing of the lesions within a few weeks. At this dose, clofazimine is generally well tolerated, although gastrointestinal intolerance can be a problem. At higher doses, clofazimine has rarely been reported to precipitate in mesenteric arteries, resulting in major abdominal catastrophes such as splenic infarction (342). A pink–brown–black skin pigmentation develops in most patients on long-term clofazimine therapy. This pigmentation resolves over months to years after discontinuing the drug. Similar discoloration of bodily secretions also frequently occurs.

Thalidomide

Thalidomide 50 to 200 mg per day, can be very effective in SCLE and DLE (343–347). We have now had considerable experience using this drug. It is highly effective in treating recalcitrant cutaneous LE. It has minimal if any effect on the systemic features other than the possibility of exacerbating a pro-coagulant state (347a). Its teratogenicity is well known, and has limited the frequency with which it is prescribed. Additionally, a predominately sensory peripheral neuropathy has been described and occurs in 10% to 25% of treated patients even with low doses 50 to 100 mg daily. Because thalidomide works quickly in SCLE, it is possible to treat recalcitrant patients with short courses of thalidomide (8 to 16 weeks) to minimize toxicity. To prevent flares after discontinuation of thalidomide, antimalarial therapy should be administered concomitantly with thalidomide and continued after thalidomide is withdrawn (M.I.C., unpublished data). Thalidomide's mechanism of action is unclear, however many have suggested TNF-α inhibition (348). If this is true, the potential efficacy of newer biologic agents that inhibit TNF is intriguing because these agents are much more potent inhibitors of TNF-α than thalidomide. In fact, one report describes improvement of SCLE in a patient with RA who was treated with etanercept (348a). However, the small number of reports of induction of LE-like illness warrants cautious use of such agents (349,350).

Gold

Oral gold (auranofin [Ridaura]) or parenteral gold (aurothiomalate [Myochrysine] and aurothioglucose [Solganal]) therapy have been successfully used in those patients with cutaneous LE whose disease is resistant to the less-toxic forms of therapy (351,352). Gold frequently has mucocutaneous toxicity and, less commonly, has hematologic, renal, and pulmonary toxicities that may require its discontinuance.

Systemic Corticosteroids and Other Immunosuppressive Agents

Systemic corticosteroids and cytotoxic agents (azathioprine, mycophenolate mofetil, cyclophosphamide, methotrexate, etc.) are reserved for patients with more severe disease who have failed to respond to the less toxic forms of therapy discussed before. A patient may occasionally be encountered whose disease is so severe that these more potent agents may be used earlier in the disease course, even before the patient is given a complete trial of the less toxic agents, or before the less toxic agents (i.e., hydroxychloroquine) reach steady-state levels.

Methylprednisolone given in "pulse doses" (1 g intravenously slowly (~ 4 hours) for 3 consecutive days) has been reported to provide improvement in patients with SCLE with systemic LE (353). Anecdotally, cyclophosphamide and methotrexate (329) as well as azathioprine (354) have been suggested to be of benefit in refractory SCLE. Due to the potential for severe immunosuppression, risk for cancer induction, and bone marrow and mucous membrane toxicities, these agents should be reserved for patients with severe disease and used only as a last resort in patients with severe cutaneous LE alone.

UVA-1 Phototherapy

Preliminary animal work has suggested that UVA might dampen the autoimmune abnormalities in experimental murine models of SLE (355). In addition, work from two centers has suggested that patients with SCLE might benefit from very low doses of whole-body UVA-1 (340 to 400 nm) irradiation (356,357). However, the true value of this somewhat controversial form of treatment ultimately remains to be confirmed by controlled studies in larger groups of patients. Caution should be taken in interpreting these data in view of the increasing evidence that UVA (190–200), including long-wave UVA (201), can play an exacerbating role in the cutaneous manifestations of SLE.

A suggested algorithm for using the various systemic agents discussed before is presented in Fig. 2.42. These recommendations are based on the authors' personal experience pertaining to the relative efficacy and safety of this group of drugs.

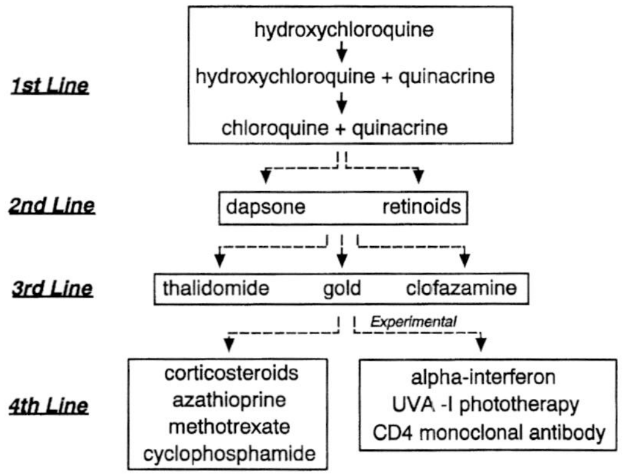

Figure 2.42. Suggested algorithm for the use of systemic medical agents in the management of subacute cutaneous lupus erythematosus (SCLE) and chronic cutaneous lupus erythematosus (LE).

CHRONIC CUTANEOUS LUPUS ERYTHEMATOSUS

The initial approach to the medical management of classic and variant forms of DLE lesions is the same as that described before for SCLE lesions. For the most part, both forms of cutaneous LE respond similarly to medical therapy. Local therapy, especially intralesional corticosteroids (e.g., triamcinolone acetonide suspension, 3 to 5 mg/mL for the face, with higher concentrations allowable elsewhere), is often more useful in the management of DLE than in SCLE because one is often treating fewer individual lesions in a patient with DLE than in a patient with SCLE. In addition, we and others (332) have been particularly impressed that combination antimalarial treatment (hydroxychloroquine or chloroquine plus quinacrine) has been more effective in a number of our patients with DLE who did not respond to hydroxychloroquine alone. As mentioned before, antimalarial agents do not appear to be efficacious in patients who smoke cigarettes. One of us (R.D.S.) was the first to informally observe several patients whose antimalarial-refractory DLE lesions improved dramatically following the cessation of cigarette smoking without any other change in their treatment regimens (160,161). This has since been confirmed by several others (348a,358–360). It is possible that the dramatic effects that cigarette smoking can have on hepatic microsomal enzyme induction (361) might alter the metabolism of the aminoquinoline antimalarials in a way that blunts their effect on cutaneous LE. Alternatively, compounds present in cigarette smoke might be capable of directly exacerbating LE-specific cutaneous inflammation.

As in SCLE, drugs such as Dapsone (362,363), retinoids (329,333,334,340,363,364), clofazimine (364–367), thalidomide (345,347,368), gold (350,351), methotrexate (369), and azathioprine (194,353,362,365), can be of value in DLE when antimalarials have failed.

Reportedly, the small number of hypertrophic DLE lesions that do not respond to single-agent or combined antimalarial therapy responds to treatment with systemic retinoids such as isotretinoin (Accutane) (339).

Untreated, LE panniculitis/profundus is indolently progressive with ulceration often eventually supervening. Intralesional corticosteroid therapy should be approached with great caution because even this minimal form of trauma can cause LE panniculitis lesions to break down and ulcerate. Even a carefully executed diagnostic skin biopsy can at times produce chronic ulceration in these lesions. Most cases of LE panniculitis/profundus can be managed successfully with single-agent or combined antimalarial therapy (370); however, some will require more aggressive treatment with systemic corticosteroids (208). Thalidomide (371) and gold (372) have also been used in patients with refractory LE panniculitis/profundus. LE panniculitis/profundus lesions that have undergone dystrophic calcification are particularly difficulty to treat. Only a few treatments for cutaneous calcification have been described (see Chapter 3) and none of them works well. Both azathioprine and mycophenolate mofetil have been advocated for those patients having antimalarial-resistant palmar/plantar DLE (342,348a,373).

Once DLE lesions have progressed to the point of irreversible dystrophic scarring, the use of properly personalized and applied corrective camouflage cosmetics (e.g., Covermark, Dermablend) and properly fitted hair pieces can offer temporary refuge from the devastating emotional impact that this disfiguring disease process can produce.

Once scarring develops within a DLE lesion, little can be done to reverse this process. Although disease activity is present, the trauma of plastic surgery procedures carries the risk for further exacerbating disease activity (the Köebner or isomorphic phenomenon). However, recent reports have suggested that procedures such as dermabrasion, hair transplantation, autologous fat transplantation, and laser surgery might occasionally be safely carried out in areas of scarring that are devoid of active inflammation (179,374–378). There is some evidence to suggest that the risk for disease reactivation is lessened if the patient is concurrently on medical therapy (e.g., antimalarials) to blunt the Köebner response (Fig. 2.27). The best overall strategy for the management of DLE, however, is always one of early, aggressive medical management to suppress the inflammatory disease process before scarring and alopecia have developed.

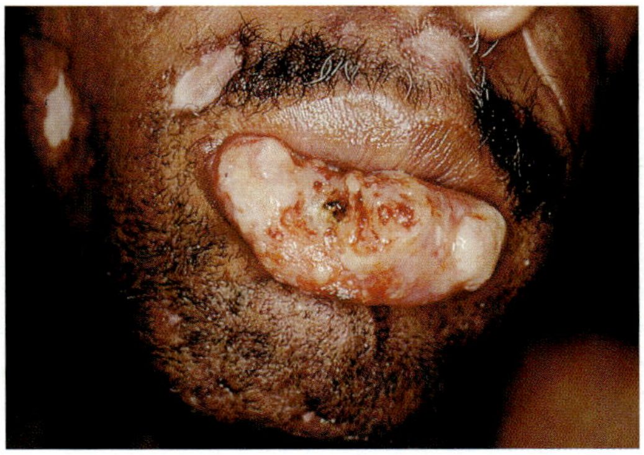

Figure 2.43. Squamous cell carcinoma developing in a discoid lupus erythematosus (DLE) lesion of the lower lip.

Prognosis

The risks of developing systemic manifestations of LE have already been discussed under the sections dealing with the relationship between the cutaneous and systemic manifestations of the various types of LE-specific skin disease. In this section, we will deal with the outcome of the skin lesions themselves and the available morbidity and mortality data concerning these forms of cutaneous LE.

ACUTE CUTANEOUS LUPUS ERYTHEMATOSUS

Localized ACLE lesions can wax and wane in parallel with the underlying SLE activity (1), often leaving pigment changes in their wake but not producing atrophic dermal scarring. The authors are unaware of mortality data associated specifically with ACLE. As previously discussed, ACLE is often considered to be an integral expression of underlying SLE and, as such, little effort has been made to determine whether such patients fare better or worse than those who do not develop ACLE.

SUBACUTE CUTANEOUS LUPUS ERYTHEMATOSUS

Having been recognized as a distinct disease entity for only 25 years, the long-term outcome associated with SCLE lesions has yet to be determined. In the authors' experience, most patients appear to have intermittent recurrences over long periods. However, some have unremitting lesions that smolder in the same location for years. A superficial form of atrophy has been noted to develop in lesions of several such patients who have sustained inflammation at the same site for years (R.D.S., personal observation) (Fig. 2.19). Other patients appear to enjoy long-term, if not permanent, remissions of their skin disease.

In short-term follow-up studies, approximately 15% of the patients with SCLE studied by one of the authors (R.D.S.) developed ACLE lesions and evidence of active SLE, including lupus nephritis (169,177). This subgroup of patients was marked by the presence of high-titer ANA, leukopenia, or anti-dsDNA (90,177). Follow-up studies by others have supported this view (378a). Long-term follow-up studies of SCLE will be required to determine the true risk for severe systemic disease in patients presenting with SCLE skin lesions. One of the authors is aware of only one death directly attributable to SLE in over 150 patients with SCLE that he has personally examined (R.D.S., personal unpublished observation).

CHRONIC CUTANEOUS LUPUS ERYTHEMATOSUS

Left untreated, most patients with classic DLE lesions tend to have an indolently progressive disease that can spread to produce large areas of dystrophic cutaneous scarring and scarring alopecia, which can be emotionally, if not physically, disabling. In one series of 86 patients with chronic cutaneous LE with mean disease duration of 15.1 years, 57% had some form of destructive or deforming scarring, whereas 35% had pigmentary disturbances (379). Spontaneous remission is occasionally observed (147) and the disease activity can recrudesce within the site of older inactive lesions. Squamous cell carcinoma occasionally develops in chronic smoldering DLE lesions (226,380–383) (Fig. 2.43).

Death from SLE disease activity is distinctly uncommon in patients who present initially with only localized DLE. As previously discussed, generalized DLE carries a greater risk for associated SLE activity.

PATHOGENESIS AND ETIOLOGIC FACTORS OF LUPUS ERYTHEMATOSUS–SPECIFIC SKIN DISEASE

The pathogenesis of LE-specific skin disease is inextricably intertwined with that of SLE. Any hypothesis concerning the etiologic factors and pathogenesis of LE-specific skin disease must take into account the fact that there are no fundamental differences between LE skin lesions that occur in the presence or absence of underlying SLE activity. For example, there are no clinical, histopathologic, or immunopathologic differences between the DLE lesions that occur as an isolated clinical phenomenon and those that develop in patients with preexisting SLE.

The theoretical model of SLE pathogenesis depicted in Fig. 2.3 may be applied to any organ system involved in LE, and we will use it as a framework to summarize the currents of thought that relate to the etiologic factors and pathogenesis of LE-specific skin disease.

Phase I: Susceptibility Phase

Recent advances in the genetics of SLE are described before. Genetic susceptibility to LE-specific skin disease has involved three main groups of candidate genes: MHC class I and II genes, MHC class III genes, and non-MHC genes. The strong association between SCLE, anti-Ro(SS-A) autoantibody production, and the HLA-A1 B8, DR3, DQ2, DRW52 haplotype has previously been discussed. HLA B8, DR3 and B7, DR2 have been associated with DLE in whites.

The MHC also includes genes for various complement components (C2, C4A, C4B and factor B) in the class III region. Genetic deficiency or polymorphism of C1q, C2, C3, or C4 has also been associated with both SCLE and SLE (40,71a,117,118). Genetic deficiency of complement components has also been described in patients with DLE (384). It is interesting to note that most patients with homozygous C2 or C4 complement deficiency have circulating Ro(SS-A) autoantibodies (40,42). Other class III genes including those encoding TNF-α and -β have also been implicated in susceptibility to LE-specific skin disease (385). Recent *in vitro* evidence suggests that IL -1 plus UVB induced a dramatic 300-fold transcription of the 308A human TNF-α promoter over baseline. This allelic form of the TNF-α promoter is found to be statistically increased in patients with SCLE and to be linked to the HLA-DR3 haplotype (71).

Heat shock proteins (Hsps) are also located within the class III MHC region, and linkage disequilibrium with other HLA genes has led several authors to investigate the role of Hsp70 genes in susceptibility to cutaneous LE. Hsp genes are activated by cellular stresses such as heat, UVR, cytokines, and chemicals, many of which exacerbate cutaneous LE. A study by Furukawa et al. (386) observed increased binding of Ro/SS-A antibodies to keratinocytes after application of a prostaglandin known to induce Hsp70, suggesting that Hsps may be involved in the expression of Ro antigen on the surfaces of cells.

Genes outside the MHC locus that have been suggested as potential candidates for cutaneous LE susceptibility include the IL-1 gene cluster, and genes encoding intercellular adhesion molecule-1 (ICAM-1), E-selectin, and Fas/FasL. Two studies have shown IL-1RA polymorphisms in patients with photosensitive SLE and in patients with DLE (387,388). Increased keratinocyte expression of ICAM-1 and increased cutaneous vascular endothelial expression of E-selectin have been noted in the skin of patients with cutaneous LE compared with controls, suggesting both of these as potential candidate genes for the development of CLE (385). Polymorphisms in a Fas promoter gene have been detected in patients with photosensitive SLE. *Fas/FasL* genes and other genes involved in apoptosis are particularly intriguing to implicate in the pathogenesis of cutaneous LE because of the correlation of apoptosis with induction of self-tolerance.

Phase II: Induction Phase

The induction of LE-specific skin disease likely involves exposure to environmental agents such as UVL and drugs (i.e., hydrochlorothiazides, procainamide, penicillamine, sulfonylureas, oxprenolol, and griseofulvin). Recent studies have drawn attention in particular to the development of SCLE lesions in anti-Ro(SSA)–positive patients treated with terbinafine. Infections such as (Epstein–Barr virus) may lead to the induction of autoreactive T cells by mechanisms such as molecular mimicry (389).

UV light may cause keratinocyte injury that exposes normally concealed, intracellular antigens or induces the expression of "neoantigens" (390,391). Investigators have demonstrated that UVB can displace Ro(SS-A) antigens from within keratinocytes to the cell surface (43,392–397). Preliminary evidence suggests that UV-induced apoptosis could be one mechanism responsible for this aberrant pattern of autoantigen expression (44). This displacement would allow Ro(SS-A) autoantibodies present in the circulation to have access to the Ro(SS-A) autoantigens normally sequestered inside cells. Antibody binding to the exposed antigens could result in tissue injury through complement-mediated lysis or antibody-dependent, cell-mediated cytotoxicity. Estrogen, when added to cultured human keratinocytes, may increase the amount of Ro(SS-A) antigens on the cell surface (393). Infection by α viruses such as Sindbis also appears to be capable of inducing cell surface expression of Ro(SS-A) antigens in cells undergoing apoptosis (74). It is also possible that humoral factors other than anti-Ro(SS-A) are involved in the pathogenesis of LE photosensitivity (396–398).

Phase III: The Expansion Phase

Gilliam first suggested the central role of autoantigen-specific T cells in the pathogenesis of LE-specific skin disease based on the infiltration of activated T cells in LE-specific skin lesions (398a). These lymphocytes are likely involved in injury via direct cytotoxicity and in the expansion phase by further recruitment of T cells that provide help to B cells. The presence of elevated serum levels of soluble IL-2 receptors in cutaneous LE subsets such as SCLE also indirectly supports a role for T cells in the pathogenesis of LE-specific skin disease (399,400). Keratinocytes are likely involved in the expansion phase of cutaneous LE lesions as well. Keratinocytes in LE-specific skin lesions often express class II HLA antigens (401,402) as well as adhesion molecules involved in T-cell binding interactions such as ICAM-1 (402). Denfeld et al. (403) have reported that most of the infiltrating T cells in skin lesions of patients with ACLE, SCLE, and DLE were CD28, B7-1 and B7-2 suggesting that the B7-CD28 costimulatory pathway may be important for the propagation of T-cell activity in LE-specific skin lesions. Insights about which cells are involved in the expansion phase of LE-specific skin disease may be gained from examination of mononuclear cells around blood vessels and dermal appendages. These cells consist predominately of CD4 T lymphocytes that express class II histocompatibility antigens (399,401,404–412). Other T-cell activation markers such as the IL-2 receptor and thymidine incorporation appear to be only variably expressed on these infiltrating T cells (401,402,413). Monocytes and macrophages are seen to a lesser extent and B cells are quite rare. One study suggests that the infiltrating T cells predominately have the helper-inducer phenotype ($CD4^+$, CD45RA, $CD45RO^+$) (410). Preliminary studies have indicated that there are no significant differences in the inflammatory infiltrate seen in DLE and SCLE lesions (401,407). There are conflicting opinions concerning the predominant type of T-cell receptor expressed by infiltrating T cells. Fivenson et al. (414) have reported that gamma/delta receptor–positive T cells are virtually nonexistent in the epidermis and dermis of chronic cutaneous LE lesions, whereas Volc-Platzer et al. (415) have suggested that T cells having a specific gamma/delta receptor phenotype (V-2/V-2) are preferentially expanded within the epidermal and dermal T-cell infiltrates of chronic cutaneous LE lesions (415).

Phase IV: The Injury Phase

Much data suggesting mechanisms of injury in LE-specific skin disease have been obtained from studying the natural and experimental pathology/immunopathology of cutaneous LE. The general pattern of cellular change in LE-specific skin disease is that of a lichenoid tissue reaction, a pattern of cutaneous injury in which epidermal basal cells are the primary focus of injury (51). Prototypes of this tissue reaction pattern are lichen planus and graft versus host skin disease. Increasing evidence suggests that lichen planus is the result of cytoxic T-lymphocyte–mediated injury within the skin (415). Graft versus host skin disease is believed to result from an attack by donor T-lymphocytes on host histocompatibility antigens within the skin (416,417). Further evidence for direct cytotoxic injury to epidermal keratinocytes is the thickened epidermal basement membrane seen often in LE-specific skin disease, more so in classic DLE than SCLE (175). Ultrastructurally, this appears to be due to reduplication of the basal lamina (413), suggesting the possibility that a process of continual premature death and regeneration of epidermal basal cells might be occurring. This possibility is consistent with the observation that hyperproliferation occurs within the epidermal compartment in DLE lesions (418). The Köebner or isomorphic phenomenon is the development of a skin lesion in an area of previously normal skin that has been traumatized in some way (419). Although this phenomenon is more typical of other skin diseases such as psoriasis and lichen planus, experienced observers recognize that it can also occur in patients with cutaneous LE (420,421) (Fig. 2.32). A classic example is the "grease burn" on the face of a homemaker that does not heal and is later recognized to represent DLE. The mechanism of this response is not known. It is tempting to speculate that the T cells present in the infiltrate of cutaneous LE lesions (415) might be capable of recognizing the products of stress response (i.e., heat shock) genes expressed on injured epidermal cells, thereby targeting that cell for further injury through cell-mediated cytotoxicity.

Autoantibodies are a hallmark of any LE-related disease process and may be directly involved in the injury phase of disease. Although Ro(SS-A) autoantibodies are common in SCLE, they are also found in a number of other autoimmune disorders as well as in some healthy individuals (306). Whether these autoantibodies play a direct role in the pathogenesis of skin disease or represent merely an epiphenomenon has not been determined. The most compelling evidence that these antibodies play a major role in the injury phase of disease comes from patients with NLE. These infants acquire maternal Ro(SS-A) antibodies transplacentally and develop skin lesions not unlike SCLE, typically within the first few days or weeks after delivery. Several months later, as the maternally acquired Ro(SS-A) antibodies are cleared from the infant's circulation, the skin lesions resolve spontaneously (300). These antibodies are probably also responsible for the congenital heart block, transient hematologic abnormalities, and hepatic injury that may occur in these infants (300). The mere presence of the Ro(SS-A) antibodies is not sufficient to induce disease, however, as many neonates who are exposed to Ro(SS-A) antibodies from their mother's circulation never develop skin, heart, hepatic, or hematologic disease. This suggests that some cofactor, such as a congenital viral infection, may be necessary for the full expression of this syndrome (for further discussion see chapter on neonatal lupus erythematosus).

The data as recorded above support the following hypothesis relevant to injury pathogenesis of DLE and SCLE lesions. The lesions of DLE most likely are a result of a T-cell autoaggressive phenomenon. However, the nature of the antigen(s) remains to be determined. The lesions of SCLE, based on the data obtained from studies of the NLE syndrome, support a hypothesis that the lesions of SCLE are the result of an antibody-dependent cellular cytotoxicity (ADCC) mechanism in which the maternal antibody binds to an antigen in the skin (most likely a Ro(SS-A)–related antigen) and the infant's mononuclear cells (presumably T cells) serve as effector cells.

It is uncertain whether autoantibodies other than Ro/SS-A are directly involved in the pathogenesis of LE-specific skin disease. Generally, various classes of immunoglobulins and complement components found at the dermal–epidermal junction have been associated with type VII collagen (422). Elution studies of lupus band immunoreactants in the skin of patients with SLE have suggested that they contain antinuclear and anti–basement membrane zone reactivity (423). A nonspecific mechanism of immune complex deposition at the dermal–epidermal junction based on charge alone has been reported (424,425). These immune deposits appear to be the result, rather than the cause, of cutaneous inflammation in cutaneous LE lesions because they clearly follow the first signs of cellular inflammation in UV-induced cutaneous LE lesions (405,426).

TABLE 2.8. Nonspecific Cutaneous Manifestations of Systemic Lupus Erythematosus (SLE)

Vasculitis
Antiphospholipid syndrome
Raynaud phenomenon
Alopecia
DLE lesions in the scalp
Telogen effluvium
"Lupus hair"
Sclerodactyly
Rheumatoid nodules
Bullous lesions
Extension of liquefaction degeneration of acute Ro (SS-A) antibody–positive SLE lesions
Anti–type VII collagen antibodies
Bullae as the result of putative immune complex vasculitis
Erythema multiforme–like lesions
Cutaneous mucinosis
Pigmentary changes
Miscellaneous
Anetoderma
Mid-dermal elastolysis
Acanthosis nigricans

DLE, discoid lupus erythematosus; SLE, systemic lupus erythematosus.

Lupus Erythematosus–Nonspecific Skin Disease

The nonspecific cutaneous manifestations of systemic lupus erythematosus are presented in Table 2.8.

CUTANEOUS VASCULAR DISEASE

Cutaneous Vasculitis

Reportedly, vasculitic lesions occur in 20% to 70% of patients with SLE (29,79,82,427–430). The morphologic manifestations of cutaneous vasculitis in SLE range from urticaria-like lesions to large ulcers. In the authors' experience, palpable and nonpalpable purpura lesions involving the lower extremities are most common. On occasion, these leg lesions may ulcerate. Vasculitic lesions involving the lower extremities are especially common in anti-Ro(SS-A) antibody–positive patients SSj/LE (90,189).

The level and intensity of the inflammatory insult of blood vessels in the skin determine the morphologic features of cutaneous vasculitis. For example, vasculitic lesions involving arterioles and veins high in the papillary portion of the dermis produce erythema and petechiae. However, if the insult is intense, epidermal necrosis is seen. Blood vessel involvement deep in the papillary dermis, as well as in the reticular portion of the dermis, may produce palpable and nonpalpable purpuric lesions or urticaria-like lesions. Intense vasculitic lesions in this area can result in bullous formation or ulcerations. The blister formation results from the destruction of the integrity of the dermal–epidermal junction. Vasculitic lesions involving the muscular arteries at the dermal subcutaneous tissue level can result in indurated nodules (polyarteritis nodosa–like lesions). If the

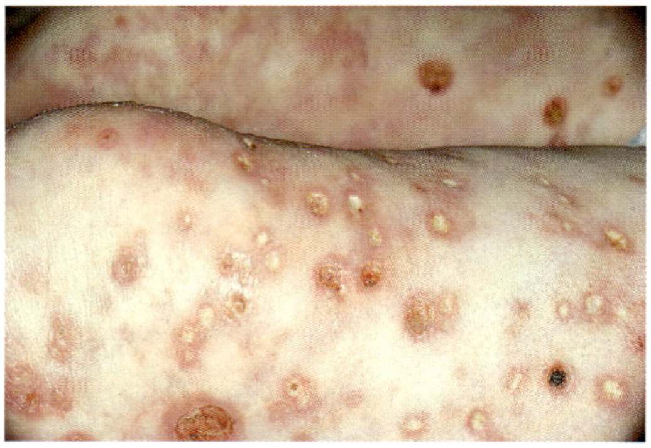

Figure 2.44. Ulcerating nodules of the legs in a patient with systemic lupus erythematosus (SLE) with polyarteritis nodosa–like systemic vasculitis. Shortly after this photograph was taken, this middle-aged woman died from bowel infarction secondary to mesenteric vasculitis. It is not known whether she was antiphospholipid antibody–positive at the time this photo was taken.

inflammatory process at this level is severe enough, and if there is not sufficient collateral circulation, ulceration may occur (Fig. 2.44). In one recent case, acute gangrenous changes of the fingertips were the presenting manifestation. These striking changes were most likely the result of digital arteritis (431). Vasculitic lesions involving the venules and arteries of the tips of the fingers can produce small tender nodules (Osler nodes). Splinter hemorrhages, cuticle nailfold injection (periungual telangiectasia), and small infarcts can also result from vasculitic lesions involving small arterioles and venules in the hands (Fig. 2.45). Nailfold erythema, telangiectasia, or both, have been reported to occur in 10% to 15% of patients with SLE (432). Furthermore, erythematous, nontender lesions involving the thenar and hyperthenar eminence (Janeway spots) can also occur.

These varied cutaneous manifestations of vasculitis are the putative manifestations of circulating immune complexes that histologically produce a generally leukocytoclastic type of vasculitis. In addition, recent evidence indicates the presence of elevated levels of activated circulating endothelial cells during flares of SLE. It is hypothesized that these activated endothelial cells represent a marker for endothelial injury. These activated endothelial cells may be capable of enhancing vascular damage by producing inflammatory and prothrombic mediators and actively participating in the aggregation of neutrophils and platelets (433). Direct immunofluorescent examination of lesional biopsies generally demonstrates granular IgG, complement, and fibrinogen depositions around blood vessels.

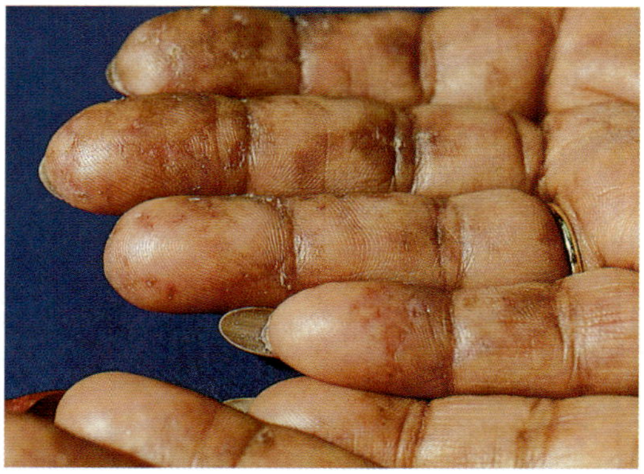

Figure 2.45. Small-vessel vasculitis in the hands and fingers of a patient with systemic lupus erythematosus (SLE). The biopsy of such lesions often shows mixed elements of vasculitis and occlusive vasculopathy.

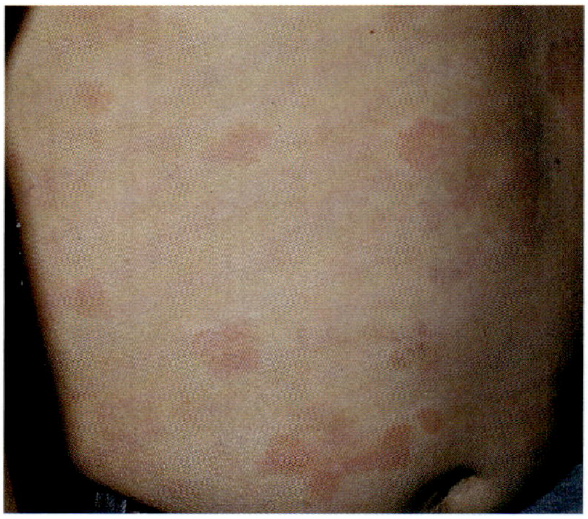

Figure 2.46. Urticarial vasculitis in a patient with systemic lupus erythematosus (SLE). These urticaria-like lesions differ from true urticaria in that they produce pain and burning rather than itching, last longer than 24 hours, and heal with residual bruising, hyperpigmentation, or telangiectasia. The urticarial vasculitis lesions seen in patients with systemic lupus erythematosus (SLE) are clinically indistinguishable from urticarial vasculitis lesions seen in patients with non–lupus erythematosus (LE).

In recent years, urticaria has been recognized as a cutaneous manifestation of vasculitis in patients with SLE (Fig. 2.46). O'Laughlin et al. (434), in a study at a tertiary referral center, detected urticaria-like lesions in 12 of 54 patients with SLE. An analysis of their patients revealed that 10 had generalized urticaria and four had associated angioedema of the face and lips; livedo reticularis was also noted in several patients. Histologically, 10 of 12 patients demonstrated a necrotizing vasculitis; one had a diffuse perivascular neutrophilic infiltrate, and the other had a perivascular lymphocytic infiltrate. Hypocomplementemia was present in seven and renal disease was present in five.

In another study of 143 consecutive patients with untreated SLE, 10 (8%) were detected with urticaria-like lesions (435). In all instances, the urticaria was characterized by persistence for greater than 24 hours, hyperpathia to light touch, and on occasion, evidence of petechiae or bruising in the urticaria-like lesions. Biopsies in seven of nine patients revealed a leukocytoclastic angiitis and a mononuclear vasculopathy in two. These urticaria-like lesions were associated with clinical disease activity (arthritis, renal disease, etc.) in nine of 10 patients. Furthermore, hypocomplementemia was detected in nine and renal disease in eight patients. Anti-dsDNA antibodies were detected in six patients, and complement-fixing anti–single-stranded DNA antibodies were detected in two. U_1RNP autoantibodies were detected in five patients, anti-Sm antibodies were detected in six, and anti-Ro(SS-A) antibodies were detected in three of these patients with SLE. Lupus patients with discoid lesions in the absence of systemic disease served as controls and failed to demonstrate these lesions.

In recent years, hypocomplementemic urticaria-like vasculitis has been detected in patients with SLE. These patients demonstrate cutaneous vasculitis, arthritis, and occasionally renal disease. Because these patients with SLE, like patients with the idiopathic hypocomplementemic urticarial vasculitis syndrome (HUVS), possess antibodies against the collagen-like region (CLR) of C1q, these two entities may be related, representing opposite ends of a spectrum of disease (436–439). Additional data indicate a strong association on anti-C1q antibodies and nephritis in patients with SLE (440,441). C1q binds to the surface blebs on apoptotic keratinocytes (442). Because there is evidence that apoptotic keratinocytes are immunogenic in SLE, the presence of

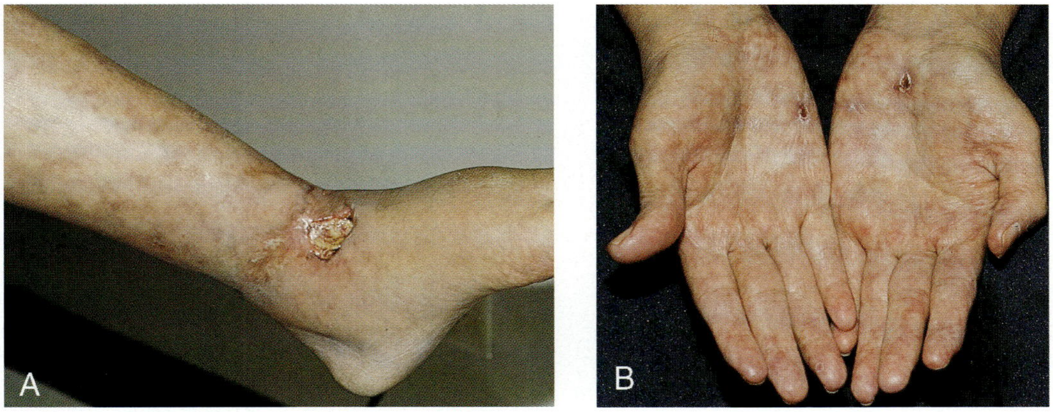

Figure 2.47. Livedo reticularis and ulceration of the leg in a patient with systemic lupus erythematosus with high-titer IgG anticardiolipin antibodies (A). B: Similar changes on the hands of this same patient.

apoptotic bound C1q might explain the frequent occurrence of anti-C1q antibodies in SLE (35%) and HUVS (100%).

These collective data indicate that urticarial-like vasculitic lesions, with or without hypocomplementemia, occur in approximately 10% of patients and are associated with clinical and serologic evidence of active disease (443). On the basis of these observations, it is recommended that all patients suspected of having LE and demonstrating urticaria-like lesions be evaluated for a vasculitis and systemic involvement.

Although angioedema has been seen in association with urticaria-like vasculitis in SLE (434), the association of angioneurotic edema with LE is rare. However, during the past 15 years it has been recognized that there is an increased frequency of LE (both cutaneous LE and SLE) in individuals with hereditary angioneurotic edema (444–447).

Antiphospholipid Syndrome

In addition to vasculitis, patients with lupus may also have an additional form of vascular insult. This vasculopathy is characterized by recurrent thrombi involving blood vessels of all sizes in the general absence of significant inflammation. This type of vascular insult is associated with the presence of antiphospholipid antibodies (i.e., anticardiolipin antibodies, lupus anticoagulant, or both). The frequency of antiphospholipid antibodies varies greatly (2% to 94%) (448). One of the current authors (T.T.P.) has detected an approximate 50% frequency of anticardiolipin antibodies in a large cohort of patients with SLE (449).

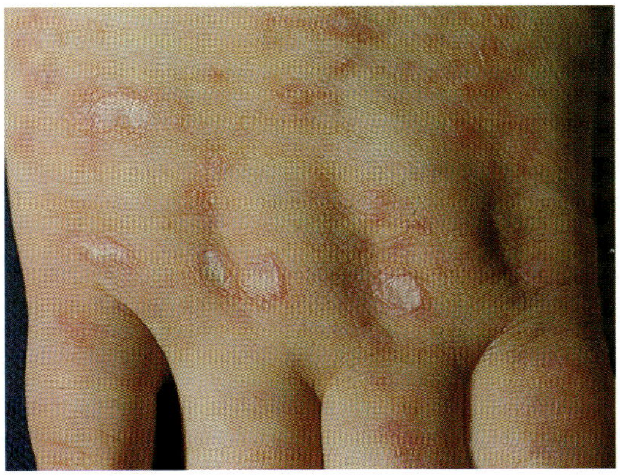

Figure 2.48. Degos-like lesions in a patient with systemic lupus erythematosus (SLE).

Anti-Ro(SS-A) antibody–positive patients with SLE have a low frequency of antiphospholipid antibodies (112,123). These patients are characterized by livedo reticularis, generally of the lower extremities (with or without ulceration) (Fig. 2.47), but at times extending to other areas of the body; recurrent arterial and venous thromboses including thrombophlebitis; thrombocytopenia; increased fetal wastage in the late first trimester; valvular heart disease; Libman–Sachs endocarditis; and pulmonary hypertension (448–454). On rare occasions, acral cyanosis, cutaneous infarction resembling Degos disease, and small-vessel infarction resulting in atrophied blanche–like lesions occur (445–462) (Fig. 2.48). Recurrent central nervous system infarction in association with livedo reticularis (Sneddon syndrome) producing neurologic defects, including postinfarct dementia, is increasingly recognized as a serious sequela (463–469). Yasue (469) reported that 11 (17%) of 66 patients with SLE demonstrated livedo reticularis and 81% of patients with SLE with livedo reticularis were anticardiolipin antibody–positive.

In addition to the cases demonstrating the common association of antiphospholipid antibodies with SLE, a group of patients without evidence of connective tissue disease, but possessing the clinical and serologic features of the antiphospholipid syndrome, has been described. This condition is termed "primary antiphospholipid syndrome" (470).

The antiphospholipid antibodies appear to be a heterogeneous group of autoantibodies generally directed against a variety of negatively charged phospholipid proteins (471–473). Most recent evidence indicates that those phospholipids in association with β_2 glycoprotein I (apolipoprotein H) are the primary targets of pathologic antiphospholipid antibodies (473–477). Antiphospholipid antibodies can occur in chronic infections (e.g., leprosy) and with certain drugs such as chlorpromazine, but these autoantibodies are directed against the phospholipid protein alone (473). The exact pathologic consequence of the antiphospholipid antibody is not known. The possible procoagulant effects of antiphospholipid antibodies are listed in Table 2.9. The consequence of these autoantibodies is *in vivo* coagulation with thrombus formation, resulting in a partial consumption of coagulation factors involved in the formation of the prothrombin complex (factor Xa, factor V, calcium, and phospholipid).

Recent evidence suggest that anti–annexin V, anti–protein S, anti–protein C and antiprothrombin antibodies may also be associated with a hypercoagulable state in SLE (478).

Antiphospholipid antibodies are measured using an anticardiolipin ELISA assay (473). One large study indicates that

TABLE 2.9. Possible Procoagulant Effects of Antiphospholipid Antibodies

Inhibition of activated protein C pathway
Up-regulation of tissue factor pathway
Inhibition of anti–thrombin III activity
Disruption of annexin V shield on membranes
Inhibition of anticoagulant activity of β_2 glycoprotein I
Enhanced expression of adhesion molecules by endothelial cells and adherence of neutrophils and leukocytes to endothelial cells
Activation and degeneration of neutrophils
Potentiation of platelet activation
Enhanced platelet aggregation
Enhanced binding of β_2 glycoprotein I to membranes
Enhanced binding of prothrombin to membranes

From Levin JS. The antiphospholipid syndrome. *N Eng J Med* 2000;346:752–763, with permission.

patients with lupus patients with anticardiolipin titers above 10 SD are at particular risk for developing clinical features (476). The other assay for measuring the presence of antiphospholipid antibodies is a functional phospholipid-dependent coagulation test (also known as the lupus anticoagulant). Prothrombin time is generally not sensitive enough to detect the presence of these antiphospholipid antibodies. The activated partial thromboplastin time has been used, but the most sensitive and most commonly used assay is a Russell viper venom test (RVVT). Failure to reconstitute the test plasma to a normal clotting time with normal plasma is diagnostic. Unfortunately, there is at least 25% discordance between the presence of anticardiolipin antibodies and the lupus anticoagulant as measured by the RVVT (477). Thus, both tests need to be used in the evaluation of patients suspected of having antiphospholipid antibodies.

Coumadin is now recommended for the treatment of antiphospholipid syndrome, keeping the degree of anticoagulation equal to or greater than an international normalized ratio (INR) of 3. Careful monitoring of these patients for bleeding complications is mandatory. However, such intense Coumadin therapy is virtually 100% effective in preventing the thrombosis of the antiphospholipid syndrome (479).

Raynaud's Phenomenon

In addition to vasculitis and thrombi formation, patients with SLE frequently have Raynaud's phenomenon. Several large studies have indicated that the frequency of Raynaud's phenomenon has ranged between 18% and 46% (29,79,82,427–430, 480,481). Raynaud's phenomenon is characterized by triphasic color changes involving the fingers, toes, or both. Initially, there is a vasospastic component characterized by blanching, then by a purplish, cyanotic discoloration, followed by a reperfusion erythema at rewarming associated commonly with pain. Most patients who develop Raynaud's phenomenon do not have an associated connective tissue disease. However, on occasion, Raynaud's phenomenon may be the initial symptom, antedating the development of SLE by years. Reports indicate that between 2% and 10% of patients with Raynaud's phenomenon evaluated by a rheumatologist have SLE (480–483).

Some lupus patients appear to be especially prone to developing Raynaud's phenomenon (484–488). For example, patients with anti-U_1RNP lupus have been reported to have an increased frequency of Raynaud's phenomenon (60–90%). Maddison et al. (484) detected that patients with U_1RNP-positive lupus had twice the frequency of Raynaud's phenomenon compared with patients with non-U_1RNP-positive lupus. In addition, Sharp et al. (487,488) have detected a group of U_1RNP-positive patients with features of sclerodactyly, Raynaud's phenomenon, esophageal dysmotility, pulmonary disease, and evidence of myositis. This condition has been called "the mixed connective tissue disease syndrome" (487,488). By comparison, in a study evaluating 50 patients with anti-Ro(SS-A) antibody–positive lupus, Raynaud's phenomenon was detected in 23 (46%) (90).

The frequency and severity of Raynaud's phenomenon are obviously environmentally dependent, being more frequent and severe in patients with SLE living in cold climates. For example, Tuffanelli and Dubois (29) reported an 18% frequency of Raynaud's phenomenon in patients seen in southern California, whereas Hochberg et al. (82) reported a 44% frequency in patients examined in Baltimore.

The pathogenesis of Raynaud's phenomenon is due to severe vasospasm involving abnormal digital arteries having intimal hyperplasia. There is no correlation between the severity of the Raynaud's phenomenon and SLE disease activity. In fact, one study has indicated there are less renal disease and fewer deaths than in unaffected patients (489).

Treatment of Raynaud's phenomenon is difficult. Raynaud's phenomenon is not steroid-responsive. The use of form-fitting gloves together with mittens and a double layer of socks may be helpful. Avoidance of β-blockers and ergot alkaloids is also helpful. In recent years, the calcium channel blocker, nifedipine, has been found to be effective in treating some patients (10 to 30 mg per day or 30 mg per day of the sustained-release form of the drug preparation) (490). Other vasodilators such as nicardipine and nitroglycerin paste have also proven effective.

ERYTHROMELALGIA (ERYTHERMALGIA)

On rare occasions, erythromelalgia has been found in association with SLE. Erythromelalgia is characterized by erythema, increased warmth, and aching pain in the hands, feet, or both following exposure to heat. A burning sensation in the involved extremities is also noted. Erythromelalgia may also be seen in association with hypertension, diabetes, and myeloproliferative disorders.

Alarcon-Segovia et al. (491) reviewed 51 cases of erythromelalgia seen at the Mayo Clinic from 1951 through 1960. One of these 51 cases had classic manifestations of SLE. Thirty of these patients had primary erythromelalgia. In 10 cases, myeloproliferative disorders, particularly polycythemia vera, were detected. A follow-up study of 168 patients with erythromelalgia from the same institution failed to detect any additional patients with erythromelalgia with SLE (492). Studies that are more recent suggest vascular instability with large-vessel vasodilatation and small-vessel vasospasm may be of etiologic significance (493).

Reportedly, one patient with erythromelalgia in association with SLE has been successfully treated with clonazepam (494).

ALOPECIA

In addition to the permanent form of alopecia associated with the scarring DLE lesion, patients with SLE may experience a diffuse, nonscarring, transient hair loss associated with exacerbations of their lupus disease process. This diffuse alopecia (telogen effluvium) is in all probability the result of the severe catabolic effects of the lupus disease flare. This diffuse alopecia can be acute, occurring 2 to 3 months after a flare of the lupus disease process, but also can be chronically associated with continuing lupus disease activity. With the onset of quiescence of the

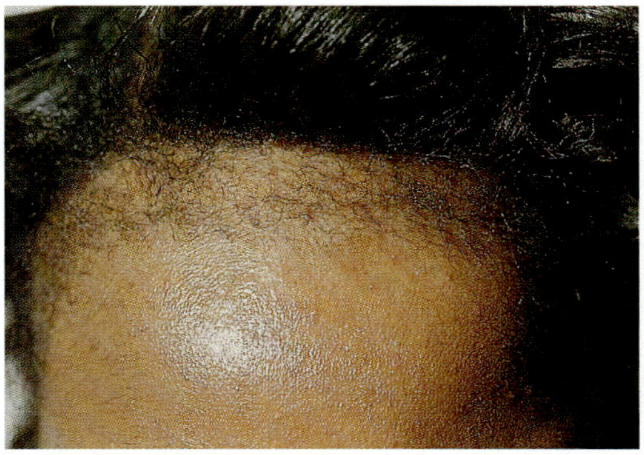

Figure 2.49. "Lupus hair." Note the sparse, unruly hair at the anterior hairline. The abnormal appearance of the hair in this area is somewhat accentuated by the fact that this patient has a hair weave, giving an artificially healthy appearance to the remainder of her hair.

SLE disease process, normal hair growth resumes and the alopecia disappears.

A third form of alopecia, also transient, is probably closely related in causation to the telogen effluvium, and is termed "lupus hair" or "wooly hair" (Fig. 2.49). During an exacerbation of the SLE disease process, or in patients with chronically active SLE, peculiar nonscarring alopecia characterized by thin, weakened hairs, especially at the periphery of the scalp, occurs. These hairs easily fragment and the hair becomes unruly, giving a characteristic appearance. This type of alopecia is not permanent. It is hypothesized that with the induction of a negative nitrogen balance, normal hair growth is interrupted leading to the production of thin, weakened hairs that easily fragment above the surface of the scalp.

On unusual occasions, alopecia areata has been detected in patients with SLE (495). This is an unusual occurrence and no causal relationship between SLE and this type of alopecia has been established. In all probability, it represents a coincidental finding.

SCLERODACTYLY

Sclerodermatous changes are uncommon in SLE. However, in recent years patients with U_1RNP-positive lupus have been detected to have sclerodermatous changes characterized by sclerotic lesions and swollen puffy hands in addition to Raynaud's phenomenon (483,484,496). One study has reported a 7% frequency of swollen hands and a 3% frequency of sclerodermatous changes in 30 patients with U_1RNP-positive SLE (483). Other studies have described sclerodermatous changes in 33% of 100 patients with anti-U_1RNP antibody–positive mixed connective tissue disease (486); 66% of these patients had swollen hands. Esophageal dysmotility was detected in 65% of 75 patients tested. In addition, pulmonary diffusion abnormalities were detected in 67% of 43 tested.

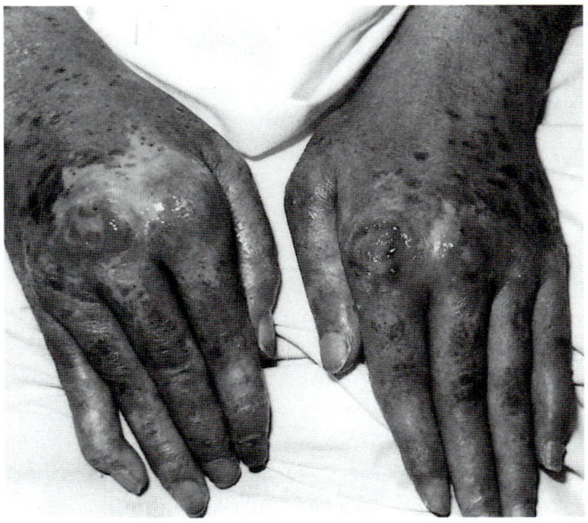

Figure 2.50. Sclerodactyly in a patient with U_1 RNP-positive systemic lupus erythematosus (SLE). This patient also had severe Raynaud phenomenon. Note the ulcers over the metacarpophalangeal joints.

Another study examining 55 patients with anti-U_1RNP–positive with a mixed connective tissue disease diagnosis reported 65% with swollen hands and 36% with esophageal dysmotility (487). In Fig. 2.50, cutaneous ulceration and prominent sclerodactyly are demonstrated in an anti-U_1RNP–positive patient, satisfying the ACR criteria for the diagnosis of SLE.

Cutaneous calcinosis is rare in LE, although calcification has been reported in DLE lesions associated with SLE (496). One of the authors (T.T.P.) has seen generalized cutaneous calciphylaxis in a U_1RNP antibody–positive patient without evidence of parathyroid dysfunction.

Recently a 22-year-old woman developed a lupus panniculitis presenting as morphea–like lesions (497).

RHEUMATOID NODULES

RA in SLE is very unusual (30,252,498). Dubois (30). described RA in 23 of 41 patients with DLE lesions. However, a review of these cases by Cohen et al. (252) indicates that approximately 10 of these patients originally described by Dubois would today be classified as having SCLE. Furthermore, Cohen et al. (252) have described an additional three patients with anti-Ro(SS-A) antibody–positive SLE with a rheumatoid-like arthritis. Boire et al. (499) described two patients with anti-Ro(SS-A) antibody–positive SCLE with RA (499). Another group has detected five lupus/RA anti-Ro(SS-A) antibody–positive patients. One of these patients had DLE lesions and one had SCLE lesions (90).

Hahn et al. (498) have described rheumatoid nodules in patients with SLE. In three of six patients reported, the diagnosis of rheumatoid nodules was confirmed by biopsy. Dermatitis was detected in three of six, and one patient had definite SSj. Rheumatoid factor activity was detected in four of six patients. In a study of 50 patients with anti-Ro(SS-A) antibody–positive lupus, two had rheumatoid nodules (90).

The arthritis in these patients is a polyarthritis characterized by significant morning stiffness. Gross deformities are very unusual. The joint deformities are a consequence of periarticular inflammation rather than erosive articular disease.

One of the authors (T.T.P.) has recently studied a large group of anti-Ro(SS-A) antibody–positive patients (90). Seventeen of these patients developed features of a rheumatoid-like arthritis over a 10-year period. The phenotypic expression of these patients was very heterogeneous. All but one were females with either SLE, an undifferentiated connective tissue disease, or SSj. It has been previously shown that all of these anti-Ro(SS-A) antibody–positive patients share an increased frequency of the HLA-B8, DR3, DQ2, and DRw52 phenotypes (113). Recently, it has been recognized that there is a small subset, approximately 5%, of patients with RA who are anti-Ro(SS-A) antibody–positive, and who are non–HLA-DR4 (499,500). These patients frequently demonstrate the concomitant presence of SSj. Although they generally have a deforming arthritis, it is of the Jaccoud type, with little or no articular erosive changes (501,502).

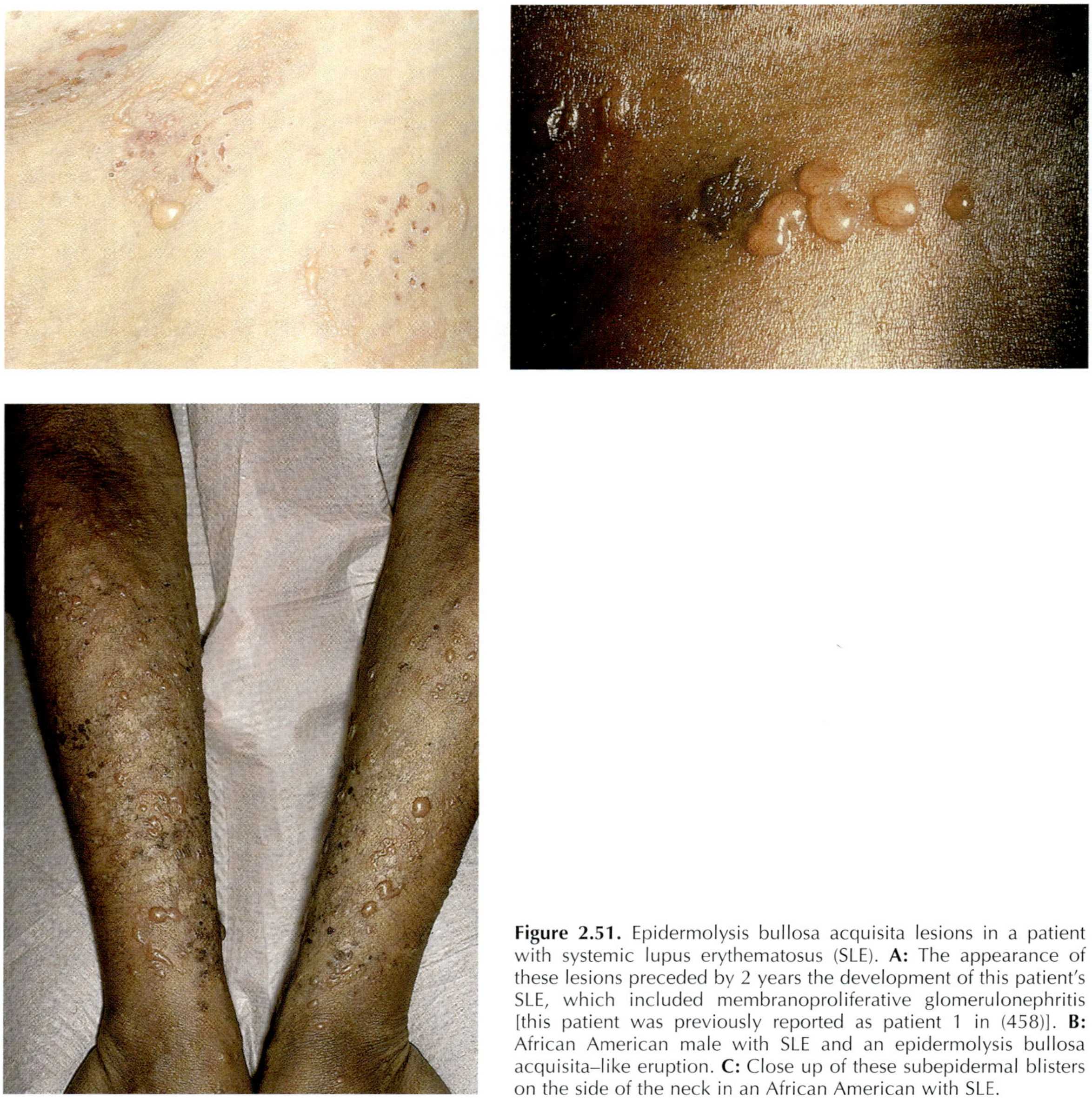

A C B

Figure 2.51. Epidermolysis bullosa acquisita lesions in a patient with systemic lupus erythematosus (SLE). **A:** The appearance of these lesions preceded by 2 years the development of this patient's SLE, which included membranoproliferative glomerulonephritis [this patient was previously reported as patient 1 in (458)]. **B:** African American male with SLE and an epidermolysis bullosa acquisita–like eruption. **C:** Close up of these subepidermal blisters on the side of the neck in an African American with SLE.

These collective studies strongly suggest that a nonerosive, but deforming arthritis similar to RA is found in a small percentage of anti-Ro(SS-A) antibody–positive, generally female, patients with SLE.

"Rheumatoid papules" have also been reported to occur in SLE patients. Such lesions present as firm red to red-purple papules distributed symmetrically on the trunk and/or extremities. The clinical lesions result from a histopathological change of extravascular necrotizing palisaded granulomatous inflammation. Such lesions have also been referred to as Churg-Strauss granuloma, superficial ulcerating rheumatoid necrobiosis, palisaded neutrophilic and granulomatous dermatitis, and interstitial granulomatous dermatitis with arthritis (502a).

LUPUS ERYTHEMATOSUS–NONSPECIFIC BULLOUS LESIONS

On unusual occasions, bullous eruptions or vesiculobullous lesions, unassociated with cutaneous lupus lesions, occur in SLE (503–508). These lesions may involve the face, neck, arms, and trunk. The bullae may approach the size of blisters in bullous pemphigoid, and in other cases, they resemble the vesiculobullous lesions of dermatitis herpetiformis. As noted before, blister formation may develop in some lupus lesions, especially the SCLE lesions associated with anti-Ro(SS-A) antibody positivity. However, in addition, several other pathophysiologic mechanisms may produce blister formation in patients with SLE. Gammon et al. (507) reported four patients with SLE with widespread vesiculobullous eruptions persisting over a 3- to 6-month period (509). These subepidermal blisters demonstrated neutrophilic microabscesses in the dermal papillae and thick linear deposits of IgA, IgG, and C3 along the basement membrane zone. Immunoelectron microscopic studies demonstrated IgG deposits at or below the lamina densa. Furthermore, indirect immunofluorescent studies demonstrated weak staining of anti–basement membrane zone antibodies in three of four patients. Using a 1-M NaCl split skin, the anti–basement membrane zone antibody titers ranged from 40 to 80 in these three patients. The staining occurred on the dermal side of the split (506,507).

Western blot analysis demonstrated that all four of the sera bound a major 290-kDa band; two also bound a minor 145-kDa band. Additional studies demonstrated that these autoantibodies bound the noncollagenous portion of type VII collagen (507). Patients possessing these autoantibodies demonstrated the HLA-DR2, DQ1 phenotypes (508). These data indicate that the autoantibodies in this bullous form of LE are similar to the autoantibodies described in epidermolysis bullosa acquista (509). Epidermolysis bullosa–like lesions may precede the development of SLE (510) (Fig. 2.51).

Before these current studies, Landry and Sams (511), and Nicholas and Gilliam (512,513) had performed acid elution studies on SLE skin, demonstrating autoantibodies reactive against human skin. It is highly likely that these investigators were dealing with autoantibodies reactive against type VII collagen.

Hall et al. (505) have described a third mechanism for the induction of blister formation in LE. They described four patients with SLE who developed vesiculobullous lesions. These lesions demonstrated neutrophilic microabscesses in the dermal papilla reminiscent of dermatitis herpetiformis. Direct immunofluorescence examination of nonultraviolet light–exposed normal-appearing skin revealed a positive LBT composed of dense granular IgA, IgE, IgM, and C3 deposition at the dermal–epidermal junction. Immune complexes were demonstrated in the sera of these patients using a Raji cell IgG radioimmunoassay and ^{125}I-C1q binding assay. In addition, anti-DNA antibodies and hypocomplementemia were detected in all four patients. It appears likely that circulating immune complexes were candidates for the pathogenesis of these lesions. All patients had a dramatic response to diaminodiphenylsulfone (Dapsone).

Porphyria cutanea tarda has been reported in association with SLE, DLE, and SCLE (514–517). In addition to porphyria cutanea tarda, acute intermittent porphyria and variegated porphyria have been found in association with LE. Callen and Ross (517) have reported one patient with SCLE in association with porphyria cutanea tarda. Following the report of Cram et al. (515) of LE and porphyria cutanea tarda coexisting in seven patients in 1973, it appeared that a causative relationship between the two diseases was likely. However, recent evaluations suggest that the association of these two conditions is not as common as was formerly believed. It has also been suggested that the hepatotoxic effect of antimalarial therapy used to treat cutaneous LE lesions may unmask latent states of porphyria.

In addition to the bullous lesions of porphyria, on occasion, LE has coexisted with bullous pemphigoid (518). SLE has also been found in association with dermatitis herpetiformis (519,520).

The Senear–Usher syndrome (pemphigus erythematosus) was described in 1926 (521). Patients demonstrate pemphigus foliaceous–like lesions, most predominantly in a seborrheic dermatitis distribution with clinical features of LE (522) (Fig. 2.52). Acantholysis and the presence of pemphigus autoantibodies have established the relationship of this entity to pemphigus. In addition, direct immunofluorescence examination of the dermal–epidermal junction has demonstrated the granular deposition of immunoglobulin and complement. These characteristic immunohistochemical findings establish the relationship of this entity to LE (523). Serologic studies generally demonstrate the presence of ANAs, but anti-DNA and anti-RNP autoantibodies are unusual. However, most of the patients reported in the literature demonstrate, by indirect immunofluorescence, autoantibodies against desmoglein I, a keratinocyte desmosomal plaque protein. Most patients demonstrate the presence of an acantholytic process at the level of the malpighian stratum. However, some cases have shown suprabasilar acantholysis consistent with a diagnosis of pemphigus vulgaris (524).

The relationship of these putative autoimmune bullous diseases with LE is intriguing. Because of their infrequent occurrence, the coexistence of these autoimmune diseases may simply represent the occurrence of two autoimmune diseases in patients who are genetically susceptible or who have been environmentally exposed to agents (e.g., drugs) capable of inducing these diseases.

On rare occasions, patients with LE possessing anti-Ro(SS-A) autoantibodies may develop cutaneous manifestations similar to toxic epidermal necrolysis (525,526). These patients are usually exquisitely photosensitive. Five of these patients with whom the authors are familiar developed their disease process following excessive UV light exposure.

ERYTHEMA MULTIFORME–LIKE LESIONS

In 1963, Rowell et al. (27) described the occurrence of erythema multiforme–like lesions in patients with LE. These lesions may initially be papular before developing into annular lesions highly reminiscent of annular SCLE. Such lesions can become vesicular or bullous, and on rare occasions, necrosis and ulceration may develop if the reaction is intense. These patients may also have lesions of pernio (236). These patients possess antibodies against a saline extract of human tissue termed "anti-SjT." The SjT antibody syndrome is named after a patient who had SSj. It is now postulated that the SjT syndrome is identical to the anti-La(SS-B) antibody system. The absence of anti-SjD antibodies in this cohort of four patients is interesting because in a 15-year period, some investigators (T.T.P. and Morris Reichlin) have never detected the presence of anti-La(SS-B) in the absence of anti-Ro(SS-A) antibodies.

On occasions, one of the authors (T.T.P.) has seen anti-Ro(SS-A)–positive patients with annular polycyclic lesions, some of which have resembled targetoid lesions. The cutaneous lesions

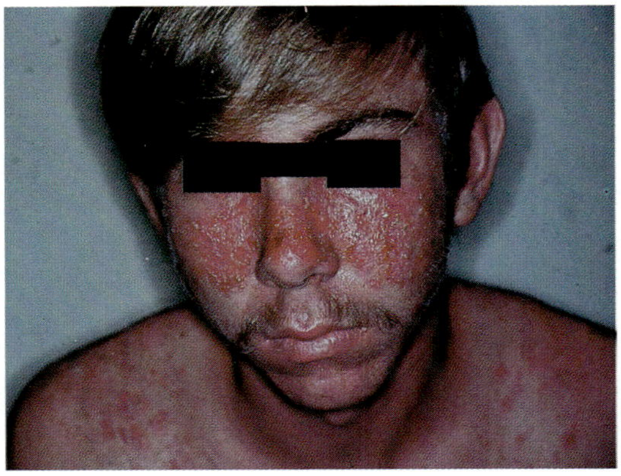

Figure 2.52. Pemphigus erythematosus.

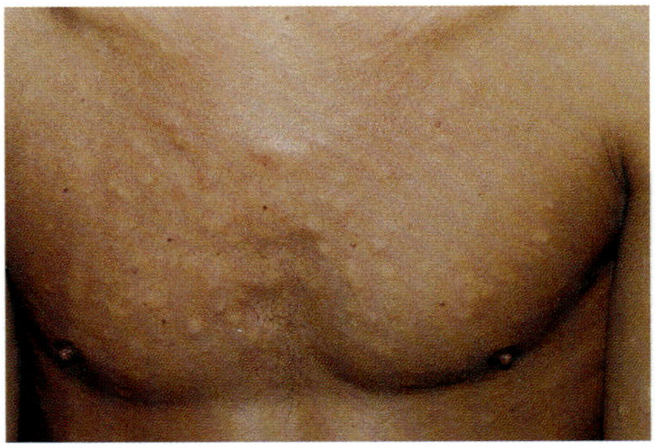

Figure 2.53. Papular and nodular dermal mucinosis in a patient with systemic lupus erythematosus (SLE), including pleural effusions and glomerulonephritis [this case was previously reported in (534a)].

of one of the neonatal lupus lesions associated with anti-U_1RNP antibodies was targetoid (527).

Recently, other investigators have reported the appearance of erythema multiforme–like lesions in anti-Ro(SS-A) antibody–positive patients (528,529).

CUTANEOUS MUCINOSIS

On very unusual occasions, flesh-colored papular and nodular cutaneous mucin depositions involving the trunk, arms, and neck have been detected in patients with SLE (530–534) (Fig. 2.53). On rare occasions, massive mucinosis may occur (533, 534). Most of these patients satisfy the ACR criteria for the diagnosis of SLE. However, on unusual occasions, these lesions can be seen in patients with only cutaneous LE. In general, these lesions appear at sites clinically free of LE-specific skin lesions.

Histopathologic examination demonstrates mucin deposition mainly in the papillary and mid-dermis among collagen bundles. A mild perivascular lymphocytic infiltrate may also be detected.

These lesions may respond to systemic therapy (prednisone and hydroxychloroquine). However, persistence of these lesions despite systemic therapy has been noted.

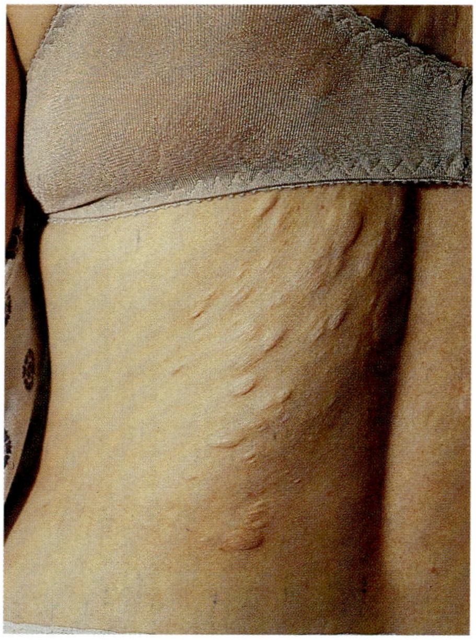

Figure 2.54. Anetoderma in a patient who had typical discoid lupus erythematosus lesions on other parts of her body.

PIGMENTARY CHANGES

Postinflammatory hypo- and hyperpigmentation at sites of previous cutaneous lesions is a common finding in patients with LE (Figs. 2.7, 2.11, 2.17, 2.22–2.24, 2.28, 2.30, 2.35). At times, depigmentation may be extensive, resulting in a significant cosmetic problem. In the authors' experience, this is an especially significant problem in black patients with scarring lupus lesions. The residua of the lesions of SCLE may either be areas of hyperpigmentation or areas of hypopigmentation.

It should be noted that antimalarial therapy has long been recognized as a cause of altered pigmentation. This therapy can result in grayness of the scalp hair, eyelashes, eyebrows, and beard. Diffuse hyperpigmentation or transverse bands of pigmentation may be seen in the nails. Mucous membrane blue–black patches of hyperpigmentation, as well as similar lesions over the anterior shins, may also be seen. These pigmentary changes are reversible if the antimalarial is stopped.

NAILS

Alterations in nails such as pitting, horizontal and longitudinal ridging, leukonychia, onycholysis, and atrophy and telangiectasia of the cuticle nailfold are commonly detected in patients with SLE (535). Urowitz et al. (535) detected nail changes in 42 (31%) of 165 patients with SLE. The most common abnormality was onycholysis.

Vaughn et al. (536) have described nail dyschromia in approximately 52% of black patients with SLE. Both diffuse and linear nail dyschromia were detected. There was no relationship to disease activity or to antimalarial therapy. Similar lesions were not detected in patients who did not have SLE. The pathogenesis of this abnormality is unknown, although it is surmised that the pigmentation is melanin.

MISCELLANEOUS

Anetoderma has been described in the presence of SLE, as well as CCLE (537,538,542) (Fig. 2.54). In addition, generalized cutis laxa has been described in association with SLE (539). Recently, two patients with mid-dermal elastolysis have been reported. One of the patients presented with flesh-colored papules and plaques on the lower extremities; the other with pink macules on arms and trunk (540).

On unusual occasions, DLE lesions have been found in an individual who also has lichen planus (166,203,541–543). White reticular oral lesions were found in association with chronic atrophic discoid lupus–like lesions. In addition, other patients had lichenoid or verrucous-like lesions. This latter type of lesion has been seen by one of the authors (T.T.P.) in association with anti-Ro(SS-A) antibodies.

Finally, there is an isolated report of acanthosis nigricans in association with lupoid hepatitis (544). This, in all probability, represents the association of chronic active hepatitis with acanthosis nigricans, and not a true case of LE. Acanthosis nigricans has also been reported to occur in patients with SLE in association with type B insulin resistance (545).

REFERENCES

1. Ropes MW. *Systemic lupus erythematosus.* Cambridge: Harvard University Press, 1976.
2. Lahita RG. *Systemic lupus erythematosus,* 2nd ed. New York: Churchill Livingstone, 1992.
3. Wallace DJ, Hahn BH, eds. *Dubois' lupus erythematosus,* 6th ed. Baltimore: Lippincott, Williams & Wilkins, 2001.
4. Lee LA, David KM. Cutaneous lupus erythematosus. In: Weston WL, Provost TT, eds. *Current problems in dermatology.* St. Louis, MO: Mosby–Year Book, 1989:161.
5. Braverman I. Connective tissue (rheumatic) diseases. In: *Cutaneous signs of systemic disease.* Philadelphia: WB Saunders, 1981:299.
6. Tuffanelli DL, Epstein J. Chronic cutaneous (discoid) lupus erythematosus. In: Wallace DJ, Dubois EL, eds. *Lupus erythematosus,* 3rd ed. Philadelphia: Lea & Febiger, 1987:283.
7. Rowell NR, Goodfield MJD. The "connective tissue diseases." In: Champion RH, Burton JL, Ebling FJG, eds. *Textbook of dermatology.* London: Blackwell Science, 1992:2163.
8. Rothfield NF. Cutaneous manifestations of multisystem diseases. In: Fitzpatrick TB, Eisen AZ, Wolff K, et al., eds. *Dermatology in general medicine.* New York: McGraw-Hill, 1993:2137.
9. Norris DA. Pathomechanisms of photosensitive lupus erythematosus. *J Invest Dermatol* 1993;100:58S.

10. Gilliam JN. The cutaneous signs of lupus erythematosus. *Cont Educ Fam Phys* 1977;6:34.
11. Gilliam JN, Sontheimer RD. Distinctive cutaneous subsets in the spectrum of lupus erythematosus. *J Am Acad Dermatol* 1981;4:471.
12. Gilliam JN, Sontheimer RD. Skin manifestations of SLE. *Clin Rheum Dis* 1982;8:207.
13. Talbott JH. Historical background of discoid and systemic lupus erythematosus. In: Wallace DJ, Hahn BH, eds. *Dubois' lupus erythematosus,* 4th ed. Philadelphia: Lea & Febiger, 1993:3.
14. Sontheimer RD. Clinical manifestations of cutaneous lupus erythematosus. In: Wallace DJ, Hahn BH, eds. *Dubois' lupus erythematosus.* 4th ed. Philadelphia: Lea & Febiger, 1993:285.
15. Cazenave PLA, Chausit M. Du lupus. *Ann Malad Peau Syph* 1852;4:113.
16. Hebra F, Kaposi M. *On diseases of the skin, including the exanthemata.* London: The New Sydenham Society, 1875.
17. Hutchinson J. On lupus and its treatment. *BMJ* 1880;1:650.
18. Osler W. On the visceral complications of erythema exudativum multiforme. *Am J Med Sci* 1895;100:629.
19. Payne JF. A postgraduate lecture on lupus erythematosus. *Clin J* 1894;4:223.
20. Friedberg CK, Gross L, Wallach K. Nonbacterial thrombotic endocarditis associated with prolonged fever, arthritis, inflammation of serous membranes and wide-spread vascular lesions. *Arch Intern Med* 1936;56:662.
21. Kiel H. Conception of lupus erythematosus and its morphologic variants: with particular references to systemic lupus erythematosus. *Arch Dermatol* 1937;36:729.
22. O'Leary PA. Disseminated lupus erythematosus. *Minn Med* 1934;17:637.
23. Hargraves M, Richmond H, Morton R. Presentation of two bone marrow elements: the "tart" cell and the "LE" cell. *Mayo Clin Proc* 1948;23:25.
24. Friou GJ. Clinical application of lupus serum: nucleoprotein reaction using fluorescent antibody technique. *J Clin Invest* 1957;36:890(abst).
25. Page F. Treatment of lupus erythematosus with mepacrine. *Lancet* 1951;ii:755.
26. Hench PS. The reversibility of certain rheumatic and nonrheumatic conditions by the use of cortisone or of the pituitary adrenocorticotrophic hormone. *Ann Intern Med* 1952;36:1.
27. Rowell NR, Swanson-Beck J, Anderson JR. Lupus erythematosus and erythema multiforme-like lesions. *Arch Dermatol* 1963;88:176.
28. Burnham TK, Neblett TR, Fine G. The application of the fluorescent antibody technique to the investigation of lupus erythematosus and various dermatoses. *J Invest Dermatol* 1963;41:451.
29. Dubois EL, Tuffanelli DL. Clinical manifestations of systemic lupus erythematosus. *JAMA* 1964;190:104.
30. Dubois E. The relationship between discoid and systemic lupus erythematosus. In: Dubois EL, ed. *Lupus erythematosus,* 1st ed. New York: McGraw-Hill, 1966:277.
31. Clark G, Reichlin M, Tomasi TB. Characterization of a soluble cytoplasmic antigen reactive with sera from a patient with systemic lupus erythematosus. *J Immunol* 1969;102:117.
32. Prystowsky SD, Gilliam JN. Discoid lupus erythematosus as part of a larger disease spectrum. *Arch Dermatol* 1975;11:1448.
33. Sontheimer RD, Thomas JR, Gilliam JN. Subacute cutaneous lupus erythematosus: a cutaneous marker for a distinct lupus erythematosus subset. *Arch Dermatol* 1979;115:1409.
34. Sontheimer RD, Stastny P, Gilliam JN. Human histocompatibility antigen associations in subacute cutaneous lupus erythematosus. *J Clin Invest* 1981;67:312.
35. Sontheimer RD, Maddison PJ, Reichlin M, et al. Serologic and HLA associations in subacute cutaneous lupus erythematosus, a clinical subset of lupus erythematosus. *Ann Intern Med* 1982;97:644.
36. Provost TT, Ahmed AR, Maddison PJ, et al. Antibodies to cytoplasmic antigens in lupus erythematosus: serologic markers for systemic disease. *Arthritis Rheum* 1977;20:1457.
37. Maddison PJ, Provost TT, Reichlin M. Serological findings in patients with "ANA-negative" systemic lupus erythematosus. *Medicine* 1981;60:87.
38. Kephart D, Hood A, Provost TT. Neonatal lupus erythematosus: new serologic findings. *J Invest Dermatol* 1981;77:331.
39. Franco HL, Weston WL, Pebble C, et al. Autoantibodies directed against sicca syndrome antigens in the neonatal lupus syndrome. *J Am Acad Dermatol* 1981;4:67.
40. Provost TT, Arnett FC, Reichlin M. Homozygous C2 deficiency, lupus erythematosus and anti-Ro (SS-A) antibodies. *Arthritis Rheum* 1983;26:1279.
41. Cataggio LF, Skinner RP, Smith G, et al. Systemic lupus erythematosus in the elderly: clinical and serologic characteristics. *J Rheumatol* 1984;11: 175–181.
42. Meyer O, Hauptmann G, Tappeiner G. Genetic deficiency of C4, C2 or C1q and lupus syndromes: association with anti-Ro(SS-A) antibodies. *Clin Exp Immunol* 1985;62:678.
43. LeFeber WP, Norris DA, Ryan SR, et al. Ultraviolet light induces binding of antibodies to selected nuclear antigens on cultured human keratinocytes. *J Clin Invest* 1984;74:1545.
44. Casciola-Rosen LA, Anhalt G, Rosen A. Autoantigens targeted in systemic lupus erythematosus are clustered in two populations of surface structures on apoptotic keratinocytes. *J Exp Med* 1994;179:1317.
44a. Gilliam J. Immunology and pathogenesis of cutaneous lupus erythematosus. In: Safai RA, Good RA, eds. *Comparative immunology: immunodermatology.* New York: Plenum Press, 1981.
44b. Provost TT. The relationship between discoid lupus erythematosus and systemic lupus erythematosus: a hypothesis. *Am J Dermatopathol* 1979;1:181–186.
45. Tam EM, Cohen As, Fries JF, et al. The 1982 revised criteria for the classification of systemic lupus erythematosus. *Arthritis Rheum* 1982;25:1271.
46. Beutner EH, Blaszcyzk M, Jablonska S, et al. Studies on criteria of the European Academy of Dermatology and Venereology for the classification of cutaneous lupus erythematosus, I: selection of clinical groups and study factors [published erratum appears in *Int J Dermatol* 1991;30:557]. *Int J Dermatol* 1991;30:411.
47. Beutner EH, Jablonska S, Whie DB, et al. Dermatologic criteria for classifying the major forms of cutaneous lupus erythematosus: methods for systematic discriminant analysis and questions on the interpretation of findings. *Clin Dermatol* 1992;10:443.
48. Beutner EH, Blaszczyk M, Jablonska S, et al. Preliminary, dermatologic first step criteria for lupus erythematosus and second step criteria for systemic lupus erythematosus. *Int J Dermatol* 1993;32:645.
49. Halmi BH. Classification of lupus erythematosus. *Int J Dermatol* 1993;32:643.
50. Rothfield NF, Braverman IM, Moschella S, et al. Classification of lupus erythematosus: an open forum. *Fitzpatrick's J Clin Dermatol* 1994; March/April:9.
51. Pinkus MD. Lichenoid tissue reactions: a speculative review of the clinical spectrum of epidermal basal cell damage with special reference to erythema dyschromicum perstans. *Arch Dermatol* 1973;107:840.
52. Kuwana M, Kaburaki J, Pandey JP, et al. HLA class II alleles in Japanese patients with immune thrombocytopenic purpura: associations with antiplatelet glycoprotein autoantibodies and responses to splenectomy. *Tissue Antigens* 2000;56:337–343.
53. Wang H, Shen B, Yan W, et al. [Study on the relations between HLA-DRB1 alleles and idiopathic thrombocytopenic purpura in children]. *Zhonghua Yi Xue Yi Chuan Xue Za Zhi* 2002;19:290–294.
53a. Ackerman B, et al. *Histologic diagnosis of inflammatory skin disease. An algorithmic method based on pattern analysis.* Baltimore: Lippincott Williams & Wilkins 1997:525–528.
54. Weinstein C, Miller MH, Axtens R, et al. Lupus and non-lupus cutaneous manifestations in systemic lupus erythematosus. *Aust N Z J Med* 1987;17:501.
55. Black AA, McCauliffe DP, Sontheimer RD. Prevalence of acne rosacea in a rheumatic skin disease subspecialty clinic. *Lupus* 1992;1:229.
56. Peterson KS, Winchester RJ. Systemic lupus erythematosus: pathogenesis. In: Koopman WJ, ed. *Arthritis and allied conditions.* Philadelphia: Lippincott Williams & Wilkins, 2000:1.
57. Tsao BP, Grossman JM. Genetics and systemic lupus erythematosus. *Curr Rheumatol Rep* 2001;3:183–190.
58. Wakeland EK, Liu K,Graham RR, et al. Delineating the genetic basis of systemic lupus erythematosus. *Immunity* 2001;15(3):397–408.
59. Kono DH, Theofilopoulos AN. The genetics of murine systemic lupus erythematosus. In: Wallace DJ, Hahn BH, eds. *Dubois' lupus erythematosus.* Baltimore: Lippincott Williams & Wilkins, 2002:121–143.
60. Sullivan KE, Wooten C, Schmeckpeper BJ, et al. A promoter polymorphism of tumor necrosis factor alpha associated with systemic lupus erythematosus in African-Americans. *Arthritis Rheum* 1997;40:2207–2211.
61. Rosen A, Casciola-Rosen L. Autoantigens as substrates for apoptotic proteases: implications for the pathogenesis of systemic autoimmune disease. *Cell Death Differ* 1999;6:6–12.
62. Nagata S. Mutations in the Fas antigen 1pr mice. *Semin Immunol* 1994;6:3–8.
63. Suda T, Takahashi T, Goldstein P, et al Molecular cloning of the Fas ligand, a novel member of the tumor necrosis factor family. *Cell* 1993;75:1169–1178.
64. Reveille JD, Moulds JM, Ahn C, et al. Systemic lupus erythematosus in three ethnic groups: the effects of HLA class II, C4, and CR1 alleles, socioeconomic factors, and ethnicity at disease onset. LUMINA Study Group. Lupus in minority populations, nature versus nurture. *Arthritis Rheum* 1998;41:1161–1172.
65. Tso BP. An update on genetic studies of systemic lupus erythematosus. *Curr Rheumatol Rep* 2002;4:359–367.
65a. Botto M, Walport MJ. C1q, autoimmunity and apoptosis. *Immunobiology.* 2002;205:395–406.
66. Boackle SA, Holers VM, Chen X, et al. Cr2, a candidate gene in the murine Sle1c lupus susceptibility locus, encodes a dysfunctional protein. *Immunity* 2201;15:775–785.
67. Korb LC, Ahearn JM. C1q binds directly and specifically to surface blebs of apoptotic human keratinocytes: complement deficiency and systemic lupus erythematosus revisited. *J Immunol* 1997;158:4525–4528.
68. Reid KBM, Turner MW. Mammalian lectius in activation and clearance mechanisms involving the complement system. *Springer Semin Immunopath* 1994; 15:307–325.
69. Garred P, Madsen HO, Holberg P, et al. Mannose-binding lectin polymorphisms and susceptibility to infection in systemic lupus erythematosus. *Arthritis Rheum* 1999;42:2145–2152.
70. Gaffney PM, Kearns GM, Shark KB, et al. A genome-wide search for susceptibility genes in human systemic lupus erythematosus sib-pair families. *Proc Natl Acad Sci U S A* 1998;95:14875–14879.
71. Werth VP, Zhang W, Dortzbach K, et al. Association of a promoter polymorphism of tumor necrosis factor-alpha with subacute cutaneous lupus erythematosus and distinct photoregulation of transcription. *J Invest Drmatol* 2000;115:726–730.
71a. Racila DM, Sontheimer CJ, Sheffield A, Wisnieski JJ, Racila E, Sontheimer RD. Homozygous single nucleotide polymorphism of the complement C1QA gene is associated with decreased levels of C1q in patients with subacute cutaneous lupus erythematosus. *Lupus.* 2003;12:124–132.
72. Emlen W, Niebur J, Kadera R. Accelerated in vitro apoptosis of lymphocytes from patients with systemic lupus erythematosus. *J Immunol* 1994;152:3685–3692.

73. Casciola-Rosen LA, Miller DA, Anhalt GJ, et al. Specific cleavage of the 70 kDa protein of the U_1 small nuclear riboprotein is a characteristic biochemical feature of apoptotic cell death. *J Biol Chem* 1994;269:30757–30760.
74. Rosen A, Casciola-Rosen L, Ahearn J. Novel packages of viral and self-antigens are generated during apoptosis. *J Exp Med* 1995;181:1557.
75. Vaishnaw AK, Toubi E, Ohsako S, et al. The spectrum of apoptotic defects and clinical manifestations including systemic lupus erythematosus, in humans with CD95 (Fas/APO-1) mutations. *Arthritis Rheum* 1999;42:1833–1842.
75a. Pickering MC, Walport MJ. Links between complement abnormalities and systemic lupus erythematosus. *Rheumatol* 2000;39:133–141.
76. Strand V. Monoclonal antibodies and other biologic therapies. *Lupus* 2002;10: 216–221.
77. Furukawa F. Antinuclear antibody-keratinocyte interactions in photosensitive cutaneous lupus erythematosus. *Histol Histopathol* 1999;14:627–633.
78. Dubois EL, Wallace DJ. Clinical and laboratory manifestations of systemic lupus erythematosus. In: Wallace DJ, Dubois EL, eds. *Lupus erythematosus,* 3rd ed. Philadelphia: Lea & Febiger, 1987:317.
79. Pistiner M, Wallace DJ, Nessim S, et al. Lupus erythematosus in the 1980s: a survey of 570 patients. *Semin Arthritis Rheum* 1991;21:55.
80. Cervera R, Khamashta MA, Font J, et al., and the European Working Party on Systemic Lupus Erythematosus. Systemic lupus erythematosus: clinical and immunologic patterns of disease expression in a cohort of 1,000 patients. *Medicine* 1993;72:113.
81. Jonsson H, Nived O, Sturfelt G. The effect of age on clinical and serological manifestations in unselected patients with systemic lupus erythematosus. *J Rheumatol* 1988;15:505.
82. Hochberg MC, Boyd RB, Ahearn JM, et al. Systemic lupus erythematosus: a review of clinicolaboratory features and immunogenetic markers in 150 patients with emphasis on demographic subsets. *Medicine* 1985;64:285.
83. Vlachoyiannopoulos PG, Karassa FB, Karakostas KX, et al. Systemic lupus erythematosus in Greece: clinical features, evolution and outcome: a descriptive analysis of 292 patients. *Lupus* 1993;2:303.
84. O'Quinn S, Cole J, Many H. Problems of disability in patients with chronic skin diseases. *Arch Dermatol* 1972;105:35.
85. Wysenbeek AJ, Guedj D, Amit M, et al. Rash in systemic lupus erythematosus: prevalence and relation to cutaneous and non-cutaneous disease manifestations. *Ann Rheum Dis* 1992;51:717.
86. Font J, Cervera R, Navarro M, et al. Systemic lupus erythematosus in men: clinical and immunological characteristics. *Ann Rheum Dis* 1992;51:1050.
87. Segasothy M, Phillips PA. Systemic lupus erythematosus in Aborigines and Caucasians in central Australia: a comparative study. *Lupus* 2001;10:439–444.
88. Rao S, Olson JM, Moser KL, et al. Linkage analysis of human systemic lupus erythematosus-related traits: a principal component approach. *Arthritis Rheum* 2001;44:2807–2818.
89. Arnett FC. Genetic aspects of human lupus. *Clin Immunol Immunopathol* 1992;63.4.
90. Simmons-O'Brien E, Chen S, Watson R, et al. 100 anti-Ro (SS-A) antibody positive patients: a 10 year follow up. *Medicine* 1995;74:109.
91. Wysenbeek AJ, Block DA, Fries JF. Prevalence and expression of photosensitivity in systemic lupus erythematosus. *Ann Rheum Dis* 1989;48:461.
92. Kuhn A, Sonntag M, Richtger-Hintz D, et al. Phototesting in lupus erythematosus: a 15 year experience. *J Am Acad Dermatol* 2001;45:86–95.
93. Mond CB, Peterson MGE, Rothfield NF. Correlation of anti-Ro antibody with photosensitivity rash in systemic lupus erythematosus patients. *Arthritis Rheum* 1989;32:202.
94. Wolska H, Blaszczyk M, Jablonska S. Phototests in patients with various forms of lupus erythematosus. *Int J Dermatol* 1989;28:98–103.
95. Furukawa F, Tokura Y, Matsushita K, et al. Selective expansions of T cells expressing V beta 8 and V beta 13 in skin lesions of patients with chronic cutaneous lupus erythematosus. *J Dermatol* 1996;23:670–676.
96. Prete PE. The mechanism of actionof L-ronavonine in inducing autoimmune phenomena [letter]. *Arch Inter Med* 1985;145:1926–1927.
97. Fritzler MJ, Rubin RL. Drug-induced lupus. In: Wallace DJ, Hahn BH, eds. *Dubois' lupus erythematosus,* 4th ed. Philadelphia: Lea & Febiger, 1993:442.
98. Wallace DJ. Infections in systemic lupus erythematosus. In: Wallace DJ, Hahn BH, eds. *Dubois' lupus erythematosus,* 4th ed. Philadelphia: Lea & Febiger, 1993:454.
99. Herrero C, Bielsa I, Font J, et al. Subacute cutaneous lupus erythematosus: clinical pathologic findings in 13 cases. *J Am Acad Dermatol* 1988;19:1057.
100. Kind P, Goetz G. Klinik und differential diagnose des cutanen lupus erythematodes. *Z Hautkr* 1987;62:1337.
101. Molad Y, Weinberger A, David M, et al. Clinical manifestations and laboratory data of subacute cutaneous lupus erythematosus. *Isr J Med Sci* 1987;23:278.
102. Mooney E, Wade TR. Subacute cutaneous lupus erythematosus in Iceland. *Int J Dermatol* 1989;28:104.
103. Cohen MR, Crosby D. Systemic disease in subacute cutaneous lupus erythematosus: a controlled comparison with systemic lupus erythematosus. *J Rheumatol* 1994;21:1665.
104. Callen JP, Klein J. Subacute cutaneous lupus erythematosus: clinical, serologic, immunogenetic, and therapeutic considerations in 72 patients. *Arthritis Rheum* 1988;31:1007.
105. Johansson-Stephansson E, Koskimes S, Partanen J, et al. Subacute cutaneous lupus erythematosus: genetic markers and clinical and immunological findings in patients. *Arch Dermatol* 1989;125:791.
106. Shou-yi S, Shu-fang F, Kang-huang L, et al. Clinical study of 30 cases of subacute cutaneous lupus erythematosus. *Chin Med J* 1987;100:45.
107. Provost TT, Talal N, Harley JB, et al. The relationship between anti-Ro(SS-A) antibody-positive Sjögren's syndrome and anti-Ro (SS-A) antibody-positive lupus erythematosus. *Arch Dermatol* 1988;124:63.
108. Vazquez-Doval J, Ruiz de Erenchun F, Sanchez-Ibarrola A, et al. Subacute cutaneous lupus erythematosus? Clinical, histopathological and immunophenotypical study of five cases. *J Invest Allerg Clin Immunol* 1992;2:27.
109. Drosos AA, Dimou GS, Siamopoulou-Mavridou A, et al. Subacute cutaneous lupus erythematosus in Greece: a clinical, serological and genetic study. *Ann Med Intern* 1990;141:421.
110. Ahearn JM, Provost TT, Dorsch CA, et al. Interrelationships of HLA-DR, MB and MT phenotypes, autoantibody expression, and clinical features in systemic lupus erythematosus. *Arthritis Rheum* 1982;25:1031.
111. Bielsa I, Herrero C, Ercilla G, et al. Immunogenetic findings in cutaneous lupus erythematosus. *J Am Acad Dermatol* 1991;25:251.
112. Watson RM, Talwar P, Alexander E, et al. Subacute cutaneous lupus erythematosus? Immunogenetic associations. *J Autoimmun* 1991;4:73.
113. Provost TT, Talal N, Bias W, et al. Ro/SS-A(SS-A) positive Sjögren's/lupus erythematosus overlap patients are associated with the HLA-DR3 and/or DRW6 phenotypes. *J Invest Dermatol* 1988;91:369.
114. Provost TT, Watson RM. Anti-Ro(SSA), HLA-DR3 positive females: the interrelationship between some ANA negative, SS, SCLE, NLE mothers and SS/LE overlap female patients. *J Invest Dermatol* 1993;100[Suppl]:14S–20S.
115. Bell DA, Maddison PJ. Serologic subsets in systemic lupus erythematosus: an examination of autoantibodies in relationship to clinical features of disease and HLA antigens. *Arthritis Rheum* 1980;23:1268.
116. Harley JP, Reichlin M, Arnett FC, et al. Gene interaction at the HLA-DQ locus enhances autoantibody production in primary Sjögren's syndrome. *Science* 1986;232:1145.
117. Partanen J, Koskimies S, Johansson E. C4 null phenotypes among lupus erythematosus patients are predominantly the result of deletions covering C4 and closely linked C21-hydroxylase A genes. *J Med Genet* 1988;25:387.
118. Van Hees CLM, Boom BW, Vermeer BJ, et al. Subacute cutaneous lupus erythematosus in a patient with inherited deficiency of the third component of complement. *Arch Dermatol* 1982;128:700.
119. Asghar SS, Venneker GT, Van Meegen M, et al. Hereditary deficiency of C5 in association with discoid lupus erythematosus. *J Am Acad Dermatol* 1991;24:376.
120. Holers MV. Complement deficiency states, disease susceptibility and infection risks in systemic lupus erythematosus. *Arthritis Rheum* 1999;42: 2023–2025.
121. Perkins W, Stables GI, Lever RS. Protein S deficiency in lupus erythematosus secondary to hereditary angio-oedema. *Br J Dermatol* 1994;130:381.
122. Pacheco TR, Weston WL, Giclas PC, et al. Three generations of patients with lupus erythematosus and hereditary angioedema. *Am J Med* 2000;109: 256–257.
123. Sontheimer RD. Subacute cutaneous lupus erythematosus: a decade's perspective. *Med Clin North Am* 1989;73:1073.
124. Nagy E, Meszaros C, Debreczeni M. Subacute lupus erythematosus of the skin: clinical aspects and laboratory findings. *Z Hautkr* 1990;65:1039.
125. David-Bajar KM, Bennion SD, DeSpain JD, et al. Clinical, histologic, and immunofluorescent distinctions between subacute cutaneous lupus erythematosus and discoid lupus erythematosus. *J Invest Dermatol* 1992;99:251.
126. Reed BR, Huff JC, Jones SK, et al. Subacute cutaneous lupus erythematosus associated with hydrochlorothiazide therapy. *Ann Intern Med* 1985;103:49.
127. Berbis P, Vernay-vaisse C, Privot Y. Lupus cutane subaigu observe au cours d'un traitement par diuretiques thiazidiques. *Ann Derm Venereol* 1986;113: 1245.
128. Darken M, McBurney EI. Subacute cutaneous lupus erythematosus-like drug eruption due to combination diuretic hydrochlorothiazide and triamterene. *J Am Acad Dermatol* 1988;18:38.
129. Fine RM. Subacute cutaneous lupus erythematosus associated with hydrochlorothiazide therapy. *Int J Dermatol* 1989;28:375.
130. Goodrich A, Kohn S. Hydrochlorothiazide induced lupus erythematosus: a new variant? *J Am Acad Dermatol* 1993;28:1001–1002.
131. Sheretz EF. Lichen planus following procainamide induced lupus erythematosus. *Cutis* 1988;42:51.
132. Gange KW, Levene GM. A distinctive eruption in patients receiving oxprenolol. *Clin Exp Dermatol* 1979;4:87.
133. Miyagawa S, Okuchi T, Shiomi Y, et al. Subacute cutaneous lupus erythematosus lesions precipitated by griseofulvin. *J Am Acad Dermatol* 1989:21:343.
134. Roura M, Lopez-Gil F, Umbert P. Systemic lupus erythematosus exacerbated by piroxicam. *Dermatologica* 1991;182:56.
135. Parodi A, Rivara G, Guarrera M. Possible naproxen-induced relapse of subacute cutaneous lupus erythematosus. *JAMA* 1992;268:51.
136. Uddin MS, Lynfield YL, Grosberg SJ, et al. Cutaneous reaction to spironolactone resembling lupus erythematosus. *Cutis* 1979;24:198.
137. Kulick KB, Mogavero H, Provost TT, et al. Serologic studies in patients with lupus erythematosus and psoriasis. *J Am Acad Dermatol* 1983;8:631–634.
138. McGrath H Jr, Scopelitis E, Nesbitt LT Jr. Subacute cutaneous lupus erythematosus during psoralen ultraviolet A therapy. *Arthritis Rheum* 1990;33:302.
139. Callen JP. Drug induced cutaneous lupus erythematosus, a distinct syndrome that is frequently unrecognized. *J Am Acad Dermatol* 2001;45:315–316.
140. Bousman G, Schiller M, Luger TA, et al. Terbinafine induced subacute cutaneous lupus erythematosus. *J Am Acad Dermatol* 2001;44:925–931.
141. Brooke R, Coulson IH, Al-Dawoud A. Terbinafine induced subacute cutaneous lupus erythematosus. *Br J Dermatol* 1998;139:1132–1133.

142. Murphy M, Barnes L. Terbinafine induced lupus erythematosus. *Br J Dermatol* 1998;138:708–709.
143. Holmes S, Kemmett D. Exacerbation of systemic lupus erythematosus induced by terbinafine. *Br J Dermatol* 1998;139:1133.
144. Crawson AN, Margo CM. Diltiazem and subacute cutaneous lupus like lesions. *N Engl J Med* 1995;333:1429.
145. Dyer V, Pluda JM, Reed E. Drug induced lupus associated with COL-3: report of 3 cases. *Arch Dermatol* 2001;137:471–474.
146. Smith CD, Marino C, Rothfield NF. The clinical utility of the lupus band test. *Arthritis Rheum* 1984;27:382.
147. Callen JP. Chronic cutaneous lupus erythematosus: clinical, laboratory, therapeutic, and prognostic examination of 62 patients. *Arch Dermatol* 1982;118:412.
148. Marten RH, Blackburn EK. Lupus erythematosus: a five year follow up of 77 cases. *Arch Dermatol* 1961;83:430.
149. Prystowsky SD, Herndon JH, Gilliam JN. Chronic cutaneous lupus erythematosus (DLE): a clinical and laboratory investigation of 80 patients. *Medicine* 1975;55:183.
150. Rothfield NF, March C, Miescher P, et al. Chronic discoid lupus erythematosus: a study of 65 patients and 65 controls. *N Engl J Med* 1963;269:1155.
151. Scott A, Rees EG. The relationship of systemic lupus erythematosus and discoid lupus erythematosus: a clinical and hematological study. *Arch Dermatol* 1959;79:422.
152. Shrank AB, Doniach D. Discoid lupus erythematosus: correlation of clinical features with serum auto-antibody pattern. *Arch Dermatol* 1963;87:677.
153. Daly D. Central nervous system in acute disseminated lupus erythematosus. *J Nerv Ment Dis* 1945;102:461.
154. Hough W. Discoid lupus erythematosus: a study of sex and age at onset. *Acta Derm Venereol (Stockh)* 1966;46:240.
155. Millard LG, Rowell NR. Abnormal laboratory test results and their relationship to prognosis in discoid lupus erythematosus: a long-term follow-up study of 92 patients. *Arch Dermatol* 1979;115:1055.
156. O'Laughlin S, Schroeter AL, Jordon RE. A study of lupus erythematosus with particular reference to generalized discoid lupus. *Br J Dermatol* 1978;991.
157. Wallace DJ. The relationship between discoid and systemic lupus erythematosus. In: Wallace DJ, Hahn BH, eds. *Dubois' lupus erythematosus,* 4th ed. Philadelphia: Lea & Febiger, 1993:310.
158. Knop J, Bonsmann G, Kind P, et al. Antigens of the major histocompatibility complex in patients with chronic discoid lupus erythematosus. *Br J Dermatol* 1990;122:723.
159. Fischer GF, Pickl WF, Fae I, et al. Association between chronic cutaneous lupus erythematosus and HLA class II alleles. *Hum Immunol* 1994;41:280.
160. Sewell ML, McCaulaffe DP. Patients with cutaneous lupus erythematosus who smoke are less responsive to antimalarial treatment. *J Am Dermatol* 2000;42:983–987.
161. Rahman P, Gladman DD, Urowitz MB. Smoking interferes with efficacy of antimalarial therapy in cutaneous lupus. *J Rheumatol* 1998;25:1716–1719.
162. Norden D, Weinberg J, Schumacher HR, et al. Bilateral periorbital edema in systemic lupus erythematosus. *J Rheumatol* 1993;20:2158.
163. McHugh NJ, Maddison PJ, MacCleod TIF, et al. Papular lesions and cutaneous lupus erythematosus: a comparative clinical and histological study using monoclonal antibodies. *J Rheumatol* 1988;15:1097.
164. Gilliam JN, Sontheimer RD. Subacute cutaneous lupus erythematosus. *Clin Rheum Dis* 1982;8:343.
165. Su WP, Alegre VA. Bullous lesions in cutaneous lupus erythematosus. *Chang Keng I Hsueh* 1991;14:15.
166. Manganoni Am, Facchetti F, Pasolini G, et al. Guess what? (Lupus erythematosus gyratum repens). *Eur J Dermatol* 1994;4:63.
167. Blaszczyk M, Magaewski S, Wasik M, et al. Natural killer cell activity of peripheral blood mononuclear cells from patients with various forms of lupus erythematosus. *Br J Dermatol* 1987;117:709.
168. Callen JP, Kulick KB, Stelzer G, et al. Subacute cutaneous lupus erythematosus: clinical, serologic, and immunogenetic studies of 49 patients seen in a non-referral setting. *J Am Acad Dermatol* 1986;15:1227.
169. David KM, Thornton JC, Davis B, et al. Morbidity and mortality in patients with subacute cutaneous lupus erythematosus. *J Invest Dermatol* 1984;82: 408(abstr).
170. Reimers CD, Schedel H, Fleckenstein JL, et al. Magnetic resonance imaging of skeletal muscles in idiopathic inflammatory myopathies of adults. *J Neurol* 1994;241:306.
171. Hymes SR, Russell TJ, Jordon RE. The anti-Ro antibody system. *Int J Dermatol* 1986;25:1.
172. Nieboer C, Tak-Diamand Z, VanLeeuwen-Wallau AG. Dust-like particles: a specific direct immunofluorescence pattern in subacute cutaneous lupus erythematosus. *Br J Dermatol* 1988;118:725.
173. Roujeau JC, Andre C, Bertoulus S, et al. Lupus cutane subaigu: etude critique.*Ann Med Interne* 1987;138:592.
174. Weinstein CL, Littlejohn GO, Thomson NM, et al. Severe visceral disease in subacute cutaneous lupus erythematosus. *Arch Dermatol* 1987;123:638.
175. Bangert JL, Freeman RG, Sontheimer RD, et al. Subacute cutaneous lupus erythematosus and discoid lupus erythematosus: comparative histopathologic findings. *Arch Dermatol* 1984;120:332.
176. Nishikawa T, Provost TT. Differences in clinical, serologic, and immunogenetic features of white versus Oriental anti-Ro/SS-A positive patients. *J Am Acad Dermatol* 1991;25:563–564.
177. Sontheimer RD. Subacute cutaneous lupus erythematosus. *Clin Dermatol* 1985;3:58.
178. Massone C, Parodi A, Rebora A. Erythema multiforme-like subacute cutaneous lupus erythematosus: a new variety? *Arch Derm Venerol* 2000;80: 308–309.
179. Grant JM. Annular vesicular lupus erythematosus. *Cutis* 1981;28:90.
180. Wechsler HL, Stavrides A. Systemic lupus erythematosus with anti-Ro antibodies: clinical, histologic and immunologic findings. *J Am Acad Dermatol* 1982;6:73.
181. Beilsa I, Herrero C, Font J, et al. Lupus erythematosus and toxic epidermal necrolysis. *J Am Acad Dermatol* 1987;16;1265.
182. DeSpain J, Clark DP. Subacute cutaneous lupus erythematosus presenting as erythroderma. *J Am Acad Dermatol* 1988;19:388.
183. Scheinman PL. Acral subacute cutaneous lupus erythematosus: an unusual variant. *J Am Acad Dermatol* 1994;30:800.
184. Caproni M, Cardinali C, Salvatore E, et al. Subacute cutaneous lupus erythematosus with pityriasis-like cutaneous manifestations. *Int J Dermatol* 2001; 40:50–66.
185. Charley MR, Sontheimer RD. Clearing of subacute cutaneous lupus erythematosus around molluscum contagiosum lesions. *J Am Acad Dermatol* 1982; 66:529.
186. Sontheimer RD. Clinical significance of subacute cutaneous lupus erythematosus skin lesions. *J Dermatol* 1985;12:205.
187. Sanchez-Perez J, Fernandez-Herrera J, Sols M, et al. Leucocytoclastic vasculitis in subacute cutaneous lupus erythematosus. *Br J Dermatol* 1993;128: 469.
188. Provost TT, Watson RM, Simmons-O'Brien E. Anti Ro (SS-A) antibody positive Sjogren's/lupus erythematosus overlap syndrome. *Lupus* 1997;6:105–111.
189. Cohen LM, Tyring SK, Rady P, et al. Human papillomavirus type 11 in multiple squamous cell carcinomas in a patient with subacute cutaneous lupus erythematosus. *J Am Acad Dermatol* 1992;26S:840.
190. George R, Mathai R, Kurian S. Cutaneous lupus erythematosus in India: immunofluorescence profile. *Int J Dermatol* 1992;31:265.
191. Abe M, Ishikowa O, Miyachi Y. Linear cutaneous lupus erythematosus following the lines of Blashko. *Br J Dermatol* 1998;139:307–310.
192. Wilson CL, Burge SM, Dean D, et al. Scarring alopecia in discoid lupus erythematosus. *Br J Dermatol* 1992;126:307.
193. Ashinoff R, Werth VP, Franks AG Jr. Resistant discoid lupus erythematosus of palms and soles: successful treatment with azathioprine. *J Am Acad Dermatol* 1988;19:961.
194. Parrish LC, Kennedy RJ, Hurley HJ. Palmar lesions in lupus erythematosus. *Arch Dermatol* 1967;96:273.
195. Wong KO. Systemic lupus erythematosus: a report of 45 cases with unusual clinical and immunological features. *Br J Dermatol* 1969;81:186–190.
196. Lodin A. Discoid lupus erythematosus and trauma. *Acta Derm Venereol (Stockh)* 1963;43:142–146.
197. Wolska H, Blaszczyk M, Jablonska S. Phototests in patients with various forms of lupus erythematosus. *Int J Dermatol* 1989;28:98.
198. Velthuis PJ, Van Weelden H, Van Wichen D, et al. Immunohistopathology of light-induced skin lesions in lupus erythematosus. *Acta Derm Venereol (Stockh)* 1990;70:93.
199. Lehmann P, Holzle E, Kind P, et al. Experimental reproduction of skin lesions in lupus erythematosus by UVA and UVB radiation. *J Am Acad Dermatol* 1990;22:181.
200. Nived O, Johansen PB, Sturfelt G. Standardized ultraviolet-A exposure provokes skin reaction in systemic lupus erythematosus. *Lupus* 1993;2:247.
201. Kanwar J, Dhar S, Ghosh S. Involvement of nails in discoid lupus erythematosus. *J Assoc Phys India* 1993;41:543.
202. Romero RW, Nesbitt LT Jr, Reed RJ. Unusual variant of lupus erythematosus on lichen planus: clinical, histopathologic and immunofluorescence studies. *Arch Dermatol* 1977;113:741.
203. Camisa C. Lichen planus and related conditions. *Adv Dermatol* 1987;2:47.
204. Perniciaro C, Randle HW, Perry HO. Hypertrophic discoid lupus erythematosus resembling squamous cell carcinoma. *Dermatol Surg* 1995;21: 255–257.
205. Dammert K. Lupus erythematosus hypertrophicus et profundus. *Acta Derm Venereol (Stockh)* 1971;52:315.
206. Otani A. Lupus erythematosus hypertrophicus et profundus. *Br J Dermatol* 1977;96:75.
207. Winkelmann RK. Panniculitis in connective tissue disease. *Arch Dermatol* 1983;119:336.
208. Irgang S. Lupus erythematosus profundus. *Arch Dermatol Syphilol* 1940;42:97.
209. Kundig TM, Trueb RM, Krasovec M. Lupus profundus/panniculitis. *Dermatology* 1997;195:99–101.
210. Peters MS, Su WPD. Lupus erythematosus panniculitis. *Med Clin North Am* 1989;73:1113.
211. Tuffanelli DL. Lupus erythematosus. *Arch Dermatol* 1972;106:553.
212. Ishikawa O, Akimoto M, Sato Y, et al. Xanthomatous reaction in lupus panniculitis. *Acta Derm Venerol* 1996;76:411–412.
213. Sheehan-Dore RA, Cunliffe WJ. Severe periorbital oedema in association with lupus erythematosus profundus. *Clin Exp Dermatol* 1988;6:406–407.
214. Magee KL, Hymes SR, Rapini RP, et al. Lupus erythematosus profundus with periorbital swelling and proptosis. *J Am Acad Drematol* 1991;24:288–290.
215. Tada J, Arata J, Katayama H. Linear lupus erythematosus profundus in a child. *J Am Acad Dermatol* 1991;24:871.
216. Stork J, Vasmik F. Lupus erythematosus panniculitis with morphea-like lesions. *Clin Exp Dermatol* 1994;19:79–82.
217. Harris RB, Winkelmann RK. Lupus mastitis. *Arch Dermatol* 1978;114:410.

218. Tuffanelli DL. Lupus erythematosus panniculitis (profundus). *Arch Dermatol* 1971;103:231.
219. Jonsson R, Heyden G, Westberg NG, et al. Oral mucosa lesions in SLE: a clinical, histopathological and immunopathological study. *J Rheumatol* 1984;11:38.
220. Schiodt M. Oral discoid lupus erythematosus, III: a histopathologic study of sixty-six patients. *Oral Surg* 1984;57:281.
221. Schiodt M. Oral manifestations of lupus erythematosus. *Int J Oral Surg* 1984;13:101.
222. Ortea CH, Buchanan JAG, Hutchinson I, et al. Systemic lupus erythematosus presenting with oral mucosal lesions: easily missed? *Br J Dermatol* 2001; 144:1219–1223.
223. Tuffanelli DL, Dubois EL. Cutaneous manifestations of systemic lupus erythematosus. *Arch Dermatol* 1964;90:377.
224. Burge SM, Frith PA, Juniper RP, et al. Mucosal involvement in systemic and chronic cutaneous lupus erythematosus. *Br J Dermatol* 1989;121:727.
225. Urman JD, et al. Oral mucosal ulceration in systemic lupus erythematosus. *Arthritis Rheum* 1978;21:58–62.
226. Andreasen JO, Poulsen HE. Oral discoid and systemic lupus erythematosus, I: clinical investigation. *Acta Odont Scand* 1964;22:295.
227. Alcala H, Alarcon-Segovia D. Ulceration and perforation of the nasal septum in systemic lupus erythematosus. *N Engl J Med* 1969;281:722.
228. Rothfield NF. Nasal septum perforation in systemic lupus erythematosus. *N Engl J Med* 1974;291:51.
229. Vachtenheim J, Grossman J. Perforation of the nasal septum in systemic lupus erythematosus. *BMJ* 1969;2:98.
230. Robson AK, Burge SM, Millard PR. Nasal mucosal involvement in lupus erythematosus. *Clin Otolaryngol* 1992;17:341.
231. Frith P, Burge SM, Millard PR, et al. External ocular findings in lupus erythematosus: a clinical and immunopathological study. *Br J Ophthalmol* 1990; 74:163.
232. Meiusi RS, Cameron JD, Holland EJ, et al. Discoid lupus erythematosus of the eyelid complicated by wound dehiscence. *Am J Ophthalmol* 1991;111:108.
233. Bettis VM, Vaughn RY, Guill MA. Erythematous plaques on the eyelids: discoid lupus erythematosus (DLE). *Arch Dermatol* 1993;129:497.
234. Raizman MB, Baum J. Discoid lupus keratitis. *Arch Ophthalmol* 1989;107:545.
235. Millard LG, Rowell NR. Chilblain lupus erythematosus (Hutchinson). *Br J Dermatol* 1978;98:497.
236. Viquier M, Pinquier L, Cavelier-Balloy B, et al. Clinical and histopathologic features and immunologic variables in patients with severe chilblains. *Medicine* 2001;80:180–188.
237. Aoki T, Ishizawa T, Hozumi Y, et al. Chilblain lupus erythematosus of Hutchinson responding to surgical treatment: a report of two patients with acute Ro/SS-A antibodies. *Br J Dermatol* 1996;134:533–537.
238. Franceschini F, Calzavara-Pinton P, Quinzanini M, et al. Chilblain lupus erythematosus is associated with antibodies to SS-A/Ro. *Lupus* 1999;8:215–219.
239. Doutre MS, Beylot C, Beylot J, et al. Chilblain lupus erythematosus: report of 15 cases. *Dermatology* 1992;184:26.
240. James DG. Sarcoidosis of the skin. In: Fitzpatrick TB, Eisen AZ, Wolff K, et al., eds. *Dermatology and general medicine.* New York: McGraw-Hill, 1987.
240a.Ruiz H, Sanchez JL. Tumid lupus erythematosus. *Am J Dermatopathol.* 1999; 21:356–360.
241. Kuhn A, Sonntag M, Richter-Hintz D, et al. Phototesting in lupus erythematosus tumidus—review of 60 patients. *Photochem Photobio* 2001;73:532–236.
242. Kuhn A, Richter-Hintz D, Oslislo C, et al. Lupus erythematosus tumidus: a neglected subset of cutaneous lupus erythematosus: report of 40 cases. *Arch Dermatol* 2000;136:1033–1041.
243. Gilliam JM, Cohen SB, Sontheimer RD, et al. Connective tissue diseases. In: Moschella SL, Hurley HJ, eds. *Dermatology.* Philadelphia: WB Saunders, 1985: 1087–1135.
244. Nagy E, Balogh E. Bullous form of chronic discoid lupus erythematodes accompanied by L.E. cell symptoms. *Dermatologica* 1961;122:6.
245. Noriko T, Katayama I, Arai H, et al. Annular erythema: a possible association with primary Sjögren's syndrome. *J Am Acad Dermatol* 1989;20:596.
246. Ruzicka T, Faes J, Bergner T, et al. Annular erythema associated with Sjögren's syndrome: a variant of systemic lupus erythematosus. *J Am Acad Dermatol* 1991;25:557.
247. Katayama I, Teramoto N, Arai H, et al. Annular erythema: a comparative study of Sjögren's syndrome with subacute cutaneous lupus erythematosus. *Int J Dermatol* 1991;30:635.
248. Katayama I, Yamamoto T, Otoyama K, et al. Clinical and immunological analysis of annular erythema associated with Sjögren's syndrome. *Dermatology* 1994;189:14.
249. Miyagawa S, Fukumoto I, Matsunaga T, et al. Annular erythema. *Br J Dermatol* 1995;133:779–782.
250. Watanabe T, Tsuchida T, Ito Y, et al. Annular erythema associated with lupus erythematosus/Sjorgen's syndrome. *J Am Acad Dermatol* 1997;36: 214–218.
251. Cohen S, Stastny P, Sontheimer RD. Concurrence of subacute cutaneous lupus erythematosus and rheumatoid arthritis. *Arthritis Rheum* 1986;29:421.
252. Boire G, Menard HA. Clinical significance of anti-Ro(SSA) antibody in rheumatoid arthritis. *J Rheumatol* 1988;15:391.
253. Konstadoulakis MM, Kroubouzos G, Tosca A, et al. Thyroid autoantibodies in the subsets of lupus erythematosus: correlation with other autoantibodies and thyroid function. *Thyroidol Clin Exp* 1993;5:1.
254. Ilan Y, Ben Yehuda A. Subacute cutaneous lupus associated with Hashimoto's thyroiditis. *Neth J Med* 1991;39:105.
255. Blanc D, Kienzler JL. Lupus erythematosus gyratus repens: report of a case associated with lung carcinoma. *Clin Exp Dermatol* 1982;7.129.
256. Kuhn A, Kaufmann I. Subakuter kutaner lupus erythematodes als paraneoplastisches syndrom. *Z Hautkr* 1986;61:581.
257. Neumann R, Schmidt JB, Niebauer G. Subacute lupus erythematosus-like gyrate erythema: report of a case associated with a breast cancer. *Dermatologica* 1986;173:146.
258. Schewach-Millet M, Shapiro D, Ziv R, et al. Subacute cutaneous lupus erythematosus associated with breast carcinoma. *J Am Acad Dermatol* 1988;19:406.
259. McKenna KE, Hayes D, McMillan JC. Subacute cutaneous lupus erythematosus-like gyrate erythema and hypertrichosis lanuginosa acquisita associated with uterine adenocarcinoma. *Br J Dermatol* 1992;127:443.
260. Goette DK. Sweet's syndrome in subacute cutaneous lupus erythematosus. *Arch Dermatol* 1985;121:789.
261. Levenstein MM, Fisher BK, Fisher LL, et al. Simultaneous occurrence of subacute cutaneous lupus erythematosus and Sweet syndrome: a marker of Sjögren syndrome? *Int J Dermatol* 1991;30:640.
262. Katayama I. Subacute lupus erythematosus and Sweet syndrome. *Int J Dermatol* 1992; 1:165.
263. Callen JP, Ross L. Subacute cutaneous lupus erythematosus and porphyria cutanea tarda; report of a case. *J Am Acad Dermatol* 1981;5:269.
264. Messenger AG, Church RE. Subacute cutaneous lupus erythematosus and malabsorption. *Br J Dermatol* 1986;115:56.
265. Ashworth J. Subacute cutaneous lupus erythematosus in a patient with Crohn's disease. *Clin Exp Dermatol* 1992;17:135.
266. Reference deleted in proof.
267. Prystowsky SD, Gilliam JN. Discoid lupus erythematosus as part of a larger disease spectrum: correlation of clinical features with laboratory findings in lupus erythematosus. *Arch Dermatol* 1975;111:1448.
268. Tebbe B, Orfanos CE. Cutaneous lupus erythematosus: an analysis of 97 patients. *Z Hautkr* 1987;15:1563(abstr).
269. Estes D, Christian CL. The natural history of systemic lupus erythematosus by prospective analysis. *Medicine* 1971;50:85.
270. Ganor S, Sagagen F. Systemic lupus erythematosus changing to the chronic discoid type. *Dermatologica* 1962;125:81(abstr).
271. Kulick K, Provost TT, Reichlin M. Antibodies to single stranded DNA in patients with discoid lupus erythematosus. *Arthritis Rheum* 1982;25:639–646.
272. Blum C, Zillikens D, Tony HP, et al. Soluble interleukin 2 receptor as activity parameter in serum of systemic and discoid lupus erythematosus. *Hautarzt* 1993;44:290.
273. Fries JF. The clinical aspects of systemic lupus erythematosus. *Med Clin North Am* 1977;61:229.
274. Spann CR, Callen JP, Klein JB, et al. Clinical, serological and immunogenetic studies in patients with chronic cutaneous (discoid) lupus erythematosus who have verrucous and/or hypertrophic skin lesions. *J Rheumatol* 1988; 15:256.
275. Burnham TK, Fine G. The immunofluorescence "band" test for lupus erythematosus, I: morphologic variations of localized immunoglobulins at the dermal-epidermal junction in lupus erythematosus. *Arch Dermatol* 1969;99:413.
276. Dahl MV, Gilliam JN. Direct immunofluorescence in lupus erythematosus. In: Beutner EH, Chorzelski TP, Kumar V, eds. *Immunopathology of the skin.* New York: John Wiley and Sons, 1987.
277. Cormane RH. Band globulin in the skin of patients with chronic discoid lupus erythematosus and systemic lupus erythematosus. *Lancet* 1964;1:534.
278. Weigand DA. Cutaneous immunofluorescence. *Med Clin North Am* 1989; 73:1263.
279. Dahl MV. Lupus erythematosus and systemic sclerosis. In: Dahl MV, ed. *Clinical immunodermatology.* Boca Raton, FL: Yearbook Medical Publishers, 1988.
280. Ueki H, Wolf HH, Braun-Falco O. Cutaneous localization of human globulins in lupus erythematosus: electron microscopy study using the peroxidase-labeled antibody technique. *Arch Dermatol* Res 1974;248:297.
281. Davis BM, Gilliam JN. Prognostic significance of subepidermal immune deposits in uninvolved skin of patients with systemic lupus erythematosus: a 10-year longitudinal study. *J Invest Dermatol* 1984;83:242.
282. Fabre VC, Lear S, Reichlin M, et al. Twenty percent of biopsy specimens from sun-exposed skin of normal young adults demonstrate positive immunofluorescence. *Arch Dermatol* 1991;127:1006.
283. Brown C, Lieu T-S, Sontheimer RD. Correlation between dermal interstitial immunoglobulin G and hypergammaglobulinemia. *J Invest Dermatol* 1991;97: 373.
284. Ahmed AR, Provost TT. Incidence of a positive lupus band test using sun exposed and unexposed skin. *Arch Dermatol* 1979;115:228?232.
285. Velthuis PJ, Kater L, Van der Tweel I, et al. Immunofluorescence microscopy of healthy skin from patients with systemic lupus erythematosus: more than just the lupus band. *Ann Rheum Dis* 1992;51:720.
286. Burnham TK, Fine G. The immunofluorescent band test for LE, III: employing clinically normal skin. *Arch Dermatol* 1971;103:24.
287. Gilliam JN, Cheatum DE, Hurd ER, et al. Immunoglobulin in clinically uninvolved skin in systemic lupus erythematosus; association with renal disease. *J Clin Invest* 1974;53:1434.
288. Provost TT, Andres G, Maddison PJ, et al. Lupus band test in untreated SLE patients: correlation of immunoglobulin deposition in the skin of the extensor forearm with clinical renal disease and serologic abnormalities. *J Invest Dermatol* 1980;74:407.

289. Rothfield N, Marino C. Studies of repeat skin biopsies of nonlesional skin in patients subacute cutaneous lupus erythematosus. *Arthritis Rheum* 1982;25:624.
290. Carvalho MF, Coelho RA. Lupus band test: diagnostic value in disseminated lupus erythematosus [in Portuguese]. *Acta Med Port* 1991;4:242.
291. Pennebaker JB, Gilliam JN, Ziff M. Immunoglobulin classes of DNA binding activity in serum and skin in systemic lupus erythematosus. *J Clin Invest* 1977;60:1331.
292. Weinstein C, Miller MH, Axtens R, et al. Lupus and non lupus cutaneous manifestations in systemic lupus erythematosus. *Aust NZ J Med* 1987;17:501.
293. Pohle EL, Tuffanelli DL. Study of cutaneous lupus erythematosus by immunohistochemical methods. *Arch Dermatol* 1968;97:520.
294. Bielsa I, Herrero C, Collado A, et al. Histopathologic findings in cutaneous lupus erythematosus. *Arch Dermatol* 1994;130:54.
295. Hood AF, Jerden MS, Moore W, et al. Histopathologic comparison of the subsets of lupus erythematosus. *Arch Dermatol* 1990;126:52.
296. Valeski JE, Kumar V, Forman AB, et al. A characteristic cutaneous direct immunofluorescent pattern associated with Ro(SS-A) antibodies in subacute cutaneous lupus erythematosus. *J Am Acad Dermatol* 1992;27:194.
297. Fabbri P, Bernacchi E, Neri R. Subacute cutaneous lupus erythematosus: review of the literature and immunological studies of 11 patients. *G Ital Dermatol Venereol* 1990;125.329.
298. Lee LA, Gaither KG, Coulter SN, et al. The pattern of cutaneous immunoglobulin G deposition in subacute cutaneous lupus erythematosus is reproduced by infusing purified anti-Ro (SSA) antibodies into human skin grafted mice. *J Clin Invest* 1989;83:1556.
299. Weigand DA. Lupus band test: anatomically regional variations in discoid lupus erythematosus. *J Am Acad Dermatol* 1986;14:426.
300. Burnham TK, Mohr RH. *Atlas of diagnostic immunofluorescence. Descriptive morphology and diagnostic significance of direct and indirect cutaneous immunofluorescence of the nuclear immunofluorescent patterns.* Evanston, IL: American Academy of Dermatology, 1991.
301. Dahl MV. Usefulness of direct immunofluorescence in patients with lupus erythematosus. *Arch Dermatol* 1983;119:1010.
302. Sanchez NP, Petrs MS, Winkelman RK. The histopathology of lupus erythematosus panniculitis. *J Am Acad Dermatol* 1981;5:673.
303. David-Bajar KM, Davis BM. Pathology, immunopathology, and immunochistochemistry in cutaneous lupus erythematosus. *Lupus* JID – 9204265 1997;6:145–157.
304. Dekle CL, Mannes KD, Kavis LS, et al. Lupus tumidus. *J Am Acad Dermatol* 1999;41[2 Pt 1]:250–253.
305. Lee LA, Roberts CM, Frank MB, et al. The autoantibody response to Ro/SSA in cutaneous lupus erythematosus. *Arch Dermatol* 1994;130:1262.
306. Yamagata H, Harley JB, Reichlin M. Molecular properties of the Ro/SS-A antigen and enzyme-linked immunosorbent assay for quantitation of antibody. *J Clin Invest* 1984;74:625.
307. Fonseca E, Alvarez R, Gonzalez MR, et al. Prevalence of anticardiolipin antibodies in subacute cutaneous lupus erythematosus. *Lupus* 1992;1:265.
308. Arnett FC, Olsen ML, Anderson KL, et al. Molecular analysis of major histocompatibility complex alleles associated with lupus anticoagulant. *J Clin Invest* 1991;87:1490–1495.
309. Marschalko M, Dobozy E, Daroczy J, et al. Subacute cutaneous lupus erythematosus: a study of 15 cases. *Orvosi Hetilap* 1989;130:2623.
310. Holtman JH, Neustadt DH, Klein J, et al. Dapsone is an effective therapy for the skin lesions of subacute cutaneous lupus erythematosus and urticarial vasculitis in a patient with C2 deficiency. *J Rheumatol* 1990;17:1222.
311. Callen JP, Fowler JF, Kulick KB. Serologic and clinical features of patients with discoid lupus erythematosus: relationship of antibodies to single-stranded deoxyribonucleic acid and of other antinuclear antibody subsets to clinical manifestations. *J Am Acad Dermatol* 1985;13:748.
312. Provost TT, Ratrie H. Autoantibodies and autoantigens in lupus erythematosus and Sjögren's syndrome. *Curr Probl Dermatol* 1990;2:150.
313. Mayou SC, Wojnarowska F, Lovell CR, et al. Anticardiolipin and antinuclear antibodies in discoid lupus erythematosus?their clinical significance. *Clin Exp Dermatol* 1988;13:389.
314. Stonecipher MR, Callen JP, Jorizzo JL. The red face: dermatomyositis. *Clin Dermatol* 1993;11:261.
315. Jablonska S, Blaszczyk-Kostanecka M, Chorzelski T, et al. The red face: lupus erythematosus. *Clin Dermatol* 1993;11:253.
316. Boyd AS, Zemtsov A, Neldner KH. Pityriasis rubra pilaris presenting as subacute cutaneous lupus erythematosus. *Cutis* 1993;52:177.
317. Chen DY, Lan JL. Crusted scabies in systematic lupus erythematosus: a case report. *Chung-Hua Min Kuo Wei Sheng Wu Chi Mien I Hsuech Tsa Chih (Chin J Microbiol Immunol (Taipei))* 1993;26:44.
318. Sehgal VN, Jain S, Jain VK. Lupus vulgaris simulating discoid lupus erythematosus. *Int J Dermatol* 1991;30:498.
319. Chung G, Kantor GR, Whipple S. Tertiary syphilis of the face. *J Am Acad Dermatol* 1991;24:832.
320. Uitto J, Santa-Cruz DJ, Eisen AJ, et al. Verrucous lesions in patients with discoid lupus erythematosus: clinical, histopathological and immunofluorescence studies. *Br J Dermatol* 1978;98:507.
321. A randomized study of the effect of withdrawing hydroxychloroquine sulfate in systemic lupus erythematosus. Canadian Hydroxychloroquine Study Group. *N Engl J Med* 1991;324:150.
321a. Ting WW and Sontheimer RD. Local therapy for cutaneous and systemic lupus erythematosus: practical and theoretical considerations. *Lupus* 2001;10: 171–184.
322. Sontheimer RD. Lupus erythematosus. In: Provost TT, Farmer ER, eds. *Current therapy in dermatology.* Philadelphia: BC Decker, 1988.
323. Lowe NJ. Photoprotection. *Semin Dermatol* 1990;9:78.
324. Callen JP, Roth DE, McGrath C, et al. Safety and efficacy of a broad-spectrum sunscreen in patients with discoid or subacute cutaneous lupus erythematosus. *Cutis* 1991;47:130.
325. Kawada A, Hiruma M, Nakada R, et al. An evaluation of broad-spectrum sunscreens against topical PUVA-induced erythema. *Acta Derm Venereol (Stockh)* 1989;69:335.
326. Sontheimer RD. Fluorescent light photosensitivity in patients with systemic lupus erythematosus: comment on the article by Rihner and McGrath. *Arthritis Rheum* 1993;36:428.
327. Furner BB. Treatment of subacute cutaneous lupus erythematosus. *Int J Dermatol* 1990;29:542.
328. Lanham JG, Hughes GRV. Antimalarial therapy in SLE. *Clin Rheum Dis* 1982;8:279.
329. Trenholme GM, Carson PE. Therapy and prophylaxis of malaria. *J Am Med Assoc* 1978;240:2293.
329a. Marmor MF, Carr Re, Easterbrook M, et al. American Academy of Ophthalmology recommendations on screening for chloroquine and hydroxychloroquine retinopathy: a report by the American Academy of Ophthalmology. *Opthalmology* 2002;109:1377–82.
330. Wallace DJ. The use of quinacrine (Atabrine) in rheumatic diseases: a reexamination. *Semin Arthritis Rheum* 1989;18:282.
330a. Dubois EL, Wallace DJ, Tuffanelli DL, Epstein JH. The relationship between discoid and systemic lupus erythematosus. In: Wallace DJ, Dubois EL, eds. *Dubois Lupus Erythematosus*. 3rd ed. Philadelphia: Lea & Febiger; 1987:302–313.
331. Feldmann R, Salomon D, Saurat J-H. The association of the two antimalarials chloroquine and quinacrine for treatment-resistant chronic and subacute cutaneous lupus erythematosus. *Dermatology* 1994;189:425.
332. Fenton DA, Black MM. Low-dose dapsone in the treatment of subacute cutaneous lupus erythematosus. *Clin Exp Dermatol* 1986;11:102.
333. McCormack LS, Elgart ML, Turner ML. Annular subacute cutaneous lupus erythematosus responsive to dapsone. *J Am Acad Dermatol* 1984;11:397.
334. Ruzicka T, Meurer M, Braun-Falco O. Treatment of cutaneous lupus erythematosus with etretinate. *Acta Derm Venereol (Stockh)* 1985;65:324.
335. Newton RC, Jorizzo JL, Solomon AR, et al. Mechanism-oriented assessment of isotretinoin in chronic or subacute lupus erythematosus. *Arch Dermatol* 1986;122:170.
336. Ruzicka T, Meurer M, Bieber T. Efficacy of acitretin in the treatment of cutaneous lupus erythematosus. *Arch Dermatol* 1988;124:897.
337. Furner BB. Subacute cutaneous lupus erythematosus response to isotretinoin. *Int J Dermatol* 1990;29:587.
338. Green SG, Piette WW. Successful treatment of hypertrophic lupus erythematosus with isotretinoin. *J Am Acad Dermatol* 1987;17:364.
339. Crovato F. Clofazimine in the treatment of annular lupus erythematosus. *Arch Dermatol* 1981;117:249.
340. McDougall AC, Horsfall WR, Hede JE, et al. Splenic infarction and tissue accumulation of crystals associated with the use of clofazimine (Lamprene B663) in the treatment of pyoderma gangrenosus. *Br J Dermatol* 1980;102:227.
341. Naafs B, Bakkers EJM, Flinterman J, et al. Thalidomide treatment of subacute cutaneous lupus erythematosus. *Br J Dermatol* 1982;107:83.
342. Knop J, Bonsmann G, Happle R, et al. Thalidomide in the treatment of sixty cases of chronic discoid lupus erythematosus. *Br J Dermatol* 1983;108:461.
343. Volc-Platzer B, Wolff K. Treatment of subacute cutaneous lupus erythematosus with thalidomide. *Der Hautarzt* 1983;34:175.
344. Holm AL, Bowers KE, McMeekin TO, et al. Chronic cutaneous lupus erythematosus treated with thalidomide. *Arch Dermatol* 1993;129:1548.
345. Ordi-Los J, Cortes F, Cucurull E, et al. Thalidomide in the treatment of cutaneous lupus refractory to conventional therapy. *J Rheumatol* 2000;27: 1429–1431.
345a. Piette JC, Sbai A, and Frances C. Warning: thalidomide-related thrombotic risk potentially concerns patients with lupus. *Lupus* 2002;11:67–70.
346. LaDuca JR, Gaspari AA. Targeting tumor necrosis factor alpha: new drugs used to modulate inflammatory diseases. *Dermal Clin* 2001;19:617–635.
346a. Fautrel B, Foltz V, Frances C, et al. Regression of subacute cutaneous lupus erythematosus in a patient with rheumatoid arthritis treated with a biologic tumor necrosis factor alpha-blocking agent: comment on the article by Pisetsky and the letter from Aringer et al. *Arthritis Rheum* 2002;46:1408–1409.
347. Shakoor N, Michalska M, Harris CA, et al. Drug-induced systemic lupus erythematosus associated with etanercept therapy. *Lancet* 2002;359:579–580.
348. Ali Y, Shah S. Infliximab-induced systemic lupus erythematosus. *Ann Intern Med* 2002;137:625–626.
349. Haxthausen H. Treatment of lupus erythematosus by intravenous injections of gold chloride. *Arch Dermatol* 1930;22:77.
350. Dalziel K, Going G, Cartwright PH, et al. Treatment of chronic discoid lupus erythematosus with an oral gold compound (Auranofin). *Br J Dermatol* 1986;115:211.
351. Goldberg JW, Lidsky MD. Pulse methylprednisolone therapy for persistent subacute cutaneous lupus. *Arthritis Rheum* 1984;27:837.
352. Callen JP, Spencer LV, Bhatnagar Burruss J, et al. Azathioprine: an effective, corticosteroid-sparing therapy for patients with recalcitrant cutaneous lupus erythematosus or with recalcitrant cutaneous leukocytoclastic vasculitis. *Arch Dermatol* 1991;127:515.
353. McGrath H Jr, Bak E, Zimny ML, et al. Fluorescent light decreases autoim-

munity and improves immunity in B/W mice. *J Clin Lab Immunol* 1990;32: 113.

354. McGrath H Jr. Ultraviolet-A1 irradiation decreases clinical disease activity and autoantibodies in patients with systemic lupus erythematosus. *Clin Exp Rheumatol* 1994;12:29.
355. Sonnichsen N, Meffert H, Kunzelmann V, et al. UV-A-1 therapy of subacute cutaneous lupus erythematosus. *Hautarzt* 1993;44:723.
356. Handy CJ, Palmer BP, Muir KR, et al. Smoking history, alcohol consumption, and systemic lupus erythematosus: a case-control study. *Ann Rheum Dis* 1998;57:451–455.
357. Jewell ML, McCauliffe DP. Patients with cutaneous lupus erythematosus who smoke are less responsive to antimalarial treatment. *J Am Acad Dermatol* 2000;42:983–987.
358. Rahman p, Gladman DD, Urowitz MB. Smoking interferes with efficacy of antimalarial therapy in cutaneous lupus. *J Rheumatol* 1998;25:1716–1719.
359. Miller LG. Cigarettes and drug therapy: pharmacokinetic and pharmacodynamic considerations. *Clin Pharmacol* 1990;9:125.
360. Ruzicka T, Goerz G. Dapsone in the treatment of lupus erythematosus. *Br J Dermatol* 1981;104:53.
361. Callen JP. Treatment of cutaneous lesions in patients with lupus erythematosus. *Dermatol Clin* 1994;12:201.
362. Shornick JK, Formica N, Parke AL. Isotretinoin for refractory lupus erythematosus. *J Am Acad Dermatol* 1991;24:49.
363. Mackey JP, Barnes J. Clofazimine in the treatment of discoid lupus erythematosus. *Br J Dermatol* 1974;91:93.
364. Krivanek KJ, Paver SK, Kossard S, et al. Clofazimine (Lamprene) in the treatment of discoid lupus erythematosus. *Aust J Dermatol* 1976;17:108.
365. Kossard S, Doherty E, McColl I, et al. Autofluorescence of clofazimine in discoid lupus erythematosus. *J Am Acad Dermatol* 1987;17:867.
366. Burrows NP, Walport MJ, Hammond AH, et al. Lupus erythematosus profundus with partial C4 deficiency responding to thalidomide. *Br J Dermatol* 1991;125:62.
367. Goldstein E, Carey W. Discoid lupus erythematosus: successful treatment with oral methotrexate. *Arch Dermatol* 1994;130:938.
368. Chung HS, Honn SK. Lupus panniculitis treated by a combination therapy of hydroxychloroquine and quinacrive. *J Dermatol* 1997;24:569–572.
369. Sorg C. Macrophages in acute and chronic inflammation. *Chest* 1991;100: 173S.
370. Irgang S. Lupus erythematosus profundus: report of an example with clinical resemblance to Darier-Roussy sarcoid. *Arch Dermatol Syphilol* 1940;42:98.
371. Goyal S, Nousari HC. Treatment of resistant discoid lupus erythematosus of the palms and soles with mycophenolate mofetil. *J Am Acad Dermatol* 2001;45:142–144.
372. Kurwa AR, Evans AJ. Discoid lupus erythematosus treated by dermabrasion. *Br J Dermatol* 1979;101:53S.
373. Roenigk HH Jr, Martin JS, Eichorn P, et al. Discoid lupus erythematosus: diagnostic features and evaluation of topical corticosteroid therapy. *Cutis* 1980;25:281.
374. Pinski KS, Roenigk HH Jr. Autologous fat transplantation: long-term follow-up. *J Dermatol Surg Oncol* 1992;18:179.
375. Tremblay JF, Carey W. Atrophic facial scars secondary to discoid lupus erythematosus: treatment using the Erbium:YAG laser. *Dermatol Surg* 2001;27: 675–677.
376. Walker SL, Harland CC. Carbon dioxide laser resurfacing of facial scarring secondary to chronic discoid lupus erythematosus. *Br J Dermatol* 2000;143: 1101–1102.

376a. Chlebus E, Wolska H, Blaszczyk M, Jablonska S. Subacute cutaneous lupus erythematosus versus systemic lupus erythematosus—diagnostic criteria and therapeutic options. *J Am Acad Dermato.* 1998;38:405–412.

377. de Berker D, Dissaneyeka M, Burge S. The sequelae of chronic cutaneous lupus erythematosus. *Lupus* 1992;1:181.
378. Wolstenholme GEW. Epithelioma arising on lupus erythematosus. *Br J Dermatol* 1949;61:126.
379. de Castelbajac D, Guillaume JC, Prost C, et al. Chronic lupus erythematosus and epidermoid carcinoma. *Ann Dermatol Venereol* 1990;117:876.
380. Voigtlander V, Boonen H. Squamous cell carcinoma of the lower lip in discoid lupus erythematosus associated with hereditary deficiency of complement 2. *Z Hautkr* 1990;65:836.
381. Sherman RN, Lee CW, Flynn KJ. Cutaneous squamous cell carcinoma in black patients with chronic discoid lupus erythematosus. *Int J Dermatol* 1993; 32:677.
382. Druz PD, Bergstresser PR. Antigen processing and presentation by epidermal Langerhans cells. *Dermatol Clin* 1990;8:633.
383. Millard TP, McGregor JM. Molecular genetics of cutaneous lupus erythematosus. *Clin Exp Dermatol* 2001;26:184–191.
384. Furukawa F, Ikai K, Matsuyoshi N, et al. Relationship between heat shock protein induction and the binding of antibodies to the extractable nuclear antigens on cultured human keratinocytes. *J Invest Dermatol* 1993;101: 191–195.
385. Blakemore AI, Tarlow JK, Cork MJ, et al. Interleukin-1 receptor antagonist gene polymorphism as a disease severity factor in systemic lupus erythematosus. *Arthritis Rheum* 1994;37:1380–1385.
386. Suzuki H, Matsui Y, Kashiwagi H. Interleukin-1 receptor antagonist gene polymorphism in Japenese patients with systemic lupus erythematosus. *Arthritis Rheum* 1997;40:389–390.
387. James JA, Kaufman KM, Farris AD, et al. An increased prevalence of Epstein-Barr virus infection in young patients suggests a possible etiology for systemic lupus erythematosus. *J Clin Invest* 1997;100:3019–3026.
388. Ioannides D, Golden BD, Buyon JP, et al. Expression of SS-A/Ro and SS-B/La antigens in skin biopsy specimens of patients with photosensitive forms of lupus erythematosus. *Arch Dermatol* 2000;136:340–346.
389. Numi Y, Ioannides D, Buyon D, et al. Heterogeneity of expression of Ro and La antigens in human skin. *Arth Rheum* 1995;38:1271–1276.
390. Furukawa F, Lyons MB, Lee L, et al. Estradiol enhances binding to cultured human keratinocytes of antibodies specific for SS-A/Ro and SS-B/la. *J Immunol* 1988;141:1480.
391. Furkawa F, Kashihara-Sawami M, Lyons MB, et al. Binding of antibodies to the extractable nuclear antigens SS-A/Ro and SS-B/la is induced on the surface of human keratinocytes by ultraviolet light (UVL): implications for the pathogenesis of photosensitive cutaneous lupus. *J Invest Dermatol* 1990;94: 77–85.
392. Jones SK. Ultraviolet radiation (UVR) induces cell-surface Ro/SSA antigen expression by human keratinocytes *in vitro*: a possible mechanism for the UVR induction of cutaneous lupus lesions. *Br J Dermatol* 1992;126:546.
393. Golan TD, Elkon KB, Gharavi AE, et al. Enhanced membrane binding of autoantibodies to cultured keratinocytes of systemic lupus erythematosus patients after ultraviolet B/ultraviolet A irradiation. *J Clin Invest* 1992;90:1067.
394. Kawashima T, Lieu T-S, Zappi E, et al. Regulation of expression of the polypeptide constituents of the Roa autoantigen complex in transformed human epidermal keratinocytes. *Lupus* 1994;3:493.
395. Davis TL, Lyde CB, Davis BM, et al. Pertubation of experimental ultraviolet light-induced erythema by passive transfer of serum from subacute cutaneous lupus erythematosus patients. *J Invest Dermatol* 1989;92:573.
396. Iacobelli D, Bianchi L, Hashimoto K. Passive transfer of photosensitivity by intradermal injection of vesculobullous lupus erythematosus serum and ultraviolet light irradiation in the guinea pig. *Photodermatology* 1987;4:288.

396a. Gilliam JN. Immunopathology and Pathogenesis of Cutaneous Lupus Erythematosus. In: Safai B, Good RA, eds. *Comparative Immunology: Immunodermatology*. New York: Plenum Publishing Corporaion; 1981:323–332.

397. Neish C, Charley M, Fertig N, et al. Elevated serum soluble interleukin-2 receptor levels in subacute cutaneous lupus erythematosus. *J Dermatol Sc* 1993;5:143.
398. Andrews BS, Schenk A, Barr R, et al. Immunopathology of cutaneous human lupus erythematosus defined by murine monoclonal antibodies. *J Am Acad Dermatol* 1986;15:474.
399. Shiohara T, Moriya N, Tanaka Y, et al. Immunopathologic study of lichenoid skin diseases: correlation between HLA-DR-positive keratinocytes or Langerhans cells and epidermotropic T cells. *J Am Acad Dermatol* 1988;18:67–74.
400. Tebbe B, Mazur L, Stadler R, et al. Immunohistochemical analysis of chronic discoid and subacute cutaneous lupus erythematosus: relation to immunopathological mechanisms. *Br J Dermatol* 1995;132:25–31.
401. Denfeld RW, Kind P, Sontheimer RD, et al. *In situ* expression of B7 and CD28 receptor families in skin lesions of patients with lupus erythematosus. *Arthritis Rheum* 1997;40:814–821.
402. Sontheimer RD, Bergstresser PR. Epidermal Langerhans cell involvement in cutaneous lupus erythematosus. *J Invest Dermatol* 1982;79:237.
403. Lehmann P, Holzle E, Kind P, et al. Experimental reproduction of skin lesions in lupus erythematosus by UVA and UVB radiation. *J Am Acad Dermatol* 1990;22:181.
404. Konttinen YT, Reitamo S, Ranki A, et al. T lymphocytes and mononuclear phagocytes in the skin infiltrate of systemic and discoid lupus erythematosus and Jessner's lymphocytic infiltrate. *Br J Dermatol* 1981;104:141.
405. Bjerke JR, Krogh H-K, Matre R. *In situ* identification of mononuclear cells in cutaneous infiltrates in discoid lupus erythematosus, sarcoidosis and secondary syphilis. *Acta Derm Venereol (Stockh)* 1981;61:371.
406. Synkowski DR, Provost TT. Characterization of the inflammatory infiltrate in lupus erythematosus lesions. *J Rheumatol* 1983;10:920.
407. Viljaranta S, Ranki A, Kariniemi A-L, et al. Distribution of natural killer cells and lymphocyte subclasses in Jessner's lymphocytic infiltration of the skin and in cutaneous lesions of discoid and systemic lupus erythematosus. *Br J Dermatol* 1987;116:831.
408. Bergroth V, Konttinen YT, Piirainen H, et al. Evaluation of lymphocyte activation in skin lesions of patients with mixed connective tissue disease and discoid lupus erythematodes. *Arch Dermatol Res* 1988;280:1.
409. Markey AC, Allen MH, Pitzalis C, et al. T-cell inducer populations in cutaneous inflammation: a predominance of T helper-inducer lymphocytes (THi) in the infiltrate of inflammatory dermatoses. *Br J Dermatol* 1990;122:325.
410. Rijlaarsdam JU, Nieboer C, de Vries E, et al. Characterization of the dermal infiltrates in Jessner's lymphocytic infiltrate of the skin, polymorphous light eruption and cutaneous lupus erythematosus: differential diagnostic and pathogenetic aspects. *J Cutan Pathol* 1990;17:2.
411. Hodge SJ, Freeman RG. The basal lamina in skin disease. *Int J Dermatol* 1978;17:261.
412. Fivenson DP, Rheins LA, Nordlund JJ, et al. Thy-1 and T-cell receptor antigen expression in mycosis fungoides and benign inflammatory dermatoses. *J Natl Cancer Inst* 1991;83:1088.
413. Volc-Platzer B, Anegg B, Milota S, Pickl W, Fischer G. Accumulation of gamma* T cells in chronic cutaneous erythematosus. *J Invest Dermatol* 1993; 100:84S.
414. Shiohara T, Moriya N, Tsuchiya K, et al. Lichenoid tissue reaction induced by local transfer of Ia-reactive T-cell clones. *J Invest Dermatol* 1986;87:33.
415. Charley MR, Bangert JL, Hamilton BL, et al. Murine graft-versus-host skin

disease: a chronologic and quantitative analysis of two histologic patterns. *J Invest Dermatol* 1983;81:412.
416. De Jong EMGJ, Van Erp PEJ, Ruiter DJ, et al. Immunohistochemical detection of proliferation and differentiation in discoid lupus erythematosus. *J Am Acad Dermatol* 1991;25:1032.
417. Boyd AS, Neldner KH. The isomorphic response of Koebner. *Int J Dermatol* 1990;29:401.
418. Barnett JH. Discoid lupus erythematosus exacerbated by contact dermatitis. *Cutis* 1990;46:430.
419. Ueki H. Koebner phenomenon in lupus erythematosus. *Hautarzt* 1994;45:154.
420. Helm KF, Peters MS. Deposition of membrane attack complex in cutaneous lesions of lupus erythematosus. *J Am Acad Dermatol* 1993;28:687.
421. Landry M, Sams WM. Systemic lupus erythematosus: studies of the antibodies bound to skin. *J Clin Invest* 1973;52:1871.
422. Joselow SA, Mannik M. Localization of preformed, circulating immune complexes in murine skin. *J Invest Dermatol* 1984;82:335.
423. Manabe M, Ogawa H. Ultrastructural demonstration of anionic sites in basement membrane zone by cationic probes. *J Invest Dermatol* 1985;84:19.
424. Cripps DJ, Rankin J. Action spectra of lupus erythematosus and experimental immunofluorescence. *Arch Dermatol* 1973;107:563.
425. Estes D, Christian CL. The natural history of systemic lupus erythematosus by prospective analysis. *Medicine* 1971;50:85–95.
426. Lee P, Urowitz MB, Bookman AA, et al. Systemic lupus erythematosus: a review of 110 cases with reference to nephritis, the nervous system, infections, aseptic necrosis and prognosis. *Q J Med* 1977;46:1–32.
427. Drenkard C, Villa AR, Reves E, et al. Vasculitis in systemic lupus erythematosus. *Lupus* 1997;6:235–242.
428. Grigor R, Edmonds J, Lewkonia R, et al. Systemic lupus erythematosus: a perspective analysis. *Ann Rheum Dis* 1978;37:121–128.
429. Yang SG, Kim KH, Park KC, et al. A case of systemic lupus erythematosus showing acute gangrenous changes of fingertips. *Br J Dermatol* 1996;34: 178–192.
430. Weinstein C, Miller MH, Athens R, et al. Lupus and non-lupus cutaneous manifestations in systemic lupus erythematosus. *Aust N Z J Med* 1987;17: 501–506.
431. Clancy R, Marder G, Martin V, et al. Circulating activated endothelial cells in systemic lupus erythematosus. *Arthritis Rheum* 2001;44:1203–1208.
432. O'Laughlin S, Schroeter AL, Jordon RE. Chronic urticaria-like lesions in systemic lupus erythematosus. *Arch Dermatol* 1978;114:879–883.
433. Provost TT, Zone JJ, Synkowski D, et al. Unusual cutaneous manifestations of systemic lupus erythematosus, I: urticaria-like lesions. *J Invest Dermatol* 1980;75:494–499.
434. Shu U, Mannik M. Low molecular weight C1q binding immunoglobulin G in patients with systemic lupus erythematosus consists of autoantibodies to the collagen-like lesion of C1q. *J Clin Invest* 1988;82: 816–824.
435. Wisnieski JJ, Jones SM. Comparison of autoantibodies to the collagen-like region of C1q in hypocomplementemic urticarial vasculitis syndrome and systemic lupus erythematosus. *J Immunol* 1992;148:1396.
436. Wisnieski JJ. Urticarial vasculitis. *Curr Opin Rheumatol* 2000;12:24–31.
437. Trendelenburg M, Courvoisier S, Spath PJ, et al. Hypo complementenic urticarial vasculitis or systemic lupus erythematosus. *Am J Kidney Dis* 1999;34:745–751.
438. Siegert C, Daha M, Westedt ML, et al. IgG autoantibodies against C1q are correlated with nephritis, hypocomplementimia and dsDNA antibodies in systemic lupus erythematosus. *J Rheumatol* 1991;18:230–234.
439. Trendelenburg M, Marfurt J, Gerber I, et al. Lack of occurrence of severe lupus nephritis among anti-C1q autoantibody negative patients. *Arthritis Rheum* 1999;42:187–188.
440. Korb LC, Ahearn JM. C1q binds directly and specifically to surface blebs on apoptotic human keratinocytes. *J Immunol* 1997;158:4525–4528.
441. Asherson RA, Cruz DD, Stephens CJM, et al. Urticarial vasculitis in a connective tissue disease clinic: patterns, presentations, and treatment. *Semin Arthritis Rheum* 1991;20:285–296.
442. Kohler PF, Percy J, Campion WM, et al. Hereditary angioedema and "familial" lupus erythematosus in identical twins. *Am J Med* 1974;56:406–411.
443. Donaldson VH, Hess EV, McAdams AJ. Lupus erythematosus-like disease in three unrelated women with hereditary angioneurotic edema. *Ann Intern Med* 1977;86:312–313.
444. Guillet G, Sassolas B, Plantin P, et al. Anti-Ro positive lupus and hereditary angioneurotic edema. *Dermatologica* 1988;177:370–375.
445. Duhra P, Holmes J, Porter DI. Discoid lupus erythematosus associated with hereditary angioneurotic edema. *Br J Dermatol* 1990;123:241–244.
446. McNeil HP, Chesterman CN, Krilis SA. Immunology and clinical importance of antiphospholipid antibodies. *Adv Immunol* 1991;49:193–281.
447. Watson R, Kang JE, May M, et al. Thrombocytopenia in the neonatal lupus syndrome. *Arch Dermatol* 1988;124:560–563.
448. Chartask EK, Lans DM, Paget SA, et al. Aortic insufficiency and mitral regurgitation in patients with systemic lupus erythematosus and the antiphospholipid syndrome. *Am J Med* 1989;86:407–412.
449. Khamashta MA, Cervera R, Asherson RA, et al. Association of antibodies against phospholipids with heart valve disease in systemic lupus erythematosus. *Lancet* 1990;335:1541?1544.
450. Rosove MH, Brewer PMC. Antiphospholipid thrombosis: clinical course after the first thrombotic event in 70 patients. *Ann Intern Med* 1992;117:303–308.
451. Ginsburg KS, Leong MH, Newcomer L, et al. Anticardiolipin antibodies and the risk of ischemic stroke and venous thrombosis. *Ann Intern Med* 1992;117: 997–1002.
452. Lockshin MD, Qamar T, Druzin ML, et al. Antibody to cardiolipin, lupus anticoagulant and fetal death. *J Rheumatol* 1987;14:259–262.
453. Ascherson RA, Mayou SC, Merry P et al. The spectrum of livido reticularis and anticardiolipin antibodies. *Br J Dermatol* 1989;120:215–221.
454. Gibson GE, Su WPD, Pittelkow MR. Antiphospholipid antibodies and the skin. *J Am Acad Dermatol* 1997;36:370–382.
455. Acland KM, Dorvay A, Wakelin SH, et al. Livedoid vasculitis: a manifestation of the antiphospholipid syndrome? *Br J Dermatol* 1999;140:131–135.
456. Englert HJ, Hawkes CH, Boey ML, et al. Degos' disease: association with anticardiolipin antibodies and the lupus anticoagulant. *BMJ* 1984;289:576.
457. Asherson RA. The catastrophic antiphospholipid syndrome [editorial]. *J Rheumatol* 1992;19:508–512.
458. Giob JJ, Bonerandi JJ. Cutaneous manifestations associated with the presence of the lupus anticoagulant. *J Am Acad Dermatol* 1986;15:211–219.
459. Black MM, Hudson PM. Atrophie blanche lesions closely resembling malignant atrophic papulosis (Degos' disease) in systemic lupus erythematosus. *Br J Dermatol* 1976;95:649–652.
460. Stevanovic DV. Atrophie blanche. *Arch Dermatol* 1974;109:858–862.
461. Trimble M, Bell DA, Brien W, et al. The antiphospholipid syndrome: prevalence among patients with stroke and transient ischemic attacks. *Am J Med* 1990;88:593–597.
462. Beck RL, Baker WF. Anticardiolipin and thrombosis. *Hematol Oncol Clin North Am* 1992;6:1287–1299.
463. Sneddon JB. Cerebrovascular lesions and livedo reticularis. *Br J Dermatol* 1965;77:180–185.
464. Levine SR, Langer SL, Albers JW, et al. Sneddon's syndrome: an antiphospholipid antibody syndrome. *Neurology* 1988;38:798–800.
465. Coull BM, Levine SR, Brey RL. The role of antiphospholipid antibodies in stroke. *Neurol Clin* 1992;10:125–143.
466. Olsen ML, O'Connor S, Arnett FC, et al. Autoantibodies and rheumatic disorders in a neurology patient population: a prospective study. *Am J Med* 1991;90:479–488.
467. Yasue T. Livedoid vasculitis and central nervous system involvement in systemic lupus erythematosus. *Arch Dermatol* 1986;122:66–70.
468. Asherson RA, Khamashta M, Ordi-Ross, et al."Primary" antiphospholipid syndrome: major clinical and serological features. *Medicine (Baltimore)* 1989; 68:366–374.
469. McNeil HP, Hunt JE, Krilis SA. Antiphospholipid antibodies: new insights into their specificity and clinical importance. *Scand J Immunol* 1992;36:647–652.
470. Viard JP, Amoura Z, Bach JF. Association of anti-β_2 glycoprotein I antibodies with lupus type circulating anticoagulant and thrombosis in systemic lupus erythematosus. *Am J Med* 1992;93:181–186.
471. Galli M, Comfurius P, Maasen C, et al. Anticardiolipin antibodies directed not to cardiolipin but to a plasma cofactor. *Lancet* 1990;335:1557.
472. Matsuura E, Igaraski Y, Yasuda T, et al. Anticardiolipin antibodies recognize beta 2 glycoprotein I structure altered by interacting with an oxygen solid phase surface. *J Exp Med* 1994;179:457?462.
473. Roubey RAD, Pratt CW, Buyon JP, et al. Lupus anticoagulant activity of autoimmune antiphospholipid antibodies is dependent upon beta 2–glycoprotein I. *J Clin Invest* 1992;90: 1100–1104.
474. Alarcon-Segovia D, Deleze M, Oria CV, et al. Antiphospholipid antibodies and the antiphospholipid syndrome in systemic lupus erythematosus. *Medicine (Baltimore)* 1989;68:353–365.
475. Brey RL, Hart GR, Sherman DG, et al. Antiphospholipid antibodies and cerebral ischemia in young people. *Neurology* 1990;40:1190–1195.
476. Levin JS. The antiphospholipid syndrome. *N Engl J Med* 2002;346:752–763.
477. Khamashta MA, Cuadrado MJ, Mujic F, et al. The management of thrombosis in the anti-phospholipid syndrome. *New Engl J Med* 1995;332:993–997.
478. Kallenberg CG, Wauda AA, The TH. Systemic involvement and immunologic findings in patients presenting with Raynaud's phenomenon. *Am J Med* 1980;69:675–679.
479. Blunt RJ, Porter JM. Raynaud's syndrome. *Semin Arthritis Rheum* 1981;10:282.
480. Velayos EE, Robinson H, Porcuincula FU, et al. Clinical correlation and analysis of 137 patients with Raynaud's phenomenon. *Am J Med Sci* 1971;262:347.
481. Dement J, Ginzler E, Schleisinger M, et al. The clinical significance of Raynaud's phenomenon in systemic lupus erythematosus. *Arthritis Rheum* 1979; 22:815–819.
482. Maddison PJ, Mogavero H, Reichlin M. Patterns of clinical disease associated with antibodies to nuclear ribonucleoprotein. *J Rheumatol* 1978;5:407–411.
483. Ginsberg WW, Conn DL, Banch TW, et al. Comparison of clinical and serologic markers in systemic lupus erythematosus and overlap syndrome: a review of 247 patients. *J Rheumatol* 1983;10:235–241.
484. Nimelstein SH, Brody S, McShane D, et al. Mixed connective tissue disease: a subsequent evaluation of the original 25 patients. *Medicine (Baltimore)* 1980;59:239–248.
485. Sharp GC, Irvin WS, May CM, et al. Association of antibodies to ribonucleoprotein and Sm antigens with mixed connective tissue disease, systemic lupus erythematosus, and other rheumatic diseases. *N Engl J Med* 1976;295: 1149–1154.
486. Sharp GC, Irvin WS, Tan EM, et al. Mixed connective tissue disease: an apparent distinct rheumatic disease syndrome associated with a specific antibody to an extractable nuclear antigen (ENA). *Am J Med* 1972;52:148–159.
487. Diment J, Ginzler E, Schlesinger M, et al. The clinical significance of Raynaud's phenomenon in systemic lupus erythematosus. *Arthritis Rheum* 1979; 22:815–819.

488. Rodeheffer RJ, Rommer JA, Wigley F, et al. Controlled, double-blind trial of nifedipine in the treatment of Raynaud's phenomenon. *N Engl J Med* 1983; 305:880–884.
489. Alarcon-Segovia D, Babb RR, Fairbairn JF. Systemic lupus erythematosus and erythromyalgias. *Arch Intern Med* 1963;112:102–106.
490. Davis MDP, O'Fallen WM, Rogers RS, et al. Natural history of erythromelalgia: presentation and outcomes of 168 patients. *Arch Dermatol* 2000;136:330–336.
491. Cohen JS. Erythromelalgia: new theories and new therapies. *J Am Acad Dermatol* 2000;43:841–847.
492. Kraus A. Erythromyalgia in a patient with systemic lupus erythematosus treated with clonazepam. *J Rheumatol* 1990;17:120–122.
493. Werth VP, Sanchez M, White W, et al. Alopecia areata with lupus erythematosus. *Arthritis Rheum* 1989;32:R17(abstr).
494. Kabir JDI, Malkinson FD. Lupus erythematosus and calcinosis cutis. *Arch Dermatol* 1969;100:17–22.
495. Storck J, Vosmik F. Lupus erythematosus panniculitis with morphea like lesions. *Clin Exp Dermatol* 1994;19:79–82.
496. Hahn BH, Yardley JH, Stevens MB. Rheumatoid nodules in systemic lupus erythematosus. *Ann Intern Med* 1970;72:49–58.
497. Boire G, Menard HA, Gendron M, et al. Rheumatoid arthritis: anti-Ro antibodies define a non-HLA-DR4 associated clinical serological cluster. *J Rheumatol* 1993;20:1654–1660.
498. Moutsopoulos HM, Skopouli FN, Sarras AK, et al. Anti-Ro(SS-A) positive rheumatoid arthritis (RA): a clinical serologic group of patients with a high incidence of D-penicillamine side effects. *Ann Rheum Dis* 1985;44:215–219.
499. Kramer LS, Ruderman JE, Dubois EL, et al. Deforming, non-erosive arthritis of the hands in chronic systemic lupus erythematosus. *Arthritis Rheum* 1970;13:329–330.
500. Russell AS, Percy JS, Rigal WM, et al. Deforming arthropathy in systemic lupus erythematosus. *Ann Rheum Dis* 1974;33:204–209.
500a. Obermoser G, Zegler B, Zangerle R, Sepp N. Extravascular necrotizing palisaded granulomas as the presenting skin sign of systemic lupus erythematosus. *Br J Dermatol.* 2002;147:371–374.
501. O'Lansky AJ, Briggaman RA, Gammon WR, et al. Bullous systemic lupus erythematosus. *J Am Acad Dermatol* 5. 511, 1982.
502. Penneys NS, Wiley HE. Herpetiform blisters is systemic lupus erythematosus. *Arch Dermatol* 1979;115:1427.
503. Hall RP, Lawley TJ, Smith HR, et al. Bullous eruption of systemic lupus erythematosus. *Ann Intern Med* 1982;97:165.
504. Gammon WR, Briggman RA. Bullous SLE: a phenotypically distinctive, but immunologic heterogeneous bullous disorder. *J Invest Dermatol* 1993; 100:28S.
505. Gammon WR, Woodley D, Dole KC, et al. Evidence that anti-basement membrane zone antibodies in bullous eruption of systemic lupus erythematosus recognized epidermolysis bullosa acquisita autoantigen. *J Invest Dermatol* 1985;84:472–476.
506. Camisa C, Sharma HM. Vesiculobullous systemic lupus erythematosus: report of two cases and review of the literature. *J Am Acad Dermatol* 1983;9:924.
507. Barton DD, Fine JD, Gammon WR, et al. Bullous systemic lupus erythematosus: an unusual clinical course and detectable circulating antibodies to the epidermolysis bullosa acquisita antigen. *J Am Acad Dermatol* 1986;16: 369.
508. Boh E, Roberts LJ, Lieu TS, et al. Epidermolysis bullous acquisita preceding the development of systemic lupus erythematosus. *J Am Acad Dermatol* 1990; 22:587.
509. Landry M, Sams WM Jr. Systemic lupus erythematosus: studies of autoantibodies bound to skin. *J Clin Invest* 1974;52:1871.
510. Nicholas BK, Gilliam JN. Counterimmunoelectrophoretic detection of epidermal basement membrane antibody in systemic lupus erythematosus serum. *Clin Res* 1982;30:600.
511. Nicholas BK, Gilliam JN. Isolated and characterization of an epidermal basement membrane zone antigen which may be involved in antibody binding at the dermal/epidermal junction in systemic lupus erythematosus. *Fed Proc* 1981;40:198.
512. Clemmensen O, Thomasen K. Porphyria cutanea tarda in systemic lupus erythematosus. *Arch Dermatol* 1982;118:160–162.
513. Cram DL, Epstein JH, Tuffanelli DL. Lupus erythematosus in porphyria: coexistence in 7 patients. *Arch Dermatol* 1973;108:779–784.
514. Weatherhead L, Adam J. Discoid lupus erythematosus: coexistence with porphyria cutanea tarda. *Int J Dermatol* 1985;24:453–455.
515. Callen J, Ross L. Subacute cutaneous lupus in porphyria cutanea tarda. *J Am Acad Dermatol* 1981;5:269–273.
516. Miller JF, Dawhan TF, Chapel TA. Coexistent bullous pemphigoid in systemic lupus erythematosus. *Cutis* 1985;21:368–373.
517. Vandersteen PR, Jordon RE. Dermatitis herpetiformis with discoid lupus erythematosus *Arch Dermatol* 1974;110:95–98.
518. Davies MG, Marks R, Waddington E. Simultaneous systemic lupus erythematosus and dermatitis herpetiformis. *Arch Dermatol* 1975;112:1292–1294.
519. Senear FE, Usher B. An unusual type of pemphigus combing features of lupus erythematosus. *Arch Dermatol* Syphilol 1926;13:761.
520. Cruz PD Jr. Coldison BM, Sontheimer RD. Concurrent features of cutaneous lupus erythematosus and pemphigus erythematosus following myasthenia gravis and thymoma. *J Am Acad Dermatol* 1987;16:472.
521. Chorzelski T, Jablonska S, Blasczyk M. Immunopathological investigations in the Senear-Usher syndrome (coexistence of pemphigus and lupus erythematosus). *Br J Dermatol* 1968;80:211–217.
522. Amerian ML, Ahmed AR. Pemphigus erythematosus. *J Am Acad Dermatol* 1984;10:215–222.
523. Bielsa I, Herrero C, Font J, et al. Lupus erythematosus and toxic epidermal necrolysis. *J Am Acad Dermatol* 1987;16:1265–1267.
524. Gilliam JM, Cohen SB, Sontheimer RD, et al. Connective tissue diseases. In: Moschella SL, Hurley HJ, eds. *Dermatology.* Philadelphia: WB Saunders, 1985:1087–1135.
525. Provost TT, Watson RM, Gammon WR, et al. The neonatal lupus syndrome associated with U_1RNP (nRNP) antibodies. *N Engl J Med* 1987;316:1135–1138.
526. Lyon CC, Blewitt R, Harrison PV. Subacute cutaneous lupus erythematosus: two cases of delayed diagnosis. *Acta Derm Venerol* 2000;78:57–59.
527. Marzano A, Berto E, Gasparini C, et al. Lupus erythematosus with antiphospholipid syndrome and erythema multiforme-like lesions. *Br J Dermatol* 1999;141:720–724.
528. Rongiolette F, Revora A. The new cutaneous mucinosis: a review with an up-todate classification of cutaneous mucinosis. *J Am Acad Dermatol* 1991;24:265.
529. Rongiolette F, Revora A. The new cutaneous mucinosis: a review with an up-todate classification of cutaneous mucinosis. *J Am Acad Dermatol* 1991;24:265.
530. Fowler JF, Callen JP. Cutaneous mucinosis associated with lupus erythematosus. *J Rheumatol* 1984;11:380.
531. Gammon WR, Caro I, Long JC, et al. Secondary cutaneous mucinosis with systemic lupus erythematosus. *Arch Dermatol* 1978;114:432.
532. Maruyama M, Miyauchi S, Haskimoto K. Massive cutaneous mucinosis associated with systemic lupus erythematosus. *Br J Dermatol* 1997;137:450–453.
533. Kanda N, Tsuchida T, Watanabe T, et al. Cutaneous lupus mucinosis: a review of our cases and the possible pathogenesis. *J Cutan Pathol* 1997;248:553–558.
533a. Pandya AG, Sontheimer RD, Cockerell CJ, et al. Papulonodular mucinosis associated with systemic lupus erythematosus: possible mechanisms of increased glycosaminoglycan accumulation. *J Am Acad Dermatol* 1995;32:199.
534. Urowitz MB, Gladman DD, Chalmers A, et al. Nail lesions in systemic lupus erythematosus. *J Rheumatol* 1978;5:551.
535. Vaughn RY, Bailey JP Jr, Field RS, et al. Diffuse nail dyschromia in black patients with systemic lupus erythematosus. *J Rheumatol* 1990;16:640.
536. Bracco MM, Bianchi CA, Bianchi O, et al. Hereditary complement (C2) deficiency with discoid lupus erythematosus and idiopathic anetoderma. *Int J Dermatol* 1979;18:713–717.
537. Ryll-Nardzewski C. Remarques sur le lupus erythemate profond et sur l'anetodermie erythematoide. *Ann Dermatol Syphilol* 1960;87:627–636.
538. Randle HW, Muller S. Generalized elastolysis associated with systemic lupus erythematosus. *J Am Acad Dermatol* 1983;8:869–873.
539. Boyd AS, King LE. Mid dermal elastolysis in two patients with lupus erythematosus. *Am J Dermatopathol* 2001;23:136–138.
540. Copeman PWM, Schroeter AL, Kierland RR. An unusual variant of lupus erythematosus or lichen planus. *Br J Dermatol* 1970;83:269-272.
541. VanDerHorst JC, Cirkel PKS, Niebore C. Mixed lichen planus: lupus erythematosus disease: a distinct entity? Clinical, histopathological, and immunopathological studies in 6 patients. *Clin Exp Dermatol* 1983;8:631–640.
542. Camisa C, Nett JC, Olsen RG. Use of indirect immunofluorescence in the lupus erythematosus/lichen planus overlap syndrome: an additional diagnostic clue. *J Am Acad Dermatol* 1984;11:1050–1059.
543. Tuffanelli DL. Acanthosis nigricans with lupoid hepatitis. *JAMA* 1964;189: 584–585.
544. Rendon MI, Cruz PD, Sontheimer RD, et al. Acanthosis nigricans: a cutaneous marker of tissue resistance to insulin. *J Am Acad Dermatol* 1989;21:461.

CHAPTER 3

Dermatomyositis

Richard D. Sontheimer, Rebecca L. Euwer, and Melissa I. Costner

HISTORICAL PERSPECTIVE

Classic Dermatomyositis

Dermatomyositis (DM) was first recognized as a distinct clinical entity during the second half of the 19th century by Wagner (1863) (1) and Unverricht (1887) (2) (i.e., Wagner–Unverricht disease). Bohan (3) indicates that the first report in the American literature was presented by Jacoby in 1888 (4). Gottron characterized the cutaneous manifestations of this disease in depth in 1930 (5). Other descriptive accounts by Gottron have been described (6,7) (Hiroaki Ueki, personal communication, June 2002). Keil provided a connoisseur's description of the classic cutaneous manifestations of DM in 1942 (8).

The rather hopeless outlook that patients with this disease faced in the presteroid era can be appreciated from the work of O'Leary and Waisman in 1940 (9). However, with the advent of corticosteroid and antibiotic therapy, DM and polymyositis (PM) have become much more manageable conditions, although many challenges still remain concerning these disorders (10–12). During the 1950s and 1960s, the work of Eaton (10), Walton and Adams (11), Williams (13), Winklemann (14), and Rose and Walton (12) served to further define this group of diseases.

Much credit must be given to Pearson for his pioneering studies in the 1960s and 1970s, which laid the groundwork for our current understanding of the spectrum of disease processes that we recognize as DM/PM (15–19). It was from the foundation of Pearson's work that subsequent workers have framed the conventional nosology of this group of disorders (3,20,21). The description of inclusion body myositis as a distinct clinical entity has led to a reformulation of classification of this group of diseases under the designation of the idiopathic inflammatory myopathies (IIMs) (21), a group designation that tends to underemphasize the importance of the cutaneous manifestations of DM. Everett and Curtis (22) in 1957 and Banker and Victor (23) in 1966 began to describe the differences between the juvenile and adult forms of DM, emphasizing that severe vasculopathy/vasculitis, calcification, and disability are more often experienced by children with this disease than adults. These differences have been subsequently emphasized by others (24–28).

As Callen (29,30) has reported, the association between DM/PM and malignancy has been the subject of intense debate since the publication of the work of Shy (31) in 1962. However, the more recent population-based data presented by several groups have strongly argued that patients with DM clearly have a higher than expected risk for malignancy (32).

Clinically Amyopathic Dermatomyositis

It is not unusual for the cutaneous manifestations of DM to precede clinical evidence of myositis; however, most patients develop muscular weakness within 6 months after the onset of cutaneous inflammation (19,33). Throughout the history of this disease process, it has been recognized that a small percentage of patients will occasionally express the classic cutaneous manifestations of DM for very long periods without accompanying clinical evidence of muscle disease (33–37). Keil (8) in 1942 was among the first to accept the concept that patients can express the classic cutaneous manifestations of DM for years without the appearance of symptomatic muscle disease.

In the past, such patients have been referred to as patients with dermatomyositis siné myositis and have not been the subject of systematic study because they fail to meet the conventional modern diagnostic criteria for DM by virtue of the absence of objective evidence of muscle involvement (38). Euwer and Sontheimer (39,40) began to focus attention on this subgroup of patients in the early 1990s by referring to this form of disease as amyopathic dermatomyositis (amyopathic DM) (39,40), a term that Pearson had introduced earlier (35). The realization that such patients do in fact have a form of DM emphasizes that the classic form of DM occupies but one position in a disease spectrum that extends from patients who have idiopathic inflammatory myositis only (PM) to those who have DM-specific skin disease only (amyopathic DM) (Fig. 3.1). Within this spectrum, skin and striated muscle are affected to variable degrees by a characteristic pattern of vasocentric inflammatory injury of unknown etiology.

Clinically amyopathic DM is considerably more common than was previously thought, can present during childhood, and can on occasion be accompanied by potentially fatal systemic complications of classic DM such as interstitial lung disease (ILD) in the complete absence of clinical evidence of muscle weakness (38,41–43).

Sontheimer (38,43) has reported the deficiencies of the traditional nomenclature used in describing the IIM with respect to cutaneous-only or cutaneous-predominant subsets of DM. He has proposed a new nomenclature and classification system in this regard, which is presented in Tables 3.1 and 3.2. This nomenclature will be used in this presentation.

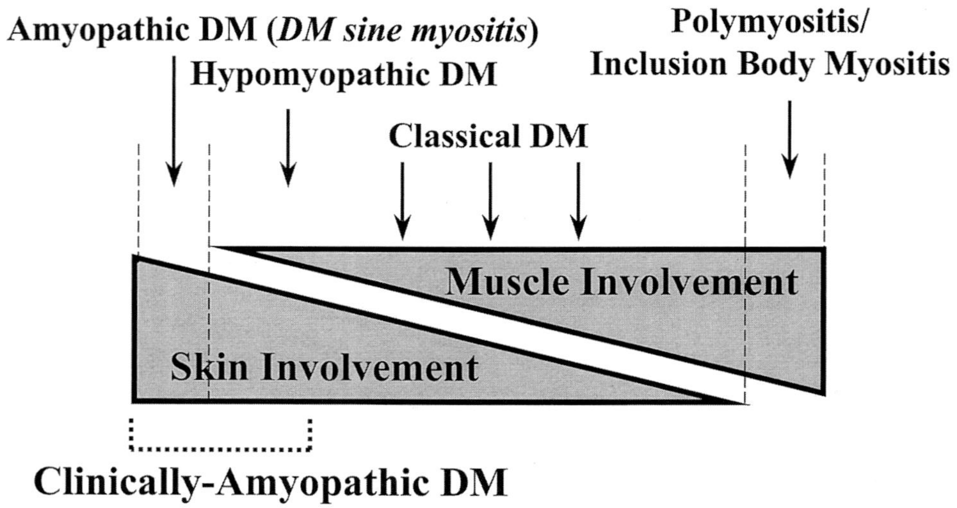

Figure 3.1. Conceptualization of the relationship that exists between clinically amyopathic dermatomyositis (DM) and classic forms of DM and polymyositis. Clinically amyopathic DM accounts for approximately 10% of patients with DM ascertained from dermatology practices in the United States. Extrapolating from the demographic characteristics of classic DM, clinically amyopathic DM likely accounts for somewhat less than 5% of patients with DM/polymyositis overall.

TABLE 3.1. Definitions of Unfamiliar/Unconventional Terms Used[a]

Terms (Abbreviation)	Definitions
Amyopathic DM[b] (ADM)	A subset of patients with DM characterized by biopsy-confirmed hallmark cutaneous manifestations of classic DM occurring for 6 months or longer with no clinical evidence of proximal muscle weakness and no serum muscle enzyme abnormalities. If more extensive muscle testing is carried out, the results should be within normal limits (if such results are positive or abnormal, the patient should be classified as having "hypomyopathic DM" [see later]). For the purpose of improved communication and future clinical studies, an approach to defining the minimal set of skin findings necessary to qualifying as "hallmark cutaneous manifestations of DM" are defined in Table 3.2. Exclusion criteria for amyopathic DM include: 1. Treatment with systemic immunosuppressive therapy for 2 consecutive months or longer within the first 6 months after skin disease onset (such therapy could prevent the development of clinically significant myositis). 2. Use of drugs known to be capable of producing isolated DM-like skin changes (e.g., hydroxyurea, "statin" cholesterol-lowering agents) at the onset of cutaneous DM changes.
Classic DM (CDM)	Patients having the hallmark cutaneous manifestations of DM, proximal muscle weakness, and objective evidence of muscle inflammation characteristic of DM.
Clinically amyopathic DM (C-ADM)	A functional designation that can be used to refer to patients with either amyopathic DM and/or hypomyopathic DM as defined here (i.e., C-ADM = amyopathic DM + hypomyopathic DM). This designation has been coined to emphasize the fact that the predominant *clinical* problem is skin disease in patients is so affected.
DM siné myositis	A term now of predominately historic significance that is synonymous for amyopathic DM.
DM-specific skin disease (DSSD)	A clinicopathologic pattern of skin change seen only in DM (analogous to the "LE-specific skin disease concept" coined by James N. Gilliam, M.D. in 1975).
Hallmark cutaneous lesions/changes of DM	Skin lesions that alone or in combination are seen only in patients with some form of DM (synonymous with DM-specific skin disease).
Hypomyopathic DM	Patients with DM-specific skin disease and no clinical evidence of muscle disease who are found to have subclinical evidence of myositis at laboratory, electrophysiologic, or radiologic evaluation.
Idiopathic inflammatory dermatomyopathies (IIDM)	A more inclusive disease group designation for the spectrum of illness that has conventionally been referred to as "idiopathic inflammatory myopathies."

[a]From Sontheimer R.D.: Would a new name hasten the acceptance of amyopathic dermatomyositis (dermatomyositis siné myositis) as a distinctive subset with the idiopathic inflammatory dermatomyopathies spectrum of clinical illness? *J Am Acad Dermatol* 46:626–636, 2002.
[b]For the purposes of clinical studies, amyopathic DM and hypomyopathic DM can be qualified as "provisional" (skin disease duration for 6–23 months) or "confirmed" (skin disease duration for 24 months or longer).

TABLE 3.2. Classification of the Idiopathic Inflammatory Dermatomyopathies

Dermatomyositis (DM)
- *Adult onset*
  - Classic DM
    - Classic DM alone
    - Classic DM with malignancy
    - Classic DM as part of an overlap connective tissue disorder
  - Clinically amyopathic DM[a]
    - Amyopathic DM
    - Hypomyopathic DM
- *Juvenile onset*
  - Classic DM
  - Clinically amyopathic DM
    - Amyopathic DM
    - Hypomyopathic DM

Polymyositis (PM)
- PM alone
- PM as part of an overlap connective tissue disorder
- PM associated with internal malignancy (?)[b]

Inclusion Body Myositis

Other Clinicopathologic Subgroups of Myositis
- Focal myositis
- Proliferative myositis
- Orbital myositis
- Eosinophilic myositis
- Granulomatous myositis

[a]Patients with adult-onset and juvenile-onset amyopathic DM and hypomyopathic DM can be further subcategorized as "provisional" and "confirmed" when patients have biopsy-confirmed hallmark cutaneous manifestations of DM without muscle weakness and with normal muscle enzymes for greater than or equal to 6 months (provisional) or 24 months (confirmed)(40).
[b]Although recent population-based European studies have clearly confirmed that adult-onset classical DM is associated with a significant risk for internal malignancy, if such a relationship exists for PM it is much weaker.
From Sontheimer RD. Cutaneous features of classical dermatomyositis and amyopathic dermatomyositis. *Curr Opin Rheumatol* 1999;11:475–482, with permission.

EPIDEMIOLOGY

Classic Dermatomyositis

Population studies of DM/PM have revealed that cutaneous disease occurs in 30% to 40% of adult patients (19,44) and 95% of children (45–48). By definition, skin disease is absent in patients with PM and present in 100% of patients with DM and amyopathic DM. Skin involvement commonly precedes the development of muscle disease in classic DM (19,33).

The incidence of hospital-based diagnoses of DM/PM among residents of Pittsburgh and Allegheny County, Pennsylvania, was determined over a 20-year period (1963 to 1982) to be 5.5 cases per million (49). Interestingly, the incidence in the first decade of this study was 2.5 per million and in the second decade, it was 8.9 per million. The greatest increase occurred in black women during their childbearing years (range, 20 to 44 years). Bridges (50) has suggested the possibility that DM might be underdiagnosed in blacks because of the more subtle coloration of the inflammatory skin changes in this setting. Juvenile-onset classic DM is reported to affect 1 to 3 million children per year annually. In whites, females are affected twice as often as males (51). Reports from Singapore, Hong Kong, and Taiwan have indicated that patients with DM of those ethnic backgrounds are more likely to be male as opposed to females. DM/PM can occur at any age from infancy to adult life, with the largest proportion of cases developing in the fifth and sixth decades.

Familial occurrence is rarely seen in adults or children (24). Concordant disease expression has been reported in identical twins (24). The rare familial occurrence of adult and juvenile DM/IIM has been noted (52–54).

An increased frequency of HLA-DR3 and HLA-DRw52 is seen in patients with classic DM/PM (55,56). HLA-DQA1 homozygosity may be a genetic risk factor for familial IIM. A single nucleotide polymorphism in the tumor necrosis factor-α (TNF-α) promoter (TNF-α-308A) has been associated with disease chronicity, calcinosis, and high levels of TNF-α in a cohort of white patients with juvenile-onset classic DM (57).

A single case of adult-onset DM occurring in a young Japanese woman who was subsequently shown to be genetically deficient in the C5 component of complement has been reported. DM-associated ILD occurs more commonly in Japanese patients with classic DM compared with other ethnic groups. Several observations have suggested the possibility that environmental triggers might be important in the elicitation of this autoimmune disease process. Seasonality has been noted in the onset of both childhood-onset (24) and adult-onset PM/DM (56,58). Such seasonality would suggest the possibility of an infectious etiology of this disorder.

Clinicians appreciate that DM-specific skin disease can be provoked or aggravated by exposure to ultraviolet (UV) radiation, although there are little published data documenting this (59). Indirect support of a link to UV radiation is the fact that the prevalence of DM is inversely related to distance from the equator (60).

The role of infectious agents such as viruses in the induction of DM has long been debated. The development of DM- and PM-like syndromes in patients with X-linked immunodeficiency (61–63), as well as the acquired immunodeficiency syndrome and human T-cell leukemia virus type I infection (64–67) further suggest the possibility for an infectious basis for this disease process. Further anecdotal evidence has been presented arguing in favor of a relationship between DM and parvovirus B19 (68,69) and Epstein–Barr virus (70).

Other environmental factors that have been suggested to be associated with DM/PM include exposure to certain drugs. Drugs such as penicillamine (71), statin lipid-lowering agents (atrovostatin, pravastatin, simvastatin) (72,73); alfuzosin (74), and phenytoin (75) appear to be capable of inducing both the cutaneous and muscle manifestations of DM.

Other implicated environmental factors include silicone breast implants (76,77), silicon (78), and bovine collagen implants (79). However, the link to bovine collagen implants has been seriously questioned (80). In addition, formal epidemiologic analysis has not supported a significant association between silicone breast implants and any classic form of autoimmune rheumatic disease.

Clinically Amyopathic Dermatomyositis

The incidence and prevalence of clinically amyopathic DM in the United States are unknown but are assumed to be extremely low; however, published data currently exist on more than 300 such patients. Most epidemiologic data relating to classic DM have been collected from hospitalized patient populations fulfilling the Bohan and Peter diagnostic criteria, thereby excluding patients with clinically amyopathic DM (19,20).

Information related to the incidence of clinically amyopathic DM in the United States derives predominately from anecdotal reports from outpatient practices of academic dermatologists, where clinically amyopathic DM has been estimated to occur with approximately 10% of the incidence of classic DM (33,39).

In Europe, a similar incidence has been observed (81), whereas in Asia, clinically amyopathic DM appears to be relatively more common. A retrospective analysis of 28 patients with DM seen at the National Skin Center in Singapore between 1996 and 1998 revealed that 13 (46%) had clinically amyopathic DM (82). In another cohort of 143 Taiwanese patients with DM/PM seen in a veteran's hospital system, clinically amyopathic DM was the second most commonly encountered subgroup (14%) following classic adult-onset DM (64%). Clinically amyopathic DM was somewhat more common than juvenile DM/PM (13%) and PM (10%) in this study (83). Very little data exist concerning the incidence of juvenile clinically amyopathic DM. In a retrospective analysis of all patients with juvenile DM seen at an academic medical center in Pennsylvania between 1968 and 1998, two (12%) of 16 patients were categorized as having clinically amyopathic DM (84).

Fortunately, larger cohorts of patients with amyopathic DM are now being reported. A retrospective analysis of all patients with DM seen at the Mayo Clinic between 1976 and 1994 revealed that 32 (4%) of 746 patients with DM conformed to the definition of clinically amyopathic DM (85). Twenty-seven of these patients had amyopathic DM and five had hypomyopathic DM (an additional group of five patients having subjective muscle weakness but no demonstrable muscle abnormalities was included in the analysis by El-Azhary et al. (85), however these patients are not included in the analysis here because they do not conform to the definition of clinically amyopathic DM presented in Table 3.1). Follow-up information was available on 16 of the patients with amyopathic DM at the Mayo Clinic. Ten patients (67%) had no muscle weakness after 2 to 10 years of follow-up, four (25%) had no weakness at 1 year, and two (13%) developed weakness within 5 years after diagnosis. None of the three patients with hypomyopathic DM who were followed up showed evidence of muscle weakness 8 to 17 years after diagnosis. Thus, of the 19 patients with clinically amyopathic DM who were followed up (16 amyopathic DM, three hypomyopathic DM), only two (11%) had developed clinical evidence of myositis after prolonged follow-up periods. Thus, the presence of subclinical muscle abnormalities at the time of diagnosis of amyopathic DM does not necessarily portend the subsequent development of clinically significant muscle disease.

In a retrospective analysis, Caproni et al. (86) identified 13 patients with amyopathic DM representing 8.2% of 157 patients with DM seen during a 10-year period by the Italian Group of Immunodermatology. The patients consisted of 12 women and one man with a mean age of 53 years. Eleven patients (85%) experienced skin disease for at least 2 years (i.e., confirmed amyopathic DM), whereas two (15%) had skin disease for longer than 6 months but less than 24 months (provisional amyopathic DM). There was one juvenile case presenting at 13 years of age. Four of these patients could be classified as having hypomyopathic DM by virtue of abnormalities noted on electromyogram (EMG) (three of eight patients tested) or muscle biopsy (one of two tested). Arthralgias were noted in two patients (15%) and Raynaud's phenomenon in four (31%). Internal malignancy was not identified in any of these 13 patients. There was no mention of any of these patients experiencing systemic complications such as ILD.

Clinically amyopathic DM appears to have an even stronger female preponderance in whites than the classic form of the disease. However, in Asian patients, clinically amyopathic DM appears to be more common in males (83). Clinically amyopathic DM affects all age groups, although it has been reported to occur more commonly in adults than children.

Female siblings with classic DM and clinically amyopathic DM have been reported (53). In addition, one of the authors (R.D.S.) has observed a curious familial constellation of clinically amyopathic DM occurring in a father and both of his adult daughters (personal unpublished observation July, 1996).

Clinically amyopathic DM appears to share HLA associations similar to those found in patients with classic DM (i.e., HLA-DQA1) (87).

Increasingly, certain drugs are being reported to induce the cutaneous or systemic manifestations of DM/PM (43,88). It has been further emphasized that chronic hydroxyurea therapy in the setting of chronic myelogenous leukemia can produce a DM-like cutaneous eruption that is clinically and histopathologically quite similar to idiopathic DM-specific skin disease (89,90). Muscle weakness and other systemic symptoms have been characteristically absent in such cases, raising the possibility that this might be a clinically amyopathic DM-like cutaneous eruption rather than a classic DM-like cutaneous eruption. Painful leg ulcers are also often seen in this setting as is xerosis and cutaneous atrophy. This form of drug-induced DM skin change usually occurs only after the patient has been on hydroxyurea for 2 to 10 years. Other drugs that have been implicated in inducing DM-like skin disease include nonsteroidal antiinflammatories (e.g., diclofenac) and D-penicillamine.

DEFINITION AND CLASSIFICATION

Classic Dermatomyositis

The IIMs are a heterogeneous group of genetically determined autoimmune disorders that characteristically target the skin and skeletal musculature, resulting in widespread cutaneous inflammatory disease and muscle weakness of the limb girdles. In a small percentage of patients, other organ systems such as the lungs (e.g., ILD), joints (arthritis), and heart (e.g., cardiomyopathy, conduction defects) can also be affected by inflammatory injury. On rare occasion, some patients can display IIM-related internal organ involvement (e.g., ILD with antisynthetase autoantibodies) without clinical evidence of myositis or skin disease (91). Significant clinical differences exist between adult-onset and juvenile-onset DM. Juvenile DM displays higher rates of the hallmark skin lesions of DM and vasculopathy/vasculitis with the resulting complication of dystrophic calcification. Classic DM and PM represent the most common clinical presentation of the IIM.

Classic DM is an inflammatory necrotizing disease of striated muscle associated with characteristic inflammatory cutaneous lesions. Patients with PM have an identical clinical pattern of muscle disease but lack skin changes. Patients with inclusion body myositis have a different type of muscle disorder and no characteristic skin lesions.

Bohan et al. (19,20) contributed significantly to our understanding of PM/DM in 1977 by separating these disorders into five clinical subgroups and establishing diagnostic criteria for classic DM that are still used today. Unfortunately, this classification scheme did not allow the inclusion of patients with amyopathic DM, a point that Euwer and Sontheimer (39) later attempted to rectify by proposing amyopathic DM as a sixth clinical subgroup within the Bohan classification scheme.

In 1991, Dalakas (21) codified thinking at that time about PM, DM, and inclusion body myositis by suggesting that they represent a spectrum of "idiopathic inflammatory myopathies." In that same year, Euwer and Sontheimer (39) proposed a set of diagnostic criteria for amyopathic DM and suggested that any classification scheme of PM/DM would be incomplete if it did not include this entity. These investigators have subsequently proposed a combined classification scheme for the IIMs that includes amyopathic DM (92). The classification criteria for clinically amyopathic DM have been further refined and a new umbrella designation for this group of diseases has been proposed (idiopathic inflammatory dermatomyopathies) (38,43) (Table 3.2). Other classification schemes have been presented (93–96).

Another recent trend in thinking concerning the classification of these disorders relates to the idea that there might be distinct prognostic subgroups that can be recognized by the patterns of myositis-specific autoantibodies (MSAs) that are produced (e.g., antisynthetase syndrome) (56,58,97).

Clinically Amyopathic Dermatomyositis

In 1975, Krain (34) described six patients who expressed the skin manifestations of DM for very long periods before ultimately developing the typical DM muscle disease. Such patients have been described anecdotally by others as well (33,35–37,98). "Dermatomyositis siné myositis" is a term often used by dermatologists in the past to refer to such patients (95,99–101). However, the published basis of the origin of this name is quite obscure. Most formally (Medline) and informally (Internet) published data on this cutaneous subset of DM currently appears under the designation "amyopathic DM" (38).

In 1991, Euwer and Sontheimer (39) described six patients (five adults and one child) with biopsy-confirmed classic cutaneous findings of DM who did not have clinical or laboratory evidence of muscle disease for at least 2 years after onset of their skin disease. These patients were referred to as having amyopathic DM in honor of Pearson, who first suggested this term in reference to several patients he had seen with classic cutaneous findings of DM but minimal to no muscle involvement (35). Issues related to such patients have been further discussed by these authors (38,40,43,92,102). Subsequently, the term "provisional amyopathic DM" was used to describe those patients who have the cutaneous manifestations of DM longer than is typical for the classic form of DM (6 months) but for less than 2 years (40). Table 3.2 presents a conceptual view of amyopathic DM in the context of the classification schemes previously offered by Bohan et al. (19) and Dalakas (21).

Caution should be taken when entertaining the diagnosis of either classic or amyopathic DM in patients who are taking drugs that have been reported to be capable of inducing DM-like skin lesions such as hydroxyurea (103), penicillamine (21,71), nonsteroidal antiinflammatory agents such as niflumic acid/diclofenac (104), tryptophan (21), practolol (105) and the statin lipid-lowering agents (atrovostatin, pravastatin, simvastatin) (72,73). In addition, it cannot be certain that patients with only DM skin lesions who are treated with systemic immunosuppressive therapy within 6 months of the onset of their disease and never develop muscle disease might not have gone on to develop myositis had they not been so treated.

Considering the large differential diagnosis of proximal muscle weakness, modern physicians influenced by the earlier work of Bohan and Pearson (19,20) are quite reticent to make a diagnosis of IIM without firm evidence that inflammatory myositis is the cause of weakness. However, this approach often results in the underappreciation of the clinical specificity of the hallmark cutaneous manifestations of DM. Because the hallmark inflammatory skin changes can be so specific, the only significant differential diagnostic consideration is cutaneous lupus erythematosus (LE) occurring in the context of an overlap syndrome that includes features of myositis.

Those who care for patients with juvenile-onset DM, a form of the disease in which the hallmark cutaneous manifestations are almost always present at the outset of the disease process, seem to have a greater appreciation of the diagnostic specificity of the cutaneous changes of DM. In one survey, a large percentage of pediatric rheumatologists indicated that they found EMG or muscle biopsy to be of little incremental value when the hallmark cutaneous manifestations of DM are present along with a typical clinical pattern of muscle weakness (106).

Stonecipher et al. (96) in 1993 proposed a classification scheme for patients having cutaneous manifestations of DM that included three groups: (a) patients with cutaneous changes only (i.e., amyopathic DM), (b) patients with cutaneous changes at baseline and subsequent evolution to myositis (i.e., delayed-onset classic DM), and (c) patients with cutaneous changes and normal muscle enzymes but in whom diagnostic evaluations showed subclinical myositis (i.e., hypomyopathic DM). This classification approach has been advocated by others (85,107).

One of the authors (R.D.S.) has recently summarized his personal perspective on disease classification in this area and has proposed a more inclusive classification scheme under the designation, "idiopathic inflammatory dermatomyopathies" (IIDMs) (38,43). This classification scheme is presented in Table 3.2. Until recently, the general medical community has been unwilling to account for patients with clinically amyopathic DM in the classification approach to clinical disorders that have traditionally been referred to as DM/PM/IIM (82,95,108–111). However, to continue to do so will further orphan patients having exclusively or predominately cutaneous subsets of DM and delay the design and completion of clinical studies needed to ascertain the overall clinical significance of skin-only patterns of disease presentation and persistence. In addition, such reticence will further delay the development of optimal management strategies for patients with clinically amyopathic DM and inhibit a more complete understanding of the immunopathogenetic relationships that exist within the myositis spectrum of clinical illness. Figure 3.1 and Table 3.2 attempt to consolidate and illustrate the ideas and concepts concerning clinically amyopathic DM that are discussed in this chapter.

Some are unfortunately using the term "amyopathic DM" to describe patients who have just been recognized to have hallmark DM skin changes but who lack clinical evidence of muscle involvement (112). Additionally, some workers have used the term "amyopathic DM" to describe the stage of classic DM in which persistent or recurrent cutaneous involvement following therapy-induced remission of muscle weakness is the predominant clinical problem. The designation, "postmyopathic DM skin disease activity" could be used to describe this phase of such a patient's illness. The authors recommend that for the purposes of various forms of clinical investigation, the term "amyopathic DM" be reserved for those individuals displaying the hallmark cutaneous manifestations of DM for at least 6 months or longer without the appearance of clinical evidence of myositis. Other diagnostic criteria for amyopathic DM are presented in Table 3.1.

The term "premyopathic" has been offered to describe patients with clinically amyopathic DM with the implication that all such patients will eventually develop clinically significant muscle involvement (113). However, there is increasing evidence that some patients who present with clinically amyopathic DM go for 10 to 20 years or longer without developing clinical evidence of muscle disease (43,85,114). Perhaps the term "premyopathic" might be used to describe those patients displaying the hallmark cutaneous manifestations of DM without muscle weakness for less than 6 months.

The term "DM-specific skin disease" has also been proposed as an alternative designation for the biopsy-confirmed hallmark cutaneous manifestations of DM (38). If adopted, perhaps this term could focus more interest and emphasis on the cutaneous manifestations of DM for their own sake, regardless of whether they are accompanied by clinically significant or insignificant abnormalities in muscles or other organ systems. The analogy between "DM-specific skin disease" and "LE-specific skin disease" is discussed elsewhere (38). The term "DM-specific skin disease" will likely be preferred by many dermatologists over terms such as "the heliotrope rash" or the "rash of DM" that have often been used in the literature in the past when referring to the hallmark cutaneous manifestations of DM.

In several reports, the term "amyotrophic" DM appears to have been used mistakenly in referring to patients with clinically amyopathic DM (115,116).

Juvenile-Onset Dermatomyositis

Unlike adult-onset IIM, virtually all children who develop inflammatory myositis also express typical cutaneous manifestations of DM that are usually evident at the time of or prior to the diagnosis of myositis (i.e., juvenile-onset PM is an extremely rare clinical situation). Although the mortality rate of juvenile-onset DM tends to be lower than adult-onset DM (in part due to the lower incidence of associated malignancy), long-term morbidity from complications such as subcutaneous calcification, muscle infarction and calcification, and contractures are increased.

Juvenile-onset classic DM differs from adult-onset classic DM in several other important aspects (24). Childhood DM often follows an upper respiratory tract infection and demonstrates a seasonal incidence. In addition, it is not significantly associated with internal malignancy. However, children with DM more commonly have widespread destructive vasculopathy, which is often expressed clinically as ischemic skin lesions, retinopathy, and bowel infarction with perforation (23). This form of vascular injury is often inappropriately referred to as a form of vasculitis. However, vascular lumen occlusion rather than inflammatory injury of vessel walls is the predominant change noted on pathology examination. The central nervous system can also be affected by this form of vasculopathy. Children with DM also more frequently develop cutaneous, subcutaneous, and muscular dystrophic calcification as a result of the widespread soft-tissue damage caused by the vasculopathy. Children are also more likely to develop muscle infarction with subsequent scarring and crippling contracture. Muscle atrophy and contractures occur more commonly in the last stages of childhood DM.

Raynaud's phenomenon and overlap with other connective tissue diseases are seen less frequently in juvenile-onset classic DM. In addition to cutaneous calcinosis, hypertrichosis and lipodystrophy are cutaneous features seen more often in juvenile-onset DM.

Clinically amyopathic DM is being increasingly recognized in children as well as adults.

Malignancy-Associated Dermatomyositis

There has long been a question of whether there is a significantly increased risk for internal malignancy in adult-onset classic DM. This has been answered by several large, well-designed, population-based epidemiologic studies from northern Europe, which have confirmed the existence of such a relationship. A high relative risk for ovarian cancer in adult women with classic DM has been reported in several of these studies. Approximately 20% to 25% of older adults with new-onset classic DM will have an associated internal malignancy. Whether there is an increased risk for internal malignancy in clinically amyopathic DM remains to be determined.

Dermatomyositis as a Component of an Overlap Connective Tissue Disease

DM/PM can overlap with other connective tissue diseases individually such a systemic lupus erythematosus (SLE), rheumatoid arthritis, and Sjögren syndrome. DM/PM overlaps with features of SLE, rheumatoid arthritis, and scleroderma in mixed connective tissue disease. U1RNP autoantibody is the serologic marker for this particular overlap constellation. The concurrence of Raynaud's phenomenon, arthritis, and ILD would be a clinical indication of DM/PM occurring in the context of an overlapping connective tissue disease. Internal malignancy is quite rare in DM/PM overlapping with other connective tissue diseases.

Polymyositis

PM is a pattern of inflammatory myositis causing a pattern of proximal muscle weakness that is identical to that seen in patients with classic DM. However, there are some immunopathologic differences in the pattern of muscle inflammation between patients with PM and those with DM, enough so that some have questioned whether the patterns of inflammatory myositis seen in PM and DM are fundamentally different. There are no characteristic cutaneous associations of PM. Patients with PM appear to have a much lower risk for internal malignancy than patients with classic DM.

Inclusion Body Myositis

Inclusion body myositis is a histopathologically distinctive type of steroid-resistant myositis that more commonly affects the distal muscle groups of older men in an asymmetric pattern. Its name is derived from the observation that there are characteristic microscopic inclusion bodies present on muscle biopsy. Characteristic skin changes are not seen with this disorder. This pattern of myositis is extremely difficult to treat.

Other Clinical Patterns of Myositis

In addition to PM and inclusion body myositis, several other rare clinicopathologic types of myositis have been described: focal myositis, proliferative myositis, orbital myositis, eosinophilic myositis, granulomatous myositis. No characteristic skin lesions are associated with any of these clinical entities.

CUTANEOUS MANIFESTATIONS

Classic Dermatomyositis

CLINICAL FEATURES AND PATTERN OF EVOLUTION OF TYPICAL SKIN LESIONS

The cutaneous manifestation of DM can be divided into those that are pathognomonic, characteristic, and compatible (39) (Table 3.3). As previously discussed, Gottron papules and Gottron sign of DM represent the pathognomic cutaneous lesions of this disorder. The specificity of Gottron papules for DM has been questioned by some experienced observers (117); however, we have been unable to identify documented cases of fully formed, pathologically confirmed Gottron papules occurring in any clinical setting other than DM or amyopathic DM. Such lesions might occur in a patient who has overlapping features of DM and other rheumatic disorders like scleroderma or SLE (37), although this appears to be quite uncommon. It is our opinion, as well as that of others (37), that Gottron papules in conjunc-

TABLE 3.3. Cutaneous Manifestations of Dermatomyositis

Pathognomic skin lesions of DM

1. Gottron papules
   Papules having a violaceous hue overlying the dorsolateral aspect of interphalangeal, or metacarpophalangeal joints, or both. When fully formed, these papules become slightly depressed at the center, which can assume a white, atrophic appearance. Associated telangiectasia can be present.
2. Gottron sign of DM
   Symmetric macular violaceous erythema with or without edema overlying the dorsal aspects of the interphalangeal/metacarpophalangeal joints, olecranon processes, patellae, and medial malleoli.

Highly characteristic skin lesions of DM

1. Periorbital violaceous (heliotrope) erythema with or without associated edema of the eyelids and periorbital tissue.
2. Grossly visible periungual telangiectasia with or without dystrophic cuticles.
3. Symmetric macular violaceous erythema overlying the dorsal aspect of the hands and fingers (where it can track the extensor tendon sheaths), extensor aspects of the arms and forearms, deltoids, posterior shoulders and neck (the shawl sign), V-area of anterior neck and upper chest, central aspect of the face and forehead.

Compatible skin lesions of DM

1. Poikiloderma atrophicans vasculare (poikilodermatomyositis)
   Circumscribed violaceous erythema with associated telangiectasia, hypopigmentation, hyperpigmentation, and superficial atrophy most commonly found over the posterior shoulders, back, buttocks, and V-area of the anterior neck and chest.
2. Calcinosis cutis

DM, dermatomyositis.
From Euwer RL, Sontheimer RD. Dermatologic aspects of myositis. *Cur Opin Rheumatol* 1994, 6:583–589.

tion with the prominent nailfold capillary abnormalities that are often seen in this disease are specific for DM or amyopathic DM. Although the periorbital heliotrope erythema is highly characteristic of cutaneous DM, this cutaneous change is not specific for this disorder (93,118). Similar changes can be caused by allergic hypersensitivity, sarcoidosis, trichinosis (119), toxoplasmosis (120), and SLE (121–123). Bilateral upper eyelid swelling has also been reported to occur in focal myositis (124), an entity that is believed to be distinct from DM/PM.

The primary lesion of classic cutaneous DM consists of symmetrically distributed, poorly marginated, nonscaling, erythematous macules and patches that initially appear most often over the face, or the extensor aspects of the upper extremities, or both (Fig. 3.2). Such changes can be characterized as patchy or confluent macular violaceous erythema. Although it can be present from the outset, the violaceous hue that is so characteristic of DM skin inflammation in light-skinned individuals becomes more evident as the disease progresses. This characteristic violaceous hue is often compared with the color of the reddish-purple flowers of heliotropes, plants of the borage family that characteristically track the course of the sun across the sky over the course of a day. There is an interesting literary parallel in that the skin involvement in many patients with DM is clearly exacerbated by exposure to the sun. This violaceous hue helps to distinguish DM lesions from the early lesions of cutaneous LE.

Pruritus is often present very early in the course of the violaceous erythema, helping to distinguish DM skin change from all clinical forms of cutaneous LE, which typically lack pruritus. Secondary changes of cutaneous DM include scale, follicular hyperkeratosis, pigmentary change, subepidermal bullous change, and ulceration. Chronic skin involvement from DM, especially in certain parts of the body such as the V-area of anterior neck and upper chest, back, flanks, and buttocks can present with poikiloderma atrophicans vasculare that can be indistinguishable from other causes of this set of skin changes (e.g., mycosis fungoides). Although characteristically affecting these areas, poikiloderma can supervene in any area of skin chronically affected by the inflammatory changes of cutaneous DM. As the disease progresses, patches of violaceous erythema frequently become confluent over rather large areas of affected skin including the face, trunk, and extremities (Figs. 3.3 and 3.4). Involvement of the face is often focused around the eyes. For many nondermatologists, heliotrope erythema affecting the eyelids (often most notable on the upper lids) and periorbital tissue represent the most characteristic cutaneous manifestations of DM (Figs. 3.3 and 3.5). However, as previously discussed, periorbital heliotrope erythema is not specific for DM. It should be noted that in some series reported by dermatologists,

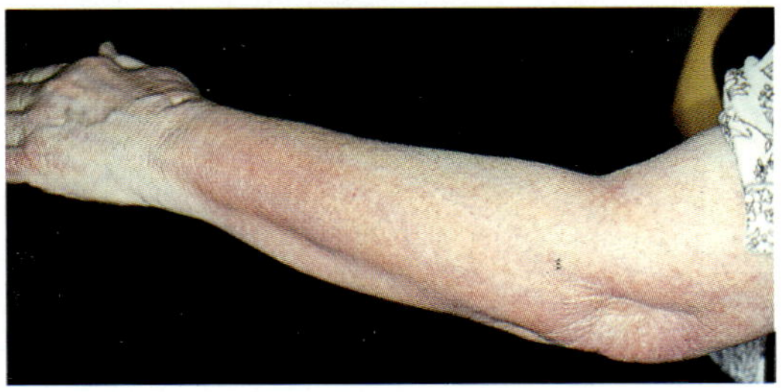

Figure 3.2. The primary lesion of cutaneous dermatomyositis is a confluent macular violaceous erythema as shown on the extensor aspect of the forearm and hand of this elderly white woman with classic dermatomyositis.

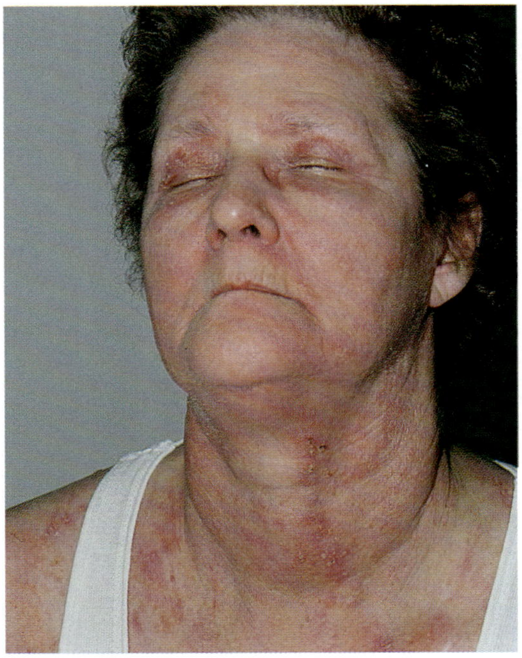

Figure 3.3. Classic dermatomyositis. Note the characteristic heliotrope (violaceous) periorbital erythema especially involving the upper lids. There is also crusting over the upper lids and anterior neck secondary to vesiculation and superficial erosion resulting from intense inflammation.

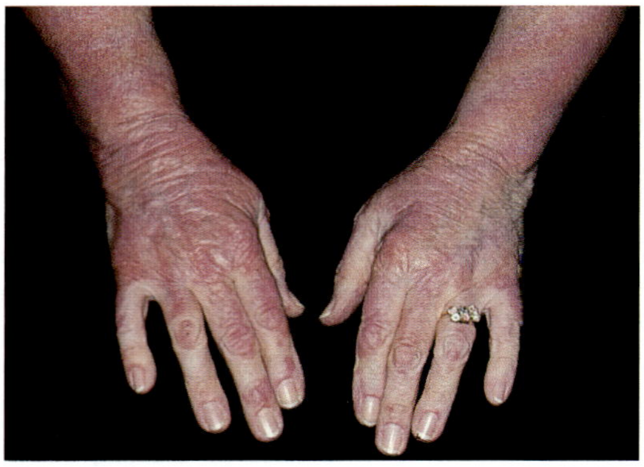

Figure 3.4. Confluent violaceous erythema over the dorsal aspects of the hands of a patient with advanced amyopathic dermatomyositis. Note the linear streaking of the violaceous erythema over the extensor tendon sheaths of the fingers that is accentuated over the knuckles.

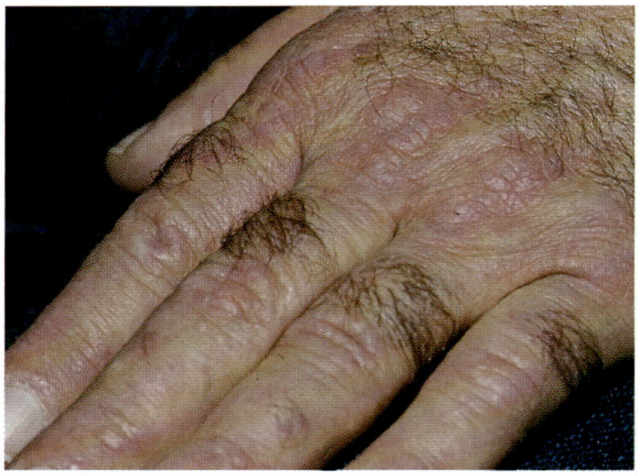

Figure 3.6. Violaceous erythema overlying the knuckles of a 45-year-old white man with amyopathic dermatomyositis representing one component of Gottron sign.

Gottron papules have been more commonly seen than heliotrope periorbital erythema (39,59). A possible explanation for this discrepancy is that the heliotrope erythema and edema of the eyelids and periorbital areas might be more common in patients who have clinical evidence of muscle disease and are therefore more likely to be managed by rheumatologists and internists rather than dermatologists. However, convincing data that address this point are not available.

The skin overlying the joints is especially targeted by the DM inflammatory process (Gottron sign of DM) (Figs. 3.6–3.8). As the inflammatory process continues to mature, Gottron papules can form over the proximal and distal interphalangeal (IP) joints as well as metacarpophalangeal (MCP) joints (Figs. 3.9–3.11). These papules most often occur over the dorsolateral aspect of these joints. Prominent periungual erythema and telangiectasia appear (Figs. 3.10–3.13) commonly as part of the hallmark cutaneous findings of DM. Pruritus is frequently the dominant symptom of the disease and can be severe enough to be disabling (i.e., sleep disturbance, interference with occupational activities and daily activities of life). As previously mentioned, cutaneous LE characteristically does not itch.

The term "Gottron sign" can be confusing in that it was initially used to describe the acral skin changes encountered in erythrokeratodermia congenitalis progressiva symmetrica of Gottron (syn., familial acrogeria, familial acromicria). To avoid confusion, perhaps it might be best to use the designation "Gottron sign of DM" when referring to the cutaneous changes of DM.

With further escalation of the disease, secondary skin changes can become evident. It is not uncommon for more established skin lesions to develop superficial induration due to the intense accumulation of mucin within the dermis. Multiloculated vesicles or subepidermal bullous lesions can develop over the dorsal surfaces of the hands or forearms and occasionally other areas, at times simulating an allergic contact dermatitis (125) (Figs. 3.14 and 3.15). Although not often described in the literature, it has been our experience that older lesions not infrequently develop white lacy areas within the areas of violaceous erythema, somewhat similar to what can be seen in lichen planus. This change can be especially evident overlying the central areas of Gottron papules (Figs. 3.10 and 3.11). Others have commented on the similarities between cutaneous DM and lichen planus, which also has a characteristic violaceous hue (126).

As the inflammation of cutaneous DM subsides, postinflammatory hypopigmentation can remain (Fig. 3.16). In dark-skinned individuals in whom the violaceous erythema can be difficult to discern early in its course, the associated postinflammatory pigmentary disturbances can suggest the diagnosis. Note that as a rule, dark-skinned patients tend to be more

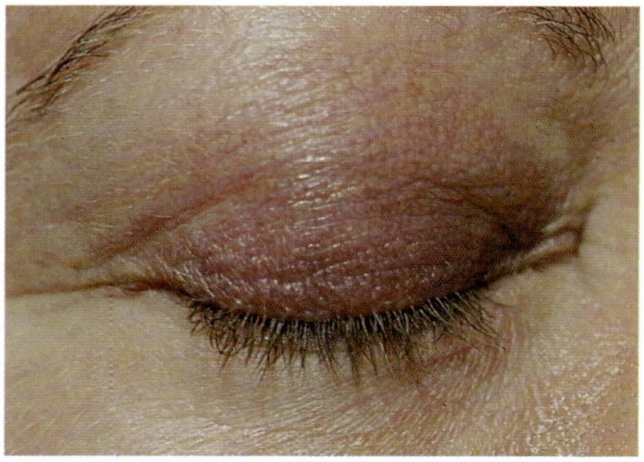

Figure 3.5. Violaceous erythema accentuated at the margins of the upper eyelids of a 47-year-old white woman with classic dermatomyositis at a time when her muscle disease was in complete remission.

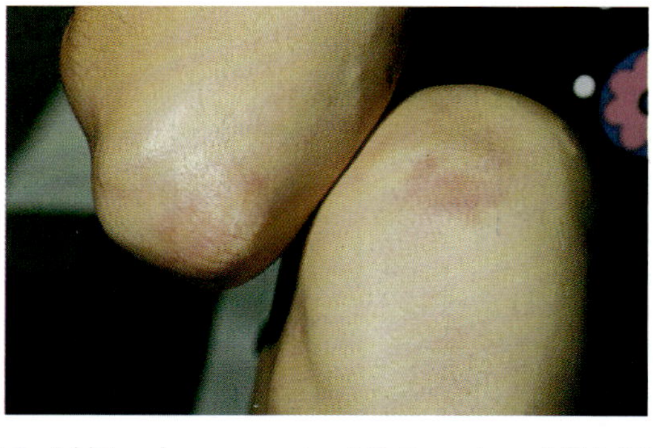

Figure 3.7. Additional components of Gottron sign of DM. Violaceous erythema overlying the olecranon process and patella of a 27-year-old white woman having the classic cutaneous manifestations of dermatomyositis without clinical evidence of myositis for 12 years. These changes were bilaterally symmetric.

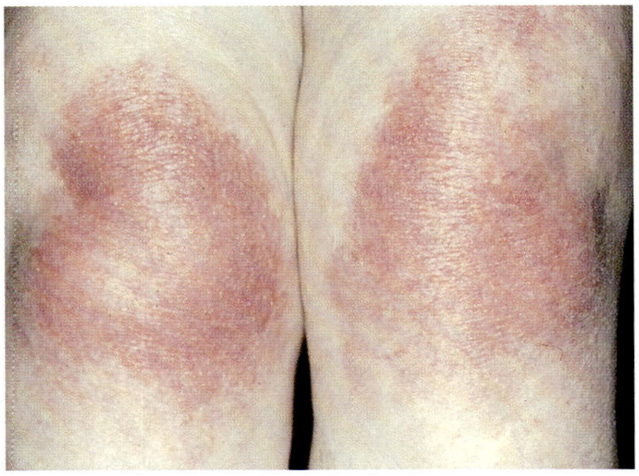

Figure 3.8. A more advanced example of Gottron sign overlying the knees of an elderly white woman with classic dermatomyositis.

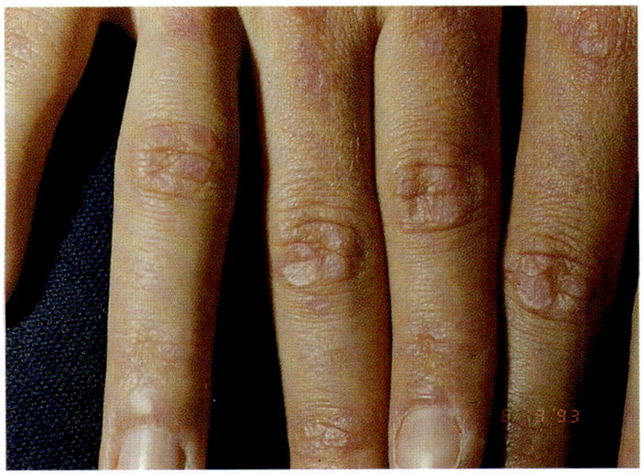

Figure 3.9. Gottron papules in the same patient described in Fig. 3.7.

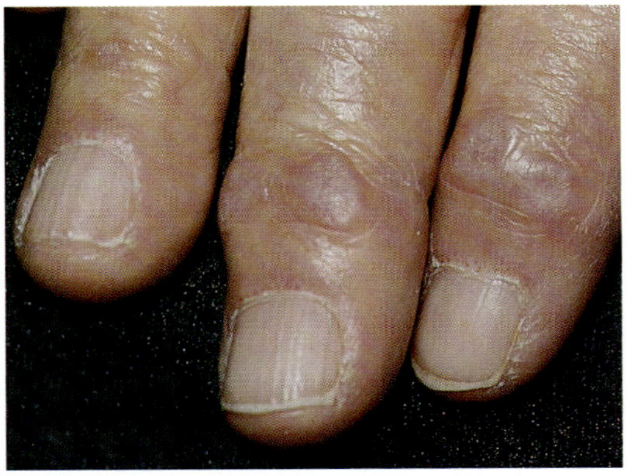

Figure 3.10. Gottron papules in a more advanced stage of evolution in a 60-year-old white woman with classic dermatomyositis. Also, note the periungual erythema and grossly visible telangiectasia. The black speck in the medial aspect of the cuticle of the index finger represents an area of hemorrhage from one of the incompetent telangiectatic capillaries.

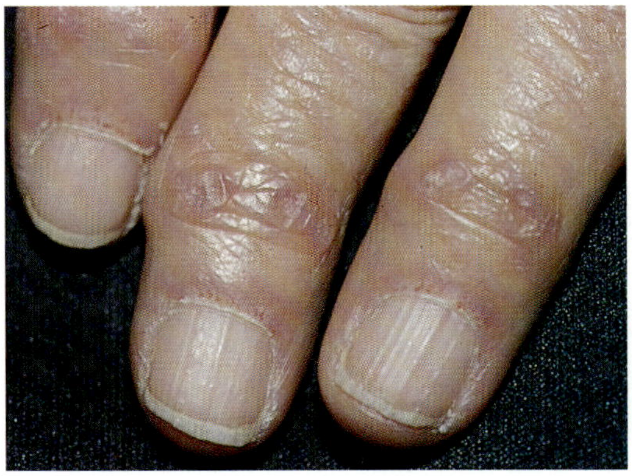

Figure 3.11. Another example of Gottron papules in a 50-year-old white woman with amyopathic dermatomyositis.

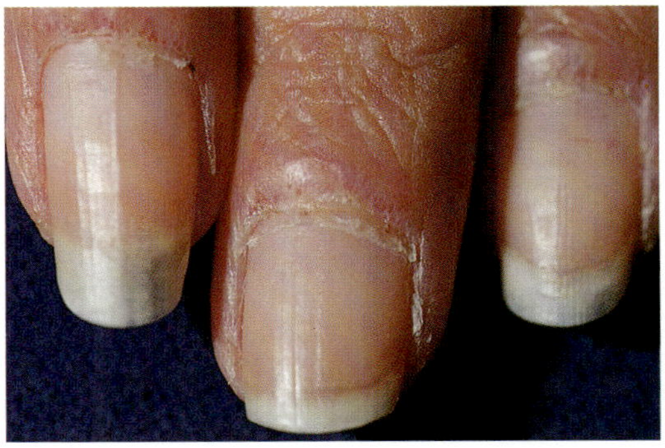

Figure 3.12. Close-up view of the periungual changes of a 35-year-old Latin American woman with classic dermatomyositis. Ragged cuticles are present in addition to erythema, grossly visible telangiectasia, and punctate cuticular hemorrhage.

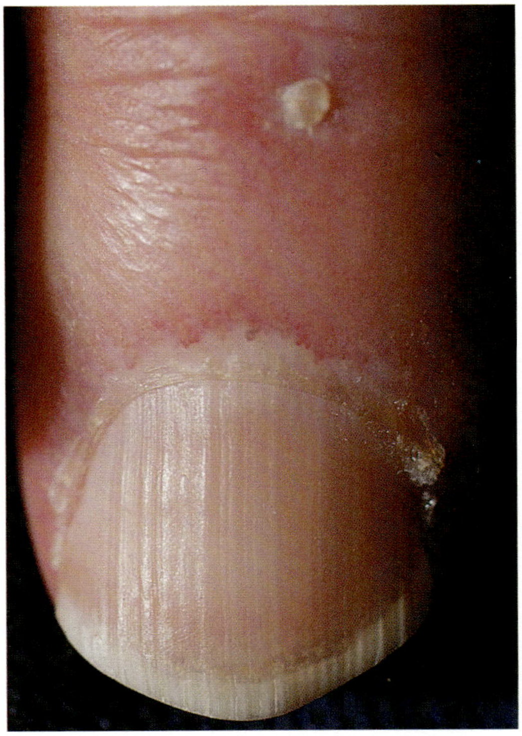

Figure 3.13. Periungual changes similar to those in Fig. 3.12 in a 33-year-old white woman with amyopathic dermatomyositis. There is also a focal scale-crust over the distal interphalangeal joint resulting from vesicle formation and erosion.

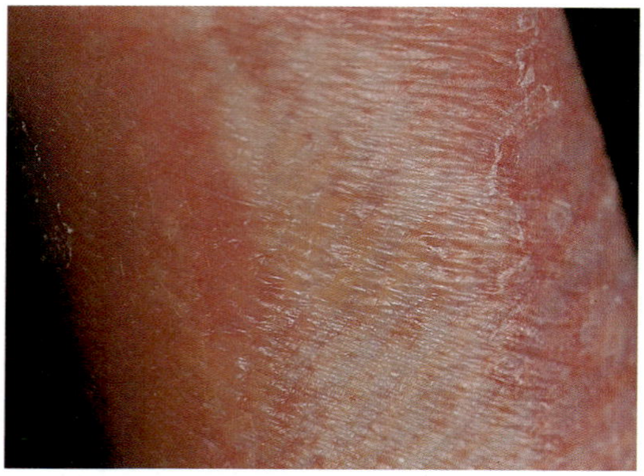

Figure 3.14. Vesiculation resulting from intensely inflamed skin overlying the volar aspect of the wrist of a 35-year-old white woman with amyopathic dermatomyositis. Biopsy showed a cleavage plane extending through the epidermal basal layer.

aware of subtle color changes in their skin than are their lighter skinned physicians.

Prominent atrophic dermal scarring as occurs in classic discoid LE does not develop in DM. Persistent inflammation at the same site for prolonged periods on any area of the body can result in poikilodermatous changes—the combination of atrophy, telangiectasia, and speckled hyperpigmentation and hypopigmentation (poikilodermatomyositis) (127). The original case of poikiloderma atrophicans vasculare reported by Jacobi actually is believed to have actually occurred in a patient with DM (128).

Superficial erosions and ulcers can subsequently develop over the face and eyelids as well as other areas affected by particularly intense and protracted inflammation (Fig. 3.15). Deeper, irregular retiform ulcers can also develop in areas of poikiloderma in both the adult (129) and childhood forms of DM (130). Lipomembranous (membranocystic) changes previously thought to be specific for panniculitis have been noted in the histopathology of punched-out ulcers of DM (131).

Left untreated, the cutaneous involvement of DM most commonly tends to be indolently progressive. However, some patients can experience explosive worsening of their skin disease over short periods, rapidly progressing to the appearance of an exfoliative erythroderma (132–134). Others display only limited degrees of skin involvement for many years without systemic therapy. Patients who had their skin and muscle

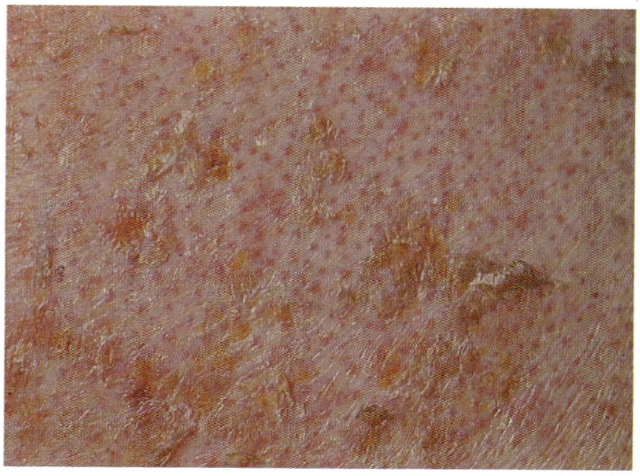

Figure 3.15. Close-up view of another area of cutaneous involvement in the same patient described in Fig. 3.14 showing areas of crusting resulting from spontaneous rupture of vesiculobullous changes.

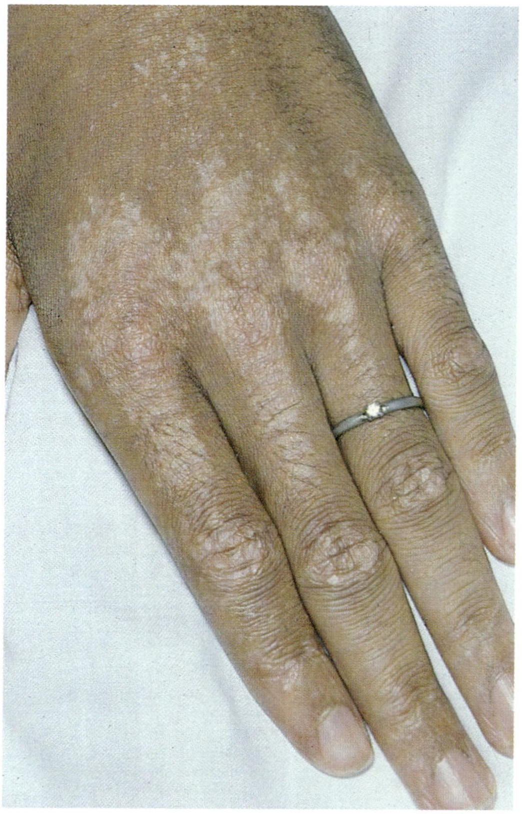

Figure 3.16. Postinflammatory hypopigmentation over the dorsal aspects of the hands and fingers of a 14-year-old black girl with classic dermatomyositis. Note the accentuation of changes over the metacarpophalangeal and interphalangeal joints. This patient was formally presented elsewhere during an earlier phase of her disease (the single pediatric case in Euwer and Sontheimer [39]).

involvement completely suppressed with systemic corticosteroid therapy can have their skin disease recur in the absence of muscle weakness or any other systemic manifestations of the disorder (as previously mentioned, the term "postmyopathic cutaneous DM activity" could be used to describe this pattern of recrudescent skin disease activity). Thus, the activity of the cutaneous manifestations of DM cannot be used as a reliable gauge of systemic disease activity in this disorder.

The hallmark cutaneous manifestations of DM typically undergo sequential change over time. DM-specific skin disease often presents nonspecifically and is often initially confused with seborrheic dermatitis, rosacea, psoriasis, atopic dermatitis, contact dermatitis, photodermatitis, or LE. As the cutaneous changes evolve to include the typical anatomic distribution, a highly characteristic or pathognomic pattern becomes evident.

REGIONAL DISTRIBUTION OF TYPICAL SKIN LESIONS

Some areas of the skin are more commonly affected by DM than are others; however, the relative frequency of such anatomic differences has not been well documented. Table 3.4 compares some of the earlier data that address this point (34,39,59,135). A similar comparison of more recent observations with similar results has been made by Caproni et al. (86). In addition, a number of reports indicate that macular violaceous erythema overlying the extensor aspect of the upper extremities with or without fully formed Gottron papules is present more frequently in both classic DM and clinically amyopathic DM than is perior-

TABLE 3.4. Anatomic Regional Differences in DM/Amyopathic DM

	Krain (n = 6)[a]	Nesbitt (n = 7)[b]	Euwer (n = 6)[c]	Cheong (n = 10)[d]
Photosensitivity	29%	100%	50%	—
Gottron papules	?	?	83%	80%
Gottron sign of DM:	?	86%	100%	?
IP, MCP joints	83%	?	100%	?
Elbows	83%	?	50%	?
Knees	83%	?	33%	?
Periorbital heliotrope	67%	100%	67%	60%
Periungual:				
Telangiectasia	67%	100%	83%	80%
Erythema	?	?	100%	?
Poikiloderma	0	71%	33%	20%
Violaceous erythema:				
Extensor arms	83%	?	83%	?
Extensor legs	83%	?	33%	?
Neck, chest, back	50%	?	100%	?
Shoulders	50%	71%	50%	?
Extensor tendons	?	?	33%	—
Generalized erythema	0	?	0	20%
Scalp inflammation	?	?	83%	?
Alopecia	?	71%	17%	?

IP, interphalangeal; MCP, metacarpophalangeal; DM, dermatomyositis.
[a]From (34).
[b]From (135).
[c]From (39).
[d]From (59).

bital heliotrope erythema (83–85,136). As has been previously mentioned, it has been traditionally thought that periorbital heliotrope erythema was the most common and most specific cutaneous manifestation of DM.

Although it is generally believed that skin involvement does not reflect systemic disease activity, systematically collected data relating to the clinical significance of different patterns of skin disease involvement with respect to systemic disease associations are lacking. In one such report, only flagellate erythema, a relatively rare cutaneous finding of DM (5%), was found to correlate with systemic disease activity (137). Some effort has been made to correlate the pattern of autoantibody production and attendant systemic disease risk with certain types of skin lesions (56,58). This issue will be discussed later in the section dealing with laboratory assessment.

It is not well understood why the cutaneous manifestations of this disorder have such a predilection for certain anatomic locations. One could speculate that physiologic changes associated with the stretching of skin over joints could serve as one such localizing factor. Relative cutaneous ischemia during skin stretching at these sites could be a localizing factor. Minor trauma would also be expected to occur over such areas and could represent another localizing factor.

Involvement of the face and extensor aspects of the arms may be related to sun exposure in some patients with DM, because the cutaneous manifestations of DM are known to be precipitated or exacerbated by natural sunlight and artificial sources of UV light (22,59,138,139). Although definitive data do not exist, some studies have suggested that approximately 50% of patients with DM experience photosensitivity (22,59). The action spectrum appears to include UVB and UVA (59). It would be interesting to know whether clinical photosensitivity in DM correlates with the presence of the TNF-α-308A of promoter polymorphism that is associated with increased TNF-α production following UVB exposure.

Some experienced clinicians have suggested that like LE, the activity of DM/PM can be precipitated or exacerbated by emotional and physical stress, although there is little objective evidence to support this idea. There is little argument that undue physical exertion could be detrimental to patients with active myositis.

Because regional anatomic localization can be so helpful in the recognition of DM skin involvement, we will use this approach to further discuss the cutaneous manifestations of this disease. This will be discussed in a "head-down" fashion.

Scalp. The scalp may be involved with patchy or confluent violaceous erythema, or scale, or both (Fig. 3.17) (140). This can occur as a generalized change throughout the scalp or can be focused in certain areas (e.g., posterior scalp and upper neck, anterior and temporal hairline). The violaceous erythema and scaling of the scalp that can be seen in patients with DM is often exceedingly pruritic and may require special therapeutic attention. Generalized, nonscarring alopecia of the scalp can also be seen, the histopathology of which has not been well studied. Scalp involvement occurs with equal frequency in patients with adult classic DM and patients with clinically amyopathic DM. This feature has recently been reported to occur in approximately 25% of patients with juvenile-onset DM as well (84).

Head and Neck. The eyelids, especially the upper lids, often display characteristic violaceous erythema often associated with edema that can extend to involve the entire periorbital region (Figs. 3.3 and 3.5). Stone (141) has suggested that the edema associated with this disease indirectly produces the violaceous hue by displacing the hyperemic cutaneous vasculature

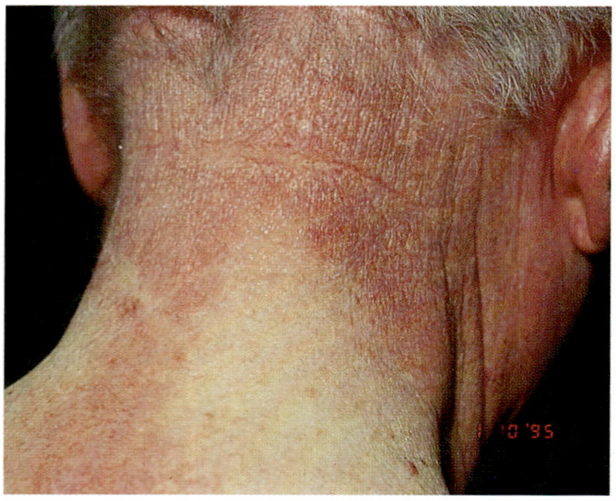

Figure 3.17. Violaceous erythema overlying the nape of the neck, hairline, and scalp in a 65-year-old white man who presented with amyopathic dermatomyositis that evolved over a 5-year period to classic dermatomyositis.

more deeply into the dermis. In some patients, the disease presents with striking periorbital and facial edema without or with only a minimal degree of the characteristic color changes (142, 143). Following the periorbital areas, facial involvement is usually most marked on the malar areas. The heliotrope discoloration can also be present on the forehead where it may or may not be associated with fine scales, telangiectasia, or hypopigmentation. As with cutaneous LE, the nasolabial folds are usually spared. Deeper dermal atrophy is never seen in the early stages of this disease as can occur in discoid LE. Poikiloderma on the central face is relatively rare. The ears are usually spared. Oral mucosal involvement has been reported but this is quite rare (8,144). The characteristic violaceous discoloration may be seen in the V area of the neck and contiguous aspects of upper chest (usually the areas that would be exposed if one were to wear a V-neck, an open collar or a t-shirt) (Fig. 3.18). Poikiloderma commonly develops in this area with long-standing inflammation. The nape of the neck is also a favored site for cutaneous DM (Fig. 3.17). Symmetric violaceous erythema that extends across the nape of the neck to the posterior aspects of the shoulders and upper back has been referred to as the shawl sign (56,58) (Fig. 3.19).

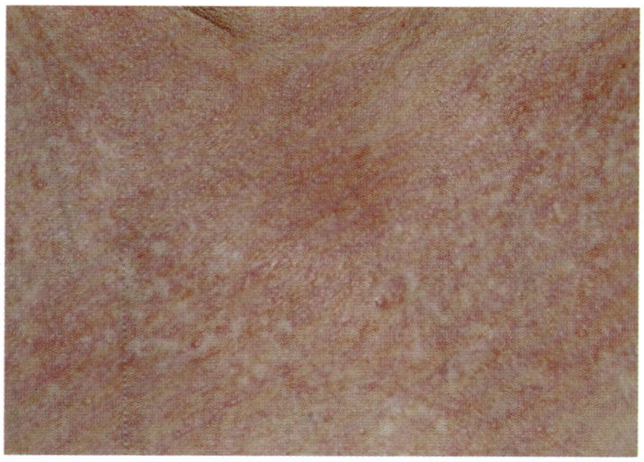

Figure 3.18. Poikilodermatous changes over the V area of the anterior neck and upper chest in a 65-year-old white woman with classic dermatomyositis.

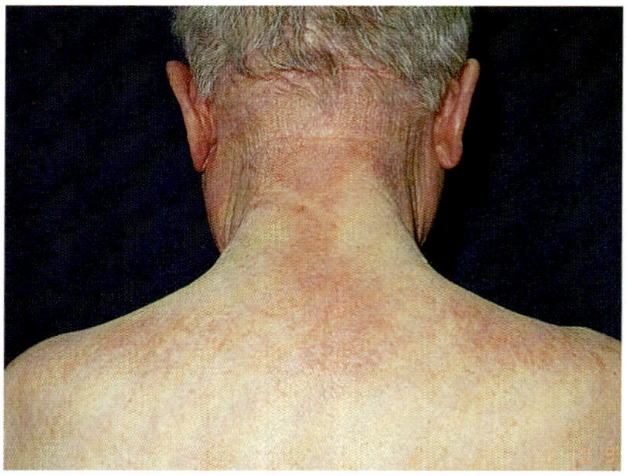

Figure 3.19. The shawl sign. Violaceous erythema over the nape of the neck and posterior aspects of the shoulders in the same patient described in Fig. 3.17.

Trunk. The trunk is less often affected by DM, although patchy or confluent macular violaceous erythema can occur on any aspect of the chest or back (Fig. 3.20A). In addition, asymmetric round or oval patches of violaceous erythema can be seen over the back or upper buttocks areas. Such lesions can progress relatively quickly to poikilodermatous skin changes (Fig. 3.20B). There are reports of a peculiar pattern of centripetal flagellate erythema (zebra-like stripes) over the back and lateral chest walls in a small percentage of patients with both classic and clinically amyopathic DM (137,145).

Upper and Lower Arms. Violaceous erythema often extends to the extensor aspects of the deltoid areas, upper arms, and forearms (Figs. 3.2 and 3.4). When the arms are affected, the violaceous erythema can be especially prominent over the olecranon processes, the knuckles, the knees, and the medial malleoli (i.e., Gottron sign of DM) (Figs. 3.6–3.9 and 3.21). Cutaneous calcification is considerably less common in adult-onset classic DM compared with juvenile onset classic DM (146). When it does occur in adults, it often presents as firm dermal or subcutaneous papules or nodules that are often most prominent around the elbows and hands (Figs. 3.22 and 3.23), although other areas can be affected. Large subcutaneous tumoral deposits can occur over the trunk of patients with DM. Such lesions may be filled with a liquid suspension of calcium crystals (i.e., "milk of calcium") (147). Cutaneous calcinosis is rare in amyopathic DM.

Hands and Wrists. The dorsal and lateral aspects of the interphalangeal (IP) and metacarpophalangeal (MCP) joints commonly display the characteristic violaceous erythema without scale. The violaceous erythema may also be seen to streak over the dorsum of the fingers as if it were tracking over the extensor tendon sheaths (Fig. 3.24). Occasionally, similar changes can be seen on the palm overlying the flexor tendon.

Gottron papules are reddish-purple papules that can develop within chronically affected skin overlying the extensor aspects of the IP, or MCP joints, or both (Figs. 3.6 and 3.9–3.11). The dorsolateral aspects of the joints are often preferentially targeted. These papules can occur on only one knuckle, several knuckles, or all knuckles. They are usually flat-topped and may or may not be associated with scale. Well-established Gottron papules may develop focal atrophy at their centers. The central areas of these papules can be hypopigmented and on occasion display a white lacy appearance similar to that of Wickham striae seen in lichen planus (Figs. 3.10 and 3.11). Telangiectasia can also be prominent in such lesions.

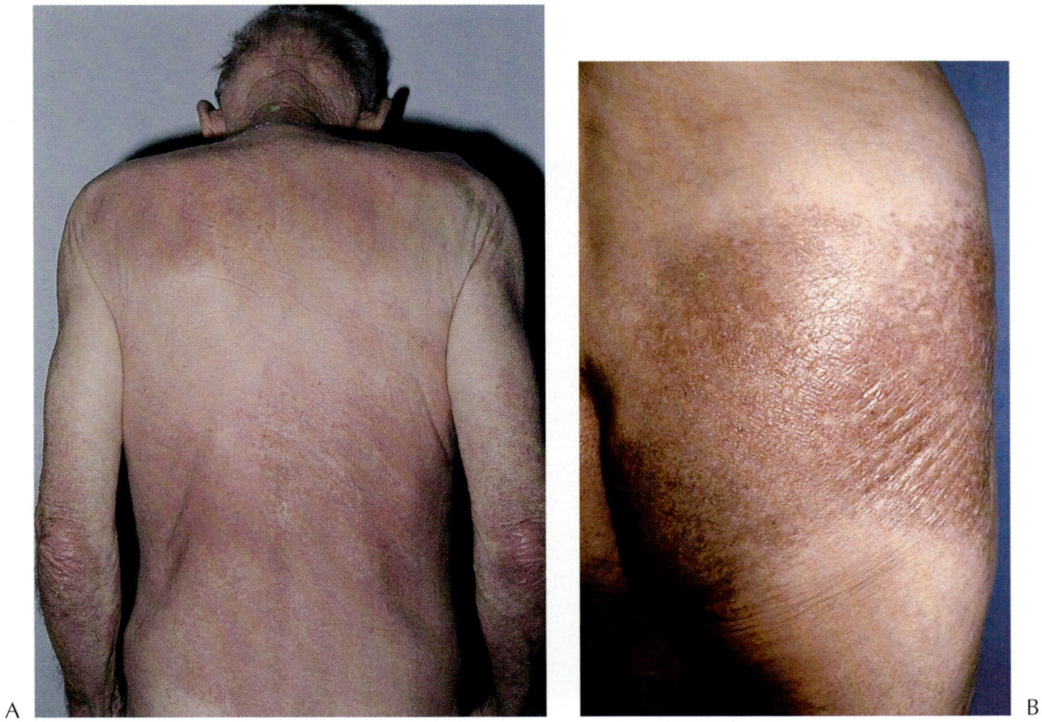

Figure 3.20. **A:** Violaceous erythema over the shoulders, back, and flanks of the same patient described in Fig. 3.17. **B:** Isolated plaque of poikilodermatous change over the flank and buttock of a different male patient having classic DM.

The periungual areas are often erythematous and the cuticles can have a ragged or dystrophic appearance (148) (Figs. 3.10–3.13). Close inspection with the naked eye of the periungual areas in light-skinned individuals can often reveal dilated capillary loops (Figs. 3.10–3.13), cuticular hemorrhages (Figs. 3.10 and 3.12), or both. When grossly visible nailfold vascular changes are not present, more subtle vascular abnormalities can be observed at the bedside with a portable dermoscopy unit such as the DermLite 3GEN (Derma Instruments, Vienna, Austria) (e.g., dilated, torturous, arborizing capillaries intermixed with capillary dropout, avascular areas, punctate cuticular hemorrhage). Similar changes can also be seen in patients with systemic sclerosis and less commonly, those with SLE.

A distinctive hyperkeratotic change, the "mechanic hands" lesion, was initially described on the hands of eight patients with polymyositis and connective tissue disease (four with mixed connective tissue disease, three with DM, and one with systemic lupus erythematosus (SLE) (149). It consists of a nonpruritic, hyperkeratotic eruption accompanied by scaling, fissuring, and hyperpigmentation giving the appearance of the calloused hands of a laborer, thus its name. The changes are bilaterally symmetric, distributed along the ulnar aspect of the thumb and radial aspect of the fingers, and are most prominent on the index and middle fingers with occasional extension to the palmar surfaces (Fig. 3.25). All of the initial patients described with this lesion had an inflammatory myopathy. In patients with myositis, Love et al. (56) subsequently found a positive correlation between these skin changes and the presence of the antisynthetase syndrome (anti-

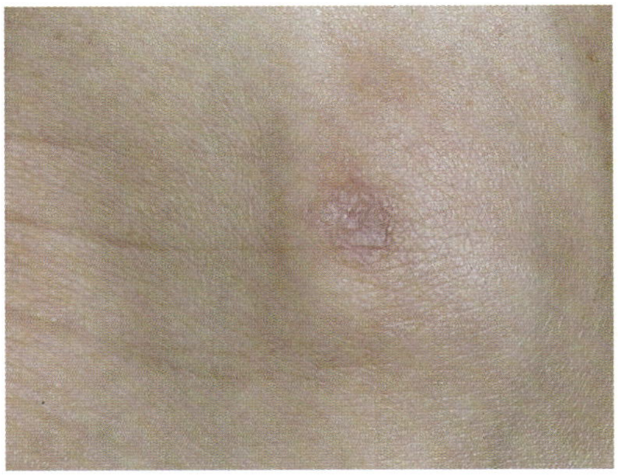

Figure 3.21. Small atrophic plaque over the medial malleolus of the same patient with amyopathic dermatomyositis described in Fig. 3.7. On close inspection the following changes were noted: violaceous erythema, telangiectasia, white striae, and central atrophy. This combination of clinical changes approaches that of fully evolved Gottron papules shown in Figs. 3.10 and 3.11. The medial malleolus is one of the less commonly affected areas by classic cutaneous dermatomyositis.

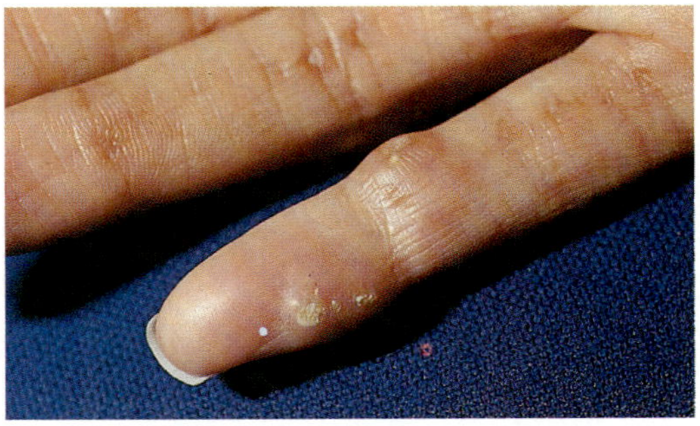

Figure 3.22. Calcinosis cutis in a 13-year-old black girl with a 7-year history of amyopathic dermatomyositis. This is the same patient described in Fig. 3.16.

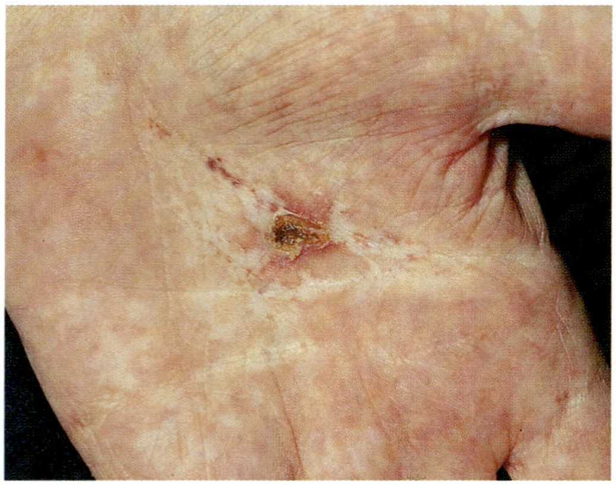

Figure 3.23. Calcinosis cutis of the palm with overlying ulceration in a 60-year-old white woman with classic dermatomyositis.

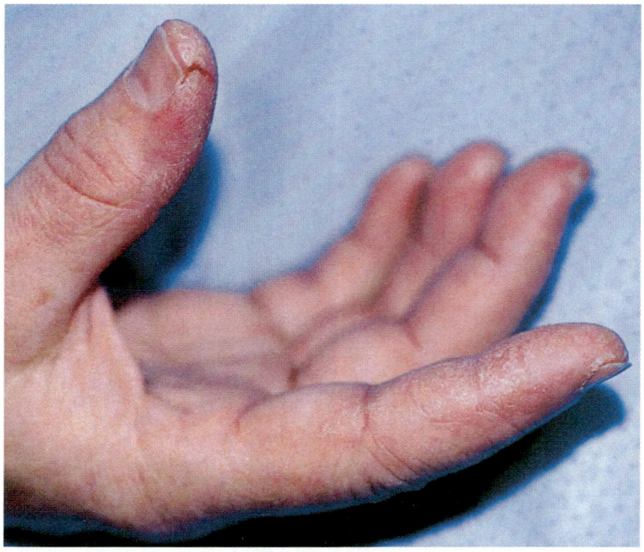

A

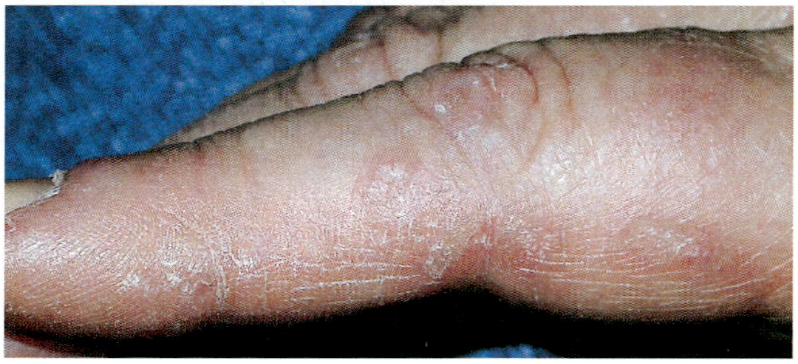

B

Figure 3.25. Mechanic's hand lesion. **A:** Note the hyperkeratotic changes of the thumb and index finger in a classic DM patient. **B:** Note hyperkeratosis on lateral aspect of index finger of a clinically amyopathic DM patient.

synthetase antibodies such as Jo-1, Raynaud's phenomenon, arthritis, and ILD). Mitra et al. (150) subsequently reiterated the association of the mechanic's hand lesion with the antisynthetase syndrome. However, further study of this skin change has failed to support such associations (151). In addition, one of the authors (R.D.S.) has observed the mechanic's hand lesion in several patients having clinically amyopathic DM without arthritis, Raynaud's phenomenon, interstitial pneumonia, or MSAs (personal unpublished observations).

Approximately 10% to 40% of patients with classic DM will experience Raynaud's phenomenon (19,152). The fingers especially at the tips may display the physical changes of Raynaud's phenomenon (i.e., tuft atrophy, pitted scars; pterygium inversus unguis). The changes of Raynaud's phenomenon are more likely to be present in those patients who have DM/PM as a component of an overlap connective tissue disease. Raynaud's phenomenon appears to occur much less frequently in clinically amyopathic DM.

It is also not uncommon for patients with classic or amyopathic DM to develop symptoms of carpal tunnel syndrome secondary to edematous compression of the median nerve (153).

Lower Extremities. In some cases, the anterior and lateral aspects of the thighs can be markedly affected (Fig. 3.26); however, more limited involvement in these areas is more typical. Patients having hallmark cutaneous manifestations of DM elsewhere may often have a bilaterally symmetric, patchy, macular violaceous erythema often displaying a reticulated or livedoid pattern and at times, a poikilodermatous pattern localized over the lateral aspects of the upper thighs and hips. These skin changes tend to be centered over and inferior to the greater trochanter of the femur and as such have some similarity to the localization of DM skin lesions elsewhere over bony prominences. This cutaneous change has been referred to as the "holster sign" as the area of skin affected roughly underlies the general area where a pistol holster is worn from a belt on the waist (41).

The suprapatellar aspects of the skin overlying the knees can display a striking violaceous erythema as a component of Got-

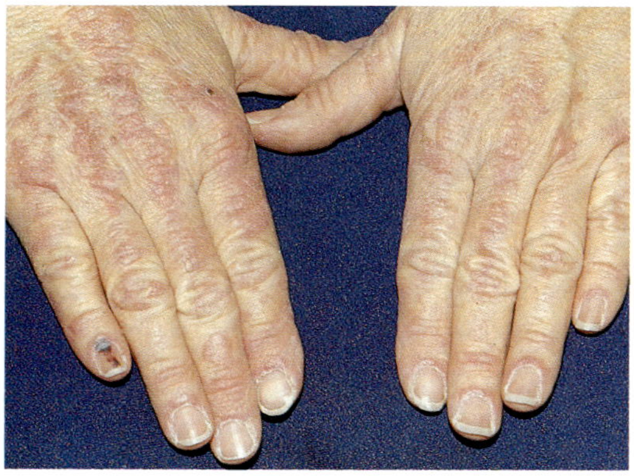

Figure 3.24. Linear streaking of violaceous erythema overlying the extensor tendons of a 45-year-old white woman with classic dermatomyositis.

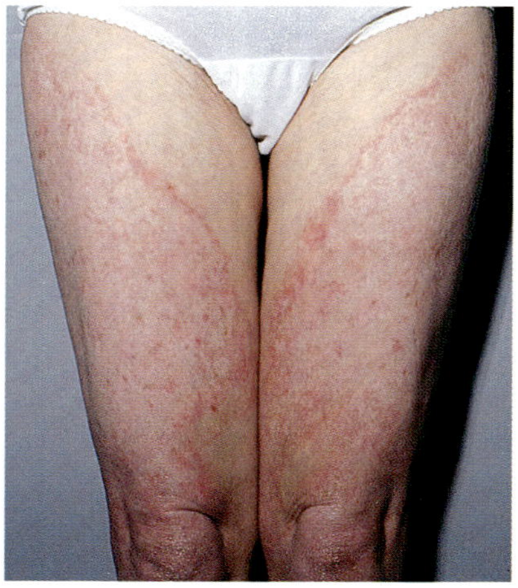

Figure 3.26. Sharply marginated violaceous erythema with early poikilodermatous changes over the thighs of a patient with classic dermatomyositis.

tron sign of DM (Fig. 3.8). In addition, small, focal macular areas of violaceous erythema can develop over the medial malleoli, sometimes progressing to focal atrophy and telangiectasia somewhat simulating Gottron papules (Fig. 3.21). Curiously, the lateral malleoli and other parts of the feet are usually spared.

There have been no documented differences in the clinical and histopathologic expression of skin disease in patients having classic DM or clinically amyopathic DM. As more information is published concerning clinically amyopathic DM, skin changes thought previously to occur only in patients with classic DM (e.g., mechanic's hand lesion) are being recognized to occur in the context of clinically amyopathic DM as well.

For the purposes of future clinical studies, a provisional minimal set of hallmark cutaneous manifestations of DM that needs to be present to define the presence of DM-specific skin disease has recently been proposed (41). Obviously, formal studies designed to validate such a criteria set will be needed.

SKIN LESIONS ENCOUNTERED ONLY RARELY IN PATIENTS WITH DERMATOMYOSITIS

A number of cutaneous changes have been reported to occur in patients with DM/PM on a rare or one-time-only basis (Table 3.5). Because of the sporadic nature of these reports, one can question whether such lesions have occurred in patients with DM only by chance. For the sake of completeness, these unusual entities are briefly summarized below:

Anasarca. Anasarca as the presenting manifestation of classic juvenile DM has again been noted to be an ominous prognostic sign (154).

Autoimmune Bullous Disease. Bullous pemphigoid and dermatitis herpetiformis have been reported to have occurred in patients with DM/PM (155–157).

Hypertrichosis. Excessive hair growth can occur on the forearms, legs, and temples of children with DM (158,159). A predilection toward infrapatellar localization of hypertrichosis in children has been noted (160). Braverman (37) has also noted that hypertrichosis can develop in areas of prior DM cutaneous involvement.

Ichthyosis, Acquired. Acquired ichthyosis developed over the flanks and the extensor surfaces of the extremities in a 65-year-old woman with DM (161). No evidence of internal malignancy was present at the time of initial evaluation and for 2 years thereafter.

Lichen Planus. Histopathologically and immunopathologically typical lichen planus developed on the dorsal hands and forearms of two patients with otherwise typical DM (126). Oral lesions were not present in either case.

Linear IgA Bullous Dermatosis. A 56-year-old woman developed linear IgA bullous dermatosis shortly before developing DM (162). High-dose corticosteroids therapy started at the time of DM onset resulted in slow resolution of both disease processes. No evidence of internal malignancy was noted.

Lipodystrophy, Acquired. Acquired lipodystrophy has been increasingly reported in patients with juvenile classic DM. One report of 20 patients indicated that 25% had evidence of lipodystrophy, whereas 50% demonstrated hypertriglyceridemia and insulin resistance (163). In another preliminary report, lipodystrophy was associated with calcinosis (164).

Malakoplakia. Malakoplakia is a rare idiopathic granulomatous skin change having a characteristic histopathology marked by the presence of Michaelis-Gutmann bodies that usually affect the urinary tract. Painful perianal abscesses and draining sinuses with histopathologic changes of malakoplakia were observed in a young man having DM of 3 years' duration (165).

Mucinosis, Cutaneous. Dermal mucin deposition is highly prominent in the histopathology of cutaneous DM and the inflammatory cutaneous lesions of DM at times have an indurated quality due in part to this mucin accumulation (166,167). Indurated plaques can sometimes develop on noninflamed skin of patients with DM that on biopsy, are found to be the result of intense accumulation of mucin within the dermis (166). Although not well documented in the literature, one of the authors (R.D.S.) has observed several cases in which mucinous papules and nodules have been present in noninflamed skin of patients with DM (Fig. 3.27). These patients appeared

TABLE 3.5. Mucocutaneous Lesions Reported to Occasionally Occur in Patients with Dermatomyositis/Polymyositis

Acquired ichthyosis (161)
Anasarca (154)
Erythroderma (133,134)
Facial swelling without erythema (142)
Follicular hyperkeratosis (185,186)
Gingival telangiectasia (189)
Hypertrichosis (37,158,159)
Ichthyosis, acquired (161)
Lichen planus (126)
Linear IgA bullous dermatosis (162)
Lipodystrophy, acquired (163)
Malakoplakia (165)
Malignant erythema (suffusion) (14)
Mechanic's hand pattern of palmar hyperkeratosis (149)
Mucinosis, cutaneous (167)
Mucous membrane lesions (8,144)
Nasal septal perforation (175)
Panniculitis (178)
Pityriasis rubra pilaris–like changes (185)
Steroid-induced acanthosis nigricans (188)
Urticaria (190)
Vasculitis, cutaneous (190,191)
Vulvar changes (192) and scrotal (193) involvement
Zebra-like stripes (centripetal flagellate erythema) (145,184)

Numbers in parentheses represent reference sources.

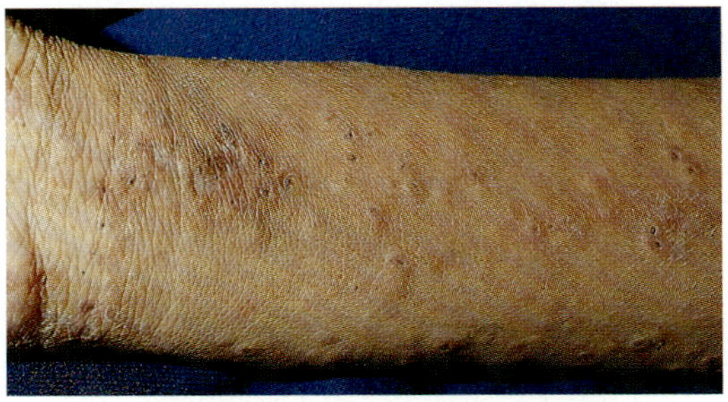

Figure 3.27. Indurated dermal papules and nodules over the flexor aspect of the forearm of a 30-year-old black woman with classic dermatomyositis with disabling muscle weakness. Biopsy revealed marked accumulation of mucin within the dermis. It was not clear whether the punctate areas of crusting that overlay many of these lesions was the result of scratching or represented a primary manifestation of the underlying disease process.

different from the few cases of scleromyxedema (lichen myxedematous) that have been observed in the past in patients with DM (168,169). A plaquelike pattern of cutaneous mucinosis has also been described in DM (170).

Mucous Membrane Involvement. Braverman (37) reported that Kiel had earlier noted erythema (Fig. 3.28) and white patches (Fig. 3.29) of the palate, buccal mucosa, and tongue in some of his patients with DM (8). Others have also noted such lesions (144). Lip ulceration has also been reported (171). Patients are often unaware that they have such oral lesions. Reportedly, the conjunctival mucosa is affected on occasion. Bilateral membranous conjunctivitis (172) and exuberant conjunctival pseudopolyposis (173) have been noted. Blepharochalasis (thin discolored eyelid skin, acquired pseudoepicanthal folds, and eyelid muscle laxity) has also been reported in a case of juvenile DM (174).

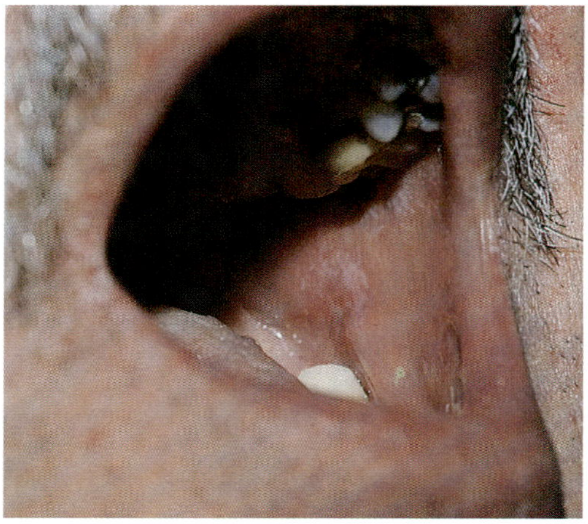

Figure 3.29. White plaques over the buccal mucosa of a 45-year-old white man with amyopathic dermatomyositis. These mucosal changes were quite reminiscent of oral lichen planus; however, this patient's skin changes were very typical of dermatomyositis (this is the same patient as in Fig. 3.6).

Nasal Septal Perforation. A young woman with DM developed a perforated nasal septum (175), a change that would be expected to occur more commonly in other rheumatic diseases such as SLE. Reportedly, other causes of nasal septal perforation were excluded in this case, although no specific indication was given that syphilis had been excluded.

Nail Dystrophy. An unusually severe case of scarring nail dystrophy resulting in complete loss of all toenails was reported as the only cutaneous finding in a single patient with DM (176).

Panniculitis. Clinical evidence of subcutaneous inflammation is very rare in DM (177,178). In one such case, tender subcutaneous nodules over the buttocks, thighs, arms, abdomen, and breast presented approximately 10 months before development of muscle weakness (178). In addition to a lobular panniculitis, hydropic degeneration of epidermal basal cells was noted on the skin biopsy. Curiously, this patient was not reported to have any of the more typical superficial inflammatory skin lesions of DM (see Table 3.3) that might be expected to be associated with this pattern of epidermal basal cell injury. This case is quite representative of the five earlier cases of panniculitis in DM that have been reported to date (data reviewed by Fusade [178]). Additional cases of panniculitis in adult and juvenile DM have been reported (179–182). One case of multifocal lipoatrophy in a child has also been reported (183).

Pityriasis Rubra Pilaris–like Lesions (i.e., type Wong DM). Dupré et al. (184) reported that hyperkeratotic follicular erythematosus papules have been observed to occur in a linear distribution over the dorsal aspects of the hands and feet in Chinese (185) and white individuals with DM (186). One of us (R.D.S.) has seen a striking example of this in a 46-year-old white woman with amyopathic DM where the hyperkeratotic follicular papules extended onto the forearms, arms, and shoulders (Fig. 3.30). Attention has been refocused more recently on this type of cutaneous change in DM (187). This variant usually presents as perifollicular keratosis over the extensor aspects of the upper extremities in adult-onset classic DM (185). This can simulate the appearance of florid keratosis pilaris and some such patients have had atopic dermatitis as well as DM. However, more widespread patterns of involvement better simulating pityriasis rubra pilaris (PRP) have also been described, although such patients have not had other classic features of PRP such a desquamative palmar plantar hyperkeratosis.

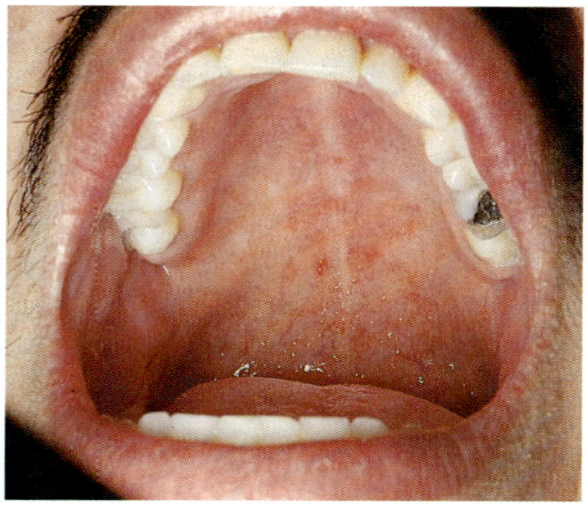

Figure 3.28. Asymptomatic, nonerosive erythema of the palatal mucosa having a sharply marginated, scalloped border. This patient was a 30-year-old Hispanic man with classic dermatomyositis.

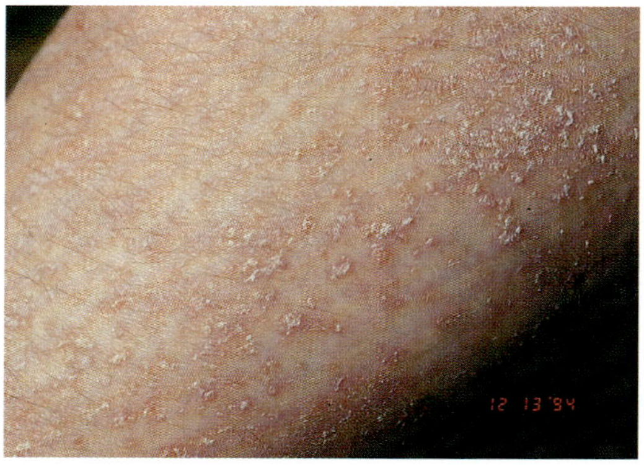

Figure 3.30. Follicular hyperkeratosis over the extensor aspect of the arms in a 38-year-old white woman with classic dermatomyositis. Typical histopathologic changes of cutaneous dermatomyositis were noted at biopsy of these hyperkeratotic lesions. This patient also had punctate follicular hyperkeratoses over noninflamed skin of the upper arms and shoulders having the appearance of typical keratosis pilaris from which the lesions shown in this photograph appeared to evolve.

Steroid-Induced Acanthosis Nigricans. Acanthosis nigricans developed in a patient with DM who had been treated with systemic corticosteroids for 8 years. These changes resolved 10 years after discontinuation of steroid therapy (188). The authors indicate that several similar cases have been reported by others.

Telangiectasia, Gingival. Gingival telangiectasia have been described as an oral mucosal manifestation of juvenile-onset classic DM (189). However, these mucosal changes are not specific for DM, having also been observed in patients with LE and systemic sclerosis.

Urticaria. Urticaria has been reported to occur in patients with DM/PM (190).

Vasculitis, Cutaneous. Seven (9.2%) of 76 patients with adult-onset DM/PM examined over an 11-year period had cutaneous vasculitis expressed clinically as subcutaneous nodules, periungual infarcts, and digital ulcers (191). These lesions occurred almost exclusively in patients with DM who had no evidence of overlap connective tissue disease. An associated malignancy was found in 28.6% of these patients, a frequency that was much higher than in those without cutaneous vasculitic skin lesions. As previously noted, a relatively noninflammatory vasculopathy that often targets the skin is quite common in juvenile DM. Urticarial vasculitis has also been reported to occur in patients with DM/PM (190). A causal relationship between urticarial vasculitis and the underlying myositis was claimed because the vasculitis recurred with each exacerbation of muscle disease activity.

Vulvar Changes. Histologically confirmed DM of the labia majora presenting as pruritic erythematous thickening was documented in a 29-year-old married woman (192). Scrotal involvement leading to necrosis and ulceration has also been reported (193).

Zebra-like Stripes (Centripetal Flagellate Erythema). Blotchy purple macules were observed over the back, shoulders, and extremities of a 14-year-old girl with DM resulting in the appearance of her having been flogged (184). This pattern of skin change has been referred to as centripetal flagellate erythema (145) and appears to occur in approximately 5% of patients with DM (137) (Fig. 3.31).

Other skin changes have anecdotally been noted to occur in patients with DM/PM, including dermatographism, erythema nodosum, erythema multiforme, hyperhidrosis, psoriasiform eruptions with nail pitting, and livedo reticularis (37,184,194). The significance of these extremely rare associations is unknown.

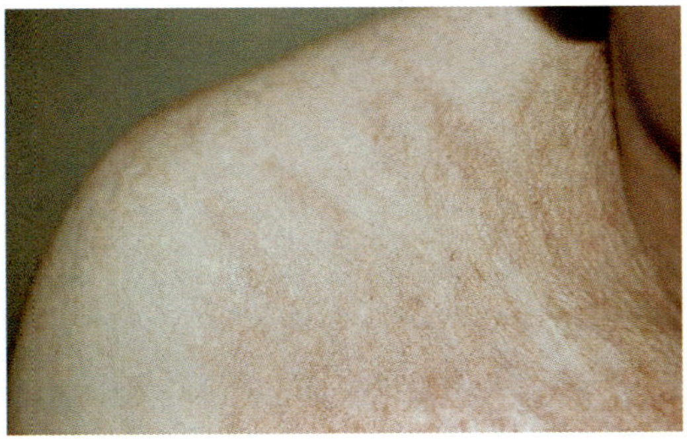

Figure 3.31. An adult patient with dermatomyositis displaying linear erythematosus and macular lesions over the upper anterior chest giving the appearance of having been flogged.

SPECIAL CONSIDERATIONS CONCERNING THE SKIN CHANGES ASSOCIATED WITH CERTAIN SUBTYPES OF IDIOPATHIC INFLAMMATORY MYOPATHY

Dermatomyositis with Malignancy. Winklemann (14) has suggested that a very bright vascular flush of the face, scalp, neck, and shoulders which he designated as "malignant erythema," is seen more commonly in patients with DM who have an associated malignancy. Cutaneous disease in malignancy-associated DM is relatively refractory to systemic corticosteroids.

Juvenile Dermatomyositis. Myositis occurring in the absence of skin disease (i.e., PM) is extremely rare in children. Cutaneous ulceration occurring as a result of infarctive vasculopathy or as a complication of underlying dystrophic calcification is more common in the childhood form of the disease. These issues are discussed further by Lee and Weston in Chapter 13 of this book. Lipodystrophy and hypertrichosis also occur more commonly in juvenile classic DM. Bowyer et al. (195) described four types of dystrophic calcification occurring in children with DM: (a) a superficial pattern consisting of small firm nodules and plaques within the skin, (b) periarticular subcutaneous nodules (calcinosis circumscripta), (c) deposition along fascial planes within muscles (calcinosis universalis), and (d) a severe "exoskeleton" pattern of deposition within the subcutaneous tissue. Calcinosis cutis or calcium deposition in muscles and tendons is more common in the late phases of the disease in children.

Dermatomyositis as Part of an Overlap Connective Tissue Disorder. Typical cutaneous changes of DM can occasionally overlap with systemic sclerosis. Raynaud's phenomenon, sclerodactyly, sclerosis of the skin, and the characteristic hyperpigmentation are present. At times, these features are so striking that the original diagnosis is forgotten. The presence of Gottron's papules, poikiloderma, and severe muscle disease will indicate the correct diagnosis. The term "sclerodermatomyositis" has been used to describe patients who present with DM and develop striking features of scleroderma 6 months to 3 years later (14,196).

As previously mentioned, DM/PM can overlap with other connective tissue diseases individually (SLE, rheumatoid arthritis, Sjögren syndrome) or in a combined fashion (mixed connective tissue disease). The presence of Raynaud's phenomenon, arthritis, or ILD is suggestive of an overlapping connective tissue disease involving DM/PM. Internal malignancy is extremely rare in DM/PM overlapping with other connective tissue diseases.

Clinically Amyopathic Dermatomyositis

It should be emphasized that the cutaneous manifestations of amyopathic DM are indistinguishable clinically and histopathologically from those of classic DM.

RELATIONSHIP BETWEEN CUTANEOUS AND SYSTEMIC FEATURES OF THE DISEASE

Classic Dermatomyositis

RELATIONSHIP BETWEEN CUTANEOUS AND MUSCLE MANIFESTATIONS OF CLASSIC DERMATOMYOSITIS

Muscle disease in patients with DM is clinically indistinguishable from that of PM patients—symmetric weakness of the proximal muscles of the extremities and esophagus. It is not unusual for the lower extremities to be involved initially, causing difficulty with activities such as rising from a chair or bathtub and climbing stairs. Weakness of the upper extremities soon develops, resulting in difficulty raising the arms above the head to perform activities such as combing the hair. In addition, the patient often notices pain or tenderness in the affected muscle groups. The onset of the weakness is usually insidious; however, some patients have a more acute course, resulting in a disabling illness within a period of a few weeks. Proximal dysphagia can also develop. The cutaneous findings have little correlation with the degree of muscular involvement. Skin lesions may be extensive in the presence of mild myositis, may be minimal in the presence of severe muscle disease, or may reflect to some degree the activity of muscle inflammation.

Confirmation that proximal muscle weakness is due to the inflammatory myositis of DM/PM can be quite challenging because there are so many other clinical settings in which proximal muscle weakness can be seen (93) (Table 3.6). The diagnosis can be supported by demonstrating the characteristic muscle enzyme elevations in the serum as well as identifying diagnostic EMG and muscle biopsy changes. The use of muscle enzymes and muscle biopsy in the diagnosis of myositis in patients with DM/PM will be addressed below in the section on laboratory assessment.

The EMG changes of myositis include myopathic pattern of the motor-unit action potential, myopathic recruitment pattern, increased insertional activity, and increased spontaneous activity (93,197). The paraspinous muscles can be abnormal on EMG when the limb girdle musculature is normal. As many as 10% of patients with biopsy-documented myositis have normal EMG findings.

Early muscle involvement in DM/PM can be very difficult to document. Magnetic resonance imaging (MRI) of muscles has been shown to correlate with clinical muscle weakness and may be more sensitive than a muscle biopsy in revealing muscle inflammation. Fraser et al. (198) have shown that fat-suppressive STIR (short tau inversion recovery) image signal intensity correlates with clinical disease activity in patients with idiopathic inflammatory myopathies and in most cases, with the presence of inflammation on muscle biopsy. Reimers et al. (199) evaluated the MRI appearance of the muscles in childhood DM and showed that involved muscles had increased signal intensity on T2-weighted images. There was a good correlation between the distribution of muscle involvement by MRI and by functional testing. Follow up MRI in patients with favorable outcome demonstrated that the affected muscles had returned to normal signal intensity, and although the MRI findings were not specific in the proper clinical context, they were concluded to be helpful in establishing the diagnosis of DM. They also concluded that MRI may be used in establishing an appropriate muscle biopsy site and may be useful for monitoring the progress of disease.

MRI is now the method of choice for diagnostic imaging of muscle abnormalities in patients with myositis (200). MRI-guided needle biopsy may obviate the need for the more costly and invasive blinded open-muscle biopsy (201). Phosphorus-31 (^{31}P) spectroscopy has also been used as a noninvasive measure of muscle inflammation (202).

In addition, MRI and ^{31}P magnetic resonance spectroscopy (MRS) can be useful in assessing the status of muscle disease activity during treatment. Unfortunately, these procedures are quite expensive and cannot be used in some individuals having metallic implants. Therefore, less costly approaches to monitoring muscle disease activity are being explored. Examples include power Doppler and gray-scale ultrasonography (203, 204).

Among the most common presenting symptoms of DM is the characteristic macular violaceous erythema over the face and upper extremities (19,33). Usually, in about half of patients with such skin findings, muscle weakness will also be present at the same time. The cutaneous manifestations can precede muscle involvement by as little as several weeks, or as much as 4 to 6 years (19,34). However, in classic DM, this interval rarely exceeds several months. Figure 3.32 illustrates the temporal sequence of onset of the cutaneous and muscular manifestations in DM observed in different patterns of disease presentation. Unfortunately, as previously noted, there is no reliable correlation between the pattern and extent of cutaneous inflammation and muscle disease activity. Some patients can have very widespread and symptomatic skin disease activity and no clinical evidence of muscle inflammation for prolonged periods (e.g., severely symptomatic clinically amyopathic DM), whereas others have disabling myositis but never develop skin disease (PM).

Considerable effort has been made to correlate the periungual microvascular changes that can be seen in DM by nailfold capillaroscopy (i.e., dilatation, tortuosity, budding or arborization, and avascularity) with the systemic manifestations of this disease process, including myositis (205). These changes can occur in both DM (classic and amyopathic) and PM, although they appear to be more prominent in DM (206). In the largest series of adult patients with classic DM/PM studied, the presence of severe avascular areas and confluent areas of capillary dilatation was seen significantly more often in those patients who had pulmonary involvement, arthritis, and Raynaud's phenomenon; however, no correlation was noted between these periungual microvascular changes and the presence or extent of myositis (206). In juvenile classic DM, these periungual microvascular changes have been correlated with more severe and chronic forms of the disease (207). However, it is also now clear that the periungual nailfold capillary changes are as marked in patients with amyopathic DM as in patients with classic DM. These microvascular changes are not specific for DM/PM in adults or children: Similar changes can be seen in systemic sclerosis and to a lesser degree in SLE and mixed connective tissue disease.

Patients with DM associated with other connective tissue disorders usually present with symptoms of joint pain and sub-

TABLE 3.6. Conditions That Can Simulate the Proximal Muscle Weakness of DM/PM

Infectious myopathies	
	HIV-1, HTLV-1, Coxsackie, Echovirus, influenza, adenovirus, hepatitis B, Epstein–Barr viruses
Other myopathies	
	Inclusion body myositis, rheumatic disease vasculitis, muscular dystrophies, metabolic myopathies, neurologic disorders, myasthenia gravis, amyotrophic lateral sclerosis, Guillain–Barré syndrome
Endocrine disorders	
	Hypothyroidism and hyperthyroidism, Cushing syndrome, diabetic neuropathy, hypokalemia
Drug-induced myopathies	
	Alcohol, antimalarials (vacuolar myopathy), colchicine, corticosteroids, cyclosporine, street drugs (cocaine, heroin), lipid-lowering agents (lovastatin, gemfibrozil, clofibrate, niacin), D-penicillamine, zidovudine

From (93).

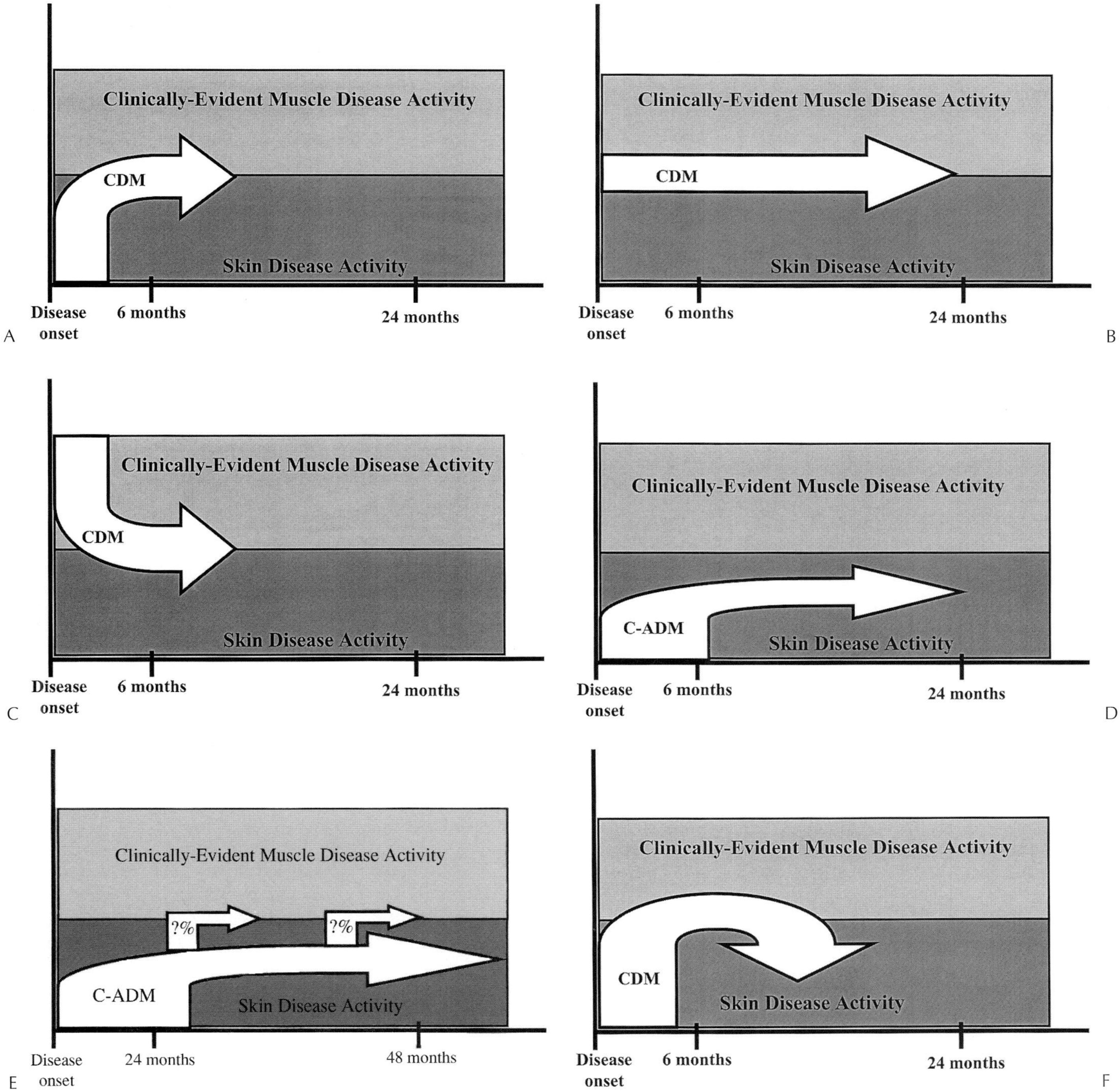

Figure 3.32. Graphic illustration of the various temporal relationships that exists between the clinical onset of the cutaneous and muscular manifestations of classic dermatomyositis (DM) and clinically amyopathic DM. **A:** Classic DM presenting with cutaneous manifestations but soon developing clinically evident muscle disease. **B:** Classic DM presenting with both cutaneous and clinically evident muscle disease simultaneously. **C:** Classic DM presenting initially with clinically evident muscle disease followed briefly by the appearance of cutaneous changes. **D:** Confirmed clinically amyopathic DM with skin disease being present for 2 years or longer without the appearance of clinically evident muscle disease. **E:** Confirmed clinically evident amyopathic DM and which clinically evident muscle disease appears in a very delayed fashion. The percentage of patients with clinically amyopathic DM that take this course is unknown. **F:** Classic DM in which symptomatic muscle disease resolves with treatment but skin disease relapses without reappearance of muscle disease muscle weakness. The skin disease–only phase of such a disease course has been erroneously labeled as "amyopathic DM." Perhaps a more appropriate term would be "postamyopathic cutaneous DM activity."

sequently develop weakness. The hallmark cutaneous manifestations of DM are seen less commonly in these patients. The incidence of Raynaud's phenomena in these patients is much higher than the other groups of patients with PM/DM.

INTERNAL ORGAN INVOLVEMENT IN CLASSIC DERMATOMYOSITIS

Organ systems other than the skin and musculature can be involved in PM/DM (208) (Table 3.7). These include lungs, joints, heart, gastrointestinal tract, and eyes. The most recent focus of interest in this area within the literature has been on pulmonary and joint disease. As with muscle involvement, there is no good correlation between the type or extent of cutaneous disease and any of the patterns of systemic organ involvement.

Pulmonary Disease. Lung function can be compromised in a number of ways in patients with classic DM (208,209): restrictive lung defect due to respiratory muscle weakness, aspiration pneumonia secondary to gastrointestinal reflux and impaired esophageal muscle function, opportunistic infections, and interstitial pneumonitis/fibrosis related to the underlying autoimmune disease process. In addition, systemic drug therapies such as methotrexate used to treat DM can also produce pulmonary complications (i.e., hypersensitivity pneumonitis).

There has been increasing interest recently in interstitial pneumonitis resulting from both classic DM and clinically amyopathic DM. Between 5% and 40% of patients with classic DM will develop ILD. The wide range of this percentage is due in part to sensitivity of techniques used for detection (e.g., spiral computed tomography [CT] scan of the chest can identify earlier lung involvement than routine chest radiograph). This complication presents clinically with symptoms of nonproductive cough and exertional dyspnea, which are accompanied by bibasilar fine crackling rales. Pulmonary function tests show a restrictive pattern with reduced diffusion capacity. Several types of ILD have been described: bronchiolitis obliterans with organizing pneumonia (BOOP), diffuse alveolar damage, desquamative interstitial pneumonia, nonspecific interstitial pneumonia, and respiratory bronchiolitis ILD. This subject has recently been reviewed comprehensively (210,211).

ILD can present with two clinical patterns: an acute/subacute type and a chronic type. In the acute/subacute type, patients present with severe, rapidly progressive dyspnea and progressive hypoxemia within a month from onset of lung involvement. Such a patient is often treatment-resistant and at risk for death. The chronic type presents with slower clinical pace of progressive dyspnea. In the absence of symptoms, ILD can be identified by chest radiographs, pulmonary function tests, or chest CT. Some authors suggest that ILD associated with the MSAs (antisynthetases) can occasionally occur in the absence of skin and muscle disease (91). In some individuals, ILD presents before the clinical appearance of myositis. In addition, as will be discussed below, ILD can occur in patients with clinically amyopathic DM.

Patients with classic DM who have the antisynthetase syndrome (Jo-1, PL-7, PL-12, or other synthetase autoantibodies; arthritis; Raynaud's phenomenon) have an increased risk for developing ILD. The antisynthetase syndrome and interstitial pneumonitis can also be seen in children with classic DM. Interstitial pneumonitis and air leakage was recently observed in a 4-year-old girl with classic juvenile DM (212).

TABLE 3.7. Systemic Manifestations/Associations of Classic DM/PM

Musculoskeletal
Myositis with proximal weakness
Muscle atrophy and contracture[a]
Muscular calcification[a]
Cardiac
Cardiomyopathy
Conduction defects
Respiratory
Dysphonia
Diffuse interstitial pneumonitis/fibrosis (also reported in amyopathic DM)
Aspiration pneumonia
Respiratory failure from muscle weakness
Gastrointestinal
Proximal dysphagia
Large-bowel infarction/perforation secondary to vasculopathy[a]
Ophthalmologic
Retinopathy[a]
Internal malignancy[b] (also reported in adult amyopathic DM)

DM, dermatomyositis; PM, polymyositis.
[a]Usually limited to juvenile DM.
[b]Not significantly increased in juvenile DM.
From Sontheimer RD. Dermatomyositis. In: Freedberg IM, Eisen AZ, Wolff K, et al., eds. *Fitzpatrick's dermatology in general medicine* 5th ed. New York: McGraw Hill, 1999:2009–2022, with permission.

Arthritis. Arthritis has been reported in 20% to 65% of juvenile- and adult-onset classic DM (213). This tends to be a nonerosive arthritis involving the knees, wrists, elbows, and fingers and is seen early in the course of the disease. For some patients, this can be a major symptomatic problem. Arthritis has also been observed in some patients with juvenile-onset clinically amyopathic DM. In one recent study, three (60%) of five patients with juvenile clinically amyopathic DM followed up over an average period of 4.9 years were reported to have arthritis, whereas 49 (61%) of 80 children with classic DM in the same study were observed to experience arthritis (213).

Other Internal Organs. It is not uncommon for patients with classic PM/DM to complain of a sore throat, dysphonia, and proximal dysphasia (difficulty initiating a swallow) as a reflection of pharyngeal, upper esophageal, and palatal muscle involvement. Bowel perforation, infarction, or both can result from vasculopathy in juvenile-onset DM. An association between DM and Crohn disease has been suggested (214). Some series reported myopathic involvement of the myocardium resulting in conduction defects (208,209). Vasculopathy in children with DM can also cause retinal injury.

DYSTROPHIC CALCIFICATION

Approximately 25% of patients with juvenile-onset classic DM have dystrophic calcification at the time of diagnosis and 40% to 50% will develop calcinosis sometime during the course of their illness. This treatment-resistant complication can be a major contributor to morbidity and, occasionally, to mortality in such patients (e.g., some individuals can die from septic complication of ulcerating dystrophic calcification long after complete resolution of the activity of their myositis). The higher rate of vasculopathy that occurs in juvenile classic DM is thought to be a forerunner of dystrophic calcification.

MRI has recently been suggested to be capable of identifying edema/inflammation in skin, subcutaneous tissue, and fascia resulting from vasculopathy in patients with classic juvenile DM (215). In approximately 80% of the 26 children studied, MRI abnormalities indicating skin, subcutaneous, or fascial edema were observed. Clinical skin disease activity scores correlated positively with MRI skin edema scores. Five children developed soft-tissue calcification in areas previously found to be edematous by MRI after 4- to 9-month follow-up intervals. These observations suggests the possibility that MRI soft-tissue assessment could be of value in predicting risk for developing dystrophic calcification and in monitoring disease treatment to prevent or minimize this complication.

Dystrophic calcification appears to be quite uncommon in both adult- and juvenile-onset clinically amyopathic DM. It is of interest in this regard that there was little relationship found between MRI indices of edema/inflammation in the superficial (skin and subcutaneous tissue) and deep (fascial and muscle) tissue compartments of patients with juvenile-onset classic DM (215). TNF-α-308A promoter polymorphism might represent a risk factor for developing calcinosis (57).

RISK FOR MALIGNANCY IN CLASSIC DERMATOMYOSITIS

In 1962, Shy (31) reported an unusually strong association between DM/PM and malignancy. In 1980, Callen et al. (216) found a relationship between DM and malignancy in 25% of their patients. The validity of such an association has been the subject of intense debate due to the retrospective nature of most of the studies that have addressed this issue (29,30,83,217–220).

In early 1990, Sigurgeirsson et al. (32) presented one of the most definitive studies to date addressing this question. They examined a population-based cohort of 788 patients with DM and PM over an average of 10 years. In this uniquely designed study, computerized hospital records (most patients suspected of having DM/PM in Sweden are hospitalized for evaluation) were matched with data from a countrywide tumor registry. Fifteen percent of 392 patients with DM had an associated malignancy (relative risk for cancer, 2.4 in males and 3.4 in females). Malignancies were found in 9% of 396 patients with PM (relative risk for cancer, 1.8 for males and 1.7 for females). The mortality rates from cancer were 3.8 in patients with DM and 0.9 for the patients with PM. During the 5-year period after the diagnosis of DM, the risk for a woman developing ovarian cancer in this study was 16.7-fold higher than that for a woman without DM. These data could argue strongly that a search for occult cancer at the time of diagnosis of DM and at regular intervals thereafter is warranted.

This pioneering work is supported by several additional population-based epidemiologic studies in European whites with classic DM (221–224). Curiously, these studies indicate marginal to no increased risk for malignancy in patients with PM. Increasing age, skin disease extent and severity (e.g., blistering, ulceration), and creatine kinase (CK) levels appear to enhance the risk for malignancy in patients with classic DM. The presence of other systemic manifestations of DM, such as ILD, appears to be negatively correlated with risk for internal malignancy (83).

A variety of solid tumors has been associated with DM, including malignancies of the skin such as melanoma (225), mycosis fungoides (226), and Kaposi sarcoma (227). In general, carcinomas are more frequent than sarcomas, and lymphoproliferative malignancies are uncommon, although they can occur. Except for ovarian cancer in women, no preponderance of specific types of cancer is seen in white patients with DM/PM. However, Oriental males with classic DM most frequently develop nasopharyngeal carcinoma (228,229). The leading cause of death in patients with DM/PM with malignancy is metastatic spread of the malignancy, rather than from complications directly related to DM or treatment of DM.

In most instances, the diagnosis of cancer is made by following up on leads discovered in a comprehensive history, review of systems, physical examination, and routine laboratory/radiologic testing. In addition, a baseline screening (e.g., chest radiograph, sigmoidoscopy/colonoscopy, complete blood count, serum chemistry levels, stool occult blood examination) with careful follow-up of any leads detected should be performed in both sexes. In addition, a sex-specific malignancy survey should be performed in females (mammography, complete pelvic examination) and males (testicular and prostate examination, prostate-specific antigen level). After that, different physicians have different approaches (230). Some pursue aggressive blind radiologic imaging studies of the entire body, whereas others advocate watchful waiting with aggressive follow-up of new signs and symptoms. Recent support for performing thoracic and abdominopelvic CT scans in all patients with classic DM/PM has been presented (231). Repeated malignancy surveillance measures need to be performed every 6 to 12 months for the first 3 to 5 years after the diagnosis of DM. After this period, the risk for malignancy appears to return to that of the age- and sex-matched population in general.

There is a consensus that serum tumor markers (e.g., carcinoembryonic antigen [CEA], cancer antigen 125 [CA-125], CA-15-3, MUC-1, TPS) are not sensitive or specific enough for malignancy screening purposes in the general population. However, some authors suggest that in a patient population (i.e., classic DM) having a higher incidence of a disease (i.e., malignancy), Bayes theorem would argue that the usefulness of tumor markers should increase (232). Thus, tumor markers such as those indicated before might be of greater value in monitoring for malignancy in classic DM, especially if a trend of changing values is noted in multiple assays obtained sequentially over time in the same patient (232). Considering the now-confirmed association between ovarian cancer and classic DM, it is curious that there have been no reports examining the role that screening for mutations in familial and sporadic cancer-associated genes such as *BRCA1* and *BRCA2* might have in stratifying risk for malignancy in women with classic classic DM.

The increased incidence of ovarian cancer in female patients with DM (32,98,233) justifies special attention because this form of malignancy can be very difficult to detect in its earlier, more treatable stages. Whitmore et al. (98) have suggested that the workup in all women with DM should include initial and frequently repeated gynecologic examinations (pelvic examination, CA-125 serum levels, and transvaginal ultrasonography) over several years.

In patients with malignancy, the myositis (and possibly the cutaneous manifestations as well) tends to be less responsive to systemic corticosteroid therapy. In a few well-documented cases, definitive therapy for the malignancy has resulted in resolution of the DM, and a recurrence of the cancer has been associated with reappearance of the DM (30). Older age at the time of onset of DM is also a risk factor for malignancy.

As previously noted, there is not a significantly increased risk for internal malignancy in juvenile-onset classic DM.

Clinically Amyopathic Dermatomyositis

POSSIBILITY OF SUBCLINICAL MUSCLE DISEASE IN AMYOPATHIC DERMATOMYOSITIS

Muscle biopsies and EMG were not obtained in the original six patients with amyopathic DM described by Euwer and Sontheimer (39) because the disabling nature of their patient's cutaneous symptoms required aggressive treatment with high-dose systemic corticosteroids. (It was believed that the results of such tests would not have altered the treatment plan considering the severity of the cutaneous symptoms suffered by these patients.) Their failure to obtain EMG and muscle biopsy data has been criticized by others who believed that a true diagnosis of amyopathic DM could not be made without those studies having been performed and confirmed to be negative (234,235).

Stonecipher et al. (96) have prospectively assessed a similar group of patients in a more systematic fashion. They characterized a group of 13 patients having clinicopathologic features of cutaneous DM who had normal muscle enzyme levels at the time of presentation. Skin disease in these patients had been present from 4 to 11 years and they were followed up from 1 to 6 years during this study. Two patients had minimal evidence of muscle weakness, whereas four others remained free of evidence of muscle involvement as documented by EMG and muscle biopsy. Seven patients having cutaneous changes only at baseline developed clinical myositis from 2 months to 3 years (median, 6 months) after onset of skin disease. Four patients in this study had confirmed amyopathic DM as defined by Euwer and Sontheimer (i.e., no evidence of muscle disease for 2 years or longer). Two patients who appeared to have amyopathic DM initially, on further investigation, were found to have evidence of muscle disease. The remaining seven patients had a more typical course of skin disease that preceded muscle disease by a relatively short time.

Cosnes et al. (152) have further analyzed these issues in their study of 12 patients with DM who did not have clinical evidence of myositis. Although muscle weakness was not evident clinically in any of their patients, all had to have at least one of the Bohan criteria for myositis for inclusion in the study (19) (thus, all of these patients could be classified as having hypomyopathic DM). Although one of these patients did have an associate malignancy, overall they enjoyed a relatively good prognosis with only conservative treatment measures such as antimalarials.

MRI is proving to be a very useful noninvasive method for evaluating muscle disease activity in DM. MRI is more sensitive than muscle biopsy in detecting clinical disease activity. Although it is not as specific as muscle biopsy, the positive predictive values of the two techniques do appear comparable (198,236). MRI may be particularly useful in the workup of a patient with amyopathic DM as the following studies suggest.

Stonecipher et al. (203) used MRI to evaluate five patients who had the cutaneous manifestations of DM with normal muscle enzymes, three of whom could be classified as having amyopathic DM. One of the patients with amyopathic DM, who had a negative EMG and muscle biopsy at baseline, was found to have positive findings at MRI, suggesting clinically silent myositis (i.e., hypomyopathic DM). The two other patients with amyopathic DM who had classic skin disease present for 5 and 12 years had normal MRI findings. This study further supports the notion that some patients may express only the cutaneous features of DM for very long periods.

MRI and ^{31}P spectroscopy (MRS) have been used to sequentially evaluate the same patient with amyopathic DM over time (202). During the patient's amyopathic phase, no inflammation was noted on MRI; however, a small degree of fatty infiltration was noted in her thigh muscles. ^{31}P-MRS was normal at rest but mildly abnormal at exercise. When this patient later developed muscle pain and increasing cutaneous inflammation, repeated MRI/MRS examinations revealed muscle inflammation even though her CK levels remained normal (her baseline muscle biopsy and EMG studies approximately 1.5 years prior to MRI/MRS were normal). After this patient's disease was suppressed with medical treatment, improvement in her MRI/MRS studies was noted. This patient would best be classified as "hypomyopathic DM" using the nomenclature and classification system used in Tables 3.1 and 3.2. This highly instructive case report demonstrates the potential usefulness of MRI/MRS in assessing the overall clinical status of patients with amyopathic DM/DM as well as monitoring the response to therapy.

Dunn and James (237) have described an additional case that further illustrates the potential for MRI in this setting. These authors suggest that an MRI-directed muscle biopsy might decrease the incidence of false-negative findings. It is conceivable that in the future, MRI-guided, closed-needle biopsy may replace the blind open-muscle biopsy in the diagnostic evaluation of patients suspected of having DM/PM (201).

The utility of MRI and MRS in documenting subclinical muscle changes in patients with clinically amyopathic DM has recently been reviewed (200). Artificial neural networks have been proposed as an effective way to analyze the multichannel functional data that results from ^{31}P-MRS examination (238). A central issue in this area is whether the subtle muscular abnormalities that can be identified with these sensitive imaging systems have real clinical value (i.e., can they predict with significant clinical utility the subsequent appearance of weakness occurring as result of clinically significant myositis?).

A retrospective analysis of all patients with DM seen at the Mayo Clinic between 1976 and 1994 revealed that 32 (4%) of 746 patients with DM conformed to the definition of clinically amyopathic DM (85). Twenty-seven of these patients had amyopathic DM and five had hypomyopathic DM (an additional group of five patients having subjective muscle weakness but no demonstrable muscle abnormalities was included in the analysis by this group.). However, these five patients are not included in the present analysis because they do not conform to the definition of clinically amyopathic DM presented in Table 3.1 (perhaps these patients had clinically amyopathic DM and fibromyalgia). Follow-up information was available on 16 of the Mayo clinic patients with amyopathic DM. Ten patients (67%) had no muscle weakness after 2 to 10 years of follow-up, four (25%) had no weakness at 1 year, and two (13%) developed weakness within 5 years after diagnosis. None of the three patients with hypomyopathic DM who were followed up showed evidence of muscle weakness 8 to 17 years after diagnosis. Thus, of the 19 patients with clinically amyopathic DM who were followed up (16 amyopathic DM, three hypomyopathic DM), only two (11%) developed clinical evidence of myositis after prolonged follow-up periods. Thus, the presence of subclinical muscle abnormalities at the time of diagnosis of amyopathic DM does not necessarily mean the subsequent development of clinically significant muscle disease.

Caproni et al. (86) identified 13 patients with amyopathic DM representing 8.2% of 157 patients with DM seen retrospectively during a 10-year period by the Italian Group of Immunodermatology. The patients comprised 12 women and 1 man (mean age, 53 years). Eleven patients (85%) experienced skin disease for at least 2 years (i.e., confirmed amyopathic DM), whereas two (15%) had skin disease for more than 6 months but less than 24 months (provisional amyopathic DM). There was one juvenile case presenting at 13 years of age. Four of these patients could be classified as having hypomyopathic DM by virtue of abnormalities noted on EMG (three of eight patients tested) or muscle biopsy (one of two tested).

Fibromyalgia is a well-known symptomatic accompaniment of classic DM. Although fatigue or myalgia without objective evidence of muscle inflammation have been described in a number of clinically amyopathic DM case descriptions, a single case report of documented fibromyalgia occurring in amyopathic DM has been presented (239). The symptoms of fatigue, muscle pain, and muscle tenderness associated with fibromyalgia could falsely imply the development of myositis in a patient with clinically amyopathic DM. Olsen et al. (200) have proposed dividing amyopathic DM into three subsets: I, pure amyopathic with skin disease only; II, skin disease with subjective myalgias; and III, skin disease with normal muscle strength but some laboratory finding abnormalities. In this classification approach, perhaps subgroup II would be synonymous with amyopathic DM with fibromyalgia, and subgroup III with hypomyopathic DM.

There continues to be debate concerning the risk for patients with juvenile-onset clinically amyopathic DM ultimately developing clinically significant myositis, with some groups seeing a relatively low risk (240) and others a relatively high risk (241).

To fulfill the definition of clinically amyopathic DM, clinical evidence of muscle weakness should not be present. Therefore, it is important that dermatologists who care for such patients are fully aware of how to do an adequate muscle physical examination to detect weakness resulting from inflammatory myositis. Muscle strength testing is graded on a 1 to 5 scale: 0, no muscle action; 1, trace contraction; 2, visible contraction but unable to overcome gravity; 3, fair contraction but can overcome gravity; 4, contraction able to offer some resistance; 5, evaluator cannot overcome contracted muscle. The focus of the examination should be on the proximal muscle groups that control the neck, shoulders, and hips. It should be realized that manual muscle testing is reproducible; however, variables such as pain, contractures, voluntary effort, and motivation may influence the ability of an individual to exert maximal muscle effort (e.g., concurrent arthritis might give one the impression that a patient has distal muscle weakness because of guarding).

RISK FOR SYSTEMIC MANIFESTATIONS OF DERMATOMYOSITIS OUTSIDE THE SKELETAL MUSCULATURE IN PATIENTS WITH CLINICALLY AMYOPATHIC DERMATOMYOSITIS

ILD is a potentially fatal complication of DM/PM, occurring in 5% to 40% of patients with classic DM. It is becoming increasingly clear that interstitial pneumonitis and pulmonary fibrosis can complicate clinically amyopathic DM as well as classic DM (114,115,242–252). El-Azhary et al. (85) reported that five patients with clinically amyopathic DM had radiographic evidence of asymptomatic pulmonary fibrosis. Although previously thought to be quite rare, among the approximately 300 cases of clinically amyopathic DM that have now been formally reported, there are 34 published cases of often-fatal ILD occurring in patients having DM-specific skin disease but no muscle weakness (42). A disproportionately high percentage of patients with clinically amyopathic DM with ILD has been reported from Japan, perhaps related to the fact that interstitial pneumonitis appears to be an especially common complication of classic DM in Japanese. In many cases, interstitial pneumonitis occurred in patients with clinically amyopathic DM in the absence of antisynthetase autoantibodies such as Jo-1, which are considered serologic markers for risk for ILD in patients with classic DM.

In addition to the 34 conventionally published cases of ILD in patients with clinically amyopathic DM, other similar cases have been reported in abstract form or on Internet websites (two cases, both fatal). Thus, there can be little doubt that clinical evidence of muscle weakness need not be present for the development of potentially fatal, DM-associated ILD. Failure to recognize this clinical constellation can delay diagnosis and institution of proper treatment and thereby contribute to disastrous consequences.

Not all of the ILD cases reported occurring in clinically amyopathic DM meet the classification criteria for clinically amyopathic DM, because DM-specific skin disease had been present for less than 6 months when the ILD presented clinically. Perhaps such cases might better be referred to as "premyopathic DM" or as individuals expressing "DM-specific skin disease without myositis." Clearly, some type of conventional designation needs to be agreed on to describe previously healthy individuals who present with DM-specific skin lesions and then die from rapidly progressive ILD without ever having developed muscle weakness.

There are two typical clinical patterns of presentation of ILD: acute/subacute and chronic. The acute/subacute pattern of disease presentation with rapidly progressive dyspnea, progressive hypoxemia, treatment-resistance, and fatal outcome occurs in a disturbingly high percentage of patients with clinically amyopathic DM developing pulmonary disease. Cyclosporine and cyclophosphamide have each been reported to be of value in severe ILD in patients with clinically amyopathic DM, especially when started before frank respiratory failure has developed (249,250). It is currently unknown whether patients with amyopathic DM might be at risk for other systemic manifestations of classic DM such as cardiac and gastrointestinal disease. However, it would appear that such findings are relatively uncommon (34,39,86,96,98,152).

RISK FOR MALIGNANCY IN CLINICALLY AMYOPATHIC DERMATOMYOSITIS

The possibility that patients with amyopathic DM, like patients with classic DM (253), might have an increased risk for occult malignancy has been addressed only recently. Braverman (37) had earlier mentioned a patient who developed only the cutaneous changes of DM as a manifestation of lung cancer. Euwer and Sontheimer (102) reported that a patient with amyopathic DM developed an intraductal carcinoma of the breast 2.5 years following the onset of her skin disease. Two patients in the study by Stonecipher et al. (96) had breast adenocarcinoma. One patient had skin disease for 3 years before developing EMG evidence of myositis and the other had developed evidence of muscle disease 4 months after onset of her skin disease. The malignancies preceded the onset of muscle disease in both patients but were not detected until after the onset of the cutaneous manifestations of DM. Whitemore et al. (98) described three patients who developed metastatic ovarian carcinoma after prolonged illnesses that were dominated by the cutaneous manifestations of DM in spite of regular gynecologic examinations. A further follow-up by this group since 1986 has detected 33 amyotrophic dermatomyositis patients; 24% have developed malignancy (breast, ovarian, lungs, cervical, prostate) (T. T. Provost, personal communication, 2002). Cosnes et al. (152) reported a case of breast cancer developing in one patient with DM who had only minimal, subclinical evidence of myositis.

In a 3-year retrospective review of patients with DM from Singapore, clinically amyopathic DM was a common presentation in that ethnic population. In addition, a clinically amyopathic DM presentation appeared to carry a lower risk for associated malignancy than classic DM (82). In a retrospective analysis of 143 Taiwanese patients with DM, no malignancies were reported in the 20 patients with amyopathic DM (83). However, six of 10 patients with amyopathic DM identified in a retrospective study in Hong Kong were found to have associated malignancy, especially nasopharyngeal carcinoma (254).

A retrospective analysis of all Mayo Clinic patients with DM seen between 1976 and 1994 revealed that 32 (4%) of 746 patients with DM conformed to the definition of clinically amyopathic DM (85). Four (25%) of the 16 patients with amyopathic DM in that study who were followed up after 2 to 10 years had an internal malignancy; all four were women. Malignancies included carcinomas of the lung, ovaries, breast, endometrium, and metastatic adenocarcinoma of unknown primary. None of the three patients with hypomyopathic DM who were available for follow-up had associated malignancy. Thus, overall a minimum of four (15%) of 27 of the patients with clinically amyopathic DM reported in that series had an associated internal malignancy, with two patients succumbing from this complication.

Caproni et al. (86) identified no malignancies in their Italian cohort of 13 patients with clinically amyopathic DM. That study had a mean follow-up period of 6.8 years.

Although there have been a number of case reports or small series of internal malignancy occurring in patients with clinically amyopathic DM, whether there is a significantly increased risk for internal malignancy in patients with clinically amyopathic DM is currently not known as there are no population-based data addressing this question. However, until such data are available, it is the opinion of the authors that patients with clinically amyopathic DM, like patients with classic DM, should be carefully evaluated for the possibility of developing occult malignancy. Because of the increasing evidence linking ovarian carcinoma to DM (32,233) and amyopathic DM (98), an argument can be made for frequent gynecologic examinations including pelvic examination, CA-125 determinations, and transvaginal ultrasonography in the workup of all female patients with amyopathic DM as well as those with classic DM for the first 3 to 5 years after diagnosis of DM.

PATHOLOGY AND IMMUNOPATHOLOGY

Skin Lesions

The histopathology of biopsy specimens from cutaneous lesions of DM is not specific for DM. Kasper et al. (255) have reviewed the histopathologic changes seen in three clinical categories of cutaneous DM: (a) lupus-like DM, (b) poikiloderma, and (c) Gottron papules.

Biopsy specimens from well-established skin lesions defined as lupus-like (i.e., scaling violaceous erythema) display changes that are similar to and sometimes indistinguishable from those seen in LE (256). Those changes include hyperkeratosis, epidermal atrophy, and effacement of the rete ridges. Also commonly present are an interface dermatitis with vacuolar degeneration of the basal keratinocytes and a sparse, superficial, patchy or bandlike perivascular lymphocytic infiltration. Thickening of the basement membrane and pigment incontinence may also be prominent features. Often, the dermis is pale, owing to the accumulation of edema and mucin.

A similar histopathologic picture may be seen in poikiloderma, except that prominent dermal vascular ectasia is present (256). The histopathologic features of Gottron is papules include hyperkeratosis, acanthosis, mild undulating papillomatosis, vacuolar alteration of basal keratinocytes, thickened basement membrane, variable lymphocytic exocytosis, and increased mucin deposition in the epidermis (257).

A fourth subset of cutaneous DM can be recognized histologically, although the pattern is quite subtle (255). Although this pattern has no clear clinical correlate, it is probably indicative of very early cutaneous involvement. The histologic appearance is similar to that of normal skin except for periodic acid–Schiff–positive thickening of basement membrane, a smudgy homogenous appearance of the papillary dermis, and increased dermal mucin and edema. No lymphocytic infiltrate is seen, and vacuolar alteration of basal keratinocytes, pigment incontinence, and colloid body formation are variably present. The histologic changes of cutaneous DM can be focal and may sometimes be found in only small areas of a biopsy. Therefore, to maximize the chance of identifying the characteristic changes, the biopsy specimen should be relatively large; assessment of several sections may be necessary. Reportedly, the cutaneous histologic changes of amyopathic DM are indistinguishable from those of classic cutaneous DM (39).

Direct and indirect immunofluorescence exam of skin lesions of DM are of no clear value diagnostically. A variety of findings can be seen including granular deposits of immunoglobulin and complement components in a bandlike array along the dermal–epidermal junction, subepidermal cytoid bodies, dermal connective tissue staining, and epidermal cytoplasmic staining (135,255,258–260). Lesional dermal–epidermal junction bands have been reported to occur in 5% to 67% of patients depending on the site of biopsy. One study suggested that dermal–epidermal junction immune deposits were found in biopsies taken from the nailfold more frequently than other anatomic regions (260). The sun-exposed skin of otherwise healthy young adults can contain nonspecific junctional immune deposits that can be a significant source of confusion if not properly interpreted (261).

Some work has suggested that antigens associated with the C5-9 membrane attack complex of complement are seen more often in the dermal microvessels compared with the dermal–epidermal junction in cutaneous DM lesions whereas the opposite was true for cutaneous LE lesions (262). However, others have been unable to identify such differences (263).

Hausmann et al. (259) characterized the immunopathology of 25 lesional biopsy specimens from patients with cutaneous DM. The dermal infiltrate consisted predominately of macrophages and CD4 T-lymphocytes, some of which demonstrated an activation phenotype. Focal HLA-DR antigen expression was noted on lesional keratinocytes; however, HLA-DR expression on dermal endothelial cells was reduced. These changes were qualitatively quite similar to those seen in cutaneous LE lesions.

Muscle Disease

The muscle biopsy in DM/PM usually shows a perivascular infiltrate of T-lymphocytes and histiocytes and on occasion B-lymphocytes, plasma cells, and eosinophils (255). Pathologic evidence of muscle fiber degeneration/regeneration, perifascicular atrophy, and capillary injury are also frequently present. $CD8^+$ T cells in some studies have been seen to be preferentially associated with damaged muscle fibers in patients with PM (264). Biopsies from patients with DM more often show $CD4^+$ T cells and B cells in the perivascular areas. It should be noted that inflammation may be absent in up to 25% of biopsy specimens from patients with otherwise typical muscle disease by clinical, EMG, or biochemical criteria (19).

Emslie-Smith et al. (265) have shown a decrease in capillary density in muscle specimens from patients with DM with minimal structural alteration. In advanced DM specimens with atypical alterations, these findings were similar but more severe. In PM and inclusion body myositis, the capillaries had a normal overall density.

Variable patterns of immunoglobulin and complement deposition occur within affected muscle tissue. However, this is not a consistent finding nor does it relate to disease activity (266,267). The presence of the complement membrane attack complex in muscle capillaries has suggested that local activation of complement with endothelial cell toxicity could be related to the microvascular abnormalities of this disorder (265,268). However, a recent case report of classic DM occurring in a young Japanese woman who was subsequently shown to be genetically deficient in the C5 component of complement argues somewhat against this hypothesis (51).

An occlusive vasculopathy is a striking part of the pathology of childhood PM/DM. Banker and Victor (23) described phlebitis and arteritis leading to intimal hyperplasia and fibrinous occlusion of vessels with infarction of the involved tissues.

The muscles, gastrointestinal tract, and nerves were particularly affected. The muscle vasculopathy is noninflammatory and occurs predominately in the capillaries. There is a spectrum of endothelial changes from swelling to obliteration to necrosis.

Differential expression patterns of adhesion molecules, cytokines, and chemokines have also been reported in inflammatory myositis (269,270).

LABORATORY MANIFESTATIONS

Muscle Enzymes

Serum levels of muscle enzymes are the most useful routine laboratory tests for diagnosing and following DM/PM. Its high sensitivity and relative specificity for muscle injury make CK the most widely used of the muscle enzymes. CK is elevated in over 90% of patients with classic DM/PM at some point in their disease course (19,44). Patient series ascertained from dermatology practices have a lower prevalence of elevated CK levels (93). By definition, CK and other muscle enzymes are negative in amyopathic DM.

Circumstances other than myositis such as those listed in Table 3.6 can on occasion be responsible for elevated CK levels (e.g., strenuous physical exertion, needle trauma [intramuscular injection, EMG needle insertion], other myopathies, hypothyroidism, and drug ingestion). Inhibitors present in the serum can sometimes interfere with the routine enzymatic detection of CK activity (271). Most of the CK elevation seen in DM/PM is due to the CK-MM isoenzyme; however, CK-MB elevations may occur, especially in the setting of chronically stressed or regenerating muscle (93).

Elevations of CK can precede the development of clinical weakness and the CK can normalize several weeks before the complete return of strength during treatment (272). Some research has suggested that patients with DM/PM who present with normal CK levels have a worse prognosis with respect to pulmonary disease and associated malignancy (273). CK levels are usually normal in patients with proximal muscle weakness due to corticosteroid myopathy.

Serum aldolase levels can also accurately reflect muscle inflammation. Although somewhat less sensitive for muscle involvement in DM/PM, on occasion aldolase levels will be elevated in the presence of a normal CK (93). This is especially true in juvenile-onset DM. Transaminase and lactic dehydrogenase levels can also be elevated in DM/PM but are much less useful because of their low degree of specificity. Care should be taken in interpreting elevations of transaminases in patients with DM/PM who are being treated with potentially hepatotoxic drugs such as methotrexate.

Autoantibodies

Abnormal levels of conventional antinuclear antibodies (ANAs) identified by indirect immunofluorescence using cultured human tumor cell substrates such as HEp-2 can be found in 40% to 60% of patients with PM/DM (274). Ouchterlony double immunodiffusion has been used to identify precipitating autoantibodies that are directed against a disparate group of nuclear and cytoplasmic antigens (Table 3.8). These individual autoantibody specificities can have diagnostic and prognostic value. More comprehensive discussions of this subject than are possible here, including in-depth characterizations of the molecular identities of the various target autoantigens, have been presented elsewhere (93,94,275–278).

Autoantibodies of known molecular specificity in DM are categorized into two groups: MSAs and myositis-associated autoantibodies (MAAs) (279). MSAs include the antisynthetases (Jo-1, PL-7, PL-12, OJ, EJ), Mi-2, and SRP. PM/Scl, Ro/SS-A (Ro52, Ro60), and U1RNP represent the major MAAs.

TABLE 3.8. Autoantibodies Encountered in the Idiopathic Inflammatory Dermatomyopathies

Autoantibody	Median Prevalence[a]	Molecular Specificity	Clinical Association
High specificity for DM/PM			
155 kD &/or Se	80%	Uncharacterized polypeptides	Clinically amyopathic DM (?)
Jo-1	20%	Histidyl tRNA synthetase	PM, anti-synthetase syndrome
Mi-2	15%	Helicase nuclear proteins	Shawl sign, cuticular overgrowth
SRP	5%	Signal recognition particle	Fulminant DM/PM, cardiac involvement
PL-7	3%	Threonyl tRNA synthetase	Antisynthetase syndrome
PL-12	3%	Alanyl tRNA synthetase	Antisynthetase syndrome
OJ	Rare	Isoleucyl tRNA synthetase	Antisynthetase syndrome
EJ	Rare	Glycyl tRNA synthetase	Antisynthetase syndrome, possibly increased frequency of skin changes
Fer	Rare	Elongation factor 1-α	—
Mas	Rare	Small RNA	—
KJ	Rare	Translation factor	—
Low specificity for DM/PM			
ANA (most common IF patterns-speckled, nucleolar)	50%		Clinically amyopathic DM (80%) Classic DM (40%–60%)
ssDNA	40%	—	SLE, SSc
PM-Scl (PM-1)	40%	Ribosomal RNA-processing enzyme	Overlap with scleroderma
Ro (52 kD Ro)	15%	RNP	Overlap with SSJ, SCLE, neonatal LE/CHB, SLE
U_1RNP	10%	U1 RNP	Overlap connective tissue disease
Ku	3%	DNA end-binding repair protein complex	Overlap with scleroderma
U2RNP	1%	U2 RNP	Overlap with scleroderma

[a]Using current assay techniques.
CHB, congenital heart block; DM, dermatomyositis; LE, lupus erythematosus; PM, polymyositis; SCLE, subacute cutaneous lupus erythematosus; SLE, systemic lupus erythematosus; SSc, systemic sclerosis; SSj, Sjögren syndrome.

The most commonly encountered autoantibodies in the myositis-specific group are those that target the various aminoacyl transfer RNA synthetases, the cytoplasmic enzymes that charge the various amino acids with their cognate transfer RNA so that they can be incorporated into polypeptides by the translational machinery within the ribosomal complex. Most prominent among these "antisynthetase" autoantibodies are autoantibodies to Jo-1 (histidyl transfer RNA synthetase), which are found in 20% of patients with DM/PM and 30% to 40% of adult patients with PM (280). Other specificities include anti-PL-7 (threnoy transfer RNA synthetase), anti-PL-12 (alynyl transfer RNA synthetase), anti-OJ (isoleucyl transfer RNA synthetase), and anti-EJ (glycyl transfer RNA synthetase). Certain clinical features including fever, ILD, polyarthritis, Raynaud's phenomenon, and incomplete response to therapy appear to be more common in those patients who produce these antibodies (i.e., the "antisynthetase syndrome" [56,58]). The clinical correlations of the MSAs that have been noted in adults can be seen in patients with juvenile DM/PM as well (97).

The prevalence of the myositis-related autoantibodies in a cohort of 181 unselected European patients with classic DM was recently reported (278). These results are similar to those previously reported for separate cohorts of patients with DM from the United States and Japan. This study also identified a very strong relationship between Ro52 and Jo-1 antibodies. The fact that none of the MSAs occurs with prevalence greater than 1 in 5 patients with DM makes routine clinical testing for these autoantibodies of very little clinical utility.

The mechanic hand skin lesion was originally reported to occur more commonly in patients with the antisynthetase syndrome (56,150). However, work that is more recent has indicated that this skin lesion can also be seen in other settings such as classic DM without antisynthetase antibodies and clinically amyopathic DM. Although patients who produce anti-Jo-1 less frequently display the classic cutaneous manifestations of DM, another of the antisynthetase autoantibodies, anti-EJ, has been suggested to be more strongly associated with the typical skin changes of DM (93).

Another cytoplasmic antigen that is specifically targeted by the autoimmune response of DM/PM patients is the signal recognition particle (SRP). The SRP is responsible for conducting newly formed polypeptides from the nbo-somes in cytoplasm into the endoplasmic reticulum. Anti-SRP antibodies occur in 5% of PM patients and have been said to occur more commonly in patients who exhibit more acute-onset, severe, and treatment-resistant forms of DM/PM in which cardiac involvement is encountered (56,58). Such patients rarely have any type of skin involvement.

Autoantibodies to Mi-2, an adenosine triphosphate (ATP)–dependent nucleosome remodeling factor, are seen almost exclusively in patients with DM. This antibody has been found in 5% to 10% of patients with DM/PM overall and in 15% to 20% of patients with DM (281). This autoantibody specificity has been associated with more treatment-responsive forms of DM. The shawl sign and prominent cuticular changes are cutaneous changes that have been suggested to be associated with this autoantibody specificity (56,58). Targoff has reported the presence of anti-Mi-2 in a patient who had the skin changes of DM but no muscle disease (93); however, none of the six patients with amyopathic DM reported by Euwer and Sontheimer (39) whose sera were screened in Dr. Targoff's laboratory had such antibodies. Targoff was also unable to identify myositis-associated autoantibodies in a study by Whitmore et al., which included several patients with amyopathic DM (98) (personal communication, Thomas Provost, December, 1994). There has been no mention of MSAs in other series of patients with amyopathic DM (42,98,152). A number of other autoantibody specificities having lesser clinical significance in DM/PM are listed in Table 3.8. Some of these specificities are seen more commonly in patients who have features of DM/PM present in conjunction with other connective tissue disease syndromes such as scleroderma (PM-Sc, Ku, U1RNP, U2RNP), SLE (U1RNP, Ro/SS-A), and Sjögren syndrome (Ro/SS-A). The initial report of a new autoantibody reactive by immunoblot with a 56-kDa autoantigen (282) has been confirmed (283). Approximately 60% of patients with juvenile classic DM produce this autoantibody. In addition, this autoantibody specificity appears to correlate positively with the presence of the HLA-DQA*0501 allele. This association has been proposed to be circumstantial evidence for a viral-induced etiology of this particular autoimmune response.

Preliminary studies using immunoprecipitation have identified a new autoantibody, named "MJ," in patients with juvenile classic DM [data reviewed by Targoff [279]). This autoantibody reacts with a 140-kDa protein of unknown molecular specificity. In addition, another new MSA, PMS1, has been described which reacts with a DNA repair enzyme (284).

Most published cases of clinically amyopathic DM are ANA-positive (an even larger majority in those studies specifying human tumor cells as the ANA substrate). However, such patients do not appear to produce myositis-specific or myositis-associated antibodies (MAAs). Thus, the molecular specificities of the autoantibodies seen in clinically amyopathic DM have been unknown. Preliminary studies have indicated that a unique pair of new autoantibody specificities (155 kDa and Se) might serve as serologic markers for this subset of patients with DM (285,286). Combining the results of immunoblot and immunoprecipitation studies using HeLa cell extracts, 16 (89%) of 18 white adult patients with clinically amyopathic DM showed autoantibodies to the 155-kDa autoantigen, Se autoantigen, or both. The molecular identities of these autoantigens have not been identified, but neither appears to be associated with RNA. If these preliminary results can be confirmed, they could provide a very useful clinical tool for confirming a diagnosis of clinically amyopathic DM.

A different group of investigators has reported finding autoantibodies reactive with a 140-kDa polypeptide in five Japanese patients adult-onset clinically amyopathic DM having interstitial pneumonia (287). It is currently not clear whether a relationship exists between this autoantibody and the 155-kDa autoantibody described by Targoff et al. (285).

Miscellaneous Laboratory Abnormalities

The erythrocyte sedimentation rate may be elevated in about half of DM/PM cases but does not correlate as well with disease activity as SLE (93). Researchers have suggested that elevated erythrocyte sedimentation rate levels correlate positively with risk for internal malignancy in classic DM (288). Rheumatoid factor is elevated in 20% of cases, more often in patients with overlap disease.

Several nonenzymatic factors can also reflect muscle damage. Elevation of urinary creatine excretion occurs in patients with DM/PM; however, this can also be seen in a number of the other causes of muscle weakness listed in Table 3.6. Some work has suggested that urinary creatine excretion is actually more sensitive than CK in DM/PM and might be useful in following those patients with myositis who do not exhibit CK elevations (289,290). However, urinary creatine excretion can also be elevated in steroid myopathy (291). Serum myoglobin can also be elevated in DM/PM, occasionally in the presence of a normal CK (292). Urinary excretion of myoglobin, which can occur in patients with DM/PM who experience severe muscle injury, can produce a dipstick test positive for occult blood in the absence of red blood cells on microscopic exam (93).

As enzymatic indicators of muscle inflammation can normalize rather quickly after onset of systemic therapy, other surrogate markers of DM disease activity are used by some to guide therapy. Such indicators have been used more in the management of patients with juvenile-onset classic DM to ensure that all systemic disease activity outside the muscles such as vasculopathy/vasculitis is fully suppressed before tapering/discontinuing therapy. Other serum factors such as neopterin (293,294) and factor VIII–related antigen (von Willebrand factor) (295,296) are thought to correlate with disease activity in patients with juvenile DM. Factor VIII–related antigen has been claimed to correlate better than CK in regard to activity of the vasculopathy in juvenile DM. Other such markers include $CD19^+$ B cells (data reviewed Pachman et al. [57]). Elevated levels of other markers of vascular activation including soluble forms of VCAM-1 and E-selectin have been reported in patients with classic DM.

KL-6 is a human MUc-1 class mucin that is preferentially expressed on type II pneumocytes. KL-6 has been proposed to be a sensitive serum marker for the presence of interstitial pneumonia in the setting of classic DM (data reviewed by Hirakata and Nagai [252]). However, this molecule is not specific for DM and ILD; elevated levels are also found in the serum of patients with various malignancies, serving as a tumor marker in this setting (297). Other authors have suggested that serum levels of KL-6 are correlated with the activity of interstitial pneumonia in patients with clinically amyopathic DM (298,299).

Patients with classic DM express VCAM-1 and E-selectin in the microvessels of inflamed muscular and cutaneous tissue. In addition, patients with classic DM reportedly display elevated blood levels of VCAM-1 and E-selectin (300). Whether these soluble vascular adhesion molecules reflect activation of the muscular or dermal microvasculature (or both) has not been determined. A preliminary study of patients with clinically amyopathic DM was carried out to address this issue (301). That study found similar rates of elevation of soluble VCAM-1 in the sera of patients with either classic DM or clinically amyopathic DM, suggesting that circulating levels of this vascular adhesion molecule could reflect activation of the muscular or dermal microvasculature (or both). Much higher levels of soluble E-selectin levels were observed in patients with clinically amyopathic DM, suggesting that circulating levels of this vascular adhesion molecule might better reflect (or be limited to) activation of the dermal microvasculature.

DIFFERENTIAL DIAGNOSIS

When the hallmark cutaneous manifestations of DM-specific skin disease are fully expressed, there really are no differential diagnostic considerations as these changes can be pathognomonic. However, early in the disease, the cutaneous signs of DM may be confused with contact dermatitis, seborrheic dermatitis, lichen planus, psoriasis, polymorphic light eruption, and atopic dermatitis (14,39). In the early stages of the disease when muscle involvement has yet to develop, it can be quite difficult to distinguish the cutaneous manifestations of DM from those of acute cutaneous LE (Table 3.9). The following clinical features would favor the diagnosis of DM in such patients:

1. Confluent patches of violaceous erythema with or without scale and edema over the face, often most prominent on the upper eyelids and in the periorbital areas

TABLE 3.9. Comparative Features of DM and LE Skin Involvement

	DM	LE
Distribution of skin involvement		
Face		
Malar eminences	+	++
Eyelids, periorbital areas	++	+
Scalp	++	++
Oral mucosa	+	++
Extensor arms, forearms	++	++
Hands		
Dorsal aspect	++	++
Palmar aspect	+	+
Dorsal fingers	+	++
Knuckles	++	+
Periungual telangiectasia	++	+
Color of skin lesions		
Violaceous	++	+
Red, pink	+	++
Alopecia	+	++
Hyperkeratosis	+	++
Gottron papules	++	0
Pruritus	++	+
Pathology		
Dermal mucinosis	++	++
Intense mononuclear cell infiltrate	+	++
Immunopathology		
D-E junction band	+	++
Laboratory findings		
ANA	++	++
Anti-Ro/SS-A	+	++
Anti-native DNA	0	++
Anti-Sm	0	++
Elevated ESR	+	++
Malignancy association	++	0

ANA, antinuclear antibody; DM, dermatomyositis; ESR, erythrocyte sedimentation rate; LE, lupus erythematosus; ++, frequently seen; +, occasionally seen; 0, absent.

2. Violaceous erythema along the frontal hairline and throughout the scalp
3. Violaceous erythema with or without scale involving the sun exposed V areas of the neck, upper chest, and extensor aspects of the arms
4. Violaceous erythema with or without associated scale over the extensor surfaces of the elbows, knees, and IP/MCP joints (Gottron's sign)
5. Gottron's papules
6. Grossly visible periungual telangiectasia, cuticular hemorrhage, or both
7. Pruritus

Usually in LE, the skin over the dorsal IP and MCP joints is initially spared, and the hair-bearing skin between these joints is involved. This is the reverse of that seen in DM. However, the linear streaking of violaceous erythema along the track of the extensor tendon sheaths (Fig. 3.23) of the hands and fingers seen in DM can sometimes obscure this differential point. The presence of prominent dermal atrophy helps distinguish generalized forms of discoid LE from DM. Poikiloderma, calcinosis, and scleroderma-like features are more common in DM than LE. When myositis is present in patients with SLE, it is usually a minor feature of the illness and profound muscle weakness is unusual in this setting. Although arthralgia and arthritis can occur in DM, polyserositis, renal disease, and central nervous system disease are unusual. Gastrointestinal symptoms such as dysphagia are encountered more frequently in DM than LE.

Scleroderma might be confused with the later stages of DM; however, the presence of Gottron papules and poikiloderma favors DM. Trichinosis, because of the associated periorbital edema and myalgia, must also be considered in the differential diagnosis of DM (119).

The contrasting features of the classic cutaneous manifestations of LE and DM have been reemphasized with outstanding color illustrations (302). One curious report indicated that skin metastasis from breast cancer appeared clinically undistinguished from the skin involvement of amyopathic DM (303). As previously noted, reportedly, certain drugs cause a DM-like eruption. Hydroxyurea was a cause of DM in at least six cases (103). Other drugs reported to cause a DM-like eruption include nonsteroidal antiinflammatory agents such as niflumic acid/diclofenac (104), tryptophan (21), penicillamine (21,71), and practolol (105). Drugs such as penicillamine (71), the statin lipid-lowering agents (atrovostatin, pravastatin, simvastatin) (72,73); alfuzosin (74), and phenytoin (75) also appear to be capable of inducing the cutaneous and muscle manifestations of DM. Certain viral infections in the context of immunodeficiency states can also produce DM- and PM-like states. Chronic echovirus infection in patients with X-linked hypogammaglobulinemia has led to a DM-like syndrome (61–63). There have been some patients infected with HTLV-1 and human immunodeficiency virus (HIV) who have been noted to have PM-like (64–66) and DM-like syndromes (67). Hence, testing for HIV infection should be considered for patients presenting with DM/PM who are in high-risk groups.

Multicentric reticulohistiocytosis has been reported to masquerade as DM (304); however, the "string of pearls" in the periungual areas that is seen in this condition on close clinical and pathologic examination can be clearly distinguished from the periungual changes of DM.

Sarcoidosis and DM have been reported to coexist in several patients (305–307). Although the granulomatous myopathy that can accompany sarcoidosis might be confused with the pattern of muscle weakness produced by DM/PM, the cutaneous manifestations of these two disorders should not be difficult to distinguish.

As previously noted, there are many causes of proximal muscle weakness other than DM/PM (see Table 3.6). The broad differential diagnosis of proximal muscle weakness has been the subject of a recent review (308).

MANAGEMENT

This discussion will focus on the management of the cutaneous manifestations of DM. Comprehensive reviews of the management of other aspects of DM/PM have been presented by others (93,309–314) and are beyond the scope of this discussion.

Local Medical Therapy

Patients with DM should be instructed to avoid excessive sun exposure and to wear sunscreens. Based on the limited phototesting data that is available, sunscreens that provide SPF 30 UVB protection and maximal UVA protection (i.e., those containing avobenzone (Parsol 1789) or micronized pigments such as zinc oxide or titanium dioxide) should be recommended. These preparations are most effective when given with specific instructions concerning optimally effective usage (in real-life settings, patients often used half the amount of a chemical sunscreen product compared with the amount used by the manufacturer to determine its sun protection factor level).

Topical corticosteroids can lessen the degree of inflammation of cutaneous DM in some patients and thereby lessen the pruritus; however, these agents alone are usually inadequate in fully suppressing the disease. We have found that superpotent class I agents such as clobetasol propionate and halcinonide as well as betamethasone dipropionate and diflorasone diacetate in optimized vehicles (e.g., ointments, foams) provide the best relief. The risk for local and systemic side effects from these agents can be minimized if they are used in 2-week intermittent treatment cycles (i.e., 2 weeks of daily treatment followed by a 2-week rest period off treatment). Occlusion under plastic wrap can enhance the effects of these agents. However, the risk for associated side effects also increases. Intralesional corticosteroid injections are not often practical in cutaneous DM because of the widespread cutaneous involvement; however, such therapy can be considered for focal areas of skin involvement that are otherwise refractory.

Scalp pruritus/burning can be quite severe in some patients. Daily use of a medicated shampoo followed by application of a potent topical corticosteroid solution, gel, spray, or foam to the affected areas soon after shampooing can provide some relief. Aggressive use of oral antihistamines including long-acting, sedating agents at bedtime (e.g., low-dose doxepin) and nonsedating agents during the day are often required in this setting.

The available topical formulations of tacrolimus have generally been of sporadic clinical value in controlling DM cutaneous inflammation and pruritus (315). Theoretically, such topical immunomodulators could be of greater clinical value for cutaneous DM if formulations become available that have improved delivery of the active agent through the stratum corneum barrier of the skin. Several adjunctive measures for the pruritus of DM can also make patients more comfortable. The skin of patients with DM is often quite dry, especially in elderly patients, and effective moisturizing regimens can be of additional benefit for the difficult pruritus often experienced by such patients. Topical antipruritic agents such as combinations of menthol/phenol/camphor and pramoxine can provide short-term relief. Topical preparations of doxepin can be of benefit in the pruritus associated with DM; however, there is a risk for allergic contact dermatitis with this topical agent.

Systemic Medical Therapy

ANTIPRURITICS

Systemic antipruritic therapy can serve as an adjunct to therapy that is more definitive for cutaneous DM. The tricyclic antidepressant, doxepin, is also an extremely potent H_1 and H_2 antihistamine, and when given at bedtime in doses of 10 to 50 mg, can ameliorate pruritus and excoriation experienced unconsciously during the evening. The only side effect of concern at these doses is "hangover" somnolence the next morning, which can be usually managed by adjusting the bedtime dose downward. It is possible to monitor blood levels of doxepin, as there is great individual variation in the absorption and metabolism of this agent. Nonsedating or conventional antihistamines can be used during the day.

ANTIMALARIALS

Hydroxychloroquine sulfate (400 mg/day) has been successfully used to treat DM skin disease (316,317). Our experience has been that only a minority of patients with DM respond well to hydroxychloroquine alone. Some of our patients who have not responded adequately to hydroxychloroquine alone have responded to the combination of hydroxychloroquine and quinacrine hydrochloride (100 mg/day). Substituting chloroquine phosphate (250 mg/day) for hydroxychloroquine in this combination might also be considered. If extrapolation from the experience gained from patients with cutaneous LE is valid, patients with DM who smoke cigarettes might be less responsive to antimalarial therapy than those who do not. Appropriate measures should be taken to minimize the risk for retinal toxicity when using hydroxychloroquine or chloroquine (adherence to maximum daily dose recommendations and regular ophthalmologic examinations). Remember that on rare occasion, antimalarials can contribute to muscular weakness by causing a vacuolar myopathy as a drug side effect. Bloom et al. (318) have interjected a note of caution by describing two children with DM whose cutaneous lesions worsened while undergoing therapy with hydroxychloroquine. Chloroquine-induced neutropenia has been reported in a patient with DM (319).

CORTICOSTEROIDS

Systemic corticosteroids are the mainstay of therapy and are the first line of treatment in most patients with classic DM. The earlier the therapy with corticosteroids is begun after disease onset, the better is the overall prognosis (320). Usually, prednisone is given orally in divided doses of 60 to 80 mg per day (1 mg/kg per day) (93). For children, dosage regimens between 1 and 2 mg/kg per day have been recommended (24). Treatment is continued until there is significant improvement of muscle strength testing, normalization of muscle enzyme levels, and improvement in the clinical appearance and pruritus of the cutaneous disease. Most patients usually require 1 to 3 months of full-dose prednisone. Once patients show improvement in severity of symptoms, the dose can be consolidated from a divided dose to a single daily dose given in the morning to reduce risk for adrenal suppression and other corticosteroid side effects. The corticosteroid dose can then be progressively decreased by 10% every 2 weeks. Patients not responding to this regimen can have their daily prednisone increased to 1.5 to 2 mg/kg per day. In unresponsive, acutely ill patients, intravenous pulse therapy with methylprednisolone can be used. Intravenous pulse therapy with methylprednisolone has become increasingly popular in the management of juvenile DM (293). Alternate-day corticosteroids usually do not provide adequate relief in this disorder. If there is no response to high-dose oral corticosteroid therapy after 2 months or if maintenance doses of corticosteroids are too high, other forms of immunosuppressive therapy can be started.

Some researchers suggest that high-dose corticosteroid therapy may exacerbate the cutaneous vasculopathy that can occur in patients with juvenile classic DM, thereby potentiating cutaneous ulceration (321). This is in contrast to the belief by others that early aggressive therapy with corticosteroids can lessen the risk for vasculopathy/vasculitis with resultant dystrophic calcification (322).

Systemic corticosteroids have also been used for disabling cutaneous disease in patients with amyopathic DM (39); however, most advocate that measures that are more conservative should be used in those having less symptomatic skin disease. Stonecipher et al. (96) reserved systemic corticosteroids and other immunosuppressives for their patients with predominately cutaneous DM who were found to have objective evidence of muscle involvement. In view of the work further confirming that early treatment of inflammatory myopathy improves prognosis in patients with DM/PM (320), the recognition that amyopathic DM can represent the earliest clinical indication of smoldering myositis could be of significant clinical value. It remains to be determined whether early aggressive immunosuppressive treatment of amyopathic DM might prevent the development of clinically significant myositis in those patients so destined.

The cutaneous manifestations of DM can be quite refractory to high-dose, long-term corticosteroids in some patients. In addition, some patients have recrudescent disease activity only in their skin following complete suppression of their muscle disease with systemic corticosteroid therapy (323). Hydroxychloroquine as well as the immunosuppressives discussed later are used in this setting.

OTHER IMMUNOSUPPRESSIVE/IMMUNOMODULATING AGENTS

Approximately 25% of patients with DM/PM do not respond adequately to systemic corticosteroids (324). Azathioprine (1 to 2 mg/kg per day) (19), cyclophosphamide (1 to 2 mg/kg per day) (19), methotrexate (312), chlorambucil (2 to 6 mg per day) (325), cyclosporine (5 mg/kg per day) (326), and mycophenolate mofetil (327) have been used in this setting and for patients who cannot tolerate the numerous side effects of high-dose corticosteroids. The data concerning the use of these and other modalities in DM/PM, including total body irradiation and thymectomy, have been reviewed by Boyd and Neldner (309). Extracorporeal photochemotherapy has also been explored as an adjunctive therapy (328).

Methotrexate appears to be the agent of choice in adults, and cyclophosphamide is the most useful in children. In adults, methotrexate 20 to 50 mg a week is given orally, subcutaneously, or intravenously. Intramuscular use should be avoided because it may produce confusion concerning the state of muscle disease activity by spuriously elevating muscle enzyme levels (329). Lower doses of oral methotrexate (7.5 to 15 mg) given in pulse fashion once weekly have been successful in some patients primarily affected by cutaneous DM (312). Oral azathioprine given at 1.5 to 2 mg/kg per day can also be of benefit. Chlorambucil has been suggested to be of considerable benefit to some patients with DM whose disease is refractory to corticosteroids (325). However, this drug can produce very severe toxicity (marrow suppression, leukemia). Combination therapy with corticosteroids, methotrexate, and chlorambucil has been advocated for such resistant cases (330). In children, cyclophosphamide is given daily in a dosage of 2 to 4 mg/kg per day.

High-dose intravenous gamma globulin has been used successfully in both adults and children who are refractory to systemic corticosteroids and other immunosuppressive agents or who develop intolerable corticosteroid side effects. This could be a promising treatment for such patients, with very few side effects (331–333). However, the ultimate role of this very expensive form of treatment remains to be determined (334,335). It has been suggested that this modality could work by blocking endomysial deposition of activated complement components (336). Although initially felt to be of some benefit, a controlled trial has indicated that plasmapheresis and leukopheresis have little additional value in the management of DM/PM (337).

Dapsone has been suggested anecdotally to be of value in patients with limited to moderately active forms of cutaneous DM (114,338). Mycophenolate mofetil has also been suggested to have steroid-sparing value for the cutaneous manifestations of DM (339).

Based on experimental evidence indicating a role for TNF-α in the pathogenesis of the classic DM muscle inflammation, anti–TNF-α therapy has recently been used on an anecdotal basis for both the muscular and cutaneous manifestations of DM. Thalidomide, a TNF-α production inhibitor, has been observed anecdotally to be of value for cutaneous DM inflammation (Warren Piette, personal communication). In addition, five cases of severe, treatment-resistant DM that have been successfully treated with etanercept (Enbrel; Amgén Thousand Oaks, CA) have been published informally (340,341). In addition, three similar cases have been successfully managed with infliximab (Remicade; Centocor, Malvern, PA) (342,343). More systematic study in this area is needed to define the value of such treatment. Such therapy would have to be used with caution concerning the possibility of its uncovering other patterns of systemic autoimmunity (e.g., SLE). Formal clinical trials of infliximab in classic DM are currently under way.

There are no systematically ascertained data to guide one in the treatment of either adults or children with clinically amyopathic DM. All current approaches are based on anecdotal observations of individual cases or relatively small case series and thus are open to question. However, it is now clear that the following considerations require vigilance in the management of such individuals: the realization that patients with clinically amyopathic DM are at risk for potentially fatal ILD (42), the possibility that patients with clinically amyopathic DM may have an increased risk for internal malignancy, and the fact that some patients with clinically amyopathic DM have developed symptomatic myositis greater than 2 years after skin disease onset. Added to these concerns is the inherently refractory nature of DM skin inflammation. These aspects taken together can present a formidable task when faced with a patient with new clinically amyopathic DM.

One approach has been to treat patients with clinically amyopathic DM aggressively from the outset with systemic corticosteroids with the hope that progression to systemic involvement might be delayed or prevented (344). This approach is supported by studies of patients with juvenile- and patients with adult-onset classic DM that indicate that early systemic immunosuppressive treatment can lessen long-term disability from muscle dysfunction and complications such as calcification. However, in most published reports concerning clinically amyopathic DM, a more conservative treatment approach has been taken, an approach that is supported by reports of some patients with clinically amyopathic DM going 10 to 20 years and longer without any sign of disease activity outside the skin (43,85,239,345). More work is needed to identify risk factors for systemic disease, malignancy development, or both in patients with clinically amyopathic DM.

Until it is confirmed that adult patients with clinically amyopathic DM do not have an increased risk for internal malignancy, such patients should be evaluated for this potential complication in a manner similar to that for patients with classic DM. Because internal malignancy has not been reported in juvenile clinically amyopathic DM, it can be assumed that as in patients with juvenile classic DM, routine evaluation for internal malignancy is not indicated.

As the cutaneous manifestations of clinically amyopathic DM and classic DM are indistinguishable clinically and pathologically, the management of skin disease activity in both clinical settings is similar. However, systemic immunosuppressive therapy is used from the outset in patients with classic DM and, as a result, symptomatic skin disease activity is generally less of a problem.

Therapy for Dystrophic Calcification

Medical treatment of dystrophic calcification in DM is extremely challenging and in most cases, quite inadequate. Numerous approaches based on various rationales have been used. Those agents mentioned anecdotally most frequently include aluminum hydroxide suspension (15 to 20 mL four times per day) (346–348), probenecid (250 mg/day) (349,350), potassium paraamino benzoic acid (15 to 25 g/day) (194), warfarin (1 mg/day) (351,352), and diltiazem (30 to 90 mg/day) (353). The efficacy of warfarin has subsequently been challenged (354). Intravenous chelating agents such as EDTA have also been tried but have mostly been unsuccessful (355). Colchicine (1.2 to 1.8 mg per day) has been used to suppress inflammation that can accompany calcinosis universalis (356). A recent report has suggested that the bisphosphonates such as alendronate might be of value (357). Surgical removal of symptomatic cutaneous or subcutaneous calcium deposits can be considered as a last resort (358).

Physical Therapy

Passive range-of-motion exercise should begin early in the disease course of classic DM to prevent disabling joint contractures—this is especially true in children with DM. After disease activity is suppressed medically, an active exercise program can facilitate the return of normal strength.

Ongoing Surveillance After Diagnosis

MALIGNANCY

Surveillance for the detection of occult malignancy should be systematically integrated into the management plan for all patients with DM and amyopathic DM. The frequency and extent of such assessments are not generally agreed on; however, most recommend reevaluation every 6 to 12 months for the first 3 to 5 years after diagnosis, focusing on areas of highest malignancy risk for the sex and age of the individual. Frequent gynecologic examination including physical examination, transvaginal ultrasonography, and CA-125 serum determinations has been recommended for the early detection of ovarian cancer in female patients with classic and clinically amyopathic DM (98).

SYSTEMIC ORGAN INVOLVEMENT

In addition, any change in the clinical status of the respiratory, cardiovascular, or gastrointestinal system in a patient with DM/PM should be evaluated carefully for the possibility of increased activity of the underlying disease process in these potential target organs.

PREGNANCY

The initial observations suggested that pregnancy outcome in patients with DM/PM could be quite risky (data reviewed by Ishii et al. [359]). However, subsequent reports have suggested that patients can do quite well under these circumstances (359,360). If possible, pregnancy should be avoided during periods of disease activity. One of the authors (R.D.S.) has observed several patients with amyopathic DM proceed throughout a normal pregnancy and delivery without difficulty (R.D.S., personal observation). In addition, the same author has observed two adult sisters with clinically amyopathic DM whose cutaneous DM lesions remitted completely during several pregnancies only to flare approximately 6 weeks following delivery.

PROGNOSIS

Mortality for classic DM/PM has varied from 25% to 80% in past series, depending partly on the number of acute and chronic cases of DM, the incidence of malignancy, and the availability of immunosuppressive therapy. However, in the past two decades, the mortality has decreased significantly because of the more aggressive use of corticosteroids and immunosuppressives and better supportive medical care. The 5- and 8-year survival rates for a group of 76 patients with DM/PM studied in the 1980s was 80% and 73%, respectively (44).

A recent examination of prognosis in 77 consecutive patients with DM/PM having a minimum of 18 months of follow-up revealed a 22% mortality rate resulting predominately from malignancy and lung disease (361). As has been previously observed in both juvenile-onset and adult-onset classic DM, a better prognosis was seen in this study in individuals who received early systemic treatment for their disease. Poor outcome is associated with older age, pulmonary and esophageal involvement, and malignancy. The early and aggressive use of corticosteroids has reduced the mortality rate in children to less than 10% (24). The most common causes of death in classic DM/PM are malignancy, infection, and cardiac and pulmonary disease.

Some patients with classic adult DM will respond quickly to treatment with systemic corticosteroids and enjoy long treatment-free intervals following steroid taper, although there is always a risk for disease recrudescence. Others do not respond fully to systemic corticosteroids or to other immunosuppressive agents and will have a long-term unremitting course. The reasons for these differences are not clear. Several factors have been suggested to be associated with a poor prognosis: older age at onset, fulminant disease onset, dysphagia, ILD, cardiac involvement, associated malignancy, corticosteroids resistance, and delay in treatment (data reviewed by Targoff [93]). It has also been suggested that certain types of skin lesions correlate with a poor outcome. Basset-Seguin et al. (129) have reported that ulcers arising over violaceous indurated plaques on the trunk with or without indurated papules were more frequent in their adult patients with DM who developed a malignancy.

It has been suggested that prognosis in both patients with adult and with juvenile DM/PM is associated with the types of autoantibodies that are produced (56,58,97). The presence of antisynthetase autoantibodies (e.g., Jo-1, PL-7, PL-12) has been correlated with incomplete response to therapy and ILD. Antibodies that react with signal-recognition particle (SRP) reportedly occur in patients who have forms of disease that are more acute in onset, severe, and treatment-resistant in which cardiac involvement is seen more frequently. Autoantibodies to Mi-2 have been associated with more treatment responsive forms of DM.

Antisynthetase antibodies and TNF-α-308A allele may represent risk factors for disease chronicity and severity in juvenile-onset classic DM (57). Black children with DM tend to have more aggressive disease than white or Hispanic children. Calcinosis remains a primary cause of both disease morbidity and mortality in patients with juvenile classic DM.

There are too little long-term follow-up data available concerning patients with amyopathic DM to assess prognosis. All six of the patients described by Krain (34) who initially presented with only skin disease and were treated conservatively ultimately developed muscle disease. (However, it is not clear that the ultimate appearance of symptomatic muscle weakness was not an entry criterion for this study.) None of the five patients with amyopathic DM treated by Euwer and Sontheimer (39) with high-dose systemic corticosteroids developed clinical evidence of myositis during the follow-up period. As previously discussed, although malignancies have been reported to occur in patients with amyopathic DM, the statistical significance of such an association has not yet been determined. One of the authors (R.D.S.) and Thomas Provost have personally observed several patients with amyopathic DM who have had classic cutaneous manifestations of DM for 15 years or longer without developing clinical evidence of muscle disease, malignancy, or systemic organ involvement. As previously discussed, on the basis of the reports to date, there appears to be a low frequency of systemic organ involvement in patients with amyopathic DM, with ILD having been observed most often.

One study has suggested that patients with juvenile DM who have only cutaneous manifestations and no muscle weakness are usually not treated aggressively and frequently develop pathologic calcifications (241). This report is contrary to other studies of clinically amyopathic DM in both children (240) and adults (85,81) that have indicated that this mode of presentation is usually not associated with a high rate of subsequent dystrophic calcification. One study indicates that rheumatologists and dermatologists tend to be quite conservative in treating patients with clinically amyopathic DM (240). Interestingly, this report indicates that a high percentage of patients with juvenile-onset clinically amyopathic DM enjoy spontaneous remission without systemic immunosuppressive treatment.

ETIOLOGIC FACTORS/PATHOGENESIS

The etiologic factors and pathogenesis of DM/PM are unknown; however, there is no lack of speculation on this subject. These issues have been addressed elsewhere recently in more depth than space will allow here (93,269,275,362–367) and only the highlights relating to this subject will be discussed later.

The following observations have led to the general belief that this pattern of musculocutaneous disease results from a genetically determined autoimmune response to environmental agents: the inflammatory nature of the skin and muscle disease patterns both clinically and histopathologically, the characteristic humoral autoimmune abnormalities, the responsiveness to corticosteroids and other immunosuppressive agents, and the overlapping relationship with other autoimmune disorders such as SLE, scleroderma, rheumatoid arthritis, and Sjögren syndrome (93). Cell-mediated immunity directed against muscle-specific autoantigens has traditionally been believed to be responsible for the muscle injury that occurs in PM, whereas humoral mechanisms involving complement activation and microvascular injury have been thought to be predominately involved in the pathogenesis of DM.

Like other systemic autoimmune diseases involving autoantibody production such as SLE, DM/PM is thought to evolve through multiple sequential phases: susceptibility phase, induction phase, expansion phase, and injury phase (see Fig. 2.1). Unfortunately, a comprehensive discussion of this sequence of susceptibilities and events is beyond the scope of this presentation.

Genetic Factors

Various degrees of association have been observed with alleles of the major histocompatibility complex. HLA-B8 and -DR3 have been found to be enriched in white patients with DM/PM more so than in other races (368–370); however, it appears that this association might be due to linkage disequilibrium with HLA-DQA1*0501 (371). Curiously, other studies have failed to confirm such associations (372). Studies evaluating the association of null genes within the C4A region with juvenile DM have been inconsistent (371,373). The production of antisynthetase antibodies such as Jo-1 is strongly linked to HLA-DR3 (374) and even more so with its supertypical specificity, HLA-DRW52 (375).

Increasingly, TNF-α is thought to play a role in the pathogenesis of muscle injury in myositis. A single nucleotide polymorphism in the TNF-α promoter (TNF-α-308A) has recently been associated with high levels of TNF-α production, disease chronicity, and calcinosis in a cohort of white patients with juvenile-onset classic DM (57). This genetic trait could be causally related to DM or could represent only an association through linkage disequilibrium with the autoimmune haplotype, HL-A1, B8, DR3, DQ2, that is known to be present with increased frequency in patients with DM.

TNF-α promoter polymorphism could potentially play a role in the photosensitivity experienced by many patients with DM. TNF-α-308A promoter polymorphism has been linked to the photosensitive LE-specific skin disease subset, subacute cutaneous LE (376,377). In these studies, epidermal keratinocytes containing this TNF-α allele have been shown to produce exaggerated levels of TNF-α in the presence of IL-1α following exposure to UVB radiation. As previously mentioned, this same TNF-α promoter polymorphism has been associated with juvenile DM. These observations raise the possibility that TNF-α-inhibiting therapy, such as thalidomide or monoclonal antibodies (infliximab, etanercept), might be of value in selected patients with photosensitive DM as well as subacute cutaneous LE.

In addition, a single case report of a young adult Japanese woman who presented with clinically amyopathic DM that evolved into classic DM over a 3-year period was shown to be genetically deficient in the C5 component of complement (51). If confirmed, this case could call into question the hypothesis that skin and muscle disease activity in classic DM is causally related to the deposition of complement membrane attack complex in cutaneous and muscular microvessels.

Immunologic Abnormalities

Most of the work relating to the autoimmune aspects of this disorder has been directed toward the characteristic muscle changes. Attempts have been made to correlate the pattern of cellular inflammation within muscle tissue to clinical pattern of illness. As has been noted earlier, cell phenotyping studies have indicated that $CD8^+$ T cells are often associated with damaged muscle fibers in PM, suggesting the possibility that cytotoxic T-cell injury might be occurring (264). Evidence suggests that lymphocytes within the endomysium of affected muscles demonstrate T-cell–receptor $V\alpha/\beta$ gene restriction, a finding that would be compatible with antigen-driven oligoclonal expansion (378). Biopsies from DM muscle more often show $CD4^+$ T cells and B cells in the perivascular areas, which in conjunction with the vasculopathic features of this form of the disease, have argued for a humoral-based mechanism of vascular injury. Studies suggesting decreased capillary density in DM muscle biopsies would support this notion (265).

As has been discussed earlier, the immunopathology of the skin lesions of DM is dominated by activated macrophages and CD4 T cells, arguing in favor of cell-mediated pattern of immune injury (259). Components of the membrane attack complex of complement have been observed in the walls of dermal microvessels. Wakino et al. (379) have noted that peripheral blood lymphocyte subpopulations in one patient with amyopathic DM were different from those reported for patients with classic DM/PM.

The MSA responses have been previously addressed in the section discussing laboratory assessment. Whether these autoantibodies participate in the causation of myositis or represent only a byproduct of muscle injury is not known. However, further evidence that the MSAs are truly specific for myositis is their general absence in patients with clinically amyopathic DM. These autoantibodies are directed against molecules that are normally expressed in the cytoplasm and nucleus. Although it has traditionally been thought that antibody molecules usually do not penetrate into healthy cells, there is increasing precedent to suggest that there are some exceptions to this rule, suggesting that these antibodies may indeed be pathogenic and not merely an epiphenomenon (380–382).

Much effort has been made to identify specific lymphocyte responses to muscle tissue in patients with DM/PM and to demonstrate that lymphocytes from such patients can specifically recognize and injure muscle cells *in vitro* (data reviewed by Targoff [93]). Effector cells from the peripheral blood and affected muscle tissue have been used. For the most part, the results of these efforts have been inconsistent. However, animal models suggest that PM is a T-cell–dependent process (383).

Further evidence has been presented recently supporting the concept that cell-mediated myocytotoxicity plays a role in the pathogenesis of myositis. Both myocytotoxic $CD3^+$ T-cell clones and non-HLA–restricted myocytotoxic cells of other lineages have been shown to be present in the peripheral blood of patients with inflammatory myopathies (384). Unfortunately, very little has been done experimentally to probe for cytotoxic epidermal or dermal cell injury in patients having DM skin disease activity.

There is not always good agreement between the degree of muscle weakness or fatigue experienced by patients with classic DM and the degree of inflammation noted on muscle biopsy or increase of serum muscle enzymes. This has led to the idea that inflammatory cytokines might be capable of mediating metabolic disturbances within muscle that can exacerbate muscle weakness and fatigue (data reviewed by Lundberg [385]).

As with other rheumatic diseases such as systemic sclerosis, maternal microchimerism has been observed in patients with juvenile classic DM (386). The pathogenetic significance of alloreactive maternal lymphoid cells present in the circulation, muscle, and skin tissue of patients with juvenile DM is not yet known.

Environmental Factors

INFECTIOUS AGENTS

Considerable attention focused on the possibility that several types of myotropic infections might be capable of focusing an autoimmune attack on muscle antigens through the mechanism of molecular mimicry (data reviewed Targoff [93]). Candidates include RNA viruses such as coxsackievirus and echovirus, human retroviruses (HTLV-1, HIV). Other types of viruses have also been implicated (Epstein–Barr, Parvovirus B19) (68). Nonviral pathogens such as *Toxoplasma gondii* have also been suggested. Attempts to definitively identify persistent myotropic virus infection have not been successful (387). An association between DM/PM and *Borrelia burgdorferi* has also been claimed (388,389).

Some authors have suggested that infection by more common bacterial organisms such as streptococci can facilitate the juvenile DM process (390). In addition, Moore et al. (391) suggested that patients with juvenile DM who develop calcinosis are more likely to have staphylococcal infections and have decreased chemotaxis to *Staphylococcus aureus,* apparently due to a serum factor (391). These children also have elevated levels of IgE as well as antistaphylococcal IgE antibodies. Whether these differences were causally related to the calcinosis was not clear.

DRUGS

As has been previously noted, a number of drugs and implantable foreign materials have been suggested to be associated with the development of and are capable of producing DM- and PM-like syndromes.

Pathogenesis of the Cutaneous Lesions of Dermatomyositis

In the past, few efforts have been directed to the pathogenesis of the cutaneous manifestations of DM in part because of the assumption that skin involvement in this disorder was only a "spill-over" manifestation of the autoimmune process within the musculature. However, the recognition that the skin can be the primary if not sole target of this disease process (by virtue of the existence of clinically amyopathic DM) considerably enhances the importance of developing a better understanding of the pathogenesis of this aspect of the disease. Further supporting this possibility is the previously discussed preliminary observation that there might be unique serologic associations of clinically amyopathic DM (155 kDa, Se autoantibodies).

Early studies identifying myxovirus-like structures observed by electron microscopy in lesional skin biopsies suggested a direct link to viral infection (153,392). However, these structures are not specific for DM and there is now general agreement that they likely represent artifacts because they have been produced in cultured cells *in vitro* by interferon stimulation (393–395).

The similarity of histopathologic change between cutaneous DM and certain forms of cutaneous LE (i.e., a relatively cell-poor lichenoid tissue reaction) can be quite striking. An informal study indicated that it was not possible to reliably discriminate between hematoxylin and eosin–stained slides of biopsies from DM and subacute cutaneous LE skin lesions in a blinded comparison (R.D.S., et al., personal unpublished observation). Preliminary studies have suggested that the epidermal Langerhans cell population is differentially altered in cutaneous LE and DM skin lesions (396). The similarity between the cutaneous histopathologies of DM and LE would suggest commonality in their underlying pathogenetic mechanisms. Unfortunately, relatively little direct evidence exists concerning the pathogenesis of LE-specific skin lesions. Circumstantial evidence suggests that some forms of photosensitive cutaneous LE such as subacute cutaneous LE and neonatal LE might be mediated or exacerbated by humoral factors like Ro/SS-A autoantibody through a mechanism of antibody-dependent cell-mediated cytotoxicity (397). One hypothesis also incriminates humoral factors in the pathogenesis of DM (268,336).

As a form of lichenoid tissue reaction, one must also consider the possibility that DM skin injury might result from antigen-specific cytotoxic T cell injury (398). A considerable amount of indirect evidence suggests that PM results from a cytotoxic T-cell attack on muscle tissue (93). With a few exceptions (399), similar studies have not been systematically carried out using skin cells as targets. One study has failed to find evidence of oligoclonal T-cell expansion of the type seen in antigen-specific responses in delayed-type hypersensitivity–induced skin lesions in a small number of patients with DM (378). The $\gamma\Delta$-receptor–positive T cells have been implicated in the pathogenesis of muscle damage in patients with PM (400). This cell type has also been implicated in the pathogenesis of chronic cutaneous LE skin lesions (401); however, no studies concerning this cell type and the cutaneous manifestations of DM have been reported.

There are some interesting parallels between the cutaneous manifestations of DM and lichen planus, a pattern of lichenoid tissue reaction that may result from cytotoxic T-cell–mediated epidermal cell injury (398). Both have a distinctive violaceous hue and both are characterized by intense pruritus. The early stages of Gottron papules can often present a lichen planus–like appearance and the other cutaneous lesions of DM can at times have a very lichenoid appearance clinically (126).

Highly prominent among the pathologic changes seen in DM skin lesions are those that occur within the dermis—a relatively noninflammatory microvasculopathy associated with a marked accumulation of mucin. The changes in the dermal microvasculature are more prominent in DM than cutaneous LE and some believe that microvascular injury might be the primary lesion of DM in both the skin and muscle (336). This argument suggests that local activation of the membrane attack complex of complement (C5-9) within the microvasculature of muscle and skin by humoral factors could play a role in the pathogenesis of this disease (268,336). One possible humoral factor could be endothelial-specific autoantibodies for which some evidence does exist (402). Other than the suggestion by Hausmann et al. (259) that class II histocompatibility antigen expression by dermal endothelial cells is decreased, little is known about the immunobiologic phenotype of this cell type in DM. Such studies, including characterization of adhesion molecule expression are needed.

As previously discussed, DM skin involvement has a proclivity for localizing to areas of skin that are frequently stretched (i.e., knuckles, elbows, and knees). It is possible that the microvascular beds in such areas are fundamentally different in some way perhaps relating to chronic low-grade, stretch-induced transient ischemia. Such differences might serve as a localizing factor for the DM disease process. This could be addressed experimentally by determining whether hypoxic dermal microvascular endothelial cells are more likely to be injured by serum factors from patients with DM.

To be complete, any explanation of the pathomechanism(s) of cutaneous DM must account for the highly prominent accumulation of mucin that occurs within the dermis. One group has suggested that this might be due to increased production of glycosaminoglycans by dermal fibroblasts as a result of immunologic stimulation (167). There is evidence suggesting that mononuclear cells from patients with DM can be cytotoxic for cultured dermal fibroblasts (399). Pandya et al. (403) have suggested the possibility that a factor present in LE patient serum can stimulate the production of glycosaminoglycans by dermal fibroblasts.

Stone (141) has presented an intriguing hypothesis concerning possible mechanisms underlying the association between internal malignancy and DM/PM. He proposes that local tumor-induced changes in the surrounding extracellular matrix (i.e., depolymerization of glycosaminoglycans) can act through the circulation to change the general extracellular matrix, including that which is present in the skin. He argues that other triggers of DM such as infections and drugs like D-penicillamine could be acting through related actions on glycosaminoglycans.

Recent work has indicated that factor XIIIa–positive dermal perivascular dendritic cells may be the source of abnormal mucin production in conditions such as the reticular erythematous mucinosis syndrome (404). It is tempting to extrapolate these observations to autoimmune conditions that involve abnormal dermal mucin accumulation such as cutaneous LE and DM.

The mechanisms responsible for the photosensitivity that occurs in many patients with DM are for the most part completely unknown. The preliminary phototesting data that are available suggest a rather broad action spectrum (59). Photochallenge testing of nonlesional skin in patients with LE has suggested that perivascular mononuclear cell accumulation is the initial pathologic change seen in this disorder (405). Similar studies have not yet been reported in DM. Studies addressing abnormalities in UV-modulated epidermal cytokine expression in DM are also needed.

A striking clinical difference between the cutaneous lesions of LE and DM is that DM lesions are much more pruritic. The presence of itching always raises the possibility of mast cell involvement. Although dermal mast cell degranulation has been implicated in the pathogenesis of less pruritic types of skin involvement in other connective tissue diseases such as scleroderma (406,407), little attention has been focused on abnormalities of this cell type in DM. Informal observations have revealed no gross alteration in mast cell density in biopsies of DM skin lesions (R.D.S., personal unpublished observation).

Virtually identical clinical and pathologic features of the skin involvement of amyopathic DM and classic DM strongly suggest a common pathogenesis.

ACKNOWLEDGMENTS

The compilation of this manuscript was supported in part by National Institutes of Health grant no. AR19101 from the National Institute of Arthritis and Musculoskeletal and Skin Diseases (NIAMS). Its contents are solely the responsibility of the authors and do not necessarily represent the official views of NIAMS. This work was also supported by a University of Iowa Dermatology Department endowment from the Herzog Foundation and the generous support of the Joseph Marshall family of Morningside, Iowa.

REFERENCES

1. Wagner E. Fall einer seltuen Muskelkranheit. *Arch Heilkd* 1863;4:282.
2. Unverricht H. Polymyositis acuta progressiva. *Zeitschrift fur Klinische Medizin* 1887;12:533.
3. Bohan A. History and classification of polymyositis and dermatomyositis. *Clin Dermatol* 1988;6:3–8.
4. Jacoby GW. Subacute progressive polymyositis. *J Nerv Ment Dis* 1888;15: 697–726.
5. Gottron, H. Haut veranderungen bei dermatomyositis. In: Lomholt S, ed. *VIII Congres International de Dermatologie; 1930; Copenhagen.* Copenhagen: Engelsen and Schroder, 1931.
6. Gottron, HA, Schonfeld W. Dermatomyositis. In: Thieme G, ed. *Dermatologie und Venerologie.* Stuttgart: Verlag, 1958.
7. Gottron HA. Zur Dermatomyositis nebst Bemerkungen zur Poikilodermie. *Dermatologische Wochenschrift* 1954;35:923–930.
8. Keil H. Manifestations in the skin and mucous membranes in dermatomyositis with special reference to the differential diagnosis from systemic lupus erythematosus. *Ann Intern Med* 1942;16:828–871.
9. O'Leary PA, Waisman M. Dermatomyositis: a study of forty cases. *Arch Dermat Syph* 1940;41:1001–1019.
10. Eaton LM. The perspective of neurology in regard to polymyositis: a study of 41 cases. *Neurology* 1954;4:245–263.
11. Walton JN, Adams RD. *Polymyositis.* E.S. Livingstone, Edinburgh 1958.
12. Rose AL, Walton JN. Polymyositis: a survey of 89 cases with particular reference to treatment and prognosis. *Brain* 1966;89:742–768.
13. Williams RC. Dermatomyositis and malignancy: a review of the literature. *Ann Intern Med* 1959;50:1174.
14. Winkelmann RK. The cutaneous diagnosis of dermatomyositis, lupus erythematosus, and scleroderma. *N Y State J Med* 1963;3080–3086.
15. Pearson CM. Rheumatic manifestations of polymyositis and dermatomyositis. *Arthritis Rheum* 1959;2:127–143.
16. Pearson CM. Patterns of polymyositis and their responses to treatment. *Ann Intern Med* 1963;59:827–838.
17. Pearson CM. Polymyositis. *Annu Rev Med* 1966;17:63–82.
18. Pearson CM, Bohan A. The spectrum of polymyositis and dermatomyositis [review]. *Med Clin North Am* 1977;61:439–457.
19. Bohan A, Peter JB, Bowman RL, et al. Computer-assisted analysis of 153 patients with polymyositis and dermatomyositis. *Medicine* 1977;56:255–286.
20. Bohan A, Peter JB. Polymyositis and dermatomyositis. *N Engl J Med* 1975;292: 344–347.
21. Dalakas MC. Polymyositis, dermatomyositis and inclusion-body myositis. *N Engl J Med* 1991;325:1487–1498.
22. Everett MA, Curtis AC. Dermatomyositis: a review of 19 cases in adolescents and children. *Arch Intern Med* 1957;100:70–76.
23. Banker BQ, Victor M. Dermatomyositis (systemic angiopathy) of childhood. *Medicine* 1966;45:261–289.
24. Roberts LJ, Fink CW. Childhood polymyositis/dermatomyositis. *Clin Dermatol* 1988;6:36–46.
25. Gamstorp I. Dermatomyositis and polymyositis in childhood [review]. *Brain Dev* 1990;12:345–348.
26. Hiketa T, Matsumoto Y, Ohashi M, et al. Juvenile dermatomyositis: a statistical study of 114 patients with dermatomyositis. *J Dermatol* 1992;19:470–476.
27. Olson JC. Juvenile dermatomyositis [review]. *Semin Dermatol* 1992;11:57–64.
28. Ansell BM. Juvenile dermatomyositis. *Rheum Dis Clin North Am* 1991; 17:931–942.
29. Callen JP. Dermatomyositis and malignancy [review]. *Clin Dermatol* 1993;11: 61–65.
30. Callen JP. Malignancy in polymyositis/dermatomyositis. *Clin Dermatol* 1988; 6:55–63.
31. Shy GM. The late onset myopathy: a clinicopathologic study of 131 patients. *World Neurol* 1962;3:149–160.
32. Sigurgeirsson B, Lindelof B, Edhag O, et al. Risk of cancer in patients with dermatomyositis or polymyositis: a population-based study. *N Engl J Med* 1992;326:363–367.
33. Rockerbie NR, Woo TY, Callen JP, et al. Cutaneous changes of dermatomyositis precede muscle weakness. *J Am Acad Dermatol* 1989;20:629–632.
34. Krain L. Dermatomyositis in six patients without initial muscle involvement. *Arch Dermatol* 1975;111:241–245.
35. Pearson CM. Polymyositis and dermatomyositis. In: McCarty, DJ, ed. *Arthritis (and allied conditions),* 9th ed. Philadelphia: Lea & Febiger 1979: 742–761.
36. Caro I. A. dermatologist's view of polymyositis/dermatomyositis [review]. *Clin Dermatol* 1988;6:9–14, 47–48.
37. Braverman I. Connective tissue (rheumatic) diseases. In: *Cutaneous Signs of Systemic Disease,* 2nd ed. Philadelphia: WB Saunders, 1981: 299–314.
38. Sontheimer RD. Would a new name hasten the acceptance of clinically amyopathic dermatomyositis (dermatomyositis sine myositis) as a distinctive subset within the idiopathic inflammatory dermatomyopathies spectrum of clinical illness? *J Am Acad Dermatol* 2002;46:626–636.
39. Euwer RL, Sontheimer RD. Amyopathic dermatomyositis (dermatomyositis siné myositis): presentation of six new cases and review of the literature. *J Am Acad Dermatol* 1991;24:959–966.
40. Euwer RL, Sontheimer RD. Amyopathic dermatomyositis: a review. *J Invest Dermatol* 1993;100:124S–127S.
41. Sontheimer RD. Dermatomyositis: an overview of recent progress with emphasis on dermatological aspects. *Dermatol Clin* 2002:387–408.
42. Sontheimer RD, Miyagawa S. Potentially fatal interstitial lung disease presenting in the context of amyopathic dermatomyositis. *J Am Acad Dermatol* 48:797–798, 2003.
43. Sontheimer RD. Cutaneous features of classical dermatomyositis and amyopathic dermatomyositis. *Curr Opin Rheumatol* 1999;11:475–482.
44. Hochberg MC, Feldman D,Stevens MB. Adult onset polymyositis/dermatomyositis: an analysis of clinical and laboratory features and survival in 76 patients with a review of the literature. *Semin Arthritis Rheum* 1986;15:168–178.
45. Hanson V. Dermatomyositis, scleroderma and polyarteritis nodosa. *Clin Rheumat Dis* 1976;2:445–467.
46. Crowe WE, Bove KE, Levinson JE, et al. Clinical and pathogenetic implications of histopathology in childhood polydermatomyositis. *Arthritis Rheum* 1982;25:126–139.
47. Pachman LM, Marykowski MC. Juvenile dermatomyositis and polymyositis. *Clin Rheumat Dis* 1984;10:95–115.
48. Taieb A, Guichard C, Salamon R, et al. Prognosis in juvenile dermatopolymyositis: a cooperative retrospective study of 70 cases. *Pediatric Dermatol* 1985;2:275–281.
49. Oddis CV, Conte CG, Steen VD, et al. Incidence of polymyositis-dermatomyositis: a 20-year study of hospital diagnosed cases in Allegheny County, PA 1963-1982. *J Rheumatol* 1990;17:1329–1334.
50. Bridges BF. The rashes of dermatomyositis in a black patient [letter]. *Am J Med* 1991;91:661–662.
51. Ichikawa E, Furuta J, Kawachi Y, et al. Hereditary complement (C9) deficiency associated with dermatomyositis. *Br J Dermatol* 2001;144:1080–1083.
52. Rider LG, Gurley RC, Pandey JP, et al. Clinical, serologic, and immunogenetic features of familial idiopathic inflammatory myopathy. *Arthritis Rheum* 1998;41:710–719.
53. Plamondon S, Dent PB, Reed AM. Familial dermatomyositis. *J Rheumatol* 1999;26:2691–2692.
54. Davies MG, Hickling P. Familial adult dermatomyositis. *Br J Dermatol* 2001; 144:415–416.
55. Arnett FC, Goldstein R, Duvic M, et al. Major histocompatibility complex genes in systemic lupus erythematosus, Sjogren's syndrome, and polymyositis. *Am J Med* 1988;85:38–41.
56. Love LA, Leff RL, Fraser DD, et al. A new approach to the classification of idiopathic inflammatory myopathy: myositis-specific autoantibodies define useful homogeneous patient groups. *Medicine (Baltimore)* 1991;70:360–374.
57. Pachman LM, Liotta-Davis MR, Hong DK, et al. TNFalpha-308A allele in juvenile dermatomyositis: association with increased production of tumor necrosis factor alpha, disease duration, and pathologic calcifications. *Arthritis Rheum* 2000;43:2368–2377.
58. Miller FW. Myositis-specific autoantibodies. *JAMA* 1993;270:1846–1849.
59. Cheong W-K, Hughes GRV, Norris PG, et al. Cutaneous photosensitivity in dermatomyositis. *Brit J Dermatol* 1994;131:205–208.
60. Hengstman GJ, Van Venrooij WJ, Vencovsky J, et al. The relative prevalence of dermatomyositis and polymyositis in Europe exhibits a latitudinal gradient. *Ann Rheum Dis* 2000;59:141–142.
61. Webster ADB. Echovirus disease in hypogammaglobulinemic patients. *Clin Rheumat Dis* 1984;10:189–203.
62. Crennan JM, VanScoy RE, McKenna CH. Echovirus polymyositis in patients with hypogammaglobulinemia: failure of high-dose intravenous gamma globulin therapy and review of the literature. *Am J Med* 1986;81:35–42.
63. Thyss A, el Baze P, Lefebvre JC, et al. Dermatomyositis-like syndrome in X-linked hypogammaglobulinemia: case-report and review of the literature. *Acta Dermato-Venereologica* 1990;70:309–313.
64. Wiley CA, Nerenberg M, Cros D. HTLV-1 polymyositis in a patient also infected with the human immunodeficiency virus. *N Engl J Med* 1989;320:992–995.

65. Morgan O, Mora C, Rodgers-Johnson P. HTLV-1 and polymyositis in Jamaica. *Lancet* 1989;2:1184–1187.
66. Leon-Monzon M, Illa I, Dalakas MC. Polymyositis in patients infected with human T-cell leukemia virus type I: the role of the virus in the cause of the disease. *Ann Neurol* 1994;36:643–649.
67. Gresh JP, Aquilar JL, Espinoza LR. Human immunodeficiency virus (HIV) infection-associated dermatomyositis [letter]. *J Rheumatol* 1989;16:1397–1398.
68. Crowson AN, Magro CM, Dawood MR. A causal role for Parvovirus B19 infection in adult dermatomyositis and other autoimmune syndromes. *J Cutan Pathol* 2000;27:505–515.
69. Chevrel G, Calvet A, Belin V, et al. Dermatomyositis associated with the presence of parvovirus B19 DNA in muscle. *Rheumatology (Oxford)* 2000;39: 1037–1039.
70. Yamashita K, Hosokawa M, Hirohashi S, et al. Epstein-Barr virus-associated gastric cancer in a patient with dermatomyositis. *Intern Med* 2001;40:96–99.
71. Simpson NB, Golding JR. Dermatomyositis induced by penicillamine. *Acta Dermato-Venereologica* 1979;59:543–544.
72. Hill C, Zeitz C, Kirkham B. Dermatomyositis with lung involvement in a patient treated with simvastatin. *Aust N Z J Med* 1995;25:745–746.
73. Khattak FH, Morris IM, Branford WA. Simvastatin-associated dermatomyositis [letter; comment]. *Brit J Rheumatol* 1994;33:199–199.
74. Vela-Casasempere P, Borras-Blasco J, Navarro-Ruiz A. Alfuzosin-associated dermatomyositis. *Br J Rheumatol* 1998;37:1135–1136.
75. Dimachkie MM, Vriesendorp FJ, Heck KA. Phenytoin-induced dermatomyositis: case report and literature review [review]. *J Child Neurol* 1998;13: 577–580.
76. Love LA, Weiner SR, Vasey FB, et al. Clinical and immunogenetic features of women who develop myositis after silicone implants. *Arthritis Rheum* 1992; 35:S46.
77. Houpt KR, Sontheimer RD. Autoimmune connective tissue disease and connective tissue disease-like illnesses after silicone gel augmentation mammoplasty. *J Am Acad Dermatol* 1994;31:626–642.
78. Koeger AC, Alcaix D, Rozenberg S, et al. Occupational exposure to silicon and dermatopolymyositis: 3 cases. *Ann Med Interne* 1991;142:409–413.
79. Cukier J, Beauchamp RA, Spindler JS, et al. Association between bovine collagen dermal implants and a dermatomyositis or a polymyositis-like syndrome. *Ann Inter Med* 1993;118:920–928.
80. Rosenberg MJ, Reichlin M. Is there an association between injectable collagen and polymyositis/dermatomyositis? *Arthritis Rheum* 1994;37:747–753.
81. Caproni M, Cardinali C, Parodi A, et al. Amyopathic dermatomyositis: a review by the Italian Group of Immunodermatology. *Arch Dermatol* 2002;
82. Ang P, Sugeng MW, Chua SH. Classical and amyopathic dermatomyositis seen at the National Skin Centre of Singapore: a 3-year retrospective review of their clinical characteristics and association with malignancy. *Ann Acad Med Singapore* 2000;29:219–223.
83. Chen YJ, Wu CY, Shen JL. Predicting factors of malignancy in dermatomyositis and polymyositis: a case-control study. *Br J Dermatol* 2001;144:825–831.
84. Peloro TM, Miller OF III, Hahn TF, et al. Juvenile dermatomyositis: a retrospective review of a 30-year experience. *J Am Acad Dermatol* 2001;45:28–34.
85. El-Azhary R, Pakzad SY. Amyopathic dermatomyositis: retrospective review of 37 cases. *J Am Acad Dermatol* 2002;46:560–565.
86. Caproni M, Cardinali C, Parodi A, et al. Amyopathic dermatomyositis - A review by the Italian group of immunodermatology. *Arch Dermatol* 2002;138: 23–27.
87. Arnett FC, Targoff IN, Mimori T, et al. Interrelationship of major histocompatibility complex class II alleles and autoantibodies in four ethnic groups with various forms of myositis. *Arthritis Rheum* 1996;39:1507–1518.
88. Dourmishev AL, Dourmishev LA. Dermatomyositis and drugs. *Adv Exp Med Biol* 1999;455:187–191.
89. Marie I, Joly P, Levesque H, et al. Pseudo-dermatomyositis as a complication of hydroxyurea therapy. *Clin Exp Rheumatol* 2000;18:536–537.
90. Rocamora V, Puig L, Alomar A. Dermatomyositis-like eruption following hydroxyurea therapy. *J Eur Acad Dermatol Venereol* 2000;14:227–228.
91. Friedman AW, Targoff IN, Arnett FC. Interstitial lung disease with autoantibodies against aminoacyl-tRNA synthetases in the absence of clinically apparent myositis. *Semin Arthritis Rheum* 1996;26:459–467.
92. Euwer RL, Sontheimer RD. Dermatologic aspects of myositis. *Cur Opin Rheumatol* 1994;6:583–589.
93. Targoff IN. Dermatomyositis and polymyositis. In: Weston WL, MacKie RM, Provost TT, eds. In: *Current problems in dermatology* 1991:131–180.
94. Miller FW. Classification and prognosis of inflammatory muscle disease. *Rheum Dis Clin N Am* 1994;20:811–826.
95. Rider LG, Miller FW. Idiopathic inflammatory muscle disease: clinical aspects. *Baillieres Best Pract Res Clin Rheumatol* 2000;14:37–54.
96. Stonecipher MR, Jorizzo JL, White WL, et al. Cutaneous changes of dermatomyositis in patients with normal muscle enzymes: dermatomyositis sine myositis? *J Am Acad Dermatol* 1993;28:951–956.
97. Rider LG, Miller FW, Targoff IN, et al. A broadened spectrum of juvenile myositis: Myositis-specific autoantibodies in children. *Arthritis Rheum* 1994; 37:1534–1538.
98. Whitmore SE, Rosenshein NB, Provost TT. Ovarian cancer in patients with dermatomyositis. *Medicine* 1994;73:153–160.
99. McHugh TR, Smith GP, Elwing TJ, et al. Seropositive rheumatoid arthritis with dermatomyositis sine myositis, angioimmunoblastic lymphadenopathy with dysproteinemia-type T cell lymphoma, and B cell lymphoma of the oropharynx. *J Phycology* 2000;27:1087–1090.
100. Olhoffer IH, Carroll C, Watsky K. Dermatomyositis sine myositis presenting with calcinosis universalis. *Br J Dermatol* 1999;141:365–366.
101. Jorrizo JL. Dermatomyositis: practical aspects. *Arch Dermatol* 2002;138: 114–116.
102. Euwer R, Sontheimer RD. Amyopathic dermatomyositis (dermatomyositis siné myositis). Reply. *J Am Acad Dermatol* 1992;26:506–508.
103. Thomas L, Ferrier E, Moulin G. Dermatomyositis-like eruption complicating hydroxyurea therapy of chronic myelogenous leukemia: report of a case and literature review. *Eur J Dermatol* 1992;2:492–495.
104. Grob JJ, Collet AM, Bonerandi JJ. Dermatomyositis-like syndrome induced by nonsteroidal anti-inflammatory agents. *Dermatologica* 1989;178:58–59.
105. Cox NH, Lawrence CM, Langtry JAA, et al. Dermatomyositis: disease associations and an evaluation of screening investigations for malignancy. *Arch Dermatol* 1990;126:61–65.
106. Moenkemoeller K, Petty RE, Malleson PN, et al. What criteria do pediatric rheumatologists use to make the diagnosis of juvenile dermatomyositis? *Arthritis Rheum* 2001;44:S293.
107. Kovacs SO, Kovacs SC. Dermatomyositis. *J Am Acad Dermatol* 1998;39:899–920.
108. Tanimoto K, Nakano K, Kano S, et al. Classification criteria for polymyositis and dermatomyositis. *J Rheumatol* 1995;22:668–674.
109. Zuber M. Tanimoto's classification and diagnostic criteria for polymyositis and dermatomyositis do not recognize the variant of amyopathic dermatomyositis. *J Rheumatol* 1996;23:191.
110. Caro I. Dermatomyositis. *Semin Cutan Med Surg* 2001;20:38–45.
111. Koler RA, Montemarano A. Dermatomyositis. *Am Fam Physician* 2001;64: 1565–1572.
112. Seno A, Tokuda M, Yamasaki H, et al. [A case of amyopathic dermatomyositis presenting blister and oral ulcer]. *Ryumachi* 1999;39:836–840.
113. Trautmann C, Abdel-Naser MB, Soehnchen R, et al. [Premyopathic versus amyopathic dermatomyositis. 2 personal cases and review of the literature]. *Hautarzt*, 1995;46:47–52.
114. Cohen JB. Cutaneous involvement of dermatomyositis can respond to Dapsone therapy. *Int J Dermatol* 2002;41:182–184.
115. Chow SK, Yeap SS. Amyopathic dermatomyositis and pulmonary fibrosis. *Clin Rheumatol* 2000;19:484–485.
116. Toll A, Villa AV, Baselga E, et al. Special feature: picture of the month. Denouement and discussion: juvenile amyopathic dermatomyositis. *Arch Pediatr Adolesc Med* 2000;154:1263–1264.
117. Fitzpatrick TB, Grevelink S. Diagnosing dermatomyositis. *Fitzpatrick's J Clin Dermatol* 1994;Mar/Apr:26–27.
118. Kagen LJ. Polymyositis/dermatomyositis. In: McCarty DJ, ed. *Arthritis and allied conditions*, 11th ed. Philadelphia: Lea & Febiger, 1989: 1092–1117.
119. Herrera R, Varela E, Morales G, et al. Dermatomyositis-like syndrome caused by trichinae: report of two cases. *J Rheumatol* 1985;12:782–784.
120. Pollock JL. Toxoplasmosis appearing to be dermatomyositis. *Arch Dermatol* 1979;115:736–737.
121. Norden D, Weinberg J, Schumacher HR, et al. Bilateral periorbital edema in systemic lupus erythematosus. *J Rheumatol* 1993;20:2158–2160.
122. Smith CA, Pinals RS. Periorbital edema in systemic lupus erythematosus. *Arch Intern Med* 1982;142:1711–1712.
123. Cyran S, Douglass MC, Silverstein JL. Chronic cutaneous lupus erythematosus presenting as periorbital edema and erythema. *J Am Acad Dermatol* 1992;26[Suppl]:334–338.
124. Kim KL, Robson K, Powell RJ. Focal myositis: an unusual cause of bilateral upper eyelid swellings. *Postgrad Med J* 1993;69:876–878.
125. Findlay GH, Price GA,Van Rinsburg CRJ. Dermatomyositis with vesicular bullous lesions. *S Afr Med J* 1951;25:60.
126. Al-Najjar A, Reilly GD, Harrington C. Dermatomyositis and lichen planus—an association or manifestation? *Clin Exp Dermatol* 1985;10:174–178.
127. Lintum JC, Goedbloed R. Poikilodermatomyositis. *Dermatologica* 1974;148: 52–55.
128. Shelly WB, Crissez JT. *Classics in clinical dermatology*. Charles C. Thomas, Springfield 1953:346–349.
129. Basset-Seguin N, Roujeau JC, Gherardi R, et al. Prognostic factors and predictive signs of malignancy in adult dermatomyositis: a study of 32 cases. *Arch Dermatol* 1990;126:633–637.
130. Medenica N, Coughlin DF. Dermatomyositis with ulceration. *Arch Dermatol* 1970;101:490–491.
131. Tamamoto T, Ohkubo H, Katayama I, et al. Dermatomyositis with multiple skin ulcers showing vasculitis and membraneo-cystic lesion. *J Dermatol* 1994; 21:687–689.
132. Ramirez G, Asherson RA, Khamashta MA, et al. Adult-onset polymyositis-dermatomyositis: description of 25 patients with emphasis on treatment. *Semin Arthritis Rheumat* 1990;20:114–120.
133. Miyagawa S, Okazaki A, Minowa R, et al. Dermatomyositis presenting as erythroderma. *J Am Acad Dermatol* 1992;26:489–490.
134. Pierson JC, Taylor JS. Erythrodermic dermatomyositis [letter]. *J Am Acad Dermatol* 1993;28:136–136.
135. Nesbitt LT Jr. Cutaneous immunofluorescence in dermatomyositis. *Int J Dermatol* 1980;19:270–278.
136. Euwer RL, Sontheimer RD. Amyopathic dermatomyositis (dermatomyositis sine myositis): presentation of six new cases and review of the literature. *J Am Acad Dermatol* 1991;24:959–966.
137. Parodi A, Caproni M, Marzano AV, et al. Dermatomyositis in 132 patients with different clinical subtypes: cutaneous signs, constitutional symptoms and circulating antibodies. *Acta Derma Venereol* 2002;82:48–51.

138. Woo TR, Rasmussen J, Callen JP. Recurrent photosensitive dermatitis preceding juvenile dermatomyositis. *Ped Dermatol* 1985;2:207–212.
139. Abdel-Nasser MB, Chun SC, Gollnick H, et al. Amyopathic dermatomyositis (dermatomyositis siné myositis myositis) in a male patient and possible induction by ultraviolet light. *Eur J Dermatol* 1993;3:367–370.
140. Kasteler JS, Callen JP. Scalp involvement in dermatomyositis: often overlooked and misdiagnosed. *JAMA* 1994;272:1939–1941.
141. Stone OJ. Dermatomyositis/polymyositis associated with internal malignancy: a consequence of how neoplasms alter generalized extracellular matrix in the host [review]. *Med Hypotheses* 1993;41:48–51.
142. Cunningham JD, Lowry LD. Head and neck manifestations of dermatomyositis-polymyositis. *Otolaryngol Head Neck Surg* 1985;5:673–677.
143. Dicken CH. Periorbital edema: an important physical finding in dermatomyositis. *Cutis* 1991;48:116–117.
144. Sabiston CB. A review and proposal for the etiology of acute necrotizing gingivitis. *J Clin Periodontol* 1986;13:727–734.
145. Nousari HC, Ha VT, Laman SD, et al."Centripetal flagellate erythema": a cutaneous manifestation associated with dermatomyositis. *J Rheumatol* 1999;26:692–695.
146. Cohen MG, Nash P, Webb J. Calcification is rare in adult-onset dermatopolymyositis. *Clin Rheumatol* 1986;5:512–516.
147. Hesla RB, Karlson LK, McCauley RG. Milk of calcium fluid collection in dermatomyositis: ultrasound findings. *Pediat Radiol* 1990;20 344–346.
148. Samitz MH. Cuticular changes in dermatomyositis: a clinical sign. *Arch Dermatol* 1974;110:866–867.
149. Stahl NI, Klippel JH, Decker JL. A cutaneous lesion associated with myositis. *Ann Intern Med* 1979;91:577–579.
150. Mitra D, Lovell CL, Macleod TIF, et al. Clinical and histological features of "mechanic's hands" in a patient with antibodies to Jo-1—a case report. *Clin Exper Dermatol* 1994;19:146–148.
151. Watanabe C, Okubo Y, Ohi T, et al. A case of dermatomyositis associated with mechanic's hand. *J Dermatol* 2000;27:711–716.
152. Cosnes A, Amaudric F, Gherardi R, et al. Dermatomyositis without muscle weakness: long-term follow-up of 12 patients without systemic steroids. *Arch Dermatol* 1995;131:1381–1385.
153. Quinones CA, Perry HO, Rushton JG. Carpal tunnel syndrome in dermatomyositis and scleroderma. *Arch Dermatol* 1966;94:20–25.
154. Mitchell JP, Dennis GJ, Rider LG. Juvenile dermatomyositis presenting with anasarca: a possible indicator of severe disease activity *J Pediatr* 2001;138:942–945.
155. Glover M, Leigh I. Dermatomyositis pemphigoides: a case with coexistent dermatomyositis and bullous pemphigoid. *J Am Acad Dermatol* 1992;27:849–852.
156. White SW, Tesar JT. Dermatomyositis and dermatitis herpetiformis. *Arch Dermatol* 1982;118:599–601.
157. Kalovidouris AE, Miller FW, Lawley TJ. Polymyositis/dermatomyositis associated with dermatitis herpetiformis. *Arthritis Rheum* 1989;32:1179–1181.
158. Reich MG, Reinhart JB. Dermatomyositis associated with hypertrichosis. *Arch Dermat Syph* 1948;57:725–732.
159. Pope DN, Strimling RB, Mallory SB. Hypertrichosis in juvenile dermatomyositis. *J Am Acad Dermatol* 1994;31:383–387.
160. Piantanida NA, Person DA, Piantanida EW. Infrapatellar hypertrichosis: an unusual cutaneous manifestation of juvenile dermatomyositis. *Pediatr Dermatol* 2002;19:132–135.
161. Urrutia S, Vazquez F, Requena L, et al. Acquired ichthyosis associated with dermatomyositis [letter]. *J Am Acad Dermatol* 1987;16:627–629.
162. Barrows-Wade L, Jordon RE, Arnett FC Jr. Linear IgA bullous dermatosis associated with dermatomyositis [letter]. *Arch Dermatol* 1992;128:413–414.
163. Huemer C, Kitson H, Malleson PN, et al. Lipodystrophy in patients with juvenile dermatomyositis—evaluation of clinical and metabolic abnormalities. *J Rheumatol* 2001;28:610–615.
164. Rider L, Ruiz-Hidalgo M, Labora J, et al. Lipodystrophy in juvenile dermatomyositis is associated with calcinosis, but not with hepatocyte differentiation factor DLK levels. *Arthritis Rheum* 2001;44:S264.
165. Singh M, Kaur S, Vajpayee BK, et al. Cutaneous malakoplakia with dermatomyositis. *Int J Dermatol* 1987;26:190–191.
166. Requena L, Aguilar A, Sanchez Yus E. A corrugated plaque on the abdominal wall: cutaneous mucinosis secondary to dermatomyositis. *Arch Dermatol* 1990;126:1639–1640, 1642–1643.
167. Igarashi M, Aizawa H, Tokudome Y, et al. Dermatomyositis with prominent mucinous skin change: histochemical and biochemical aspects of glycosaminoglycans. *Dermatologica* 1985;170:6–11.
168. Johnson BL, Horowitz IR, Charles CR, et al. Dermatomyositis and lichen myxedematosus: a. clinical, histopathological and electron microscopic study. *Dermatologica* 1973;147:109–122.
169. Launay D, Hatron PY, Delaporte E, et al. Scleromyxedema (lichen myxedematosus) associated with dermatomyositis. *Br J Dermatol* 2001;144:359–362.
170. Kaufmann R, Greiner D, Schmidt P, et al. Dermatomyositis presenting as plaque-like mucinosis. *Br J Dermatol* 1998;138:889–892.
171. Agbo-Godeau S, Bertrand JC. [Lip ulceration in paraneoplastic dermatomyositis. Apropos of a case. Review of the literature] [review] [French] propos d'un cas. *Revue de la litterature. Revue de Stomatologie et de Chirurgie Maxillo-Faciale* 1993;94:287–289.
172. Sammartino A, Lucariello A, Esposito L, et al. A rare presentation of bilateral membranous conjunctivitis in dermatomyositis in young age. *J Pediatr Ophthalmol Strabismus* 1981;18:47–50.
173. Ibanez HE, Bardenstein DS, Korman NJ, et al. Exuberant conjunctival pseudopolyposis in a patient with dermatomyositis. *Ann Ophthal* 1993;25:326–327.
174. Bartley GB, Gibson LE. Blepharochalasis associated with dermatomyositis and acute lymphocytic leukemia [letter]. *Am J Ophthalmol* 1992;113:727–728.
175. Martinez-Cordero E, Lasky D, Katona G. Nasal septal perforation in dermatomyositis. *J Rheumatol* 1986;13:231–232.
176. Tosti A, De Padova MP, Fanti P, et al. Unusual severe nail involvement in dermatomyositis. *Cutis* 1987;40:261–262.
177. Winkelman WJ, Billick RC, Srolovitz H. Dermatomyositis presenting as panniculitis. *J Am Acad Dermatol* 1990;23:127–128.
178. Fusade T, Belanyi P, Joly P, et al. Subcutaneous changes in dermatomyositis. *Br J Dermatol* 1993;128:451–453.
179. Solans R, Cortes J, Selva A, et al. Panniculitis: a cutaneous manifestation of dermatomyositis. *J Am Acad Dermatol* 2002;46:S148–S150.
180. Chao YY, Yang LJ. Dermatomyositis presenting as panniculitis. *Int J Dermatol* 2000;39:141–144.
181. Ghali FE, Reed AM, Groben PA, et al. Panniculitis in juvenile dermatomyositis. *Pediatr Dermatol* 1999;16:270–272.
182. Molnar K, Kemeny L, Korom I, et al. Panniculitis in dermatomyositis: report of two cases [letter]. *Br J Dermatol* 1998;139:161–163.
183. Commens C, O'Neill P, Walker G. Dermatomyositis associated with multifocal lipoatrophy. *J Am Acad Dermatol* 1990;22:966–969.
184. Dupre A, Viraben R, Bonafe JL, et al. Zebra-like dermatomyositis [letter]. *Arch Dermatol* 1981;117:63–64.
185. Wong KO. Dermatomyositis: a clinical investigation of 23 cases in Hong Kong. *Br J Dermatol* 1969;81:544–547.
186. Dupre A, Floutard M, Christol B, et al. Dermatomyosite avec spinulosisme (dermatomyosite type Wong): Etude histologique. Essai d'interpretation pathogenique. *Ann Dermatol Syphil* 1976;103:141–149.
187. Lupton JR, Figueroa P, Berberian BJ, et al. An unusual presentation of dermatomyositis: the type Wong variant revisited. *J Am Acad Dermatol* 2000;43:908–912.
188. Randle HW, Winkelmann RK. Steroid-induced acanthosis nigricans in dermatomyositis. *Arch Dermatol* 1979;115:587–588.
189. Ghali FE, Stein LD, Fine JD, et al. Gingival telangiectases: an underappreciated physical sign of juvenile dermatomyositis. *Arch Dermatol* 1999;135:1370–1374.
190. Callen JP, Dubin HV. Urticaria and polymyositis. *Arch Dermatol* 1978;114:1545–1546.
191. Feldman D, Hochberg MC, Zizic TM, et al. Cutaneous vasculitis in adult polymyositis/dermatomyositis. *J Rheumatol* 1983;10:85–89.
192. Lavery HA, Pinkerton JH, Roberts SD, et al. Dermatomyositis of the vulva—first reported case. *Br J Dermatol* 1985;113:349–352.
193. Albert NE, Lytton B. Case report: dermatomyositis of the scrotum. *J Urol* 1977;118:491–491.
194. Rowell NR, Goodfield MJD. The 'connective tissue diseases.' In: Champion RH, Burton JL, Ebling FJG, eds. *Textbook of dermatology*, 5th ed. London: Blackwell Science, 1992: 2163–2294.
195. Bowyer SL, Blane CE, Sullivan DB. Childhood dermatomyositis: factors predicting functional outcome and development of dystrophic calcification. *J Pediatr* 1983;103:882–888.
196. Corson JK. Sclerodermatomyositis. *Arch Dermatol* 1967;96:596–597.
197. Greenlee R Jr. The neurologist's approach to polymyositis. *Clin Dermatol* 1988;6:23–35.
198. Fraser DD, Frank JA, Dalakus M, et al. Magnetic resonance imaging in the idiopathic inflammatory myopathies. *J Rheumatol* 1991;18:1693–1700.
199. Reimers CD, Schedel H, Fleckenstein JL, et al. Magnetic resonance imaging of skeletal muscles in idiopathic inflammatory myopathies of adults. *J Neurol* 1994;241:306–314.
200. Park JH, Olsen NJ. Utility of magnetic resonance imaging in the evaluation of patients with inflammatory myopathies. *Curr Rheumatol Rep* 2001;3:334–345.
201. Pitt AM, Fleckenstein JL, Greenlee RG Jr, et al. MRI-guided biopsy in inflammatory myopathy: initial results. *Magn Reson Imaging* 1993;11:1093–1099.
202. King LE Jr, Park JH, Adams L, et al. Evaluation of muscles in a patient with suspected amyopathic dermatomyositis by magnetic resonance imaging and phosphorus-31-spectroscopy. *J Am Acad Dermatol* 1994;30:137–138.
203. Stonecipher MR, Jorizzo JL, Monu J, et al. Dermatomyositis with normal muscle enzyme concentrations: a single-blind study of the diagnostic value of magnetic resonance imaging and ultrasound. *Arch Dermatol* 1994;130:1294–1299.
204. Meng C, Adler R, Peterson M, et al. Combined use of power Doppler and gray-scale sonography: a new technique for the assessment of inflammatory myopathy. *J Rheumatol* 2001;28:1271–1282.
205. Maricq HR, Maize JC. Nailfold capillary abnormalities [review]. *Clin Rheumat Dis* 1982;8:455–478.
206. Ganczarczyk ML, Lee P, Armstrong SK. Nailfold capillary microscopy in polymyositis and dermatomyositis. *Arthritis Rheum* 1988;31:116–119.
207. Spencer-Green G, Crowe WE, Levinson JE. Nailfold capillary abnormalities and clinical outcome in childhood dermatomyositis. *Arthritis Rheum* 1982;25:954–958.
208. Romans B, Cohen S. A rheumatologist's view of polymyositis/dermatomyositis: extracutaneous and extramuscular involvement and overlap syndromes [review]. *Clin Dermatol* 1988;6:15–22.
209. Schwarz MI. Pulmonary and cardiac manifestations of polymyositis-dermatomyositis [review]. *J Thorac Imaging* 1992;7:46–54.

210. Hirakata M, Nagai S. Interstitial lung disease in polymyositis and dermatomyositis [review]. *Cur Opin Rheumatol* 2000;12:501–508.
211. Douglas WW, Tazelaar HD, Hartman TE, et al. Polymyositis-dermatomyositis-associated interstitial lung disease. *Am J Respir Crit Care Med* 2001;164: 1182–1185.
212. al-Mayouf SM, Silverman ED, Feldman BM, et al. Cyclosporine in the treatment of an unusual case of juvenile systemic sclerosis. *J Rheumatol* 1998;25: 791–793.
213. Tse S, Lubelsky S, Gordon M, et al. The arthritis of inflammatory childhood myositis syndromes. *J Rheumatol* 2001;28:192–197.
214. Leibowitz G, Eliakim R, Amir G, et al. Dermatomyositis associated with Crohn's disease [review]. *J Clin Gastroent* 1994;18:48–52.
215. Kimball AB, Summers RM, Turner M, et al. Magnetic resonance imaging detection of occult skin and subcutaneous abnormalities in juvenile dermatomyositis: implications for diagnosis and therapy. *Arthritis Rheum* 2000; 43:1866–1873.
216. Callen JP, Hyla JF, Bole GG Jr, et al. The relationship of dermatomyositis and polymyositis to internal malignancy. *Arch Dermatol* 1980;116:295–298.
217. Bernard P, Bonnetblanc JM. Dermatomyositis and malignancy. *J Invest Dermatol* 1993;100:128S–132S.
218. Stockton D, Doherty VR, Brewster DH. Risk of cancer in patients with dermatomyositis or polymyositis, and follow-up implications: a Scottish population-based cohort study. *Br J Cancer* 2001;85:41–45.
219. Leandro MJ, Isenberg DA. Rheumatic diseases and malignancy—is there an association? *Scand J Rheumatol* 2001;30:185–188.
220. Callen JP. Relation between dermatomyositis and polymyositis and cancer. *Lancet* 2001;357:85–86.
221. Airio A, Pukkala E, Isomäki H. Elevated cancer incidence in patients with dermatomyositis: a population based study. *J Rheumatol* 1995;22:1300–1303.
222. Leow YH, Goh CL. Malignancy in adult dermatomyositis. *Int J Dermatol* 1997;36:904–907.
223. Yazici Y, Kagen LJ. The association of malignancy with myositis [review]. *Cur Opin Rheumatol* 2000;12:498–500.
224. Stockton D, Doherty VR, Brewster DH. Risk of cancer in patients with dermatomyositis or polymyositis, and follow-up implications: a Scottish population-based cohort study. *Br J Cancer* 2001;85:41–45.
225. Sunnenberg TD, Kitchens CS. Dermatomyositis associated with malignant melanoma: parallel occurrence, remission, and relapse of the two processes in a patient. *Cancer* 1983;51:2157–2158.
226. Connor B. Mycosis fungoides with dermatomyositis. *Proc R S Med* 1972;65: 251–252.
227. Weiss VC, Serushan M. Kaposi's sarcoma in a patient with dermatomyositis receiving immunosuppressive therapy. *Arch Dermatol* 1982;118:183–185.
228. Hu WJ, Chen DL, Min HQ. Study of 45 cases of nasopharyngeal carcinoma with dermatomyositis. *Am J Clin Oncol* 1996;19:35–38.
229. Fung WK, Chan HL, Lam WM. Amyopathic dermatomyositis in Hong Kong: association with nasopharyngeal carcinoma. *Int J Dermatol* 1998;37:659–663.
230. Till SH, Jones AC. Dermatomyositis—how far to go [review]. *Ann Rheum Dis* 1998;57:198–200.
231. Sparsa A, Liozon E, Herrmann F, et al. Routine vs extensive malignancy search for adult dermatomyositis and polymyositis: a study of 40 patients. *Arch Dermatol* 2002;138:885–890.
232. O'Gradaigh D, Merry P. Tumour markers in dermatomyositis: useful or useless? [letter]. *Br J Rheumatol* 1998;37:914.
233. Cherin P, Piette JC, Herson S, et al. Dermatomyositis and ovarian cancer: a report of 7 cases and literature review. *J Rheumatol* 1993;20:1897–1899.
234. Grau JM, Hausmann G, Casademont J, et al. Amyopathic dermatomyositis. *J Am Acad Dermatol* 1992;26:505.
235. Callen JP, Jorizzo JL. Amyopathic dermatomyositis (dermatomyositis sine myositis) [letter; comment]. *J Am Acad Dermatol* 1992;26:505–56.
236. Park JH, Vital TL, Ryder NM, et al. Magnetic resonance imaging and P-31 magnetic resonance spectroscopy provide unique quantitative data useful in the longitudinal management of patients with dermatomyositis. *Arthritis Rheum* 1994;37:736–746.
237. Dunn CL, James WD. The role of magnetic resonance imaging in the diagnostic evaluation of dermatomyositis. *Arch Dermatol* 1993;129:1104–1106.
238. Park JH, Kari S, King LE Jr, et al. Analysis of 31P MR spectroscopy data using artificial neural networks for longitudinal evaluation of muscle diseases: dermatomyositis. *NMR Biomed* 1998;11:245–256.
239. Thune P. The coexistence of amyopathic dermatomyositis and fibromyalgia. *Acta Derm Venereol* 2000;80:453–454.
240. Plamondon S, Dent PB. Juvenile amyopathic dermatomyositis: results of a case finding descriptive survey. *J Rheumatol* 2000;27:2031–2034.
241. Eisenstein DM, Paller AS, Pachman LM. Juvenile dermatomyositis presenting with rash alone. *Pediatrics* 1997;100:391–392.
242. Fernandes L, Goodwill CJ. Dermatomyositis without apparent myositis, complicated by fibrosing alveolitis. *J R Soc Med* 1979;72:777–779.
243. Tokiyama K, Tagawa H, Yokota E, et al. Two cases of amyopathic dermatomyositis with fatal rapidly progressive interstitial pneumonitis. *Ryumachi* 1990;30:204–211.
244. Wakino S, Kuwana M, Tojo T, et al. Serial lymphocyte subpopulation analysis in peripheral blood from a patient with amyopathic dermatomyositis [letter]. *Br J Rheumatol* 1994;33:498–499.
245. Takizawa H, Suzuki N, Yanagawa T, et al. Outcome in patients with interstitial lung disease and polymyositis-dermatomyositis—a subgroup with poor prognosis. *Nihon Kyobu Shikkan Gakkai Zasshi* 1996;34:1093–1097.
246. Toyoshima M, Sato A, Chida K, et al. [Clinicopathological features of interstitial pneumonia associated with amyopathic dermatomyositis]. *Nihon Kyobu Shikkan Gakkai Zasshi* 1997;35:281–287.
247. Tahara K, Nishiya K, Hisakawa N, et al. [A case of amyopathic dermatomyositis associated with interstitial pneumonitis]. *Ryumachi* 1997;37:714–718.
248. Mijailovic B, Karadaglic D, Dostanic I, et al. [Amyopathic dermatomyositis with interstitial lung disease]. *Vojnosanit Pregl* 1997;54:269–271.
249. Takashi S, Okubo Y, Yamazaki Y, et al. [Amyopathic dermatomyositis with interstitial pneumonia: effective treatment with cyclophosphamide pulse therapy]. *Nihon Kokyuki Gakkai Zasshi* 1999;37:647–651.
250. Ozawa Y, Kurosaka D, Yokoyama T, et al. [Therapeutic efficacy of cyclosporin A in four cases of amyopathic dermatomyositis with rapidly progressive interstitial pneumonia]. *Ryumachi* 2000;40:798–809.
251. Nanke Y, Tateisi M, Yamagata H, et al. [A case of amyopathic dermatomyositis with rapidly progressive interstitial pneumonia]. *Ryumachi* 2000;40: 705–710.
252. Hirakata M, Nagai S. Interstitial lung disease in polymyositis and dermatomyositis. *Curr Opin Rheumatol* 2000;12:501–508.
253. McLachlan SM, Rapoport B. The molecular biology of thyroid peroxidase: cloning, expression and role as autoantigen in autoimmune thyroid disease. *Endocr Rev* 1992;13:192–206.
254. Fung WK, Chan HL, Lam WM. Amyopathic dermatomyositis in Hong Kong: association with nasopharyngeal carcinoma [review]. *Int J Dermatol* 1998;37: 659–663.
255. Kasper CS, White CL, Freeman RG. Pathology and immunopathology of polymyositis/dermatomyositis. *Clin Dermatol* 1988;6:64–75.
256. Janis JF, Winkelman RK. Histopathology of the skin in dermatomyositis: a histopathologic study of 55 cases. *Arch Dermatol* 1968;97:640–650.
257. Hanno R, Callen JP. Histopathology of Gottron's papules. *J Cutan Pathol* 1985; 12:389–394.
258. Winkelmann RK, Jordon RE, Moragas JM. Immunofluorescent studies of dermatomyositis. *Dermatologica* 1972;145:42–47.
259. Hausmann G, Herrero C, Cinta Cid M, et al. Immunopathologic study of skin lesions in dermatomyositis. *J Am Acad Dermatol* 1991;25:225–230.
260. Chen Z, Maize JC, Silver RM, et al. Direct and indirect immunofluorescent findings in dermatomyositis. *J Cutan Pathol* 1985;12:18–27.
261. Fabré VC, Lear S, Reichlin M, et al. Twenty percent of biopsy specimens from sun-exposed skin of normal young adults demonstrate positive immunofluorescence. *Arch Dermatol* 1991;127:1006–1011.
262. Crowson AN, Magro CM. The role of microvascular injury in the pathogenesis of cutaneous lesions of dermatomyositis. *Hum Pathol* 1996;27:15–19.
263. Mascaro JM, Jr., Hausmann G, Herrero C, et al. Membrane attack complex deposits in cutaneous lesions of dermatomyositis. *Arch Dermatol* 1995;131: 1386–1392.
264. Engel AG, Arahata K. Monoclonal antibody analysis of mononuclear cells in myopathies, II: phenotypes of autoinvasive cells in polymyositis and inclusion body myositis. *Ann Neurol* 1984;16:209–215.
265. Emslie-Smith AM, Engel AG. Microvascular changes in early and advanced dermatomyositis: a quantitative study. *Ann Neurol* 1990;27:343–356.
266. Isenberg DA. Immunoglobulin deposition in skeletal muscle in primary muscle disease. *Q J Med* 1983;207:297–310.
267. Whitaker JN, Engel WK. Vascular deposits of immunoglobulin and complement in idiopathic inflammatory myopathy. *N Engl J Med* 1972;286:333–338.
268. Kissel JT, Mendell JR, Rammohan KW. Microvascular deposition of complement membrane attack complex in dermatomyositis. *N Engl J Med* 1986;314: 329–334.
269. Lundberg IE. The role of cytokines, chemokines, and adhesion molecules in the pathogenesis of idiopathic inflammatory myopathies. *Curr Rheumatol Rep* 2000;2:216–224.
270. De Bleecker JL, De Paepe B, Vanwalleghem IE, et al. Differential expression of chemokines in inflammatory myopathies. *Neurology* 2002;58:1779–1785.
271. Kagen LJ, Aram S. Creatine kinase activity inhibitor in sera from patients with muscle disease. *Arthritis Rheum* 1987;30:213–217.
272. Kroll M, Otis J, Kagen LJ. Serum enzyme, myoglobin and muscle strength relationships in polymyositis and dermatomyositis. *J Rheumatol* 1986;13: 349–355.
273. Fudman EJ, Schnitzer TJ. Dermatomyositis without creatine kinase elevation: a poor prognostic sign. *Am J Med* 1986;80:329–332.
274. Reichlin M, Arnett FC. Multiplicity of antibodies in myositis sera. *Arthritis Rheum* 1984;27:1150–1156.
275. Targoff IN. Humoral immunity in polymyositis/dermatomyositis. *J Invest Dermatol* 1993;100:116S–123S.
276. Targoff IN. Laboratory manifestations of polymyositis/dermatomyositis. *Clin Dermatol* 1988;6:76–92.
277. Sontheimer RD, McCauliffe DP, Zappi E, et al. Antinuclear antibodies: clinical correlations and biologic significance [review]. *Adv Dermatol* 1992; 7:3–52.
278. Brouwer R, Hengstman GJ, Vree EW, et al. Autoantibody profiles in the sera of European patients with myositis. *Ann Rheum Dis* 2001;60:116–123.
279. Targoff IN. Update on myositis-specific and myositis-associated autoantibodies. *Curr Opin Rheumatol* 2000;12:475–481.
280. Targoff IN, Reichlin M. Measurement of antibody to Jo-1 by ELISA and comparison to enzyme inhibitory activity. *J Immunol* 1987;138:2874–2882.
281. Targoff IN, Reichlin M. The association between Mi-2 antibodies and dermatomyositis. *Arthritis Rheum* 1985;28:796–803.
282. Arad-Dann H, Isenberg D, Ovadia E. Autoantibodies against a nuclear

56-kDa protein: A marker for inflammatory muscle disease. *J Autoimmunity* 1989;2:877–888.
283. Lutz JL, Fedcznya TO, Isenberg D, et al. The association of the DQA*0501 allele and antibody to a 56 KD nuclear proteins in sera from patients with juvenile dermatomyositis. *Arthritis Rheum* 2001;44:S293.
284. Rosen A, Casciola-Rosen L. Clearing the way to mechanisms of autoimmunity. *Nature Med* 2001;7:664–665.
285. Targoff IN, Trieu EP, Sontheimer RD. Autoantibodies to 155 KD and Se antigens in patients with clinically amyopathic dermatomyositis. *Arthritis Rheum* 2000;43:S194–S194.
286. Sontheimer RD, Targoff I, Trieu E, et al. Autoantibodies to 155 KD and Se antigens in patients with clinically amyopathic dermatomyositis. *J Invest Dermatol* 2001;117:466–466.
287. Satoh S, Hirakata M, Suwa A, et al. Antibodies to 140 kDa proteins in Japanese patients with amyopathic dermatomyositis. *Arthritis Rheum* 2001;44:S205.
288. Amerio P, Girardelli CR, Proietto G, et al. Usefulness of erythrocyte sedimentation rate as tumor marker in cancer associated dermatomyositis. *Eur J Dermatol* 2002;12:165–169.
289. Vignos PJ Jr., Goldwyn J. Evaluation of laboratory tests in diagnosis and management of polymyositis. *Am J Med Sci* 1972;263:291–308.
290. Rowell NR, Fairris GM. Biochemical markers of myositis in dermatomyositis. *Clin Exper Dermatol* 1986;11:69–72.
291. Askari AD, Vignos PJ Jr, Moskowitz LW. Steroid myopathy in connective tissue disease. *Am J Med* 1978;81:485–492.
292. Kagen LJ. Myoglobinemia in inflammatory myopathies. *JAMA* 1977;237: 1448–1452.
293. Malleson PN. Controversies in juvenile dermatomyositis. *J Rheumatol* 1990;23 [Suppl]:1–2.
294. De Benedetti F, De Amici M, Aramini L, et al. Correlation of serum neopterin concentrations with disease activity in juvenile dermatomyositis. *Arch Dis Child* 1993;69:232–235.
295. Bowyer SL, Ragsdale CG, Sullivan DB. Factor VIII related antigen and childhood rheumatic diseases. *J Rheumatol* 1989;16:1093–1097.
296. Guzman J, Petty RE, Malleson PN. Monitoring disease activity in juvenile dermatomyositis: the role of von Willebrand factor and muscle enzymes. *J Rheumatol* 1994:21:739–743.
297. Takubo T, Kumura T, Nakao T, et al. Serum KL-6 levels in haematologic malignancies and their clinical application. *Haematologia (Budap)* 2001;31: 61–67.
298. Kubo M, Ihn H, Yamane K, et al. Serum KL-6 in adult patients with polymyositis and dermatomyositis. *Rheumatology (Oxford)* 2000;39:632–636.
299. Kobayashi I, Ono S, Kawamura N, et al. KL-6 is a potential marker for interstitial lung disease associated with juvenile dermatomyositis. *J Pediatr* 2001;138:274–276.
300. Kubo M, Ihn H, Yamane K, et al. Increased serum levels of soluble vascular cell adhesion molecule-1 and soluble E-selectin in patients with polymyositis/dermatomyositis. *Br J Dermatol* 2000;143:392–398.
301. Sontheimer RD, Racila D. Blood levels of soluble vascular adhesion molecules, VCAM-1 and E-selectin, are increased in clinically amyopathic dermatomyositis. *J Invest Dermatol* 2001;117:440–440.
302. Eisner JM, English JC. Photo quiz: what are your diagnoses? The diagnoses: lupus erythematosus and dermatomyositis. *Cutis* 2001;67 58.
303. Seishima M, Shimizu H, Oyama Z. Skin metastasis of breast cancer clinically undistinguished from amyopathic dermatomyositis. *Eur J Dermatol* 2001;11: 131–133.
304. Tait TJ, Bird HA, Ford GP. Multicentric reticulohistiocytosis: presentation with the cutaneous features of dermatomyositis [letter]. *Er J Rheumatol* 1994; 33:100–101.
305. Itoh J, Akiguchi I, Midorikawa R, et al. Sarcoid myopathy with typical rash of dermatomyositis. *Neurology* 1980;30:1118–1121.
306. Lipton JH, McLeod BD, Brownell AK. Dermatomyositis and granulomatous myopathy associated with sarcoidosis. *Can J Neurol Sci* 1988;15:426–429.
307. Hart Y, Schwartz MS, Bruckner F, et al. Relapsing dermatomyositis associated with sarcoidosis [letter]. *J Neurol Neurosurg Psychiatry* 1988;51:311–313.
308. Rendt K. Inflammatory myopathies: narrowing the differential diagnosis [review]. *Cleve Clin J Med* 2001;68:505–519.
309. Boyd AS, Neldner KH. Therapeutic options in dermatomyositis/polymyositis. *Int J Dermatol* 1994;33:240–250.
310. Henriksson KG, Lindvall B. Polymyositis and dermatomyositis 1990—diagnosis, treatment and prognosis [review]. *Prog Neurobiol* 1990;35:181–193.
311. Rosenzweig BA, Rotmensch S, Binette SP, et al. Primary idiopathic polymyositis and dermatomyositis complicating pregnancy: diagnosis and management [review]. *Obstet Gynecol Surv* 1989;44:162–170.
312. Zieglschmid-Adams ME, Pandya AG, Cohen SB, et al. Treatment of dermatomyositis with methotrexate: presentation of ten cases and review of the literature. *J Am Acad Dermatol* 1995;32:754–757.
313. Choy EHS, Isenberg DA. Treatment of dermatomyositis and polymyositis [review]. *Rheumatology* 2002;41:7–13.
314. Pestronk A. Inflammatory and immune myopathies: concepts in diagnosis and treatment. *J Child Neurol* 2002;17:205–216.
315. Yoshimasu T, Ohtani T, Sakamoto T, et al. Topical FK506 (tacrolimus) therapy for facial erythematous lesions of cutaneous lupus erythematosus and dermatomyositis. *Eur J Dermatol* 2002;12:50–52.
316. Woo TY, Callen JP, Voorhees JJ, et al. Cutaneous lesions of dermatomyositis are improved by hydroxychloroquine. *J Am Acad Dermatol* 1984;10:592–600.
317. Olson NY, Lindsley CB. Adjunctive use of hydroxychloroquine in childhood dermatomyositis. *J Rheumatol* 1989;16:1545–1547.
318. Bloom BJ, Tucker LB, Klein-Gitelman M, et al. Worsening of the rash of juvenile dermatomyositis with hydroxychloroquine therapy. *J Rheumatol* 1994; 21:2171–2171.
319. Don PC, Kahn TA, Bickers DR. Chloroquine-induced neutropenia in a patient with dermatomyositis [letter]. *J Am Acad Dermatol* 1987;16:629–630.
320. Fafalak RG, Peterson MG, Kagen LJ. Strength in polymyositis and dermatomyositis: best outcome in patients treated early. *J Rheumatol* 1994;21:643–648.
321. Bukulmez H, Wargula JC, Bove K, et al. High dose corticosteroids may aggravate the vasculopathy that underlies ulcerative juvenile dermatomyositis. *Arthritis Rheum* 2001;44:S293.
322. Pachman LM, Hayford JR, Chung A, et al. Juvenile dermatomyositis at diagnosis: clinical characteristics of 79 children. *J Rheumatol* 1998;25:1198–1204.
323. Gertner E, Urowitz MB. Discordance of skin and muscle involvement in dermatomyositis. *Int J Dermatol* 1985;24:518–519.
324. Oddis CV, Medsger TA Jr. Current management of polymyositis and dermatomyositis. *Drugs* 1989;37:382–390.
325. Sinoway PA, Callen JP. Chlorambucil: an effective corticosteroid-sparing agent for patients with recalcitrant dermatomyositis [see comments]. *Arthritis Rheum* 1993;36:319–324.
326. Grau JM, Herrero C, Casademont J, et al. Cyclosporine A as first choice therapy for dermatomyositis. *J Rheumatol* 1994;21:381–382.
327. Gelber AC, Nousari HC, Wigley FM. Mycophenolate mofetil in the treatment of severe skin manifestations of dermatomyositis: a series of 4 cases. *J Rheumatol* 2000;27:1542–1545.
328. De Wilde A, DiSpaltro FX, Geller A, et al. Extracorporeal photochemotherapy as adjunctive treatment in juvenile dermatomyositis: a case report [letter]. *Arch Dermatol* 1992;128:1656–1657.
329. Metzger AL, Bohan A, Goldberg LS. Polymyositis and dermatomyositis: Combined methotrexate and corticosteroid therapy. *Ann Intern Med* 1974;81: 182–189.
330. Cagnoli M, Marchesoni A, Tosi S. Combined steroid, methotrexate and chlorambucil therapy for steroid-resistant dermatomyositis [letter]. *Clin Exp Rheumatol* 1991;9:658–659.
331. Dalakas MC, Illa I, Dambrosia JM, et al. A controlled trial of high-dose intravenous immune globulin infusions as treatment for dermatomyositis [see comments]. *N Engl J Med* 1993;329:1993–2000.
332. Esteve E, Cambie MP, Serpier H, et al. Paraneoplastic dermatomyositis: efficacy of intravenous gammaglobulin. *Br J Dermatol* 1994;131:917–918.
333. Collet E, Dalac S, Maerens B, et al. Juvenile dermatomyositis: treatment with intravenous gammaglobulin. *Br J Dermatol* 1994;130:231–234.
334. Cherin P, Piete JC, Wechsler B, et al. Intravenous gamma globulin as first line therapy in polymyositis and dermatomyositis: an open study in 11 adult patients. *J Rheumatol* 1994;21:1092–1097.
335. Reimold AM, Weinblatt ME. Tachyphylaxis of intravenous immunoglobulin in refractory inflammatory myopathy. *J Rheumatol* 1994;21:1144–1146.
336. Basta M, Dalakas MC. High-dose intravenous immunoglobulin exerts its beneficial effect in patients with dermatomyositis by blocking endomysial deposition of activated complement fragments. *J Clin Invest* 1994;94: 1729–1735.
337. Miller FW, Leitman SF, Cronin ME, et al. Controlled trial of plasma exchange and leukapheresis in polymyositis and dermatomyositis. *N Engl J Med* 1992; 326:1380–1384.
338. Konohana A, Kawashima J. Successful treatment of dermatomyositis with dapsone. *Clin Exp Dermatol* 1994;19:367–367.
339. Gelber AC, Nousari HC, Wigley FM. Mycophenolate mofetil in the treatment of severe skin manifestations of dermatomyositis: a series of 4 cases. *J Rheumatol* 2000;27:1542–1545.
340. One member's story: Enbrel use restored his strength: The Outlook for the Inflammatory Myopathies *Myositis Association of America* 2000:11.
341. Saadeh CK. Etanercept effective in polymyositis, dermatomyositis refractory to conventional therapy: the outlook for the inflammatory myopathies. *Myositis Association of America* 2001:17.
342. Hengstman G, Van den Hoogen F, van Engelen B, et al. Anti-TNF blockade with infliximab (Remicade) in polymyositis and dermatomyositis. The Outlook for the Inflammatory Myopathies *Myositis Association of America* 2001:17.
343. Nzeusseu A, Durez P, Houssiau F, et al. Successful use of infliximab in a case of refractory juvenile dermatomyositis. *Arthritis Rheum* 2001;44:S90–S90.
344. Euwer RL, Sontheimer RD. Amyopathic dermatomyositis (dermatomyositis sine myositis). Presentation of six new cases and review of the literature. *J Am Acad Dermatol* 1991;24:959–966.
345. Schmid MH, Trueb RM. Juvenile amyopathic dermatomyositis. *Br J Dermatol* 1997;136:431–433.
346. Nassim JR, Connolly CK. Treatment of calcinosis universalis with aluminium hydroxide. *Arch Dis Child* 1970;45:118–121.
347. Wang WJ, Lo WL, Wong CK. Calcinosis cutis in juvenile dermatomyositis: remarkable response to aluminum hydroxide therapy. *Arch Dermatol* 1988; 124:1721–1722.
348. Nakagawa T, Takaiwa T. Calcinosis cutis in juvenile dermatomyositis responsive to aluminum hydroxide treatment. *J Dermatol* 1993;20:558–560.
349. Dent CE, Stamp TCB. Treatment of calcinosis circumscripta with probenecid. *Br Med J* 1972;i:216.
350. Skuterud E, Sydnes OA, Haavik TK. Calcinosis in dermatomyositis treated with probenecid. *Scand J Rheumatol* 1981;10:92–94.
351. Berger RG, Featherston GL, Raason RH. Treatment of calcinosis universalis with low dose warfarin. *Am J Med* 1987;83:72–76.
352. Martinez-Cordero E, Lopez-Zepeda J, Choza-Romero F. Calcinosis in childhood dermatomyositis [letter]. *Clin Exp Rheumatol* 1990;8:198–200.

353. Oliveri MB, Palermo R, Mautalen C, et al. Regression of calcinosis during diltiazem treatment in juvenile dermatomyositis. *J Rheumatol* 1996;23: 2152–2155.
354. Lassoued K, Saiag P, Anglade MC, et al. Failure of warfarin in treatment of calcinosis universalis. *Am J Med* 1988;84:795–796.
355. Herd JK, Vaughan JH. Calcinosis universalis complicating dermatomyositis. *Arthritis Rheum* 1964;7:259–271.
356. Taborn J, Bole GG,Thompson GR. Colchicine suppression of local and systemic inflammation due to calcinosis universalis in chronic dermatomyositis. *Ann Intern Med* 1978;89:648–649.
357. Mukamel M, Horev G, Mimouni M. New insight into calcinosis of juvenile dermatomyositis: a study of composition and treatment. *J Pediatr* 2001;138: 763–766.
358. Shearin JC, Pickrell K. Surgical treatment of subcutaneous calcifications of polymyositis or dermatomyositis. *Ann Plast Surg* 1980;5:381–385.
359. Ishii N, Ono H, Kawaguchi T, et al. Dermatomyositis and pregnancy: case report and review of the literature [review]. *Dermatologica* 1991;183:146–149.
360. Ohno T, Imai A, Tamaya T. Successful outcomes of pregnancy complicated with dermatomyositis: case reports. *Gynecol Obstet Invest* 1992;33:187–189.
361. Marie I, Hachulla E, Hatron PY, et al. Polymyositis and dermatomyositis: short term and longterm outcome, and predictive factors of prognosis. *J Rheumatol* 2001;28:2230–2237.
362. Sontheimer RD, Ziff M. Questions pertaining to the etiology and pathophysiology of polymyositis/dermatomyositis [review]. *Clin Dermatol* 1988;6: 105–119.
363. De Bleecker JL, De Paepe B, Vanwalleghem IE, et al. Differential expression of chemokines in inflammatory myopathies. *Neurology* 2002;58:1779–1785.
364. Bank I, Miranda AF, Chess L. Mechanisms of cell-mediated myocytotoxicity in the peripheral blood of patients with inflammatory myopathies. *J Clin Immunol* 2001;21:328–334.
365. Dalakas MC. The molecular and cellular pathology of inflammatory muscle diseases. *Curr Opin Pharmacol* 2001;1:300–306.
366. Nagaraju K, Raben N, Villalba ML, et al. Costimulatory markers in muscle of patients with idiopathic inflammatory myopathies and in cultured muscle cells. *Clin Immunol* 1999;92:161–169.
367. Hohlfeld R, Engel AG, Goebels N, et al. Cellular immune mechanisms in inflammatory myopathies. *Curr Opin Rheumatol* 1997;9:520–526.
368. Hirsch TJ, Enlow RW, Bias WB, et al. HLA-D related (DR) antigens in various kinds of myositis. *Hum Immunol* 1981;3:181–186.
369. Plotz PH, Dalakas M, Leff RL, et al. Current concepts in the idiopathic inflammatory myopathies: polymyositis, dermatomyositis, and related disorders. *Ann Intern Med* 1989;111:143–157.
370. Pachman LM, Friedman JM, Maryjowski-Sweeney ML, et al. Immunogenetic studies of juvenile dermatomyositis, III: study of antibody to organ-specific and nuclear antigens. *Arthritis Rheum* 1985;28:151–157.
371. Reed AM, Pachman L, Ober C. Molecular genetic studies of major histocompatibility complex genes in children with juvenile dermatomyositis: increased risk associated with HLA-DQA1*0501. *Hum Immunol* 1991;32: 235–240.
372. Vavrincova P, Havelka S, Cerna M, et al. HLA class II alleles in juvenile dermatomyositis. *J Rheumatol* 1993;37[Suppl]:S17–S18.
373. Robb SA, Fielder AH, Saunders CE, et al. C4 complement allotypes in juvenile dermatomyositis. *Hum Immunol* 1988;22:31–38.
374. Arnett FC, Hirsch TJ, Bias WB, et al. The Jo-1 antibody system in myositis: relationships to clinical features and HLA. *J Rheumatol* 1981;8:925–930.
375. Goldstein R, Duvic M, Targoff IN, et al. HLA-D region genes associated with autoantibody responses to Jo-1 (histidyl-tRNA synthetase) and other translation-related factors in myositis. *Arthritis Rheum* 1990;33:1240–1248.
376. Werth VP, Zhang W, Dortzbach K, et al. Association of a promoter polymorphism of tumor necrosis factor-alpha with subacute cutaneous lupus erythematosus and distinct photoregulation of transcription. *J Invest Dermatol* 2000;115:726–730.
377. Millard TP, Kondeatis E, Cox A, et al. A candidate gene analysis of three related photosensitivity disorders: cutaneous lupus erythematosus, polymorphic light eruption and actinic prurigo. *Br J Dermatol* 2001;145:229–236.
378. Lindberg C, Oldfors A, Tarkowski A. Restricted use of T cell receptor V genes in endomysial infiltrates of patients with inflammatory myopathies. *Eur J Immunol* 1994;24:2659–2663.
379. Wakino S, Kuwana M, Tojo T, et al. Serial lymphocyte subpopulation analysis in peripheral blood from a patient with amyopathic dermatomyositis [letter]. *Br J Rheumatol* 1994;33:498–499.
380. Sontheimer RD. Antibodies inside our keratinocytes? [editorial; comment]. *Arch Dermatol* 1993;129:1184–1187.
381. Alberdi F, Dadone J, Ryazanov A, et al. Cross-reaction of lupus Anti-dsDNA antibodies with protein translation factor EF-2. *Clin Immunol* 2001;98: 293–300.
382. Reichlin M. Cell injury mediated by autoantibodies to intracellular antigens. *Clin Immunol Immunopathol* 1995;76:215–219.
383. Ytterberg SR. Cellular immunity in polymyositis/dermatomyositis [review]. *Mt Sinai J Med* 1988;55:494–500.
384. Bank I, Miranda AF, Chess L. Mechanisms of cell-mediated myocytotoxicity in the peripheral blood of patients with inflammatory myopathies. *J Clin Immunol* 2001;21:328–334.
385. Lundberg IE. Idiopathic inflammatory myopathies: why do the muscles become weak? *Cur Opin Rheumatol* 2001;13:457–460.
386. Reed AM, Picornell YJ, Harwood A, et al. Chimerism in children with juvenile dermatomyositis. *Lancet* 2000;356:2156–2157.
387. Jongen PJ, Zoll GJ, Beaumont M, et al. Polymyositis and dermatomyositis: no persistence of enterovirus or encephalomyocarditis virus RNA in muscle. *Ann Rheumat Dis* 1993;52:575–578.
388. Fraser DD, Kong LI, Miller FW. Molecular detection of persistent *Borrelia burgdorferi* in a man with dermatomyositis. *Clin Exp Rheumatol* 1992;10: 387–390.
389. Horowitz HW, Sanghera K, Goldberg N, et al. Dermatomyositis associated with Lyme disease: case report and review of Lyme myositis [review]. *Clin Inf Dis* 1994;18:166–171.
390. Martini A, Ravelli A, Albani S, et al. Recurrent juvenile dermatomyositis and cutaneous necrotizing arteritis with molecular mimicry between streptococcal type 5 M protein and human skeletal myosin. *J Pediatr* 1992;121:739–742.
391. Moore EC, Cohen F, Douglas SD, et al. Staphylococcal infections in childhood dermatomyositis—association with the development of calcinosis, raised IgE concentrations and granulocyte chemotactic defect. *Ann Rheum Dis* 1992;51: 378–383.
392. Hashimoto K, Robison L, Velayos E, et al. Dermatomyositis: electron microscopic, immunologic, and tissue culture studies of paramyxovirus-like inclusions. *Arch Dermatol* 1971;103:120–135.
393. Rich S. Human lupus inclusions and interferon. *Science* 1981;213:772–775.
394. Rich SA, Owens TR, Anzola MC, et al. Induction of lupus inclusions by sera from patients with systemic lupus erythematosus. *Arthritis Rheum* 1986;29: 501–507.
395. Luu J, Bockus D, Remington F, et al. Tubuloreticular structures and cylindrical confronting cisternae: a review. *Hum Pathol* 1989;_0:617–627.
396. Sontheimer RD, Bergstresser PR. Epidermal Langerhans cell involvement in cutaneous lupus erythematosus. *J Invest Dermatol* 1982;79:237–243.
397. Norris DA. Pathomechanisms of photosensitive lupus erythematosus. *J Invest Dermatol* 1993;100:58S–68S.
398. Shiohara T, Moriya N, Nagashima M. The lichenoid tissue reaction: a new concept of pathogenesis. *Int J Dermatol* 1988;27:365–374.
399. Saito E, Kinoshita M, Oshima H, et al. Damaging effect of peripheral mononuclear cells of dermatomyositis on cultured human skin fibroblasts. *J Rheumatol* 1987;14:936–941.
400. Hohlfeld R, Engel AG, Ii K, et al. Polymyositis mediated by T lymphocytes that express the gamma/δ receptor. *N Engl J Med* 1991;324:877–881.
401. Volc-Platzer B, Anegg B, Milota S, et al. Accumulation of gammaδ T cells in chronic cutaneous lupus erythematosus. *J Invest Dermatol* 1993;100:84S–91S.
402. Cervera R, Ramirez G, Fernandez-Sola J, et al. Antibodies to endothelial cells in dermatomyositis: association with interstitial lung disease. *BMJ* 1991;302: 880–881.
403. Pandya AG, Sontheimer RD, Cockerell CJ, et al. Papulonodular mucinosis associated with systemic lupus erythematosus: possible mechanisms of increased glycosaminoglycan accumulation. *J Am Acad Dermatol* 1995;32: 199–205.
404. Tominaga A, Tajima S, Ishibashi A, et al. Reticular erythematous mucinosis syndrome with an infiltration of factor XIIIa+ and hyaluronan synthase 2+ dermal dendrocytes. *Br J Dermatol* 2001;145:141–145.
405. Cripps DJ, Rankin J. Action spectra of lupus erythematosus and experimental immunofluorescence. *Arch Dermatol* 1973;107:563–567.
406. Claman HN. On scleroderma: mast cells, endothelial cells, and fibroblasts. *JAMA* 1989;262:1206–1209.
407. Gruber BL, Kaufman LD. Ketotifen-induced remission in progressive early diffuse scleroderma: evidence for the role of mast cells in disease pathogenesis. *Am J Med* 1990;89:392–395.

CHAPTER 4

Systemic Sclerosis

M. Kari Connolly and Denny L. Tuffanelli

HISTORICAL PERSPECTIVE

Curzio of Naples wrote the first definitive description of scleroderma in a 17-year-old girl in 1754 (1). The term "scleroderma" was introduced almost 100 years later in 1847 (2). In 1862, Maurice Raynaud (1834–1881) described the digital vasospastic phenomenon that bears his name (3). William Osler gave the best description of scleroderma in 1898: "In its more aggravated form, diffuse scleroderma is one of the most terrible of all illnesses. Like Tithonius to wither slowly, and like him to be beaten down and marred and wasted until one is literally a mummy, encased in an ever shrinking, slowly contracting, skin of steel" (4).

The concept of a collagen disease was proposed by Klemperer, Pollack, and Baehr in 1942 and began the modern era of scleroderma research (5). Although initially recognized for its cutaneous manifestations, internal organ involvement was appreciated by the mid 1900s. The term "progressive systemic sclerosis" was introduced by Goetz (6) in 1945 to emphasize the systemic nature of the disease. It was subsequently recognized that not every patient had a progressive course and therefore the preferred designation became "systemic sclerosis" (SSc) (7).

Many investigators, too numerous to be cited here, have contributed to the understanding of this complex and compelling disease. Medsger and Steen and their colleagues at the University of Pittsburgh built the Pittsburgh Scleroderma Databank. This is the largest clinical database, with more than 2,500 entries spanning a 30-year period. Much of what we know about the clinical phenotype of SSc comes from studies using this invaluable database. In 1996, a textbook, *Systemic Sclerosis,* edited by Drs. Philip Clements and Daniel Furst, was published (8). This work is a tour de force collection of topics on scleroderma from leading experts from all over the world. Jablonska et al. (9,10) have contributed significantly to our understanding of the cutaneous aspects of this disease.

The history of the drug therapy for SSc has been one of disappointment and failure. Many drugs have been tried, and many claims have been made. Nonetheless, when put to the test of a randomized, double-blinded, placebo-controlled trial, few drugs have shown a survival benefit in patients with SSc. Despite this poor track record, the future looks brighter. Support from the National Institutes of Health, the pharmaceutical and biotechnology industries, and private foundations is fueling advances in basic research and clinical trials to develop new therapies for patients with SSc. The confluence of these factors promises a brighter future for patients with SSc.

EPIDEMIOLOGY

Epidemiologic studies in scleroderma have been hindered by the relative rarity of the disease together with its clinical heterogeneity. Earlier studies underestimated the prevalence of the disease because they relied on hospital records and death certificates (11). In 1989, a population-based survey reported the prevalence of SSc among adults in South Carolina to be 29 to 113 per 100,000 (12). The more broadly defined "scleroderma spectrum disorders" were estimated to affect 67 to 265 per 100,000 ("not less than 226/100,000"). A population-based survey of the Detroit metropolitan area found a prevalence of 240 per million (13). A conservative estimate would place the number of patients with SSc in the United States at around 100,000. Other estimates place the figure four to five times higher (14). Scleroderma has a worldwide distribution; however, the incidence rates are different in different countries, with a higher rate in the United States (13). All ethnic groups are affected; however, there is a small increase in blacks (11). All studies show a female predominance. Tuffanelli and Winkelmann (5) reported one of the earliest and largest case series of 727 patients from the Mayo Clinic. In that study, 75% of patients were female. Other studies have confirmed a three to four times higher incidence in women. The median age of onset is 45 to 50 years, although it can occur in children and the elderly.

CLASSIFICATION AND NOMENCLATURE

Different classification systems have been used by different physicians and in different countries (15,16). The full spectrum of scleroderma disorders is listed in Table 4.1. *Scleroderma* is a general term describing hardening of the skin. *Systemic sclerosis* is a specific term for the systemic variant of the disease. In 1980, the American College of Rheumatology (formerly the American Rheumatism Association) published preliminary criteria for the *classification* of systemic sclerosis (Table 4.2) (17). They studied 797 patients from 29 medical centers and identified one major and three minor criteria that differentiated SSc from other connective tissue diseases and primary Raynaud phenomenon. From that study, the sole major criterion is "proximal scleroderma" defined as symmetric thickening, tightening, and induration of the skin of the fingers proximal to the metacarpophalangeal (MCP) and metatarsophalangeal (MTP) joints. The minor criteria are (a) sclerodactyly, (b) digital pits and loss

TABLE 4.1. The Scleroderma Spectrum

I. Systemic sclerosis with:
- A. *Diffuse scleroderma:* fibrotic skin changes above the elbows and including the trunk (formerly called progressive systemic sclerosis)
- B. *Limited scleroderma:* fibrotic skin changes limited to the hands (acrosclerosis) and face. Also referred to as the "CREST syndrome": calcinosis, RP, esophageal dysmotility, sclerodactyly, and telangiectasias
- C. *Sine scleroderma:* without fibrotic skin changes has RP, internal organ involvement, and positive serologies
- D. Intermediate cutaneous systemic scleroderma
- E. Undifferentiated connective tissue diseases
- F. Overlap syndromes
  - 1. Mixed connective tissue disease
  - 2. Sclerodermatomyositis
  - 3. Any other connective tissue disease

II. Localized scleroderma
- A. Morphea
  - 1. Plaque
  - 2. Guttate
  - 3. Bullous
  - 4. Profundus or deep
- B. Linear scleroderma
  - 1. En coup de sabre
  - 2. With facial atrophy (Romberg disease)
- C. Generalized morphea
  - 1. Pansclerotic
  - 2. With lichen sclerosus et atrophicus
- D. Eosinophilic fasciitis

III. Scleroderma variants
- A. Scleredema
- B. Scleromyxedema

IV. Pseudoscleroderma conditions
- A. Genetic
  - 1. Phenylketonuria
  - 2. Progeria
  - 3. Werner syndrome
  - 4. Rothmund–Thomson syndrome
  - 5. Stiff skin syndrome: congenital fascial dystrophy
- B. Environmental and occupational
  - 1. Vibration syndrome
    - a. Jackhammer operator
    - b. Chain saw operator
  - 2. Polyvinyl chloride
  - 3. Silicosis, silica dust
  - 4. Organic solvents
    - a. Aromatic hydrocarbons
    - b. Aliphatic hydrocarbons
  - 5. Epoxy resins
  - 6. Spanish rapeseed oil disease
  - 7. L-Tryptophan (eosinophilia-myalgia syndrome)
- C. Metabolic
  - 1. Congenital porphyria
  - 2. Porphyria cutanea tarda
  - 3. Primary systemic amyloidosis
  - 4. Hashimoto's thyroiditis
  - 5. Diabetes, childhood
  - 6. Crow-Fukase (POEMS) syndrome
  - 7. Scleredema (secondary to diabetes)
- D. Immunologic
  - 1. Chronic graft versus host disease
  - 2. Scleromyxedema
- E. Drugs
  - 1. Bleomycin
  - 2. Isoniazid
  - 3. Pentazocine
  - 4. Valproate sodium
  - 5. L-5-hydroxytryptophane and carbidopa
  - 6. Phytonadione (vitamin K) injections
  - 7. Bromocriptine
  - 8. Nitrofurantoin
  - 9. L-tryptophan
- F. Malignancy
  - 1. Carcinoid syndrome
  - 2. Metastatic melanoma
  - 3. Bronchoalveolar carcinoma
  - 4. Paraneoplastic
    - a. Palmar fasciitis
    - b. Fibroblastic arthritis
- G. Postinfections
  - 1. Scleredema of Buschke
  - 2. Acrodermatitis chronica atrophicans
  - 3. Partial lipodystrophy
  - 4. Hypodermitis sclerodermiformis
  - 5. Morphea secondary to *Borrelia* species?
- H. Neurologic
  - 1. Dermal fibrosis in spinal injury
  - 2. Limb immobilization
- I. Radiation
  - 1. Radiation therapy (breast cancer)
  - 2. Chernobyl nuclear accident

RP, Raynaud's phenomenon.

TABLE 4.2. American College of Rheumatology Preliminary Classification Criteria

1. Major criterion
   - a. Proximal scleroderma
     Indurated, hard skin. Often the skin is shiny with loss of cutaneous surface markings. Loss of elasticity occurs. Hyper- and hypopigmentation are common.
2. Minor criteria
   - a. Sclerodactyly
   - b. Digital pitted scars or loss of substance of the finger pad
   - c. Bibasilar pulmonary fibrosis

Diagnosis is 97% certain with one major or two or more minor criteria present. There are no specific diagnostic criteria for localized cutaneous scleroderma, scleroderma variants, overlap syndromes, and environmentally induced scleroderma at this time.
From Steen VD, Medsger TA. Severe organ involvement in systemic sclerosis with diffuse scleroderma. *Arthritis Rheum* 2000;43:2437, with permission.

of substance from the finger pad, and (c) bibasilar pulmonary fibrosis. When applied to their study population, these criteria were 97% sensitive and 98% specific. This classification system has some limitations. They are not *diagnostic* criteria. Raynaud phenomenon and autoantibodies are not included because they are too nonspecific. Furthermore, the classification criteria do not define disease subsets. The two most widely recognized subsets in the United States are (a) *limited* cutaneous scleroderma and (b) *diffuse* cutaneous scleroderma as proposed by LeRoy et al. (18).

Systemic sclerosis with limited cutaneous scleroderma describes a patient with a long prodrome with Raynaud phenomenon that begins in their 30s or 40s. The fibrotic skin involvement may be minimal and is limited to the fingers (sclerodactyly), hands, and face (hence the term *limited*). The limited form is associated with the anticentromere antibody and has a good prognosis. O'Leary and Waisman (19) at the Mayo Clinic used the term "acroscle-

TABLE 4.3. Systemic Sclerosis Subsets

	Diffuse Scleroderma	Limited Scleroderma (CREST)
Skin	Diffuse (above the elbow or knee)	Sclerodactyly Calcinosis Telangiectasia
Raynaud phenomenon	At disease onset	Precedes disease by 5 to 10 years
GI tract	Entire GI tract	Esophagus
Lungs	Interstitial lung disease	Pulmonary HTN
Renal	SD renal crisis	—
Cardiac	Arrhythmias	—
Liver	—	Primary biliary cirrhosis
Serologies	Anti-DNA topoisomerase I (anti-Scl 70)	Anti-centromere

GI, gastrointestinal; HTN, hypertension; scleroderma.

rosis" to describe this subset. The association of calcinosis with patients with scleroderma was first recorded in 1911 by Thibierge and Weissenbach (20). The limited subset has also been referred to as the *CREST syndrome* (calcinosis, Raynaud phenomenon, esophageal dysmotility, sclerodactyly, telangiectasias). Although the *CREST syndrome* is clinically useful because of its descriptive quality, the designation *limited* is preferred because not every patient in the subset has every feature of the syndrome. Approximately 60% of patients with SSc are in the limited subset.

In contrast to the limited subset, *systemic sclerosis with diffuse cutaneous scleroderma* describes a patient with a rapid onset and progressive course with cutaneous fibrosis extending from the hands up the forearms, arms, trunk, face, and lower extremities (hence the term "diffuse") (Table 4.3). The skin involvement is rapidly progressive in the first few years, tends to stabilize around years 4 to 5, and then may regress (15). The first 2 to 3 years are especially difficult for the patient experiencing diffuse disease because skin involvement may progress despite therapy. Internal organ involvement is virtually universal within the first 5 years of disease, and the prognosis is worse than that for limited disease.

Systemic sclerosis sine cutaneous scleroderma affects a rare subset of patients without evidence of cutaneous sclerosis, but with Raynaud phenomenon, esophageal dysmotility, and autoantibodies. This subset represents about 5% to 10% of all patients. The phenotype is stable (i.e., these patients do not evolve into the limited or diffuse subsets). Medsger et al. (21) have studied this subset and found that the morbidity and mortality of this group were similar to those of patients with the limited subset.

Although the two-subset system is useful, some advocate the addition of a third, or *intermediate,* subset. Initially, Barnett et al. (22) proposed a classification system based on three subsets that correlated well with survival. More recently, two studies, a large Italian cohort (14) and a French-Canadian study (23), used an intermediate cutaneous subset. They demonstrated corresponding survival data that correlated with the additional subset. This may represent a more refined classification system. It will be interesting to see whether it is adopted more broadly.

Although the nomenclature and classification system is effective for the investigators of SSc, it is not ideal. It is cumbersome and nonintuitive for colleagues outside the field and thus hampers interactions among investigators across different disciplines. More important, it is a problem for patients and a public relations problem for the disease. "Systemic sclerosis" is difficult to pronounce with five S's. If patients cannot clearly state the name of their disease, they cannot communicate effectively with their families, friends, and the community about it. This difficulty impedes public awareness, which translates to less understanding and support. There is no reason why "systemic sclerosis" should not be as widely recognized as multiple sclerosis, muscular dystrophy, or cystic fibrosis. Yet, the level of public awareness of SSc is considerably less than those diseases. Although the term "scleroderma" is often used, this term also has some limitations. We propose a new name: "total tissue dystrophy." This name more accurately reflects the complex tissue changes, is easier to say, and, like muscular dystrophy, has multiple subtypes.

PERIPHERAL VASCULAR MANIFESTATIONS

Raynaud phenomenon occurs in most patients with SSc. It is characterized by digital artery vasospasm and is precipitated by cold or emotional stress. The hands and feet are most commonly involved, but occasionally the nose, ears, and tongue are affected. The three color phases necessary for the diagnosis of Raynaud phenomenon consist of (a) white or pallor due to vasoconstriction (Fig. 4.1), (b) blue or cyanosis due to stasis of deoxygenated blood, and (c) red or erythema due to vasodilatation and reactive hyperemia. Many patients have "cold hands and feet" or "poor circulation," but do not have true Raynaud phenomenon. Primary Raynaud phenomenon has a prevalence of 3% to 4% in the general population (24). The incidence in young women may be as high as 20% to 30%.

The term "primary Raynaud phenomenon" is used when there is no underlying cause or associated condition. "Secondary Raynaud phenomenon" is used when it occurs in asso-

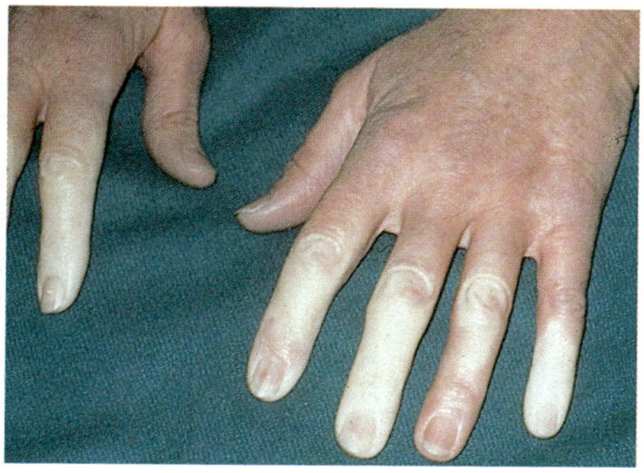

Figure 4.1. Raynaud phenomenon with vasoconstriction.

ciation with another disease. "Undifferentiated connective tissue disease" is the term that describes patients with puffy fingers, digital pitting scars, and nailfold capillary findings and may portend progression to SSc (16).

Capillary microscopy reveals abnormal nailfold capillary patterns in patients with SSc (25). Enlarged and deformed capillary loops surrounded by avascular areas, most prominently on the nailfolds, are found in 90% of patients with scleroderma (26). Different techniques can be used to visualize the nailfold capillaries in the outpatient setting. Dermatoscopy (or epiluminescence microscopy) is especially well suited to visualizing the nailfold capillaries. Immersion oil is applied to the fourth nondominant nailfold (the choice of this digit is to minimize traumatic artifacts), which is then viewed with the small, hand-held, 10× Dermatoscope. The combination of surface illumination, magnification, and large aperture allows excellent inspection of the entire nailfold. These nailfold capillary changes can sometimes be appreciated on gross inspection.

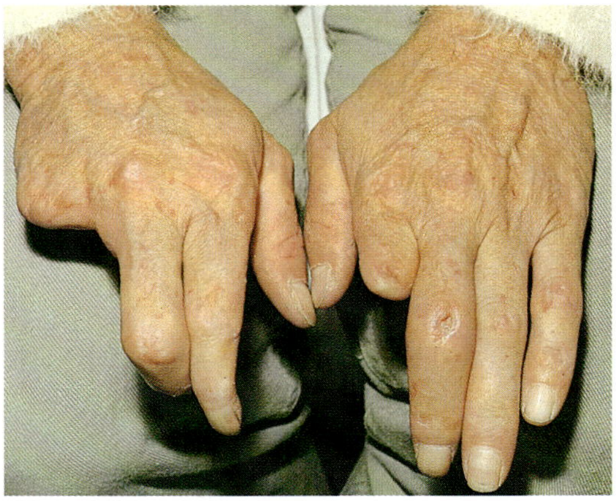

Figure 4.3. Ulcers with secondary infection and loss of digits.

CUTANEOUS MANIFESTATIONS

Sclerosis of the skin is the hallmark of this disease. The most common presenting sign is symmetric edema of the hands. The edema is followed by sclerosis. The skin becomes smooth, waxy, and bound down. It cannot be picked up (tethering). When these changes are confined to the fingers, it is known as sclerodactyly (Fig. 4.2). Pitted scars and pinhole-sized depressions, usually associated with hyperkeratosis, are observed on the tips and sides of the fingers. Painful ulcers (Fig. 4.3) can develop around the fingertips and in areas of digital calcinosis (Fig. 4.4). Severe flexion contractures of the hands and resorption of the terminal phalanges can follow (Fig. 4.5). Secondary infection, gangrene, and loss of digits can result.

Digital ulcerations occur in 35% of patients (5). In addition, ulcers over the elbows, knees, hips, and ankles can occur. The lesions are usually painful and heal extremely slowly. Secondary bacterial infection can dramatically increase the pain.

Several disorders of the nails and periungual tissues occur, including onycholysis, onychorrhexis, onychogryphosis, absence of lunula, development of deep longitudinal sulci, hapalonychia, and pterygium unguis (27,28). Pterygium inversum unguis results (characterized by adherence of the distal portion of the nail bed to the ventral surface of the nail plate, thereby obliterating the normal distal separation of the structures) and cuticular thickening is commonly present (Fig. 4.6).

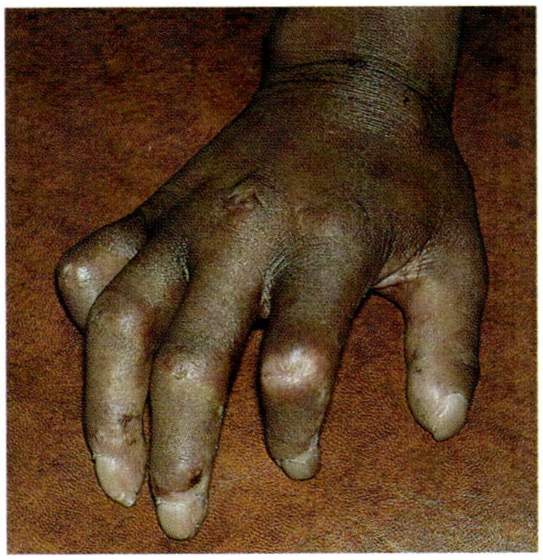

Figure 4.2. Sclerodactyly.

There are three phases of skin involvement: an early edematous phase (Fig. 4.7), a sclerotic or indurated phase (Fig. 4.8), and a late atrophic phase (Fig. 4.9). Sometimes, but not invariably, erythema accompanies the early edematous phase. Most commonly, acral areas are involved, particularly the hands and arms. Rarely, scleroderma of the skin appears first on the trunk and then spreads to involve the entire integument. Anhidrosis in affected and unaffected areas is common.

The face has a characteristic appearance with drawn, stretched skin and "masklike" or "expressionless" features (Fig. 4.10). The lips are thin and the nose looks pinched. The opening of the mouth (oral aperture) is diminished. There is exaggerated

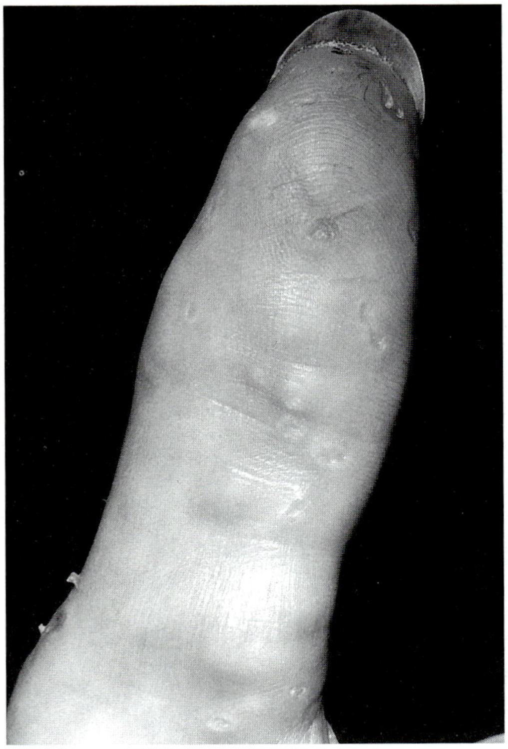

Figure 4.4. Digital calcinosis.

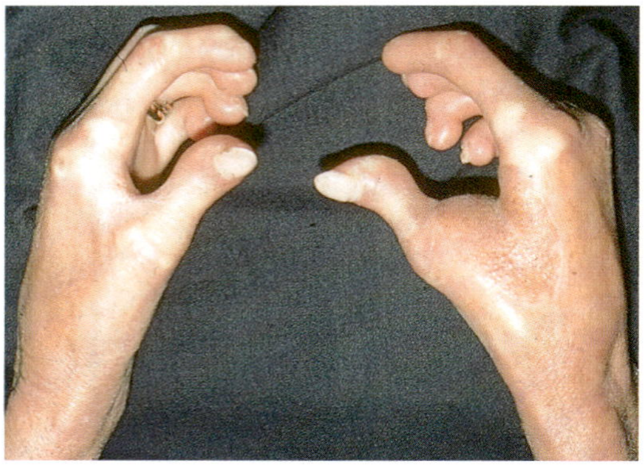

Figure 4.5. Severe articular deformities with resorption of terminal phalanges.

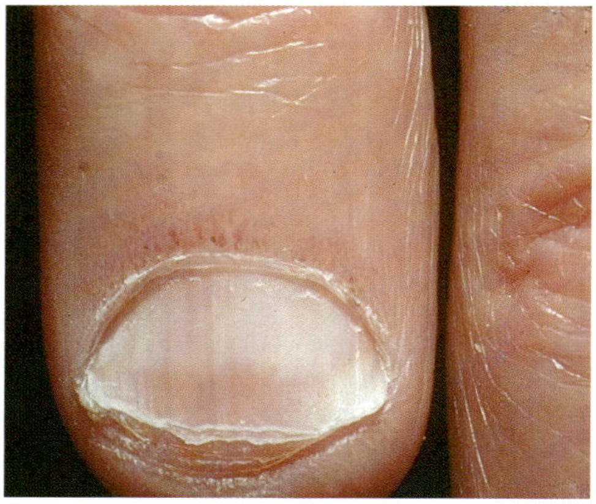

Figure 4.6. Cuticular thickening of the nail. Nailfold capillary changes can be appreciated.

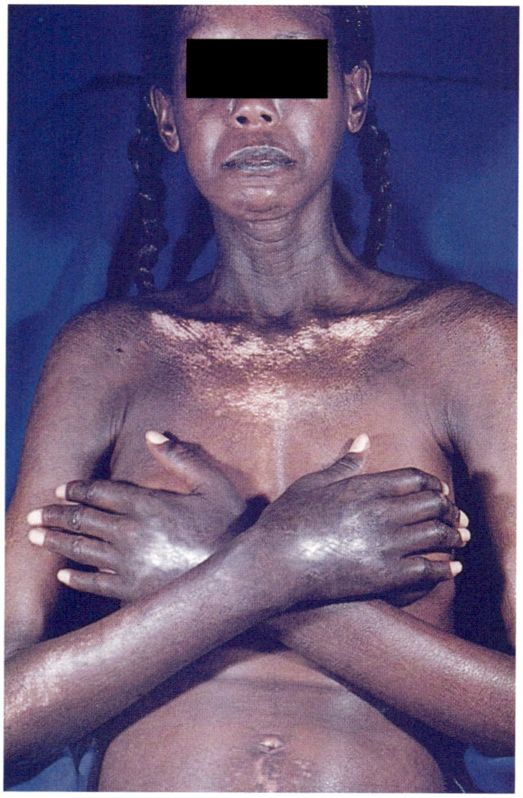

Figure 4.7. Systemic sclerosis with diffuse cutaneous scleroderma: early edematous phase. Note pigmentary changes: hypopigmentation with preserved pigment around the hair follicles.

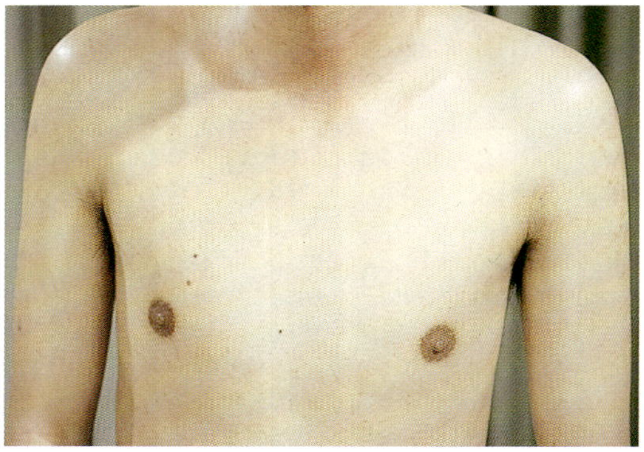

Figure 4.8. Indurated phase.

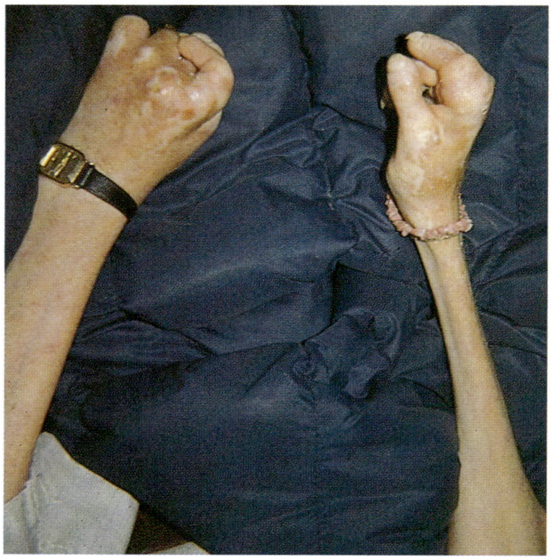

Figure 4.9. Late atrophic phase.

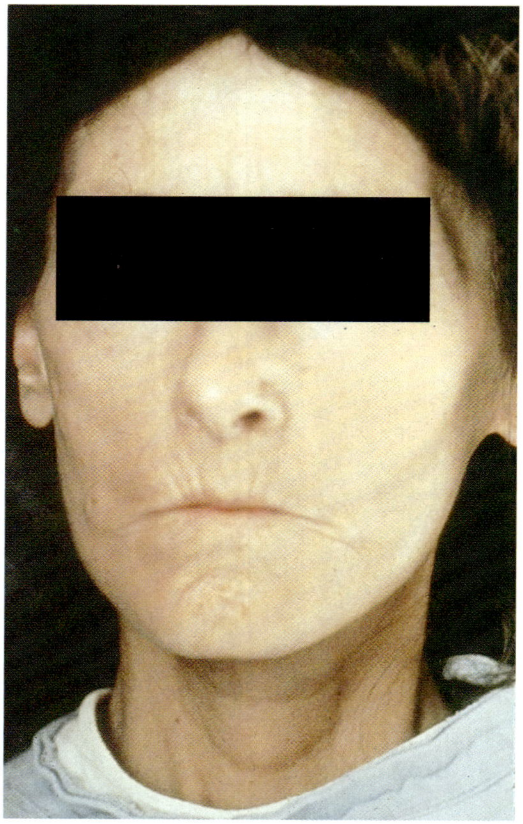

Figure 4.10. Scleroderma facies.

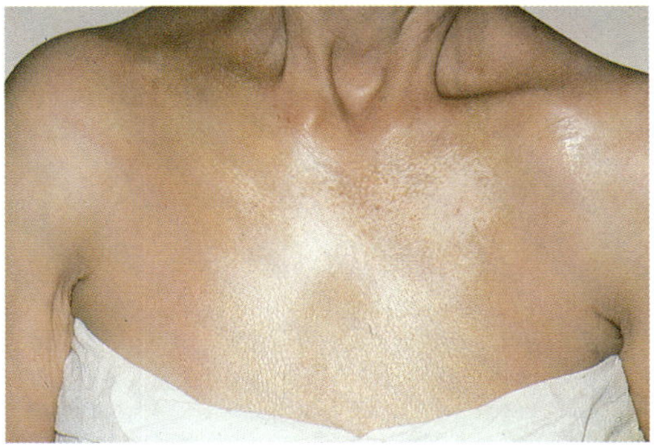

Figure 4.11. Longitudinal beading or ridging of the neck and chest.

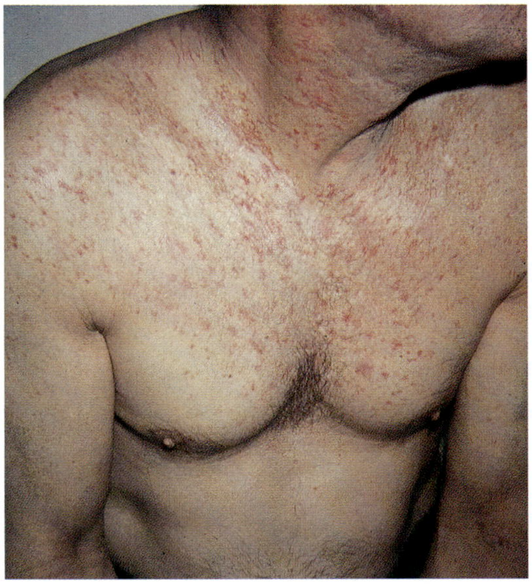

Figure 4.13. Telangiectasia of the chest.

radial fissuring around the mouth and a "mouselike" face. The neck sign consists of "ridging and tightening" of the skin of the neck and is perceived on extending the head (29). Longitudinal beading or ridging of the neck is frequently observed in patients with scleroderma (Fig. 4.11).

Characteristic, squared-off, telangiectasias are common. These occur earlier in about 70% of persons in the limited subset and later in about 50% of persons in the diffuse subset (15). Some are matted macular dilatations of superficial vessels that collapse on pressure. More commonly, dilated capillaries, venules, and arterioles are seen. Telangiectasias occur most prominently on the face, lips, tongue, chest, palms, and fingers (Figs. 4.12 and 4.13). They can also occur internally along the gastrointestinal (GI) tract and rarely be a cause of bleeding and anemia (see gastrointestinal involvement section).

Calcinosis cutis occurs in approximately one third of patients with limited scleroderma and 10% of patients with diffuse disease (15). Calcinosis cutis is a late sequela of scleroderma occurring, on average, 11 years after the onset of the disease (30). The deposits themselves are composed of calcium hydroxyapatite crystals (15). Deposits are usually small, appearing on the hands, elbows, hips, ankles, and knees (Figs. 4.4, 4.14, and 4.15). Calcinosis also presents commonly on the volar aspects of the fingertips and over the metacarpal, phalangeal, and interphalangeal joints. Occasionally a chalky white discharge may drain from a deposit and put the patient at risk for infection. Ulcers may complicate a calcium deposit.

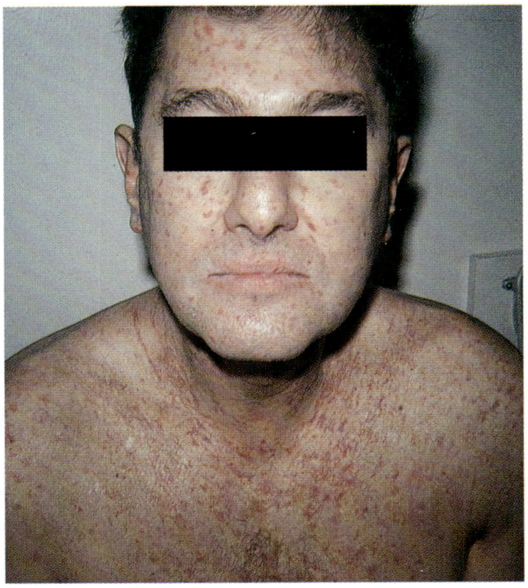

Figure 4.12. Systemic sclerosis with limited cutaneous scleroderma: squared-off telangiectasia of the face.

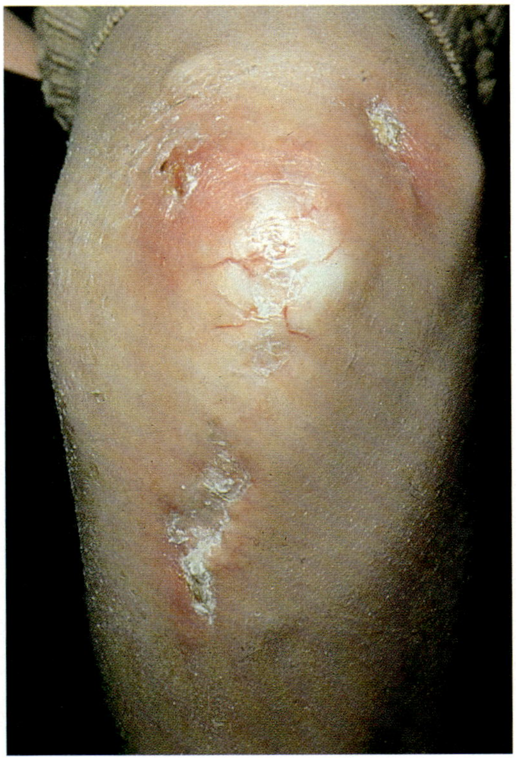

Figure 4.14. Calcinosis of the knee.

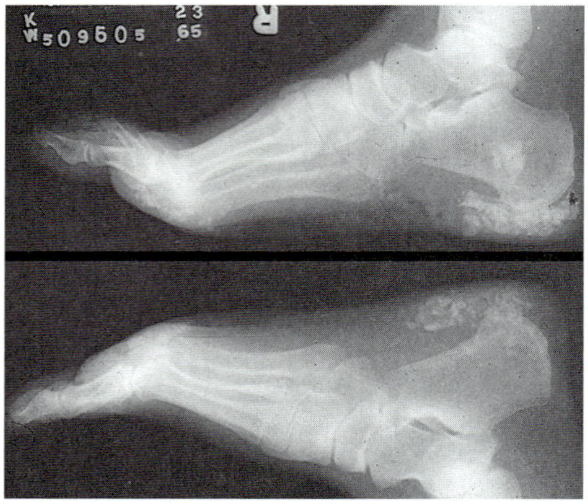

Figure 4.15. Radiograph of calcinosis of the feet.

Pigmentary abnormalities, both hypopigmentation and hyperpigmentation, can be very pronounced in patients with SSc. The cause is unclear. Initially, fair-skinned patients note a generalized hyperpigmentation with accentuation in sun-exposed areas as well as areas of friction or pressure, such as a waist band. The face may be relatively spared or even hypopigmented. Later, in areas of sclerosis and hyperpigmentation, a vitiligo-like depigmentation occurs with perifollicular pigment retention, giving rise to a "salt and pepper" pattern (Fig. 4.16). This clinical pattern can resemble vitiligo. Hypopigmentation of the forehead near the hairline can also occur. Jawitz et al. (31) observed pigment retention over superficial blood vessels within a larger field of depigmentation. Histologically, these changes are not consistent with postinflammatory pigment alteration. Sanchez et al. (32) reported the histology of complete pigment loss and associated perifollicular hyperpigmentation as resembling patches of repigmenting vitiligo.

ASSESSMENT OF CUTANEOUS INVOLVEMENT

The extent of skin involvement correlates with internal organ disease and survival in patients with SSc (33–35). Moreover, improvement in skin scores is correlated with improved survival (36). For this reason, accurate measurements of skin involvement are important.

The modified Rodnan skin score (MRSS) is one of the more commonly used measurements (16). The MRSS is determined by measuring cutaneous thickening or tethering clinically on a scale of 0 to 3 in 17 body areas for a total possible score of 51 (37). This method has been validated for inter- and intraobserver variability (38). The natural history of skin scores in patients with diffuse disease is to increase rapidly during the first 1 to 2 years of disease, reach a peak, and then slowly decline as the affected skin becomes thinner and more atrophic over time. Thus, a "decreased" skin score may reflect the natural history of the disease. This natural tendency has to be taken into account when assessing therapeutic agents.

Alternative methods proposed for assessing skin thickness include ultrasound (39), durometer (40), and the BTC-2000 suction device (SRLI Technologies, Nashville, TN) that has been shown to be a safe, sensitive noninvasive way to measure skin changes in scleroderma (41). There is still a need for is an objective, quantitative measurement that is sensitive to small changes over short periods of time.

MISCELLANEOUS CUTANEOUS FINDINGS

Bullous lesions have been reported rarely in scleroderma (42,43). Tuffanelli (44) described bullae in patients with early edematous SSc that demonstrated dilated lymphatic channels in the dermis on histology.

In general, patients with scleroderma do not have problems with keloids, hypertrophic scars, or wound healing. They tolerate biopsies or surgical procedures without significant wound healing problems. Rarely, keloid-like nodules occur in patients

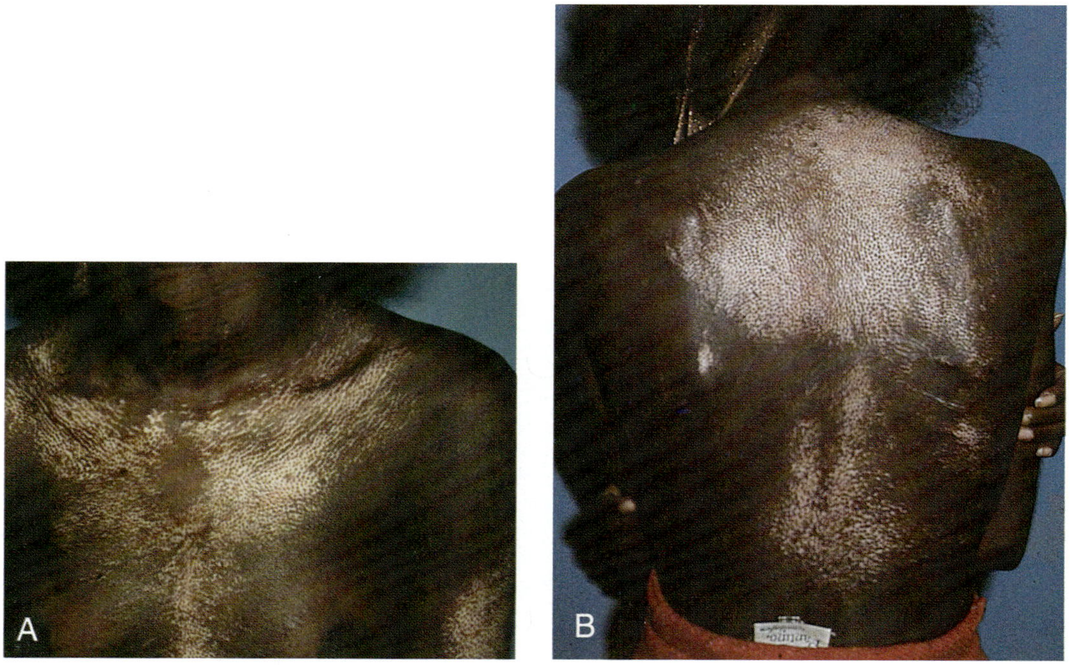

Figure 4.16. Hypopigmentation of the chest (**A**) and back (**B**).

with SSc who were either genetically at risk for keloid formation or in areas that had a high predilection for keloid formation, such as the chest (45). Panniculitis is seen rarely in scleroderma. Clinically, panniculitis can be difficult to differentiate from large nodules of calcinosis. Radiographs and biopsies can differentiate these conditions. Panniculitis is seen occasionally in patients with overlap syndromes.

MUSCULOSKELETAL INVOLVEMENT

Arthralgias are common in the early phase of the disease. Hands, wrists, elbows, shoulders, hips, knees, and ankles can be involved. Although joint pain is common, overt inflammatory synovitis and joint effusions are rare. Joint contractions, muscular atrophy, and periarticular subcutaneous calcifications occur. Tendon friction rubs are a poor prognostic sign. Fibrosis of tendons may lead to proliferative entrapment neuropathy and carpal tunnel syndrome.

Muscle involvement occurs in two ways. One is a bland myopathy, which occurs in approximately 80% of patients. The second is an inflammatory myositis similar to polymyositis with elevated muscle enzymes and electromyography abnormalities. Some authors reported that the presence of inflammatory myositis was correlated with the presence of the anti–PM-Scl antibody (46).

SYSTEMIC INVOLVEMENT

The GI tract, lungs, kidney, and heart are the most frequently affected internal organs in SSc. It is the occurrence and extent of internal organ involvement that determines the morbidity and mortality of this disease. Patients with diffuse disease are at greater risk for internal organ involvement in the first 3 to 5 years of disease (35). In contrast, the limited subset is at risk for internal organ complications later in the disease course (after 10 to 20 years). Some patients are asymptomatic when they develop internal organ involvement. For these reasons, all patients with SSc should undergo regular medical evaluations and screening for internal organ involvement.

GASTROINTESTINAL INVOLVEMENT

The GI tract is affected in 90% of patients with SSc (47). The fundamental defect that occurs in the GI tract is hypomotility with decreased peristalsis. The esophagus is the most commonly affected part of the GI tract (15). In addition to loss of motility in the esophagus, there is decreased tone in the lower esophageal sphincter predisposing to reflux. Gastroesophageal reflux disease (GERD) causes esophagitis, erosive esophagitis, Barrett esophagus, and strictures. Symptoms include dysphagia and heartburn. Patients with scleroderma with GERD report fewer symptoms associated with their reflux events (48). Therefore, screening based only on symptoms may be misleading. A number of studies can document abnormal function, including barium swallow, cine-esophagram, manometry, pH monitoring and endoscopy.

Gastroparesis with delayed gastric emptying can lead to nausea and early satiety. Telangiectasias can occur in the GI tract and can rarely be a cause of GI bleeding and anemia. Gastric antral vascular ectasia, also known as watermelon stomach, can occur in patients with scleroderma (49,50); this can be managed with endoscopic laser treatments.

Hypomotility of the small intestine occurs and is associated with bacterial overgrowth leading to bloating, pseudoobstruction, diarrhea, malabsorption, and steatorrhea. Hypomotility of the colon results in constipation. The combination of hypomotility with bacterial overgrowth can give rise to alternating episodes of constipation and diarrhea. The anorectal area is the second most common GI site to be affected and gives rise to fecal incontinence and rectal prolapse.

In general, the liver is spared in scleroderma; however, a small number of patients with late, limited disease develop primary biliary cirrhosis. This may manifest as pruritus with jaundice and an elevated alkaline phosphatase levels with positive antimitochondrial antibodies (47).

PULMONARY INVOLVEMENT

The lungs are an important target of disease in SSc. Pulmonary involvement is estimated to occur in about 70% of patients and it is the most common cause of mortality in SSc (15). The lungs are affected in two ways: (a) interstitial lung disease leading to pulmonary fibrosis and (b) pulmonary artery hypertension (PAH) (51). Interstitial lung disease can affect both diffuse and limited subsets. Isolated pulmonary hypertension occurs more often in the patient with late, limited disease. Pulmonary symptoms include progressive exertional dyspnea and dry cough, although some patients can be asymptomatic. For this reason, it is important to get pulmonary function tests, high-resolution computerized tomography, and Doppler echocardiograms at baseline, and then every 6 to 12 months during the first few years to document possible pulmonary involvement. Steen et al. (52) have demonstrated that the greatest pulmonary volume loss occurs in the first 2 years of disease. If abnormalities are found, bronchoalveolar lavage can help characterize the inflammatory infiltrate and influence prognostic and therapeutic decisions.

PAH occurs in 35% to 85% of patients with SSc (51). It should be suspected in any patient with late, limited disease who develops dyspnea on exertion. Annual screening echocardiograms are recommended to estimate pulmonary artery pressure. If there is evidence of abnormalities (pressure above 25 mm Hg at rest or 30 mm Hg with exercise), right-heart catheterization is recommended to guide new therapeutic options. PAH is associated with a very poor prognosis, with 2-year survival rates of 40% to 55%.

RENAL INVOLVEMENT

Renal disease from scleroderma renal crisis (SRC) occurs in 10% to 15% of patients with SSc (53). It occurs almost exclusively in the diffuse subset and within the first 4 years of disease (35). It is important to recognize SRC because early intervention (specifically with an angiotensin-converting enzyme [ACE] inhibitor) can be lifesaving. SRC is manifest by acute-onset arterial hypertension and renal insufficiency. Symptoms include headache, blurred vision, and seizures. It is associated with high plasma renin levels. In the past, renal involvement was associated with a poor prognosis. Patients with clinically evident renal disease usually died within 1 year; however, with the advent of ACE inhibitors, survival has improved significantly (54,55).

CARDIAC INVOLVEMENT

Despite the high prevalence of cardiac involvement in autopsy studies (80%), clinically overt manifestations are uncommon (56). If cardiac symptoms are present, the prognosis is worse. Pericarditis, myocarditis, conduction defects, and arrhythmias can occur. Cor pulmonale and right-sided heart failure are usually secondary to PAH. Myocardial fibrosis is a histopathologic hallmark. The fibrosis is patchy and distributed throughout the myocardium, and endothelial damage to small coronary arteries may be present. Raynaud phenomenon precipitated by cold exposure may adversely affect myocardial perfusion (57).

NEUROLOGIC INVOLVEMENT

Neurologic involvement is thought to be rare in SSc (5,15,16). Only 5% of the patients in the original series by Tuffanelli and Winkelmann (5) had neurologic involvement. Central nervous system involvement occurs rarely, if at all. Peripheral nervous system involvement is usually attributed to entrapment syndromes. Trigeminal neuropathies and carpal tunnel syndrome are well described in case reports (58). We have been impressed by the number of patients who present with unexplained paresthesias, dyasthesias, and neuropathic pain, typically in the hands, at the onset of their disease and often, prior to the onset of Raynaud phenomenon. Results of conventional neurophysiologic testing such as nerve conduction studies and electromyography are usually normal. We found that a significant percentage of these patients have abnormalities on quantitative sensory testing (QST) (59). A combination of large-fiber (vibration) and small-fiber (cold threshold detection) testing was abnormal in more than half of the 12 patients in one small study.

Dyshidrosis would implicate autonomic nervous system dysfunction. Sandroni and Connolly (60) found abnormal thermal sweat testing results in six of 10 patients with diffuse SSc. None of the patients reported abnormal sweating in the questionnaires they completed prior to testing. Extensive patchy anhidrosis occurred in proximal nonfibrotic skin and was normal in the hands. The dissociation between sweating and fibrosis is important because it argues against the widely held notion that overproduction of collagen is responsible for eccrine dysfunction. An alternate mechanism for sweat dysfunction must be entertained. There was an association between pruritus and abnormal sweating. Although pruritus is regarded as primary skin irritation caused by immune-mediated IgE receptor cross-linking on mast cells, neurogenic itch can be associated with peripheral and central neuropathies (61). Pruritus is common in patients with SSc early in the disease (15).

GI involvement, as discussed in a preceding section, is common in SSc, and is viewed by some to be neuropathic in origin (47,48,62). Impotence is prevalent among men with SSc (63–65). The presence of postural hypotension (66), anhidrosis (60), alternating diarrhea and constipation, diminished sphincter tone (67), and impotence (63–65) is consistent with autonomic dysfunction in patients with SSc. Whether these symptoms are secondary to microvascular insufficiency and ischemia remains unclear.

Although the combination of the patient's lack of awareness of certain symptoms and the absence of abnormalities on routine neurologic examinations and testing has resulted in the conventional view that the nervous systemic is not involved in SSc, this may not be correct. Nerve testing that is more specialized, such as QST and autonomic testing, has shown abnormal nerve function in a significant percentage of patients with SSc. The relationship of these findings to disease pathogenesis is unknown and larger studies are needed.

DISEASE ASSOCIATIONS

Thyroid disease has been reported in up to one fourth of patients with SSc (15). Most commonly, hypothyroidism and antithyroid antibodies are present. Hashimoto thyroiditis is less common. Xerostomia (dry mouth) and xerophthalmia (dry eyes), or the sicca complex, are seen in 20% to 30% of patients with SSc (15). Sjögren syndrome with positive anti–SS-A (anti-Ro) and anti–SS-B (anti-La and antibodies) and minor salivary gland infiltrates can occur with SSc.

An association of scleroderma with cancer has been reported (15). Cases of breast and lung cancer have been reported (68,69). Initially, it was believed that the lung cancers were alveolar cell carcinomas, but a variety of different cell types has been subsequently identified.

PATHOLOGY AND PATHOGENESIS

Although fibrosis of the internal organs occurs in SSc (15,16), it is not as extensive as often stated. The largest autopsy series, reported by D'Angelo et al. (70) in the late 1960s, found only mild fibrosis. They reported on 58 patients with SSc compared with 58 controls and confirmed the high frequency of skin and internal organ involvement. They noted, however, that the GI tract and skeletal muscle findings was characterized more by atrophy than fibrosis. They concluded that "fibrosis seemed to be present as a replacement for, rather than addition to, the normal muscular tissues of the gastrointestinal tract," and that "scarring represents fibrotic replacement rather than fibrotic proliferation." Goetz (71) reported a similar pattern in the heart, where the heart was smaller than normal and fibrosis had replaced the normal tissue. Investigations into the causes of the underlying tissue atrophy may prove informative

Although well recognized, atrophy in SSc is not well understood. It is regarded as an endproduct of fibrosis and malnutrition. Missing or atrophic tissues in scleroderma skin include: eccrine sweat glands (72), blood vessels (73), vascular smooth muscle (70), and subcutaneous fat (74). Attributing all of these changes to the overproduction of collagen may be a misleading oversimplification.

There are widespread vascular changes in SSc (73,75). Microvascular changes present in the nailfold capillaries and have been characterized as "leaky," giant telangiectasias with avascular areas. The small to medium arteries of the lungs, kidneys, and peripheral vascular system are involved. The findings include concentric intimal proliferation, medial hypertrophy, and adventitial fibrosis. Larger arteries such as the aorta are spared. The central nervous system vasculature is not involved. Coronary artery involvement is not different than the general population. The inflammatory destructive changes of vasculitis are notably absent. The intravascular deposition of clot is not seen.

The dermatopathology of SSc is influenced by the stage of the disease (i.e., edematous, indurated, or atrophic). Although it is generally stated that the pathology cannot differentiate between the different scleroderma subtypes (76), there are some distinguishing features. One of the more obvious differences is the degree of inflammation present in localized scleroderma as compared with SSc (77).

Early in the edematous phase, there is mucoid edema with acid mucopolysaccharide deposition. A sparse mononuclear cell infiltrate occurs primarily around the small capillaries, at the interface between the dermis and subcutaneous tissue, and in the adipose tissue (77). The infiltrate consists of lymphocytes, plasma cells, monocytes, and macrophages.

Later in the sclerotic phase, homogenous, hyalinized bundles of collagen are seen in the dermis and subcutaneous tissue. There is atrophy of the appendages. The eccrine sweat glands appear atrophic and become surrounded by a fibrous collagenous matrix. The subcutaneous fat is markedly decreased or absent. The inflammatory infiltrate around the blood vessels decreases. The elastic fibers are preserved. Results of direct immunofluorescence testing are usually negative in SSc (73,78). Electron microscopy reveals thin irregular collagen fibrils present in the early stages of the disease (74).

LABORATORY STUDIES

The diagnosis of SSc is primarily clinical. Nonetheless, laboratory studies are used to evaluate internal organ involvement, and to determine the disease subset and prognosis. Typically, complete blood cell counts and complement levels are normal. Anemia should be evaluated. Creatinine and blood urea nitrogen levels and urine analysis must be determined to evaluate for the presence of renal insufficiency. Creatine kinase levels should be monitored intermittently for the presence of myositis. Approximately 25% of patients have evidence of hypergammaglobulinemia without a monoclonal spike (16). Approximately one third of patients have low-positive rheumatoid factors. Elevated sedimentation rates may indicate interstitial lung disease with active alveolitis and are associated with a worse prognosis.

Ninety percent of patients with SSc have positive antinuclear antibodies (ANA). Speckled and nucleolar patterns are somewhat specific for scleroderma. In addition to a positive ANA, a significant proportion of patients will have disease-specific autoantibodies (79). The anti–topoisomerase I antibodies (also called Scl-70) are found in approximately 20% to 30% of the diffuse subset and are associated with a higher risk for pulmonary disease (80). In contrast, about 40% to 50% of patients with limited disease have positive anticentromere autoantibodies (81). There is a high degree of fidelity of the autoantibodies with these subsets: the anti–topoisomerase I antibodies do not occur in the limited subset and the anticentromere antibodies do not occur in the diffuse subset. Autoantibodies reported in patients with SSc are listed in Table 4.4. Despite these important associations, a significant number of patients will have neither of these autoantibodies.

DIFFERENTIAL DIAGNOSIS

Once the characteristic cutaneous fibrosis ("scleroderma") is evident, the diagnosis of SSc is relatively straightforward. In the early stage, edema of the hands can resemble rheumatoid arthritis, systemic lupus erythematosus, or mixed connective tissue disease. Distinguishing features of SSc include the typically cool edema that is not restricted to the joints. Some patients may have numbness and tingling in their hands that suggest carpal tunnel syndrome.

TABLE 4.4. Systemic Sclerosis Autoantibodies

Limited subset
Anticentromere
Anti-Th
Diffuse subset
Anti-DNA-topoisomerase I (Scl-70)
Anti-RNA polymerase I, III
U_3-RNP (fibrillarin)
Overlap
U_1-RNP
PM-Scl

An important differential diagnosis is between primary and secondary *Raynaud phenomenon* (82). This differential is particularly relevant when considering the patient with limited disease who may present with a long prodrome of Raynaud phenomenon in the absence of other obvious disease manifestations. Primary Raynaud phenomenon (formerly called Raynaud disease) occurs in the absence of an associated disease. These patients are generally younger (teens and 20s) and do not have tissue changes or positive autoantibody serologies. In contrast, secondary Raynaud phenomenon is associated with an underlying disease and tends to affect older individuals (those in their 30s and 40s). The list of secondary causes of Raynaud phenomenon goes beyond the scope of this chapter (reviewed by Wigley [82]). In the case of SSc, nailfold capillary examination, autoantibodies, and an elevated erythrocyte sedimentation rates are helpful in identifying SSc. If a patient with Raynaud phenomenon has a normal examination and laboratory results for 2 years, he or she is regarded as having primary Raynaud phenomenon and a low risk for subsequently developing a connective tissue disease.

The localized forms of scleroderma, including *morphea, generalized morphea, linear scleroderma, and eosinophilic fasciitis* are rarely confused with SSc. For the most part, these entities are readily distinguished from SSc by the focal nature of their lesions together with the absence of systemic symptoms and Raynaud phenomenon. Nonetheless, occasional confusion arises in cases of generalized morphea. In generalized morphea, lesions usually occur first on the trunk and then move peripherally. In contrast, in SSc lesions usually occur first on the hands and then move centrally. A significant percentage (from 50% to 100%) of patients with localized scleroderma has positive ANA (83,84); therefore, serologies alone cannot differentiate localized scleroderma from SSc. Furthermore, the nuclear staining can include diffuse, speckled, and nucleolar patterns similar to those seen in SSc. In one study, one child of 27 tested positive for the anti–Scl-70 antibody (84). These shared serologic features might suggest some shared pathogenic mechanisms between the localized and systemic forms of this disease.

Sclerodermoid Conditions

There are a number of sclerodermoid conditions (also referred to as pseudoscleroderma or scleroderma-like disorders) that mimic the fibrotic skin changes seen in SSc. These disorders are listed in Table 4.1 and only a few will be reviewed here.

Scleredema is classified as a cutaneous mucinosis and exists in three distinct forms: acute, chronic, and chronic associated with diabetes (85,86). The classic scleredema of Buschke occurs after a febrile respiratory infection and presents as rapid onset of nonpitting edema in the skin of the face, nape of the neck, upper back, shoulders, and chest. The acral areas are spared and Raynaud phenomenon is absent. Most will have rapid, spontaneous, resolution of edema. Another group will resolve over 1 to 2 years, and a final group will have chronic lesions. There is an association with diabetes and insulin resistance. There is also an association with a monoclonal gammapathy, typically IgG κ or λ.

Digital sclerosis of diabetes mellitus is a distinct fibrotic disorder, typically found in patients with juvenile onset diabetes. Joint contractures accompanied by fibrotic skin changes are found in one third of patients with juvenile diabetes with long-standing disease (10). Some patients respond to tighter glucose control with an insulin pump.

Papular mucinosis (synonymous with *lichen myxedematosus*) presents as 2- to 3-mm, firm, dermal papules, which on biopsy show mucin in the upper dermis, associated with a paraproteinemia, typically IgG λ light chains (87). The dorsal aspect of the hands, arms, axillae, and face are the most commonly involved sites. *Scleromyxedema* is a variant of papular mucinosis. Skin changes are generalized and sometimes erythematous. In contrast to SSc, where the skin is tight and tethered, scleromyxedema is characterized by firm skin that remains loose, often with accentuated skin folds. Involvement of the hands can occur with flexion contractures and sclerodactyly that mimic SSc (without Raynaud phenomenon) (10). A spectrum of neurologic complications can occur (88). A newly recognized association with renal transplantation and hemodialysis has been described (89,90). Treatment with immunosuppression may be beneficial.

Chronic graft versus host disease (GVHD) has a fibrotic skin component that can resemble SSc. One study reported that six long-term bone marrow transplantation survivors developed a syndrome similar to SSc (91). Cutaneous involvement, pulmonary disease, muscular involvement, keratoconjunctivitis, positive Schirmer test, Raynaud phenomenon, and cardiac disease were similar to findings in patients with SSc.

Fibrotic skin lesions can occur with ***paraneoplastic syndromes***. Sclerodermoid cutaneous lesions seen in association with ***carcinoid syndrome*** may be mediated by serotonin. A patient with metastatic melanoma developed sclerodactyly, contractions of the fingers and thickening of the skin of the hands (92). This patient did not have Raynaud phenomenon. The association of palmar fasciitis and ovarian carcinoma of the ovary has been reported (93). Another patient with arthritis and palmar fasciitis was reported with small cell carcinoma. We have seen similar patients with bronchoalveolar carcinoma (Fig. 4.17).

Patients with spinal cord injuries have been described with brawny induration of the skin and dermal fibrosis (94). The authors suggested that spinal cord injury with autonomic hyperreflexia may be associated with dermal fibrosis, establishing a scleroderma variant.

The role of trauma and immobilization and fibrotic skin reactions has been raised. Varga and Jimenez (95) reported on the development of exaggerated cutaneous fibrosis in a limb of patients with Raynaud phenomenon after immobilization by cast or secondary to trauma.

MANAGEMENT

Treatment of SSc is challenging. Despite the lack of definitive therapies, or in the parlance of rheumatic therapy, "disease modifying antirheumatic drugs," management of affected individual organ systems is improving. Survival rates are improving and this trend probably reflects a combination of earlier diagnosis together with improved supportive therapy (15,16). Although true disease remissions are rare, disease stabilization can occur and patients can live long, productive lives with this disease.

The list of drugs that have been tried and failed in scleroderma is long and fills many chapters (96,97). Drugs or procedures that have been found to be of little or no use in SSc include aminocaproic acid, *N*-acetylcysteine, chorambucil, colchicine, cyclofenil, dimethyl sulfoxide, dipyridamole, EDTA, 5-flurouracil, griseofulvin, ketanserin, ketotifen, penicillin, photopheresis, potassium aminobenzoate, novocaine, relaxin, stanazol, sympathectomy, total lymphoid radiation, and vitamin E. Drugs for which there is ongoing controversy regarding efficacy include D-penicillamine, methotrexate, and minocycline. Uncertainties regarding the underlying pathogenesis of SSc seem directly related to the numbers of experimental strategies.

Clinical trials in patients with SSc are challenging. An agent that works in early disease may not be effective in late disease. An agent that works in one organ system may not be effective in others. Ideally, randomized, placebo-controlled, double-blind trials should be done. There is an ongoing need for better primary and secondary outcome measures. The gold standard of survival rates has become impractical, given a background survival of 85% at 5 years. Studies would have to be very large and patients followed up for many years to observe significant differences. The cost of this type of study would be prohibitive. Guidelines for clinical trials in SSc have been published (98). The recommendations include use of patients with early disease (<2 years) in the diffuse subset. Treatment intervention should be for at least 18 to 36 months and a variety of internal organ involvement and skin scores should be monitored. A scleroderma health assessment questionnaire score has been validated. A "scleroderma disease activity index" with a severity score of 0 to 4 is being developed that follows nine different organ systems (99). These types of validated instruments will greatly facilitate the study of drug therapy in SSc.

Supportive Therapy

PATIENT EDUCATION

Given the extraordinary challenges that every patient with SSc faces, early patient education is essential. A variety of excellent resources are available. The Scleroderma Foundation (1-800-422-1113 or www.scleroderma.org) is a good starting point. The Scleroderma Research Foundation (1-800-441-CURE or

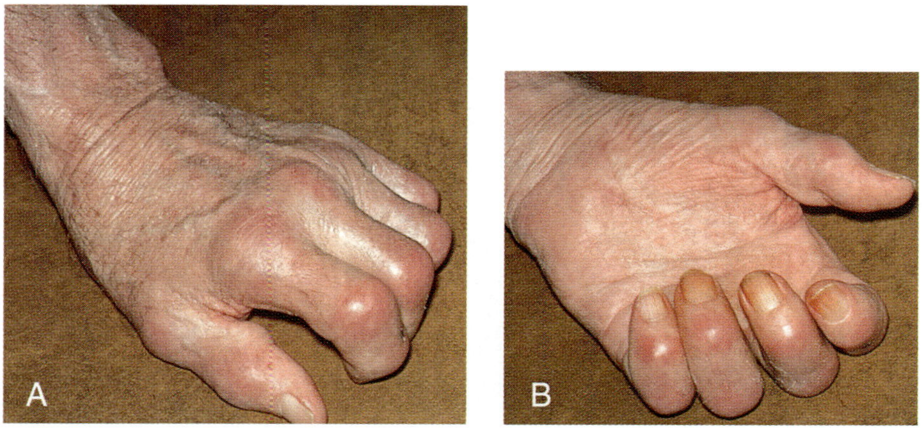

Figure 4.17. Sclerodactyly and palmar fasciitis in a patient with bronchoalveolar carcinoma.

www.srfcure.org) has an emphasis on raising funds for research. The University of California at San Francisco is developing a database and tissue bank collection (information can be downloaded online at www.dermatology.ucsf.edu/autoimmune/). Patients should be encouraged to participate in clinical trials and research programs whenever feasible. The Scleroderma Clinical Trials Consortium is an international group of physicians and medical institutions interested in therapeutic trials in scleroderma. Their website (www.sctc-online.org) lists the different ongoing trials and the contact information at different sites.

WARM ENVIRONMENT

Cold exposure induces Raynaud phenomenon and increases the incidence of digital ulcerations. Patients are advised to keep their total bodies warm. Dressing in warm clothing in layers including the trunk, head and hands is helpful. Heat therapy (putting the patient in hot room for 3 to 5 hours daily) has been advocated. An occupational history may reveal exposures at work that need to be altered. Some patients may choose to move to a warmer climate, however, problems with air conditioning may arise. Other stimuli that precipitate vasospastic reactions, including smoking, caffeine, and emotional stress, should be minimized. Beta-blockers can aggravate Raynaud phenomenon and should be avoided.

PHYSICAL THERAPY

This is useful in selected patients and can include warm whirlpool baths, hot water baths, and molten paraffin applications to the hands. Range-of-motion exercises are helpful for maintaining flexibility and minimizing joint contractures. Graduated muscle exercises may be beneficial. In certain patients, biofeedback can work. Massage can help the skin feel more supple and pliable.

TOPICAL THERAPY

Topical therapies provide adjunct support and increase patient comfort. Liberal and frequent application of emollients to keep the skin lubricated to minimize xerosis, cracking, and pruritus is helpful. For more intense pruritus, a course of topical corticosteroids can help. Ultrapotent class I topical steroids in an ointment formulation can be very helpful for the hands or a focal area twice a day with occlusion at bedtime for 2-week intervals (and then rotated off for 2-week intervals). Alternatively, for more generalized pruritus, application of Pramosone lotion 2.5%, with both topical anesthetic and a mild topical steroid, can be tried. Minor cuts and abrasions can be treated with topical antibiotics. Mupirocin (Bactroban) or MetroGel (flagyl) can be used for digital ulcers. Topical nitroglycerin ointment may improve local blood flow and can be used around an ulcer or a preulcer.

Systemic Medications

VASOACTIVE AGENTS

Calcium channel blockers are the mainstay of therapy for Raynaud phenomenon and should be used in all patients able to tolerate them (100). Nifedipine 10 to 30 mg three to four times daily is one regimen. Slow-release preparations (such as Procardia XL, 30 to 90 mg once daily) have been advocated because of convenience and the ability to increase the dose with fewer side effects (16). Amlodipine (Norvasc, 5 to 10 mg daily) is a newer calcium channel blocker that is better tolerated and can be given once a day. Side effects include flushing, headaches, and ankle edema. Calcium channel blockers may aggravate esophageal reflux, and this needs to be monitored. Other calcium channel blockers such as verapamil and diltiazem are not as effective for secondary Raynaud phenomenon. It is important to advise patients that they may not get complete resolution of their Raynaud attacks, but can still benefit from the medication.

For more severe symptoms including ischemic tissue changes and digital ulceration, additional agents can be added. If systemic blood pressure remain adequate, combination therapy may offer benefit. Prazosin (Minipress, 1 to 10 mg twice daily) can be added. One study found that the ACE inhibitor, losartan (Cozaar), 50 mg daily, was more effective than nifedipine, 40 mg daily, in treating secondary Raynaud phenomenon (101). Prostaglandins such as epoprostenol (Flolan) and iloprost can be effective in the short term. Although the intravenous form of iloprost was effective, the oral form was not (102). A new endothelin receptor antagonist, bosentan (Tracleer), has been shown to be effective in pulmonary arterial hypertension (103) and has shown some promising preliminary results in treating digital ulcerations. Other agents that theoretically improve blood flow (or minimize clot) such as aspirin 81 mg daily may be advisable (104). Pentoxifyline (Trental), 400 mg three times a day, can be tried, although formal studies demonstrating its benefit are lacking.

IMMUNOSUPPRESSIVES

Although immunosuppressive therapy may be effective for active alveolitis (see pulmonary section later) and myositis, it has been disappointing for overall disease control and survival. A well-designed randomized, placebo-controlled trial of chlorambucil for 3 years failed to show an improvement in several outcome measures or survival (105). A smaller study looking at 5-fluorouracil did not show a benefit (106). These studies have been criticized for studying patients with advanced disease (7 and 5 years, respectively). Cyclosporine showed some skin softening in an open-label trial of 10 patients; however, its use was limited by renal toxicity (107). Methotrexate treatment for 1 year in a randomized controlled trial failed to show significant differences in skin scores, physician global assessments, and DLCOs in patients with early diffuse SSc (108).

CORTICOSTEROIDS

The use of systemic glucocorticosteroids predisposes patients to an increased risk for scleroderma renal crisis (109,110) and should be used with caution. In select cases, systemic corticosteroids may be tried with close observation (such as twice-weekly blood pressure checks). Low-dose prednisone (< 10 mg daily) may be helpful for arthralgias and myalgias. Moderate-doses of prednisone 40 mg daily for polymyositis or interstitial lung disease with active alveolitis may be warranted.

This disappointing track record of immunosuppressive and antiinflammatory therapy in SSc needs to be acknowledged. SSc is different from other autoimmune diseases, including systemic lupus erythematosus, dermatomyositis/polymyositis, or rheumatoid arthritis, in this regard. Therapies that work in those disorders have not worked in SSc and vice versa. The scientific basis for this difference is not known, but the clinical reality is clear. Immune-mediated damage may occur early in scleroderma, setting the stage for downstream tissue damage that is then either irreversible or unresponsive to subsequent immunosuppression. Whatever the explanation, it is important to consider this so that patients are not subjected to increasingly dangerous regimens that ultimately prove ineffective. High-dose ablative immunosuppressive therapies with stem cell rescue or bone marrow transplantation are currently being studied in patients with severe SSc (111,112). These interventions have significant mortality rates and need to be studied carefully in double-blind, placebo-controlled trials.

ANTIFIBROTICS

Numerous agents have been tried with disappointing results. On the basis of earlier case studies and retrospective analyses, D-penicillamine has been advocated as softening skin, reducing new-onset visceral involvement, and improving survival (113). Others, however, have not been impressed with its clinical utility. In 1999, a randomized controlled trial, comparing low-dose (125 mg every other day) to high-dose (750 to 1,000 mg every day) D-penicillamine, in 134 patients with early, diffuse SSc over 2 years failed to identify any significance difference in outcome measures between the two groups (114). The high-dose group experienced increased toxicity. Although this trial was designed to definitively answer the question of D-penicillamine utility in SSc, the controversy continues. Those who think the drug *does not* work, argue that the data support that conclusion (115). Those who think the drug *does* work, argue the data support that conclusion (116). Given the refractory nature of this disease, and in the absence of better information, D-penicillamine should be considered on a case-by-case basis. If there is not clinically evident internal organ involvement, and the patient has rapidly progressive cutaneous involvement, D-penicillamine can be used in lower doses. Side effects include hematologic abnormalities and induction of autoimmune disorders, myopathy, proteinuria, and renal failure.

Interest in interferon-gamma (IFN-γ) as an antifibrotic agent comes from studies showing decreased collagen production in fibroblasts *in vitro*. In addition, a small trial in idiopathic pulmonary fibrosis showed improvement in the IFN-γ group (117). Nonetheless, experience in SSc has not been encouraging. Three small pilot studies showed improvement in skin scores, however, there were also new-onset renal disease (118), worsening Raynaud phenomenon (119), and decreased quality of life (120). A fourth study did not find improved skin scores or decreased collagen I messenger RNA synthesis (121). Interferon-alpha (IFN-α) has also been tried in SSc (122). That trial reported a decrease in pulmonary function tests and three deaths in the treated group and was stopped early. Taken together, these results suggest at best a modest benefit with significant toxicity for interferons in SSc.

Minocycline has antiinflammatory properties in addition to antimicrobial properties and has been evaluated in patients with rheumatoid arthritis. A small pilot study in SSc showed skin softening; however, three patients experienced new-onset renal crisis, suggesting that it is not protective for the vascular effects (123). Thalidomide has also been reported to result in skin softening in some patients with SSc (124).

EXPERIMENTAL THERAPIES

There is a limited experience with the biologics, such as etanercept and infliximab, in SSc. Concern over inducing a lupus-like syndrome has been raised. Halofuginone is an anticoccidioidal agent used in chickens. Some chickens developed weakened skin with increased skin tearing while on this agent. Although several animal models have shown promising results, human trials have not been published. A topical preparation is being investigated in chronic GVHD and may show utility in scleroderma. Oral tolerance to collagen I is under study in SSc. Phototherapy is another approach under investigation for both localized scleroderma and the cutaneous fibrosis component of SSc (125).

The most novel antifibrotic trials involve monoclonal antibody therapy against growth factors known to be active in fibrosis. Phase 1 anti-transforming growth factor (TGF)-β trials are currently in progress.

Organ-Specific Treatment

CUTANEOUS INVOLVEMENT

After fibrosis (see antifibrotics section), the next most troubling symptom is often intense *pruritus* in the first 1 or 2 years of disease. Pruritus can be managed topically with emollients and topical corticosteroids (see topical section). The addition of a systemic antihistamine (nonsedating during the day) and doxepin 10 to 50 mg at bedtime can provide relief.

CALCINOSIS CUTIS

There is no systemic therapy of proven value for calcinosis cutis. Early reports suggested a favorable effect of the calcium channel blocker, diltiazem (126,127); however, this finding was not confirmed in a later study (128). Particularly large and troublesome deposits can be excised surgically.

RAYNAUD PHENOMENON

See vasodilation section.

DIGITAL ULCERATIONS

The end-stage complication of vascular insufficiency is a digital ulceration. Every effort to prevent digital ulceration should be used, including putting the patient on disability. All the strategies used in Raynaud phenomenon should be used, including the use of a calcium channel blocker. The art of protecting the digit from external trauma and cold without compromising blood flow should be used. Mittens are preferable to gloves. A variety of warming devices are available that can be inserted into the mitten. Soaking the hand in warm water for 20 minutes followed by the application of MetroGel to the wound bed, DuoDerm, and loose paper tape is one regimen that works. This cycle can be repeated every few days. Application of becaplermin gel (Regranex) may also help.

Intravenous prostaglandins can help for severe ulcerations, gangrene, and threatened digit loss. There is preliminary evidence that bosentan (Tracleer) may be effective for digital ulceration. Sympathectomies either central or peripheral may be useful in select cases with select surgeons. The problem with sympathectomies is that the results are rarely long-lived and patients have a recurrence of symptoms. Rarely, surgery is required usually because of intractable pain.

When ulcers occur on the lower extremities, do not assume they are entirely due to SSc. Venous and arterial insufficiency ulcers occur in this population and they should be evaluated with noninvasive vascular studies. Underlying venous insufficiency can be managed in patients with SSc with good results.

JOINTS

Salicylates and nonsteroidal antiinflammatory drugs are first-line therapy for arthralgias. Acetaminophen can be used alone or in combination with other pain medication. Occasionally, low-dose prednisone (< 10 mg daily) can provide relief and assist with mobility. Although the methotrexate trial did not show a significant improvement in patients with early SSc (108), there may be a subset of patients with features of rheumatoid arthritis or polymyositis who do respond. Physical therapy with range-of-motion exercises can be helpful in minimizing joint contractures, particularly at the wrists and fingers. In a rare patient, reconstructive hand surgery by an experienced surgeon may restore partial function.

MUSCLES

For patients with a polymyositis variant, including elevated creatine kinase level and characteristic electromyelogram findings, treatment with methotrexate 15 to 25 mg weekly and low-dose prednisone daily or every other day, can be effective.

Unfortunately, for the larger group of patients who have the bland myopathy of scleroderma, antiinflammatory drugs are not effective. Overall, general supportive therapy with physical therapy, gentle daily exercise, good nutrition, and pain control may help.

PAIN

In addition to classic inflammatory joint and muscle pain, patients with SSc often experience neuropathic pain. Neuropathic pain can be described as sharp, shooting, and lancinating or characterized by numbness and tingling. It may occur at night and be refractory to standard pain medications. Amitriptyline (Elavil) 10 to 50 mg at bedtime can be helpful. If the amitriptyline is not effective, gabapentin (Neurontin) may help (59).

GASTROINTESTINAL INVOLVEMENT

Frequent small meals, no eating or drinking 2 to 3 hours before lying down, and raising the head of the bed to prevent gastric regurgitation are useful behavioral interventions. A number of different antacid regimens can be used, including antacids and H2 blockers. Proton-pump inhibitors (such as omeprazole) have proven particularly effective to minimize GERD and, ultimately, to prevent esophageal strictures. Prokinetic agents can be helpful in aiding peristalsis and digestion. Metoclopramide (Reglan) or low-dose erythromycin (250 mg daily) can be helpful. Cisapride (Propulsid) is an effective prokinetic agent; however, it was taken off the market because of drug interactions that led to fatal adverse events. A newer serotonin receptor agonist, prucalopride, is under investigation (129). For severe small-bowel stasis, an injectable somatostatin agonist, octreotide can be used at bedtime (130). Bowel stasis results in bacterial overgrowth, which can lead to intermittent diarrhea and malabsorption. It is best treated with rotational broad-spectrum antibiotics. Rectal prolapse and fecal incontinence are manifestations of long-standing disease that can be very difficult to treat either medically or surgically. Nutritional support is important. In severe cases, total parenteral nutrition may be indicated.

PULMONARY INVOLVEMENT

Several studies have shown that cyclophosphamide (Cytoxan) may be effective in treating interstitial lung disease in patients with SSc (131–135). Both daily oral and monthly intravenous cyclophosphamide regimens have been used, and it is not clear if one regimen has an advantage over the other. A multicenter, randomized, prospective study comparing oral cyclophosphamide (2 mg/kg/day) to placebo for 1 year is under way. Side effects of cyclophosphamide are significant and require close monitoring. Cytopenias, infections, hemorrhagic cystitis, sterility, and increased risk for long-term malignancies are concerns. The concurrent use of systemic corticosteroids is controversial. They are used for idiopathic interstitial lung disease. Nonetheless, there is concern about precipitating SRC with these agents in patients with SSc. For this reason, modified regimens using lower doses of systemic corticosteroids have been proposed (such as prednisone 0.5 mg/kg every other day for 1 month and then taper off over 2 months). Substitution of other immunosuppressive agents such as azathioprine (Imuran) or mycophenolate mofetil (CellCept) may be possible.

PULMONARY ARTERY HYPERTENSION

PAH should be suspected in any patient with SSc who develops dyspnea on exertion. Patients should be referred to centers with experience managing PAH. Calcium channel blockers can be effective in mild disease or in combinations in some patients and should be initiated. Anticoagulation should be considered. There are three Food and Drug Administration–approved drugs for the treatment of PAH: epoprostenol (Flolan), bosentan (Tracleer), and treprostinil (Remodulin). There are some differences between the drugs, the most obvious of which is that only bosentan can be taken orally (103). This new therapy represents excellent progress in the treatment of a life-threatening complication of this disease. Whether this benefit will generalize to other organs and translate into improved overall survival remains to be seen.

Lung transplantation is an option for patients with SSc. Their survival rates are comparable to the group as a whole.

Aspiration pneumonia can complicate pulmonary problems in patients with SSc. Interventions to prevent aspiration pneumonia should be initiated and treated with antibiotics where appropriate.

RENAL INVOLVEMENT

Prior to the availability of ACE inhibitor therapy, *scleroderma renal crisis* was the most common cause of death among patients with scleroderma (54,55). It is important to educate patients about this potential complication and where appropriate teach them to check their own blood pressure. New-onset hypertension in a patient with scleroderma should be taken very seriously. In general, patients with scleroderma run low blood pressures; therefore, even relatively modest increases may implicate an impending crisis and should be treated. The treatment of choice is a short-acting ACE inhibitor such as captopril. Start at 6.25 to 12.5 mg every 8 hours and increase to maximum of 100 mg three times a day over a 72-hour period. If blood pressure control has not been achieved, add a calcium channel blocker. It is important to continue the ACE inhibitor along with other antihypertensives even after the patient goes on to dialysis. About half of the patients who go onto dialysis will eventually recover renal function and be able to discontinue dialysis (55). There is some concern that the newer angiotensin receptor antagonists may not be as effective in preventing SRC. Kidney transplants can be performed in patients with scleroderma.

CARDIAC INVOLVEMENT

Treatment guidelines for cardiac disease are the same as those for all cardiac patients (56). Atherosclerotic coronary artery disease does not appear to be a significant risk for patients with SSc. Nonetheless, they do get vasospasm of the coronary arteries that can be treated with vasodilators, either ACE inhibitors or calcium channel blockers. For pericarditis that is not hemodynamically significant, nonsteroidal antiinflammatory drugs can be tried. Rarely, and with close follow up, prednisone can be used. Pericardiocenteses is indicated for hemodynamically significant pericardial effusions. Arrhythmias are managed the same as for any cardiac patient.

NATURAL HISTORY AND PROGNOSIS

There is a wide-spectrum of clinical variability and severity in the disease in patients with SSc. At one end of the spectrum, a patient may have a relatively benign course characterized by Raynaud phenomenon, sclerodactyly, and dyspepsia for many years. At the other extreme, a patient may have a rapidly progressive course with internal organ involvement and death within a few years despite aggressive therapy. Where any one patient will fall on this spectrum is difficult to predict. Nonetheless, there are certain features that portend a worse prognosis. These features include older age at disease onset, male sex, black or Native American race, the diffuse subset, skin thickening involving the trunk, visceral involvement at time of diagnosis, elevated erythrocyte sedimentation rate, and anemia (15,16).

In their 1962 study, Tuffanelli and Winkelmann (5) reported a 5-year survival rate of 70% and a 10-year survival rate of 59%. More recently, Medsger (15) reported a 5-year survival rate of 80% in the diffuse subset and 90% in the limited subset and 10-year survival of 68% in the diffuse subset and 78% in the limited subset. These numbers reflect an improvement in survival over the past few decades.

ETIOLOGIC FACTORS AND PATHOGENESIS

Environmental Agents

Most diseases reflect a combination of environmental and genetic factors. Environmental factors and occupational exposures have received considerable attention in SSc. Environmental agents and drugs that have been reported to induce scleroderma are listed in Table 4.1. Scleroderma-like conditions can be induced by polyvinyl chloride, organic solvents, silica dust, toxic oil syndrome, polyvinyl chloride, and L-tryptophan (136,137). Recent epidemiologic studies and meta-analyses, however, have called into question the strength of some of these presumed environmental associations (138,139).

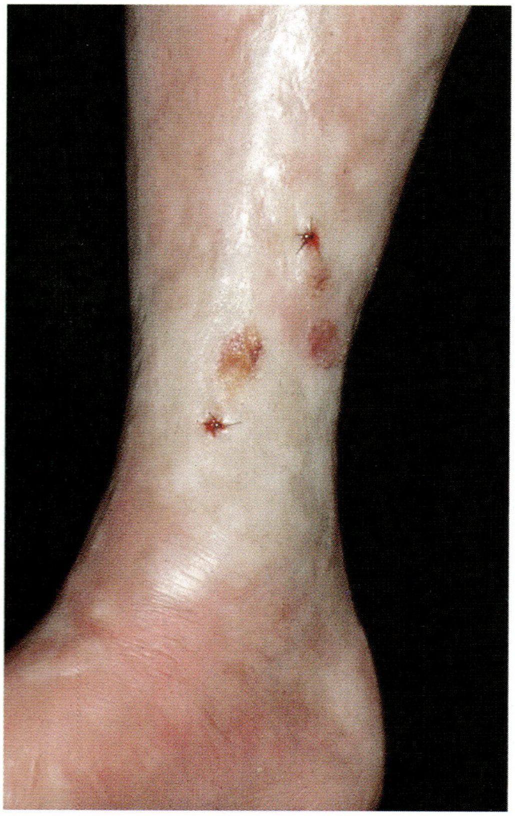

Figure 4.18. Scleroderma. Lesion on the leg secondary to L-tryptophan ingestion.

The Spanish toxic oil syndrome began in 1981. Contaminated cooking oil containing industrial-grade rapeseed oil that was known to be toxic was sold illegally. The outbreak affected over 20,000 people and more than 800 died (140). Initially, the patients developed malaise, fever, pulmonary edema, and GI symptoms, with marked eosinophilia. The illness progressed in approximately 30% of patients to include a scleroderma-like disease. Cutaneous sclerosis usually involved the arms and legs, and occasionally the hands. Severe neuropathy and pulmonary hypertension were late symptoms.

Eosinophilia myalgia syndrome (EMS) secondary to L-tryptophan occurred in 1989 (141). The patients ingested a certain brand of L-tryptophan, produced by Showa-Denka, a Japanese corporation. Ultimately, over 1,600 cases of eosinophilia myalgia syndrome were reported. One third required hospitalization and 27 died. Early signs of the EMS included severe myalgias, rash, edema, fever, respiratory illness, and an eosinophil count greater than 1,000/mm^3. Late problems included weight loss, muscle weakness, paresthesias, sclerodermoid cutaneous lesions, xerostomia, and hair loss (142). Clinically, the sclerodermoid features of EMS resemble morphea or eosinophilic fasciitis (Fig. 4.18).

The cause of the epidemic is still unknown. Initially, a contaminant in L-tryptophan was suspected, however, no contaminant was ever identified. Subsequently, a dimer of L-tryptophan was implicated. Because only a few individuals who ingested the L-tryptophan developed the syndrome, host susceptibility factors have been considered. One possibility is individual variation in tryptophan metabolism. Abnormal tryptophan metabolism in patients with SSc had been suspected long before the EMS outbreak. The "matoke"-eating natives of East Africa have a diet rich in tryptophan (bananas and plantains), have increased urinary hydroxyindole acetic acid levels, and develop a scleroderma-like syndrome. Carcinoid patients have increased urinary hydroxyindole acetic acid levels and develop skin induration with proximal fibrosis. Tuffanelli (143) did not find abnormal urinary hydroxyindole acetic acid excretion in patients with scleroderma. Jablonska and Blaszczyk (10) found elevated tryptamine/indoleacetic acid ratios in patients with scleroderma and in patients with phenylketonuria.

Phenylketonuria is an inborn error of metabolism that results from a mutation in phenylalanine hydroxylase gene or its cofactors (e.g., dihydrobiopterin). The principle phenotype is mental retardation and pigment dilution; however, fibrotic skin changes resembling scleroderma are often seen (144). Treatment with a low phenylalanine diet early in life can prevent and even reverse the fibrotic skin changes (10).

A role for dietary factors in idiopathic SSc has not been identified. It seems unlikely that a metabolic defect could explain idiopathic SSc. The relatively late onset (mean age, 45 years) would argue against an inborn error in metabolism. Furthermore, the lack of a heritable trait in the offspring makes a single spontaneous mutation unlikely. Nonetheless, perhaps patients with scleroderma have more than one genetic defect (thereby obscuring classic Mendelian inheritance patterns and making extended family pedigrees virtually unknown), involving the metabolism of some noncritical amino acid, cofactor, or other substrate. In that case, it may be that early in life, there is no discernible phenotype, but after a lifetime exposure to a particular diet, amino acid, or toxin, they manifest the phenotype. Although this seems farfetched, and the tools available to test these hypotheses are limited, in the absence of better explanations for this complex disease, it seems reasonable to leave it on the list of possible etiologic factors.

One of the more interesting stories of the intersection of environment, society, and disease involved silicone breast implants and scleroderma. This story, and the medical and legal debates that ensued, is the basis of a book entitled "Science on Trial: The Clash of Medical Evidence and the Law in the Breast Implant Case," published in 1997 by Dr. Marcia Angell (145). Angell was editor-in-chief of the *New England Journal of Medicine* when these events took place.

Augmentation mammoplasty with silicone implants was once thought to be a risk factor for scleroderma on the basis of case reports and small series (146–150). Despite these early studies, several subsequent large, well-designed, controlled epidemiologic studies consistently failed to find any link between scleroderma, or any other connective tissue diseases, and silicone breast implants (151–153). Admittedly, the impetus and funding for these large studies came from silicone breast manufacturers, plastic surgeons, and trial lawyers: all parties with a vested interest in the outcome. Nonetheless, they acknowledged this conflict of interest, and the funds were given to independent academic institutions (e.g., the Harvard School of Public Health) and the results published in the *New England Journal of Medicine*. The outcome of this story should serve as a cautionary tale not to jump to conclusions on the basis of small series and chance associations.

Infectious agents have been proposed as potential environmental triggers for SSc for many years; however, definitive data to support this idea are lacking. Although there have been numerous articles demonstrating *Borrelia* species as the possible etiology of morphea in Europe, demonstration of this association in the United States is lacking (154).

Latent cytomegalovirus infection as a possible cause of the vascular abnormalities in SSc has been suggested (155). Cross-reacting cytomegalovirus antibodies present in some patients with SSc can induce endothelial cell apoptosis (156). It is intriguing to consider a vasotrophic pathogen in SSc; however, larger studies will be needed to prove this connection.

Drug-Induced Scleroderma

A few drugs have been associated with the induction of scleroderma-like disease. These are listed in Table 4.1. Sclerodermatous skin lesions, Raynaud phenomenon, and sclerodactyly were observed following systemic bleomycin therapy (157). Intralesional bleomycin for wart therapy has been associated with digital vasoconstrictions, Raynaud phenomenon, and cutaneous sclerosis. Amphetamines have been associated with SSc. There are at least three case reports of patients who developed scleroderma-like illness associated with the ingestion of hydroxytryptophan and carbidopa (158,159). Drugs such as phytonadione (vitamin K) (160), valproate sodium (161), and bromocriptine (162) have also been associated with cutaneous sclerosis.

Radiation-Induced Scleroderma

Patients with SSc may have an increased sensitivity to radiation therapy (15). There are several reports of radiation inducing exaggerated cutaneous fibrosis in patients with SSc (163,164). Varga et al. (165) reported on four patients with stable SSc and limited skin involvement who received radiation for the treatment of solid malignant neoplasms. Following local radiation, each patient developed an exaggerated cutaneous and internal organ fibrotic reaction. The surface areas of fibrosis extended beyond the radiation portals. Four cases of pseudosclerodermatous panniculitis developed after megavoltage radiation of breast carcinoma (166). We have seen a patient develop generalized morphea following radiation therapy for breast carcinoma. Patients with SSc should be advised of this potential response when considering radiation therapy. This sensitivity to radiation may be responsible for the increased toxicities seen in patients undergoing bone marrow or stem cell therapy, where radiation is used as part of the conditioning regimen.

Genetics

From a traditional standpoint, the contribution to scleroderma from genetics is weak. Most cases occur sporadically without a positive family history. Nonetheless, familial cases occur at a frequency of 1.5% (167). Although this is a small number, when compared with the expected frequency in the population at large (0.026%), the relative risk is significant. Similarly, concordant rates among monozygotic twins are higher than dizygotic twins (168). Studies on twins have been hindered by a paucity of cases. An increased prevalence of SSc has been reported among the southeastern Oklahoma Choctaw Indians (169,170). Studies show an association with a region on chromosome 15q that could implicate the fibrillin-1 gene. Studying the Choctaw population may serve as a model for the interaction between environmental and genetic factors in scleroderma. Although there are some human lymphocyte antigen (HLA) associations with various subsets, HLA associations are weak for the group as a whole.

In the absence of convincing genetic and environmental underpinnings for most patients with SSc, attention has turned to hypotheses that might account for the pathologic findings. Hypotheses regarding the pathogenesis of SSc focus on three areas: the vascular system, the immune system, and the extracellular matrix (16,171). A significant number of abnormalities have been reported in each of these areas in patients with SSc.

THE VASCULAR SYSTEM

Microvascular changes occur early in patients with SSc (73,75). In a sequential analysis, Prescott et al. (73) identified endothelial cell dysfunction by electron microscopy and reported decreased adenosine uptake as the earliest manifestation of SSc in clinically normal skin from the flexor surface of the forearm. Similar findings were present in both limited and diffuse subsets. Vascular leak occurred with perivascular edema with a "proteinaceous fluid" in the papillary dermis seen early on. The next event was intravascular platelet plugging. Platelets are sacks of growth factors that may further influence the vasculature and the extracellular matrix. A perivascular infiltrate with mast cells, CD4 and CD8 lymphocytes, macrophages, and Langerhans cells was identified next. This infiltrate was present during the middle phase, but not in the earliest or the latest phase of the disease.

The cause of this early endothelial cell dysfunction in SSc is unknown. It could represent some intrinsic derangement of the endothelium. Alternatively, it could be a circulating toxic factor (172,173). It could result from an immunologic attack of the endothelium mediated by antibody-dependent cell-mediated cytotoxicity (156,174). It is important to note that neither vasculitis nor immunoglobulin or C3 deposition is seen, making the latter possibility less likely (73,78). Although venous thrombosis may occur in patients with SSc, it is uncommon to see thrombi in the small arterioles of the skin.

The endothelium is coordinately regulated with the vascular smooth muscle that surrounds it. Abnormalities in the vascular smooth muscle might be anticipated given the high prevalence of Raynaud phenomenon, as well as vascular lesions in the kidney and lungs of patients with SSc. Of note, atrophy of the smooth muscle of the viscera was the most prominent finding in the autopsy series by D'Angelo et al. (70), more remarkable than fibrosis. Flavahan et al. (175) found a selective increase in the α_2-adrenergic constriction in small arterioles isolated from skin in the upper arms of patients with scleroderma. It is difficult to know which changes are primary and which may be secondary. One of the difficulties in interpreting vascular abnormalities in SSc is the fact that some are found in both the primary and secondary forms of Raynaud phenomenon (176,177). This feature makes determination of their direct contribution to pathogenesis of SSc unclear. Therefore, a critical control to include in any vascular study are patients with primary Raynaud phenomenon.

Finally, the affect of the autonomic nervous system on the vasculature in SSc needs to be considered. This system controls thermoregulation and tissue perfusion; however, this area has not been well studied in scleroderma. There are a few reports that suggest generalized autonomic dysfunction (68,178–181). Nonetheless, these reports involve small numbers of patients, use different methods, and have different outcomes, making a unified understanding of the problem elusive. We found a combination of small-fiber (cold) and large-fiber (vibration) defects in patients with scleroderma using QST (59). In addition, we found decreased sweating in patients with early diffuse SSc in areas proximal to fibrosis (60). Although these findings are preliminary, they do point to a possible role of the peripheral nervous system in SSc that has not been previously appreciated.

THE IMMUNE SYSTEM

A role for the immune system in SSc is supported by the presence of autoantibodies, inflammatory infiltrates in target organs, and disease associations with other autoimmune disorders. The frequencies and specificities of some of the autoantibodies are reviewed above and listed in Table 4.4. Autoantibodies are common in patients with SSc (15). The specificities are unique to scleroderma and different from those seen in other autoimmune diseases such as systemic lupus erythematosus. Whether the autoantibodies are directly pathogenic or simply a marker of immune activation remains unclear Casciola-Rosen et al. (182) found that scleroderma serum autoantibodies reacted with antigens that were cleaved by metal-ion dependent oxidation reactions. They proposed that episodic perfusion–reperfusion injury, as exemplified by Raynaud phenomenon, uniquely damages or alters certain proteins such that they become susceptible to autoantibody reactions Because of the requirement for metal ions, and because supranormal levels of iron and copper cause the same fragmentation patterns in healthy individuals, the authors have speculated about the role of abnormal metal accumulation in scleroderma. An attractive feature of this hypothesis is that it links the vascular system to the immune system in SSc and offers an explanation for the unique autoantibody profiles.

The evidence for cellular immune involvement in SSc is mixed. Although emphasis has been placed on the cellular infiltrates in the skin of patients with SSc (167), these are not impressive. Clearly, in localized scleroderma, morphea and linear scleroderma, there is an intense and persistent lymphocytic infiltrate around blood vessels and at the deep dermal subcutaneous layer (72,77). In contrast, the infiltrates in SSc are described as "sparse," "slight," "minimal," or "absent" (72,77). In 1971, Winkelmann (183) wrote:

> A major feature of systemic scleroderma is the minimal or absent cellular inflammation in the skin, muscle, joint, and visceral lesions. Similarly, there is no evidence of proliferation of fibroblasts from which the collagen changes originate. Such a banal microscopic appearance differentiates scleroderma from necrotizing vasculitis, lupus erythematosus, and dermatomyositis in which inflammation and tissue degeneration are the obvious and immediate cause of the clinical disease.

Failure to appreciate these findings has led to generations of clinical trials targeting inflammatory cells (or fibroblasts) that are not there. Although inflammatory events may occur early, they are no longer obvious by the time patients present. Alveolitis in the lungs in scleroderma is the exception, where persistent inflammatory damage can be documented. The skin findings, or the lack of skin findings, are distinct from other autoimmune connective tissue diseases characterized by persistent inflammatory changes.

Microchimerism has been proposed as a mechanism for autoimmune diseases, particularly scleroderma, by Nelson et al. (184,185). Retention of fetal cells in the maternal circulation for extended periods of time (years) occurs commonly. Potential HLA-incompatible relationships might induce a chronic GVHD reaction as seen after bone marrow transplantation. Clinical parallels between chronic GVHD and scleroderma have been made (91,186,187). Artlett et al. (188) found male fetal DNA (as indicated by a segment of the Y chromosome) in peripheral blood and involved skin of mothers with SSc. Although this is an intriguing hypothesis, it has the problem of establishing causality from associations between common findings (microchimerism) and rare diseases (scleroderma). Substantially larger studies will be needed to confirm whether microchimerism is pathogenetically linked to scleroderma or other autoimmune diseases.

THE EXTRACELLULAR MATRIX

Sclerosis is the tissue hallmark of scleroderma (189), albeit an endstage one. Changes in collagen, the major structural protein of connective tissue, are central to this process. A myriad of cytokines (IL-1, IL-4, and IL-6) and growth factors (TGF-β, platelet-derived growth factor, and CTGF) affect collagen production by fibroblasts *in vitro* and some have been implicated by association in SSc (190). Nonetheless, despite a multitude of hypotheses and abnormalities and decades of study, the precise mechanism by which this occurs in scleroderma remains obscure.

A number of investigations have concluded that dermal collagen is normal in its genetic, molecular, and biochemical composition (16,72,191). The time-honored notion that the scleroderma occurs because fibroblasts make too much collagen remains an oversimplification of a complex process. Scleroderma is not a tumor of fibroblasts or of collagen or a keloid.

Although one might think it would be relatively straightforward to quantitate the amount of collagen in skin biopsies, the literature is replete with contradictory reports. Starting with O'Leary et al. (72) in 1957, a number of investigators have failed to identify increased collagen in the skin of SSc patients (192,193). In 1979, Rodnan et al. (194) published one of the few skin biopsy studies that show increased dermal collagen. They reported a 50% increase in dermal collagen content in patients with diffuse disease compared with patients with limited disease and healthy controls. They found the same increases in four patients with acromegaly, despite the obvious differences among the latter patients and those with diffuse SSc. A subsequent biopsy study in 1986 failed to find a correlation between dry weights, which correlate with collagen content, and either early or late diffuse or early or late limited subsets (195). Studies before and after the early study failed to confirm the finding of increased collagen in the skin.

The study by Seibold et al. (195) did find a correlation between wet weights and skin scores in patients with scleroderma. Wet weights of skin biopsies correspond to water content, or edema, and correlate with clinical measurements of skin thickness (or skin scores) in early disease. A common mistake is to equate "thick skin" with "increased collagen." A more likely scenario is that edema results in thickened skin in the acute setting. Unfortunately, the extent of the edema is often not appreciated by routine histology, because the tissue undergoes multiple dehydration steps during the paraffin embedding. This processing removes excess water and results in dissociation between skin thickening on physical examination (or by skin score or wet weights) and what is rather unimpressive under the microscope. The use of frozen sections enhances the ability to document tissue edema.

It is likely that early microvascular injury induces a host of growth factors and cytokines that affect fibroblasts and the matrix in complex ways that resemble chronic wound healing and scar formation. In such settings, compaction of collagen leads to retraction and hardening of the skin. Drugs that block collagen production *in vitro* have, in general, not been effective *in vivo,* consistent with a lack of general support for the central role for increased collagen synthesis

The question of whether there is a primary defect in the scleroderma wound healing is answered by our experience doing hundreds of skin biopsies in involved and uninvolved skin of patients with scleroderma, without any wound healing complications. Neither hypertrophic scars nor keloids nor failure to heal with ulcerations have been observed. This would argue that the scleroderma wound response is intact and active and that fibroblasts can respond normally to physical trauma.

Ultimately, patients with scleroderma shrink. This is not simply cachexia from malabsorption or malnutrition. Children with linear scleroderma can have the defect confined to a single limb that stops growing. The possibility remains that scleroderma results in the loss of a critical trophic factor(s) or growth factor(s) that eludes identification.

We examined scleroderma dermal fibroblasts *in vitro* using complementary DNA microarrays (196). Although we did not observe increases in TGF-β transcripts in the fibroblasts themselves, we did see gene expression profiles consistent with chronic TGF-β exposure including increased collagen IV and TIMP-3. Although these genes have been reported in scleroderma fibroblasts before, we found an increase in a novel transcript endoglin. Endoglin is a TGF-β receptor III normally found on endothelial cells. We confirmed these findings at the protein level. If endoglin is expressed in excess of TGF-βRI and TGF-βRII, it does not signal when it binds TGF-β. We demonstrated that overexpression of endoglin could block TGF-β-induced Smad-3 expression in normal fibroblasts. We propose that the overexpression of endoglin might be one mechanism by which scleroderma fibroblasts appropriately down-regulate their sensitivity to TGF-β during chronic TGF-β exposure.

An alternate view, and one that assumes the hypersensitivity to growth factor model, is that something inherent in the fibroblast signaling pathway is abnormal in patients with scleroderma rendering them more susceptible to growth factor stimulation and collagen production. Dong et al. (197) described a decrease in Smad-7 expression in scleroderma fibroblasts. The lack of this inhibitory signaling molecule would allow up-regulation of downstream factors such as collagen in response to TGF-β. This finding needs to be confirmed by other methods and in a larger number of patients.

Although fibroblasts are an important tool in the study of scleroderma, they do have certain limitations. Depending on the assay, results may be modest, variable, and transient. In addition, information from other relevant cell types is missing. With these limitations in mind, we began a series of investigations looking at whole-skin extracts from patients with scleroderma using DNA microarrays. These preliminary results revealed significant differences in gene expression profiles between patients with diffuse SSc and healthy controls. Whitfield et al. (198) found over 2,000 genes that were twofold different in their expression intensity between patients with scleroderma and healthy controls (198). In the future, functional genomics analysis of skin promises to be useful in a variety of diseases.

Critical pieces of this complex puzzle are still missing. With the abundance of abnormalities, and the lack of definitive therapies, many of these findings may prove to be epiphenomena and the true nature or underlying cause of this disease remains frustratingly elusive. Current paradigms are inadequate to fully explain the disease and new paradigms are needed. Basic research applying emerging technologies to this disease will lead to new insights and new targets. New ideas must be put to the test of well-designed clinical trials. Working together, basic scientists, clinicians, and patients will find better treatments and eventually a cure for this devastating disease.

ACKNOWLEDGMENTS

Support for this manuscript was provided by the Scleroderma Research Foundation. In lasting memory of Sharon L. Monsky who passed away on May 11, 2002, from systemic sclerosis, but whose dreams for a cure for scleroderma live on.

REFERENCES

1. Curzio C. An account of an extraordinary disease of the skin and its cure. Translated from Italian by R. Watson. *Philos Trans* 1754;48:579.
2. Gintrac M. Note sur la sclerodermie. *Rev Med Chir Paris* 1847;2:263.
3. Jackson R. Raynaud and Moliére. *Arch Dermatol* 1983;119:263.
4. Osler W. On diffuse scleroderma; with special reference to diagnosis, and to use of the thyroid gland extract. *J Cutan Dis* 1898;16:49.
5. Tuffanelli DL, Winkelmann RK. Systemic scleroderma. A clinical study of 727 cases. *Arch Dermatol* 1961;84:359–371.
6. Goetz RH. The pathology of progressive systemic sclerosis (generalized scleroderma) with special references to changes in the viscera. *Clin Proc* 1945;4:337.
7. Barnett AJ. History of scleroderma. In: Clements PJ, Furst DE, eds. *Systemic sclerosis.* Baltimore: Williams & Wilkins, 1996:3–22.
8. Clements PJ, Furst DE, eds. *Systemic sclerosis.* Baltimore: Williams & Wilkins, 1996.
9. Jablonska S, ed. *Scleroderma and pseudoscleroderma,* 2nd ed. Warsaw: Polish Medical Publishers, 1975.
10. Jablonska S, Blaszczyk M. Differential diagnosis of scleroderma-like disorders. In: Clements PJ, Furst DE, eds. *Systemic sclerosis.* Baltimore: Williams & Wilkins, 1996:99–120.
11. Medsger TA, Masi AT. Epidemiology of systemic sclerosis (scleroderma). *Ann Intern Med* 1971;74:714.
12. Maricq HR, Weinrich MC, Keil JE, et al. Prevalence of scleroderma spectrum disorders in the general population of South Carolina. *Arthritis Rheum* 1989; 32:998.
13. Mayes MD. Classification and epidemiology of scleroderma. *Semin Cutan Med Surg* 1998;17:22.
14. Ferri C, Valentini G, Cozzi F, et al. Systemic sclerosis. *Medicine* 2002;81:139.
15. Medsger TA. Systemic sclerosis (scleroderma): clinical aspects. In: Koopman, WJ, ed. *Arthritis and allied conditions,* 14th ed. Philadelphia: Lippincott Williams & Wilkins, 2001:1590.
16. Seibold JR. Scleroderma. In: Ruddy S, Harris ED, Sledge CB, eds. *Kelley's textbook of rheumatology,* 6th ed. Philadelphia: WB Saunders, 2001:1211.
17. Anonymous. Preliminary criteria for the classification of systemic sclerosis (scleroderma). Subcommittee for Scleroderma Criteria of the American Rheumatism Association Diagnostic and Therapeutic Criteria Committee. *Arthritis Rheum* 1980;23:581.
18. LeRoy EC, Black C, Fleischmajer R, et al. Scleroderma (systemic sclerosis): classification, subsets, and pathogenesis. *J Rheumatol* 1980;152:202.
19. O'Leary PA, Waisman M. Acrosclerosis. *Proc Mayo Clin* 1940;15:702.
20. Thibiérge G, Weissenbach RJ. Concretions calcaires sous-cutanees et sclerodermis. *Ann Derm Syphilol* 1911;42:129.

21. Poormoghim H, Lucas M, Fertig N, et al. Systemic sclerosis sine scleroderma: demographics, clinical, and serologic features and survival in forty-eight patients. *Arthritis Rheum* 2000;43:444.
22. Barnett AJ, Miller MH, Littlejohn GO. A survival study of the patients diagnosed over 30 years (1953–1983): the value of a simple cutaneous classification in the early stages of the disease. *J Rheumatol* 1988;15:276.
23. Scussel-Lonzetti L, Joyal F, Raynauld JP, et al. Predicting mortality in systemic sclerosis. *Medicine* 2002;81:154.
24. Maricq HR, Weinrich MC, Keil JE, et al. Prevalence of Raynaud's phenomenon in the general population. *J Chron Dis* 1986;39:423.
25. Maricq HR, LeRoy EC, D'Angelo WA, et al. Diagnostic potential of *in vivo* capillary microscopy in scleroderma and related disorders. *Arthritis Rheum* 1980;23:183.
26. Grassi W, Medico PD, Izzo F, et al. Microvascular involvement in systemic sclerosis: capillaroscopic findings. *Semin Arthritis Rheum* 2001;30:397.
27. Patterson JW. Pterygium inversum unguis-like changes in scleroderma. *Arch Dermatol* 1977;113:1429.
28. DeNicola P, Zavagli G. *Nail diseases in internal medicine*. Springfield, IL: Charles C Thomas, 1974.
29. Barnett AJ. The "neck sign" in scleroderma. *Arthritis Rheum* 1989;32:209.
30. Tuffanelli DL. Systemic scleroderma. *Med Clin North Am* 1989;73:1167.
31. Jawitz JC, Albert MK, Nigra TP, et al. A new skin manifestation of progressive systemic sclerosis. *J Am Acad Dermatol* 1984;11:265.
32. Sanchez JL, Vazquez M, Sanchez NP. Vitiligolike macules in systemic scleroderma. *Arch Dermatol* 1983;119:129.
33. Seibold JR, McCloskey DA. Skin involvement as a relevant outcome measure in clinical trials of systemic sclerosis. *Curr Opin Rheumatol* 1997;9:571
34. Clements PJ, Hurwitz EL, Wong WK, et al. Skin thickness score as a predictor and correlate of outcome in systemic sclerosis. *Arthritis Rheum* 2000;43: 2445.
35. Steen VD, Medsger TA. Severe organ involvement in systemic sclerosis with diffuse scleroderma. *Arthritis Rheum* 2000;43:2437.
36. Steen VD, Medsger TA. Improvement in skin thickening in systemic sclerosis associated with improved survival. *Arthritis Rheum* 2001;44:2828.
37. Clements PJ, Lachenbruch PA, Ng SC, et al. Skin score: a semiquantitative measure of cutaneous involvement that improves prediction of prognosis in systemic sclerosis. *Arthritis Rheum* 1990;33:1256.
38. Clements PJ, Lachenbruch PA, Seibold JR, et al. Inter- and intraobserver variability of total skin thickness score (modified Rodnan TSS) in systemic sclerosis. *J Rheumatol* 1995;22:1281.
39. Myers SL, Cohen JS, Sheets PW, et al. B-mode ultrasound evaluation of skin thickness in progressive systemic sclerosis. *J Rheumatol* 1986;13:577.
40. Falanga V, Bucalo B. The use of a durometer to assess skin hardness. *J Am Acad Dermatol* 1993;29:47.
41. Balbir-Gurman A, Denton CP, Nichols B, et al. Non-invasive measurement of biomechanical skin properties in systemic sclerosis. *Ann Rheum Dis* 2002;61: 237.
42. Synkowski DR, Lobitz WC Jr, Provost TT. Bullous scleroderma. *Arch Dermatol* 1981;117:135.
43. Rencic A, Goyal S, Mofid M, et al. Bullous lesions in scleroderma. *Int J Dermatol* 2002;41:335.
44. Tuffanelli DL. Lymphagiectasis due to scleroderma. *Arch Dermatol* 1975;111: 1216.
45. James WD, Berger TG, Butler DF, et al. Nodular (keloidal) scleroderma. *J Am Acad Dermatol* 1984;11:1111.
46. Mathews MB, Bernstein RM. Myositis autoantibody inhibits histidyl tRNA synthetase: a model for autoimmunity. *Nature* 1983;304:177.
47. Young MA, Rose S, Reynolds JC. Gastrointestinal manifestations of scleroderma. *Rheum Dis Clin N Am* 1996;22:797–823.
48. Sjogren RW. Gastrointestinal motility disorders in scleroderma. *Arthritis Rheum* 1994;37:1265.
49. Marie I, Levesque H, Ducrotte P, et al. Gastric involvement in systemic sclerosis: a prospective study. *Am J Gastroenterol* 2001;96:77.
50. Elkayam O, Oumanski M, Yaron M, et al. Watermelon stomach following and preceding systemic sclerosis. *Semin Arthritis Rheum* 2000,30:127.
51. Silver RM. Clinical problems: the lungs. *Rheum Dis Clin North Am* 1996;22: 825.
52. Steen VD, Conte C, Owens GR, et al. Severe restrictive lung disease in systemic sclerosis. *Arthritis Rheum* 1994;37:1283.
53. Traub XM, Shapiro AP, Rodnam GP, et al. Hypertension and renal failure (scleroderma renal crisis) in progressive systemic sclerosis: review of a 25-year experience with 68 cases. *Medicine* 1983;62:335.
54. Steen VD, Constantino JP, Shapiro AP, et al. Outcome of renal crisis in systemic sclerosis: relation to availability of angiotensin converting enzyme (ACE) inhibitors. *Ann Intern Med* 1990;113:352.
55. Steen VD, Medsger TA. Long-term outcomes of scleroderma renal crisis. *Ann Intern Med* 2000;17:600.
56. Deswal A, Follansbee WP. Cardiac involvement in scleroderma. *Rheum Dis Clin N Am* 1996;22:841.
57. Alexander EL, Firestein GS, Weiss JL, et al. Reversible cold-induced abnormalities in myocardial perfusion and function in systemic sclerosis. *Ann Intern Med* 1986;105:661.
58. Herrick AL, Jayson MIV. Organ involvement: nervous system. In: Clements PF, Furst DE, eds. *Systemic sclerosis.* Baltimore: Williams & Wilkins, 1996: 441–452.
59. Poncelet AN, Connolly MK. Peripheral neuropathy in scleroderma. *Muscle Nerve* (submitted) 2003.
60. Sandroni P, Connolly MK. Dyshidrosis in scleroderma patients. *Mayo Clin Proc* (manuscript in preparation).
61. Magerl W. Neural mechanisms of itch sensation. *IASP Newsletter* 1996. International Assoc. for the Study of Pain Sept/Oct 1996:1–10.
62. Lock G, Straub RH, Zeuner M, et al. Association of autonomic nervous dysfunction and esophageal dysmotility in systemic sclerosis. *J Rheumatol* 1998;25:1330–1335.
63. Lally EV, Jimenez SA. Impotence in progressive systemic sclerosis. *Ann Intern Med* 1981;95:150.
64. Klein LE, Posner MS. Progressive systemic sclerosis and impotence. *Ann Intern Med* 1981;95:658.
65. Nowlin NS, Brick JE, Weaver DJ, et al. Impotence in scleroderma. *Ann Intern Med* 1986;104:794.
66. Sonnex C, Paice E, White AG. Autonomic neuropathy in systemic sclerosis: a case report and evaluation of six patients. *Ann Rheum Dis* 1986;45:957–960.
67. Leighton JA, Valdovinos MA, Pemberton JH, et al. Anorectal dysfunction and rectal prolapse in progressive systemic sclerosis. *Dis Colon Rectum* 1993;36:182.
68. Roumm AD, Medsger TA. Cancer and systemic sclerosis. *Arthritis Rheum* 1985;28;1336.
69. Abu-Shakra M, Guillemin F, Lee P. Cancer and systemic sclerosis. *Arthritis Rheum* 1993;36:460.
70. D'Angelo WA, Fries JF, Masi AT, et al. Pathology observations in systemic sclerosis (scleroderma). *Am J Med* 1969;46:428–440.
71. Goetz RH. The heart in generalised scleroderma. *Angiology* 1951;2:555–578.
72. O'Leary PA, Montgomery H, Ragsdale WE. Dermatohistopathology of various types of scleroderma. *Arch Dermatol* 1957;75:75–87.
73. Prescott RJ, Freemont AJ, Jones CJP, et al. Sequential dermal microvascular and perivascular changes in the development of scleroderma. *J Pathol* 1992: 255–263.
74. Fleischmajer R, Damiano V, Nedwich A, et al. Scleroderma and subcutaneous tissue. *Science* 1971;171:1019.
75. Maricq HR, Smith EA. Organ involvement: peripheral vascular. In: Clements PF, Furst DE, eds. *Systemic sclerosis.* Baltimore: Williams & Wilkins, 1996: 365–387.
76. Lever WF, Schaumburg-Lever G. Connective tissue diseases. In: *Histopathology of the skin,* 7th ed. Philadelphia: JB Lippincott Co., 1990:494–522.
77. Hood AF, Kwan TH, Mihm MC, et al. Disorders of collagen and elastic tissue. In: Hood AF, Kwan TH, Mihm MC, et al., eds. *Primer of dermatopathology,* Boston: Little, Brown and Co., 1993:309–323.
78. Connolly SM, Winkelmann RK. Direct immunofluorescent findings in scleroderma syndromes. *Acta Derm Venereol (Stockh)* 1981;61:29–36.
79. Tuffanelli DL. Antinuclear antibody subsets: clinical and prognostic features. *Dermatol Clin* 1983;1:517.
80. Shero JH, Bordwell NF, Rothfield NF, et al. High titers of autoantibodies to topoisomerase I (Scl-70) in sera from scleroderma patients. *Science* 1986;231: 737.
81. Moroi Y, Peebles C, Fritzler M, et al. Autoantibody to centromere (kinetochore) in scleroderma sera. *Proc Natl Acad Sci USA* 1980;77:1627.
82. Wigley FM. Raynaud's phenomenon. *N Engl J Med* 2002;347:1001–1008.
83. Takehara K, Moroi Y, Nakabayashi Y, et al. Antinuclear antibodies in localized scleroderma. *Arthritis Rheum* 1983;26:612–616.
84. Rosenberg AM, Uziel L, Krafchik BR, et al. Antinuclear antibodies in children with localized scleroderma. *J Rheumatol* 1995;22:2337–2343.
85. Lever WF, Schaumburg-Lever. Metabolic diseases. In: *Histopathology of the skin,* 7th ed. Philadelphia: JB Lippincott, 1990:452–487.
86. Venencie PY, Powell FC, Su WPD, et al. Scleredema: a review of thirty-three cases.*J Am Acad Dermatol* 1984;11:128.
87. Fleischmajer R. Papular mucinosis. In: *Fitzpatrick's dermatology in general medicine,* 5th ed. 1999:2129–2131. ed. Freedberg IM, et al. McGraw-Hill NY, NY.
88. Berger JR, Dobbs MR, Terhune MH, et al. The neurologic complications of scleroyxedema. *Medicine* 2001;80:313–319.
89. Cowper SE, Su LD, Bhawan J, et al. Nephrogenic fibrosing dermopathy. *Am J Dermatopathol* 2001;23:383–393.
90. Fibrosing skin condition among patients with renal disease—United States and Europe, 1997—2002. *MMWR Morb Mortal Wkly Rep* 2002;51:25–26.
91. Furst DE, Clements PJ, Graze P, et al. A syndrome resembling progressive systemic sclerosis after bone marrow transplantation. *Arthritis Rheum* 1979;22:904.
92. Schwartz RA, Burgess GH, Fox MD. Sclerodermoid changes in a patient with metastatic malignant melanoma. *J Dermatol Surg Oncol* 1980;6:112.
93. Shiel WC Jr, Prete PE, Jason M, et al. Carcinoma-associated fasciitis and arthritis. *Am J Med* 1985;79:640.
94. Stover SL, Gay RE, Koopman W, et al. Dermal fibrosis in spinal cord injury patients. *Arthritis Rheum* 1980;23:1312.
95. Varga J, Jimenez SA. Development of severe limited scleroderma in complicated Raynaud's phenomenon after limb immobilization: report of two cases and study of collagen biosynthesis. *Arthritis Rheum* 1986;29:1160.
96. Seibold JR, Furst DE, Clements PJ. Treatment of systemic sclerosis by disease modifying agents. In: Clements PJ, Furst DE, eds. *Systemic sclerosis.* Baltimore: Williams & Wilkins, 1996:535–548.
97. Zaidi F, Altman RD. Therapy of systemic sclerosis with unproven remedies. In: Clements PJ, Furst DE, eds. *Systemic sclerosis.* Baltimore: Williams & Wilkins, 1996:549–568.

98. White B, Bauer EA, Goldsmith LA, et al. Guidelines for clinical trials in systemic sclerosis (scleroderma). *Arthritis Rheum* 1995;38:351–360.
99. Medsger TA, Silman AJ, Steen VD, et al. A disease severity scale for systemic sclerosis: development and testing. *J Rheumatol* 1999;26:2159–2167.
100. Sturgill MG, Siebold JR. Rational use of calcium-channel antagonists in Raynaud's phenomenon. *Curr Opin Rheumatol* 1998;10:584–588.
101. Dziadzio M, Denton CP, Smith R, et al. Losartan therapy for Raynaud's phenomenon and scleroderma: clinical and biochemical findings in a fifteen-week, randomized, parallel-group, controlled trial. *Arthritis Rheum* 1999;42: 264.
102. Wigley FM, Korn JH, Csuka ME, et al. Oral iloprost in patients with Raynaud phenomenon secondary to systemic sclerosis: a multicenter, placebo-controlled, double-blind study. *Arthritis Rheum* 1998;41:670.
103. Rubin LJ, Badesch DB, Barst RJ, et al. Bosentan therapy for pulmonary artery hypertension. *N Engl J Med* 2002;346:896–903.
104. Sule SD, Wigley FM. Update on management of scleroderma. *Bull Rheum Dis* 2000;49:1–4.
105. Furst DE, Clements PJ, Hillis S, et al. Immunosuppression with chlorambucil versus placebo for scleroderma: results of a three-year, parallel, randomized, double-blind study. *Arthritis Rheum* 1989;32:584–593.
106. Casas JA, Saway PA, Villareal I, et al. Five fluorouracil in the treatment of scleroderma: a randomized, double-blind, placebo controlled international collaborative study. *Ann Rheum Dis* 1990;49:926–928.
107. Clements PJ, Lachenbruch PA, Sterz M, et al. Cyclosporine in systemic sclerosis: results of a 48-week open safety study in 10 patients. *Arthritis Rheum* 1993;36:75–83.
108. Pope JE, Bellamy N, Seibold JR, et al. A randomized, controlled trial of methotrexate versus placebo in early diffuse scleroderma. *Arthritis Rheum* 2001;44:1351–1358.
109. Steen VD, Medsger TA. Case-controlled study of corticosteroids and other drugs that either precipitate or protect from the development of scleroderma renal crisis. *Arthritis Rheum* 1998;41:1613–1619.
110. DeMarco PJ, Weisman MH, Seibold JR, et al. Predictors and outcomes of scleroderma renal crisis: the high-dose versus low-dose D-penicillamine in early diffuse systemic sclerosis trial. *Arthritis Rheum* 2002;46:2983–2989.
111. Binks M, Passweg JR, Furst D, et al. Phase I/II trial of autologous stem cell transplantation in systemic sclerosis: procedure related mortality and impact on skin disease. *Ann Rheum Dis* 2001;60:548–549.
112. McSweeney PA, Nash RA, Sullivan KM, et al. High-dose immunosuppressive therapy for severe systemic sclerosis: initial outcomes. *Blood* 2002;100: 1602–1610.
113. Steen VD, Medsger TA, Rodnan GP. D-penicillamine therapy in progressive systemic sclerosis (scleroderma): a retrospective analysis. *Ann Intern Med* 1982;97:652–659.
114. Clements PJ, Furst DE, Wong WK, et al. High-dose versus low-dose D-penicillamine in early diffuse systemic sclerosis: analysis of a two-year, double-blind, randomized, controlled clinical trial. *Arthritis Rheum* 1999;42:1194–1203.
115. Furst DE, Clements PJ. D-penicillamine is not effective treatment in systemic sclerosis. *Scand J Rheumatol* 2001;30:189–191.
116. Medsger TA, Lucas M, Wildly KS, Baker C. D-penicillamine in systemic sclerosis? Yes! *Scand J Rheumatol* 2001;30:192–194.
117. Ziesche R, Hofbauer E, Wittman K, et al. A preliminary study of long-term treatment with interferon gamma-1-b and low-dose prednisolone in patients with idiopathic pulmonary fibrosis. *N Engl J Med* 2000;341:1264–1269.
118. Freundlich B, Jimenez SA, Steen VD, et al. Treatment of systemic sclerosis with recombinant interferon-gamma. *Arthritis Rheum* 1992;35:1134–1142.
119. Polisson RP, Gilkeson GS, Pyun EH, et al. A multicenter trial of recombinant human interferon gamma in systemic sclerosis: effects on cutaneous fibrosis and interleukin 2 receptor levels. *J Rheumatol* 1996;23:654–658.
120. Grassegger A, Schuler G, Hessenberger G, et al. Interferon-gamma in the treatment of systemic sclerosis: a randomized controlled multicentre trial. *Br J Dermatol* 1998;139:639–648.
121. Hunzelmann N, Anders S, Fierlbeck G, et al. Systemic scleroderma. Multicenter trial of 1 year of treatment with recombinant interferon gamma. *Arch Dermatol* 1997;133:637–642.
122. Black CM, Silman AJ, Herrick AI, et al. Interferon-alpha does not improve outcome at one year in patients with diffuse cutaneous scleroderma: results of a randomized, double-blind, placebo-controlled trial. *Arthritis Rheum* 1999; 42:299–305.
123. Le CH, Morales A, Trentham DE. Minocycline in early diffuse scleroderma. *Lancet* 1998;28:1755–1756.
124. Oliver SJ, Moreira A, Kaplan G. Immune stimulation in scleroderma patients treated with thalidomide. *Clin Immunol* 2000;97:109–120.
125. Fisher GJ, Kang S. Phototherapy for scleroderma: biologic rationale, results and promise. *Curr Opin Rheumatol* 2002;14:723–726.
126. Dolan AL, Kassimos D, Gibson T, et al. Diltiazem induces remissions of calcinosis in scleroderm. *Br J Rheumatol* 1995;34:576–578.
127. Palmieri GMA, Sebes JI, Aelion JA, et al. Treatment of calcinosis with diltiazem. *Arthritis Rheum* 1995;38:1646–1654.
128. Vayssairat M, Hidouche D, Abdoucheli-Baudot N, et al. Clinical significance of subcutaneous calcinosis in patients with systemic sclerosis: does diltiazem induce its regression? *Ann Rheum Dis* 1998;57:252–254.
129. Boeckxstaens GE, Bartelsman JF, Lauwers L, et al. Treatment of GI dysmotility in scleroderma with the new enterokinetic agent prucalopride. *Am J Gastroenterol* 2002;97:194–197.
130. Soudah HC, Hasler WL, Owyang C. Effect of octreotide on intestinal motility and bacterial overgrowth in scleroderma. *N Engl J Med* 1991;325: 1461–1467.
131. Silver RM, Warrick JH, Kinsella MB, et al. Cyclophosphamide and low-dose prednisone therapy in patients systemic sclerosis (scleroderma) with interstitial lung disease. *J Rheumatol* 1993;20:838–844.
132. Steen VD, Lanz JK, Conte C, et al. Therapy for severe interstitial lung disease in systemic sclerosis: a retrospective study. *Arthritis Rheum* 1994;37: 1290–1296.
133. Akesson A, Scheja A, Lundin A, et al. Improved pulmonary function in systemic sclerosis after treatment with cyclophosphamide. *Arthritis Rheum* 1994; 37:729–735.
134. Schnabel A, Reuter M, Gross W, et al. Intravenous pulse cyclophosphamide in the treatment of interstitial lung disease due to collagen vascular disease. *Arthritis Rheum* 1998;41:1215–1220.
135. White B, Moore WC, Wigley FM, et al. Cyclophosphamide is associated with pulmonary function and survival benefit in patients with scleroderma and alveolitis. *Ann Intern Med* 2000;132:947–954.
136. Welsh KI, Black CM. Environmental and genetic factors in scleroderma. In: Jayson, MIV, Black CM, eds. *Systemic sclerosis: scleroderma.* London: John Wiley and Sons, 1988.
137. Kipervarg Y, Connolly K. Chemically induced scleroderma. In: Arndt KA, LeBoit LE, Wintroub BU, eds. *Cutaneous medicine and surgery.* Philadelphia: WB Saunders, 1996.
138. Steen VD. Occupational scleroderma. *Curr Opin Rheumatol* 1999:11:490.
139. Mayes MD. Epidemiologic studies of environmental agents and systemic autoimmune diseases. *Environ Health Perspect* 1999;107:743.
140. Varga J, Jimenez SA. Chemical exposure-induced cutaneous fibrosis. *Arch Dermatol* 1994;130:97.
141. Varga J, Jimenez SA, Uitto J. L-tryptophan and the eosinophilia-myalgia syndrome: current understanding of the etiology and pathogenesis. *J Invest Dermatol* 1993;100:97S.
142. Kamb ML, Murphy JJ, Casten JC, et al. Eosinophilia-myalgia syndrome in L-tryptophan-exposed patients. *JAMA* 1992;267:77.
143. Tuffanelli DL. Urinary 5-hydroxyindole acetic acid excretion in scleroderma. *J Invest Dermatol* 1963;41:139.
144. Nova MP, Kaufman M, Halperin A. Scleroderma-like skin indurations in a child with phenylketonuria: a clinicopathologic correlation and review of the literature. *J Am Acad Dermatol* 1992;26:329.
145. Angell M. Science on trial: the clash of medical evidence and the law in breast implant case. W.W. Norton & Company, London 1997.
146. Varga J, Schumacher HR, Jimenez SA. Systemic sclerosis after augmentation mammoplasty with silicone implants. *Ann Intern Med* 1989;111:377.
147. Spiera H. Scleroderma after silicone augmentation mammoplasty. *JAMA* 1988;260:236.
148. Spiera H, Kerr LD. Scleroderma following silicone implantation: a cumulative experience of 11 cases. *J Rheumatol* 1993;20:958.
149. Lazar AP, Lazar P. Localized morphea after silicone gel breast implantation: more evidence of a cause-and-effect relationship. *Arch Dermatol* 1991;127:263.
150. Levine JJ, Ilowite NT. Scleroderma-like esophageal disease in children breast-fed by mothers with silicone breast implants. *JAMA* 1994;271:213.
151. Gabriel SE, O'Fallen WM, Kurland LT, et al. Risk of connective-tissue diseases and other disorders after breast implantation. *N Engl J Med* 1994;330:1697.
152. Sanchez-Guerrero J, Colditz GA, Karlson EW, et al. Silicone breast implants and the risk of connective-tissue diseases and symptoms. *N Engl J Med* 1995; 332:1666.
153. Janowsky EC, Kupper LL, Hulka BS. Meta-analyses of the relation between silicone breast implants and the risk of connective-tissue diseases. *N Engl J Med* 2000;342:781.
154. Tuffanelli DL. Morphea is not a borreliosis in California. In: Burgdorf WHC, Katz SI, eds. *Dermatology: progress and perspectives.* Proceedings of the 18th World Congress of Dermatology. New York, June 12–18, 1992.
155. Pandey JP, LeRoy EC. Human cytomegalovirus and the vasculopathies of autoimmune diseases (especially scleroderma), allograft rejection and coronary restenosis. *Arthritis Rheum* 1998;41:10–15.
156. Lunardi C, Bason C, Navone R, et al. Systemic sclerosis immunoglobulin G autoantibodies bind the cytomegalovirus late protein UL94 and induce apoptosis in human endothelial cells. *Nature Med* 2000;6:1183–1186.
157. Kerr LD, Spiera H. Scleroderma in association with the use of bleomycin: a report of 3 cases. *J Rheumatol* 1992;19:294.
158. Sternberg EM, Van Woert MH, Young SN, et al.: Development of a scleroderma-like illness during therapy with L-5-hydroxytryptophan and carbidopa. *N Engl J Med* 1980;303:782.
159. Joly P, Lampert A, Thomine E, Lauret P. Development of pseudobullous morphea and scleroderma-like illness during therapy with L-5-hydroxytryptophan and carbidopa. *J Am Acad Dermatol* 1991;25:332.
160. Pujol RM, Puig L, Moreno A, et al. Pseudoscleroderma secondary to phytonadione (vitamin K1) injections. *Cutis* 1989;43:365.
161. Goihman-Yahr M, Leal G, Essenfeld-Yahr E. Generalized morphea: a side effect of valproate sodium? *Arch Dermatol* 1980;116:621.
162. Leshin B, Piette WW, Caplan RM. Morphea after bromocriptine therapy. *Int J Dermatol* 1989;28:177.
163. Robertson JM, Clarke DH, Pevzner MM, et al. Breast conservation therapy: severe breast fibrosis after radiation therapy in patients with collagen vascular disease. *Cancer* 1991;68:502–508.

164. Trattner A, Figer A, David M, et al. Circumscribed scleroderma induced by postlumpectomy radiation therapy. *Cancer* 1991;68:2131
165. Varga J, Haustein VF, Creech RH, et al. Exaggerated radiation-induced fibrosis in patients with systemic sclerosis. *JAMA* 1991;265:3292.
166. Winkelmann RK, Grado GI, Quimby SR, Connolly SM. Pseudosclerodermatous panniculitis after irradiation: an unusual complication of megavoltage treatment of breast carcinoma. *Mayo Clin Proc* 1993;68:122.
167. Arnett FC, Cho M, Chatterjee S, et al. Familial occurrence frequencies and relative risks for systemic sclerosis (scleroderma) in three United States cohorts. *Arthritis Rheum* 2001;44:1359.
168. Feghali CA, Wright TM. Epidemiology and clinical study of twins with scleroderma (abstract). *Arthritis Rheum* 1995;38[Suppl 9]:S308.
169. Arnett FC, Howard RF, Tan F, et al. Increased prevalence of systemic sclerosis in a native American tribe in Oklahoma: association with an Amerindian HLA haplotype. *Arthritis Rheum* 1996;39:1362.
170. Tan FK, Stivers DN, Foster MW, et al. Association of microsatellite markers near the fibrillin 1 gene on human chromosome 15q with scleroderma in a native American population. *Arthritis Rheum* 1998;41:1729.
171. Furst DE, Clements PJ. Pathogenesis, fusion (summary). In: Clements PJ, Furst DE, eds. *Systemic sclerosis.* Baltimore: Williams & Wilkins, 1996:275–284.
172. Kahaleh MB, LeRoy EC. Endothelial injury in scleroderma: a protease mechanism. *J Lab Clin Med* 1983;101:553–560.
173. Majewski S, Blaszczyk M, Jablonska S, et al. Cytotoxic effects of sera from patients with systemic scleroderma: comparison of three different *in vitro* methods. *Rheumatol Int* 1990;10:65–70.
174. Sgonc R, Gruschwitz MS, Boeck G, et al. Endothelial cell apoptosis in systemic sclerosis is induced by antibody-dependent cell-mediated cytotoxicity via CD95. *Arthritis Rheum* 2000;43:2550–2562.
175. Flavahan NA, Flavahn S, Liu Q, et al. Increased alpha2-adrenergic constriction of isolated arterioles in diffuse scleroderma. *Arthritis Rheum* 200;43:1886–1890.
176. Kahaleh MB, Osborn I, LeRoy EC. Increased factor VIII/von Willebrand factor antigen and von Willebrand factor activity in scleroderma and in Raynaud's phenomenon. *Ann Intern Med* 1981;94:482–484.
177. Blann AD, Illingworth K, Jayson MIV. Mechanisms of endothelial cell damage in systemic sclerosis and Raynaud's phenomenon. *J Rheumatol* 1993;20: 1325–1330.
178. Klimiuk PS, Taylor L, Baker RD, et al. Autonomic neuropathy in systemic sclerosis. *Ann Rheum Dis* 1988;47:542–545.
179. Dessein PH, Joffe BI, Metz RM, et al. Autonomic dysfunction in systemic sclerosis: sympathetic overactivity and instability. *Am J Med* 1992;93:143–150.
180. Averbach-Heller L, Steiner I, Abramsky O. Neurologic manifestations of progressive systemic sclerosis. *Arch Neurol* 1992;49:1292–1295.
181. Ferri C, Emdin M, Giuggioli D, et al. Autonomic dysfunction in systemic sclerosis: time and frequency domain 24 hour heart rate variability analysis. *Br J Rheum* 1997;36:669–676.
182. Casciola-Rosen L, Wigley F, Rosen A. Scleroderma autoantigens are uniquely fragmented by metal-catalyzed oxidation reactions: implications for pathogenesis. *J Exp Med* 1997;185:71–79.
183. Winkelmann RK. Classification and pathogenesis of scleroderma. *Mayo Clin Proc* 1971;46:83–91.
184. Nelson JL. Maternal-fetal immunology and autoimmune disease: is some autoimmune disease auto-alloimmune or allo-autoimmune? *Arthritis Rheum* 1996;39:191–194.
185. Nelson JL, Furst DE, Maloney S, et al. Microchimerism and HLA-compatible relationships of pregnancy in scleroderma. *Lancet* 1998;351:559–562.
186. Lawley TJ, Peck GL, Muotsopoulos HM, et al. Scleroderma, Sjogren-like syndrome and chronic graft-vs-host disease. *Ann Intern Med* 1977;87:707.
187. Hood AF, Soter NA, Rappeport J, et al. Graft-vs-host reaction. *Arch Dermatol* 1977;113:1087.
188. Artlett CM, Smith JB, Jimenez SA. Identification of fetal DNA and cells in skin lesions from women with systemic sclerosis. *N Engl J Med* 1998;338: 1186–1191.
189. Liu B, Connolly MK. The pathogenesis of cutaneous fibrosis. *Sem Cutan Med Surg* 1998;17:3.
190. Ihn H. Pathogenesis of fibrosis: role of TGF-β and CTGF. *Curr Opin Rheumatol* 2002;14:681–685.
191. Fisher ER, Rodnan GP. Pathologic observations concerning the cutaneous lesions in progressive systemic sclerosis: an electron microscopic, histochemical and immunohistochemical study. *Arthritis Rheum* 1960;3:536–545.
192. Black MM, Bottoms M, Shuster S. Skin collagen content and thickness in systemic sclerosis. *Br J Dermatol* 1970;83:552–555.
193. Fleischmajer R. The collagen in scleroderma. *Arch Dermatol* 1964;89:437–441.
194. Rodnan GP, Lipinsky E, Luksick J. Skin thickness and collagen content in progressive systemic sclerosis and localized scleroderma. *Arthritis Rheum* 1979;22:130–140.
195. Siebold JR, Harris JN, De Angelo WAD, et al. Skin thickness and skin edema in systemic sclerosis (SS) (abstract). *Arthritis Rheum* 1986:29[suppl];S3.
196. Leask A, Abraham DJ, Finlay DR, et al. Dysregulation of transforming growth factor β signaling in scleroderma. *Arthritis Rheum* 2002;46: 1857–1865.
197. Dong C, Zhu S, Wang T, et al. Deficient Smad7 expression: a putative molecular defect in sclerodema. *Proc Natl Acad Sci U S A* 2002;99:3908–3913.
198. Whitfield ML, Finlay DR, Murray JI, et al. Gene expression patterns in scleroderma. *Proc Natl Acad Sci USA* 2003 (submitted).

CHAPTER 5

Localized Cutaneous Sclerosis

Thomas T. Provost, Adam S. Greenberg, and Vincent Falanga

Scleroderma is classified into three distinct groups (see Wigley et al. [1] for review). These are progressive systemic sclerosis, limited scleroderma (previously termed "acrosclerotic"), and localized scleroderma (morphea) and its variants. This chapter will make use of the figures and some of the data in the first edition of this book (2).

Localized scleroderma is characterized by fibrosis of the skin. Fibroblasts of patients with scleroderma overproduce collagen, including collagens type I, III, and VII; glycosaminoglycans; and fibronectin. The localized form of scleroderma may be transient, spontaneously disappearing, or may produce lifelong deformities. It is distinguished from systemic sclerosis by the absence of sclerodactyly, Raynaud phenomenon, periungual telangiectasia, and, generally, by the lack of internal organ involvement.

Localized scleroderma can be classified as primary or secondary (3). Primary localized scleroderma is an idiopathic inflammatory condition that may or may not be associated with features of autoimmunity (Table 5.1). Secondary localized scleroderma arises in association with another disease process (e.g., eosinophilic myalgia syndrome, following irradiation, certain drugs, and so on) (Table 5.2). Primary localized scleroderma exists in several distinct forms (Table 5.1) (reviewed by Tuffanelli [4]). These forms include plaque morphea, guttate morphea, morphea profundus, bullous or vesicular morphea, linear scleroderma, and generalized morphea. Very rare forms of localized scleroderma include a nodular (keloidal) scleroderma and atrophoderma of Pasini and Pierini.

MORPHEA

Morphea generally presents as a patch of erythema and edema. In the early development of morphea, a violaceous or erythematous border, indicative of activity, may be present (Fig. 5.1). However, the initial presentation may be quite subtle, presenting as hyperpigmented macules or ill-defined yellowish patches. As the lesions progress, they develop into porcelain white or yellowish, indurated plaques (Fig. 5.2). Lesions of morphea are more common on the trunk than the extremities. They may vary in size from 0.5 cm to as much as 30 cm in diameter (5). It also should be noted that solitary, small morphea lesions might be overlooked by the patient. With time, the lesions may become atrophic, depigmented, or hyperpigmented (Fig. 5.3). One of the authors has seen a number of patients with histologically proven morphea who, with time, developed nonindurated hyperpigmented patches as residua of their disease.

Occasionally, morphea may be associated with autoimmune features. For example, anti-U_3RNP fibrillin antibodies have been detected in a patient with morphea (6). In one case, anti-Ro(SS-A) and anti-La(SS-B) antibodies were detected in a child with morphea and the neonatal lupus erythematosus syndrome (7). Morphea has been detected in patients with dermatomyositis (2), polymyositis (4), progressive systemic sclerosis (8,8a), primary biliary cirrhosis (9), and, most recently in a patient with Schmidt syndrome (type II polyglandular autoimmune disease characterized by the universal presence of Addison's disease, either thyroid autoimmune disease [primary hypothyroidism] or insulin-dependant diabetes mellitus). Other components of this autoimmune syndrome include vitiligo, alopecia, ovarian failure, and chronic atrophic gastritis with or without pernicious anemia (10).

Guttate Morphea

At times, lesions of morphea may have a droplike (guttate) appearance (< 10 mm in size) (11). .

Morphea Profundus

These lesions involve the dermis and subcutaneous tissue and, on occasion, the muscle layers are indurated; with time, atrophy occurs (11,12). The classic cutaneous features of morphea (i.e., sclerotic hypopigmented patches) are generally absent. These lesions must be differentiated from other forms of panniculitis; they may be associated with systemic features (see later) and may respond to systemic steroids (4,13).

Bullous and Vesicular Morphea

Bullous and vesicular lesions may occur in plaques of morphea. These lesions arise from lymphatic obstruction, producing subepidermal edema with subsequent subepidermal blister formation (14,14a) (Fig. 5.4A,B).

Linear Scleroderma

This form of scleroderma is characterized by linear sclerosis and hyperpigmentation. At times, muscle and bone involvement may occur. These lesions generally occur on the extremities or face and scalp (Fig. 5.5). Linear scleroderma involving tissue

TABLE 5.1. Morphologic Variants of Localized Scleroderma

Plaque morphea
Guttate morphea
Morphea profundus
Bullous or vesicular morphea
Linear scleroderma
  "En coup de sabre"
  Parry–Romberg syndrome
Generalized morphea
Nodular (keloidal) morphea
Atrophoderma of Pasini and Pierini

TABLE 5.2. Cutaneous Scleroderma–like Disease Associated with Nonautoimmune Diseases

Drug-associated: bleomycin, pentazocine, isoniazid, valproate sodium, L-tryptophan contamination (see text), carbidopa, bromocriptine, and nitrofurantoin.
Chemical exposure–associated: toxic oil syndrome (see text), polyvinyl chloride, silicosis, organic solvents, epoxy resins.
Trauma-associated: chain saw and jack hammer operation.
Metabolic disorder–associated: porphyria, amyloidosis, Hashimoto thyroiditis, POEMS syndrome (Crow–Fukas syndrome), diabetes mellitus.
Genetic disorder–associated: progeria, Werner syndrome, Rothmund–Thompson syndrome, phenylketonuria, stiff skin syndrome.
Mucinosis-associated: scleredema of Buschke, scleromyxedema.
Malignancy-associated: carcinoid, breast cancer, metastatic melanoma, bronchioalveolar carcinoma.
Radiation associated: breast cancer irradiation.

From Tuffanelli DL. Localized scleroderma. *Semin Cutan Med Surg* 1998;17:27–33, with permission.

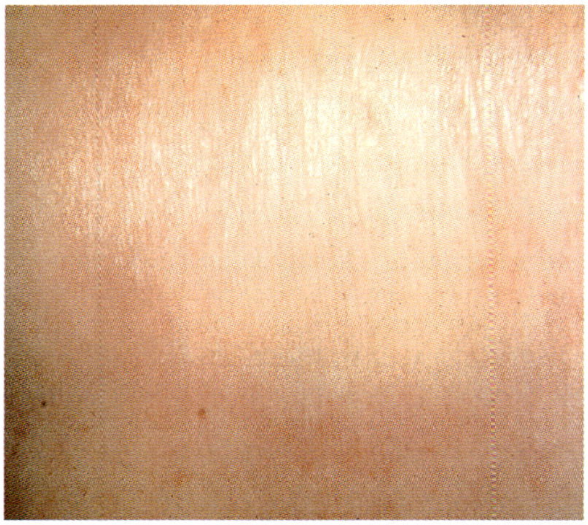

Figure 5.1. Early plaque of morphea surrounded by a red, violaceous halo. The area is only minimally indurated.

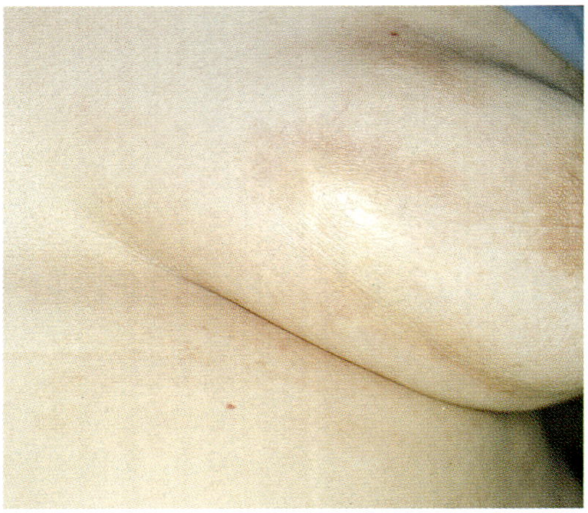

Figure 5.2. Advanced plaque of morphea on the breast next to the nipple. The center is hard, has a yellowish hue; the border is slightly hyperpigmented.

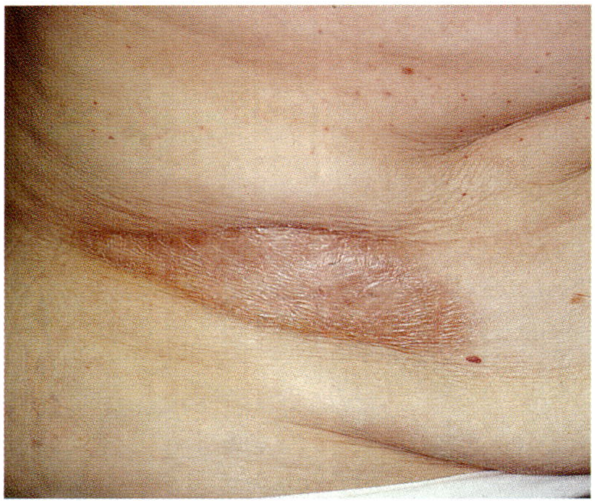

Figure 5.3. Very advanced plaque of morphea. Considerable atrophy of underlying tissue is present.

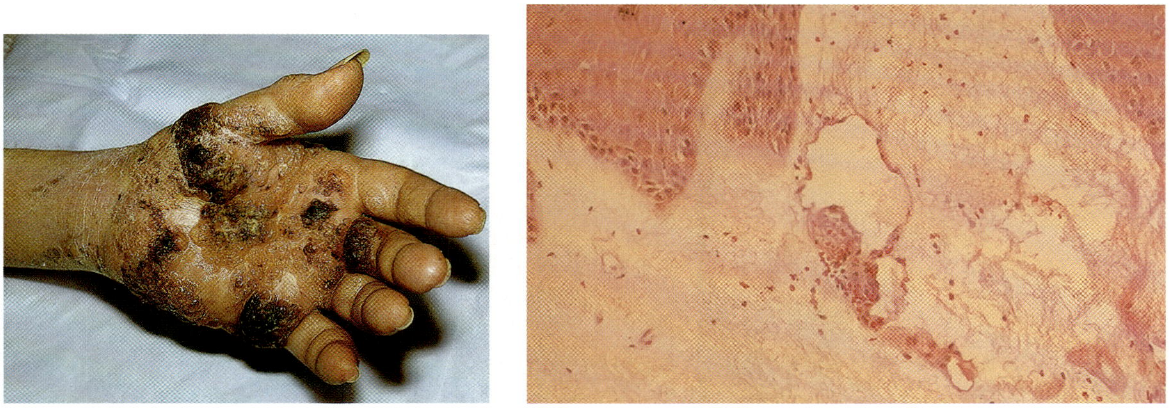

A B

Figure 5.4. A: Blister formation occurring in sclerotic lesions of hands. **B:** Biopsy showing dilated lymphatic channel at dermal/epidermal junction of skin from the sclerodermatous bullous lesion.

surrounding joints may produce crippling articular deformities, including growth retardation with shortening of the extremities (Fig. 5.6) (15). Rarely, the extremity may become functionless.

Involvement of the face may produce an "en coup de sabre" deformity. Facial atrophy may occur in these lesions.

The term "Parry–Romberg syndrome" is applied to patients who develop progressive hemifacial atrophy. This may or may not occur with other features of scleroderma (16). These patients may develop neurologic complications, including epilepsy, and should be evaluated with skull films, electroencephalography, computed tomography, and magnetic resonance imaging. It is controversial whether Parry–Romberg and linear scleroderma are variants of the same disease. However, Tuffanelli (4) has noted that all patients with Parry–Romberg syndrome who he has examined demonstrated cutaneous sclerodermoid features

Patients with linear scleroderma frequently demonstrate antinuclear antibodies, rheumatoid factor, as well as anti–single-stranded DNA (ssDNA) antibodies. Those patients with linear scleroderma with ssDNA antibodies appear to have more extensive disease (17,18). More recently, anti-U_1RNP antibodies have been described in two patients with linear scleroderma without evidence of Raynaud phenomenon (19). Recently, eight of 27 patients with linear scleroderma were detected to have anti–fibrillin-1 antibodies (20). No correlation between the presence of these antibodies and active disease were detected. Other reports indicate anti-U_3RNP antibodies and anti–p-80 coilin antibodies have been described in patients with linear scleroderma with mild disease (6,21).

Although unusual, linear scleroderma may evolve into systemic sclerosis (15). It has been found to coexist with systemic lupus erythematosus (22,23).

Generalized Morphea

Generalized morphea involves widespread areas of the body and is characterized by multiple plaques of morphea that may coalesce, producing large sclerosing areas that can involve all areas of the body (Fig. 5.7) (2,4). However, the face is generally spared. Despite the extensive morphea, Raynaud phenomenon, sclerodactyly, and periungual telangiectasia, internal organs are generally not involved. However, Dr. Provost has seen one patient who developed bullae and vesicles in the plaques of generalized morphea and had patchy

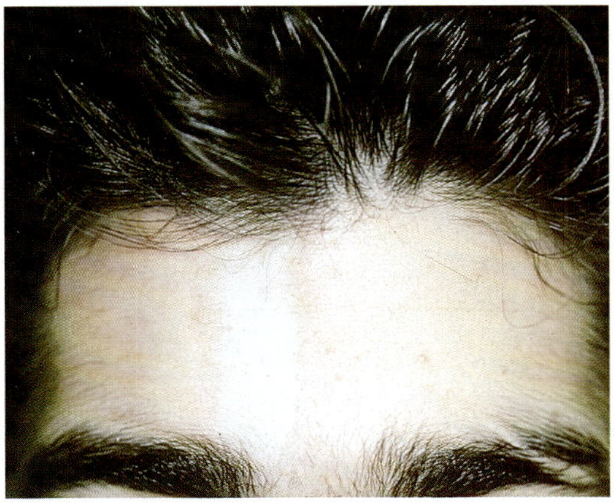

Figure 5.5. "En coup de sabre" of the forehead. The white atrophic band is characteristic of the condition.

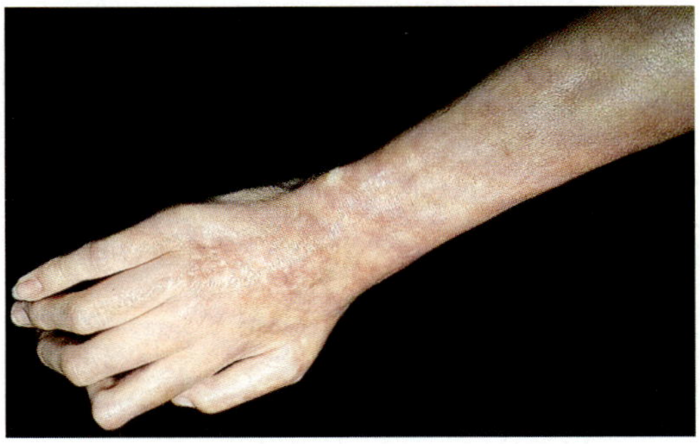

Figure 5.6. Severe linear scleroderma of the upper extremity. This has caused cutaneous fibrosis, atrophy of underlying tissues, and disabling wrist and hand contractures.

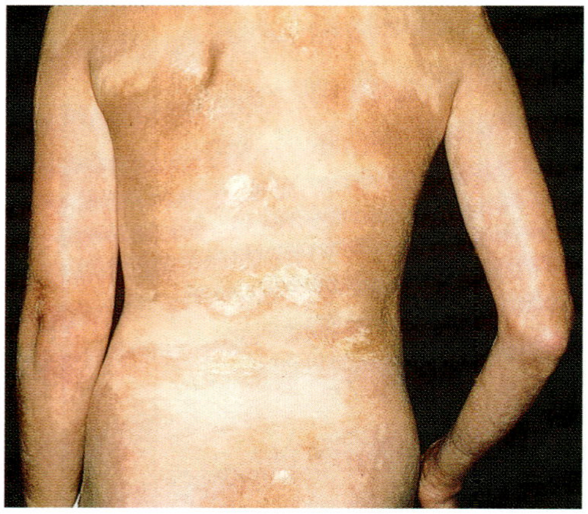

Figure 5.7. Generalized morphea. Numerous indurated lesions with varying degrees of hyperpigmentation are shown. Confluence of lesions is a hallmark of generalized morphea.

sclerodermatous involvement of her gastrointestinal tract associated with lymphatic obstruction and a protein-losing enteropathy (14).

Nodular (Keloidal) Scleroderma

On unusual occasions, patients with systemic sclerosis with generalized or localized morphea may demonstrate sharply defined sclerotic papules and plaques indistinguishable from keloid scars (Fig. 5.8) (24).

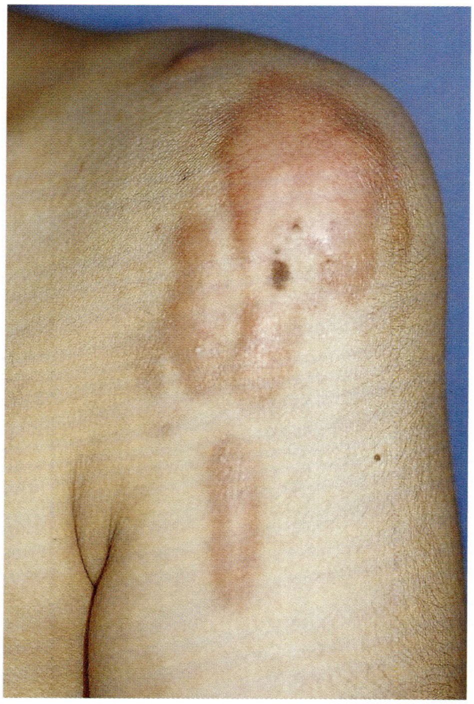

Figure 5.8. Keloidal scleroderma lesions on the shoulcer of a patient with anti-U, RNP antibodies and limited scleroderma.

ATROPHODERMA OF PASINI AND PIERINI

This disease process is a putative variant of early morphea. It is characterized by depressed patches demonstrating a sharp "cliff drop" border. These patches generally occur on the trunk or proximal extremities. They may be gray, blue–brown, or violaceous in color. Jablonska and Szczepanski (10) presented 10-year follow-up on a large group of adults and children with classic atrophoderma of Pasini and Pierini (25). They described development of induration in the patches as well as plaques of morphea in other cutaneous areas in approximately 20% of the patients. Clinicians with a good deal of experience have concluded that atrophoderma of Pasini and Pierini is an abortive form of morphea in which induration has failed to occur (4,26).

EPIDEMIOLOGY

Linear scleroderma most often occurs in the first or second decade of life. Morphea and generalized morphea generally occur in mid life. The female-to-male ratio with localized scleroderma is approximately three to one. All races appear to be affected. On unusual occasions, it occurs in families (27,28).

In a large study from the Mayo Clinic of 235 patients with localized scleroderma, morphea was described in 35%, generalized morphea in 19%, and linear scleroderma in 46% (5). Another study of 115 patients with localized scleroderma reported an occurrence of morphea in 57% patients and a 35% frequency of linear scleroderma (29).

An epidemiologic study of localized scleroderma (Olmstead County, MN) in which the diagnosis was documented by a dermatologist and/or a rheumatologist and confirmed by skin biopsy, showed a female-to-male ratio of 2.6 to 1 except in the linear group, in which there was no sex predilection (30). The overall mean and median ages at diagnosis were 33 and 30 years, respectively. However, the linear group had the lowest mean and median age at diagnosis (18 and 11 years, respectively). Plaque morphea occurred in 56% of cases, generalized morphea in 13%, linear morphea in 20%, and deep morphea in 11%. One patient had guttate morphea and two demonstrated atrophoderma of Pasini and Pierini.

The linear morphea group consisted of 10 patients; 4 patients with en coup de sabre and 2 patients with Parry–Romberg syndrome. The incidence of localized scleroderma was 2.7 per 100,000 population. The prevalence of morphea by age of 18 was judged to be 50 per 100,000 population.

This study revealed that morphea was more common than previously thought (probably because small lesions are ignored by patients but are detected by physicians) and that the number of those in the deep morphea group had increased over the past decade. It also indicated a high frequency of arthralgia, synovitis, uveitis, vertebral abnormalities, contractures, and carpal tunnel syndrome in the linear and deep subtypes of morphea. This study did not observe internal organ damage among patients with morphea. Also, they observed no case of morphea progressing to systemic sclerosis.

However, other studies have reported patients with morphea rarely progressing to systemic sclerosis. In one study, six of 106 patients with localized scleroderma progressed to systemic sclerosis (30a). Other studies indicate that systemic manifestations do occur in a small percentage of patients with morphea. For instance, in a study of 67 patients with morphea at the Mayo Clinic, systemic findings occurred in eight (31). One study indicated that nine of 135 patients with systemic sclerosis had cutaneous lesions of morphea (8). Furthermore, one report indicated that two of 27 patients with localized scleroderma had abnormal cuticle nailfold capillaroscopy. These two patients subsequently developed progressive systemic sclerosis (32).

Other studies have demonstrated that arthralgias have occurred in as many as 44% of patients with localized scleroderma (5). Arthralgias have been noted to precede the cutaneous involvement and have a tendency to disappear with progression of the disease (2). Morphea may also be associated with fever and regional lymphadenopathy on unusual occasions. In addition, migraine headaches, abdominal pain, tinnitus, neuralgias, and spinal column abnormalities are infrequently detected.

Neurologic abnormalities have been detected in patients with facial involvement with linear scleroderma (2). These include uveitis and inflammatory lesions of the cortical and subcortical regions. Rarely, the gastrointestinal tract, lung, muscle, kidney, and heart have been involved in localized scleroderma. One study reported that one patient with morphea and linear scleroderma developed cardiomyopathy (33).

After reviewing the literature, and based on Dr. Provost's 30-year experience as a dermatoimmunologist specializing in connective tissue diseases, it is evident that patients with localized scleroderma generally have a benign self-limited disease, which generally may be active for 3 to 5 years before undergoing a spontaneous resolution. Other investigators have observed a few patients with localized scleroderma to continue to develop new lesions for much longer periods (2).

Few patients with morphea demonstrate or progress to systemic sclerosis. However, patients with linear scleroderma may demonstrate a more aggressive disease, with prominent cutaneous, subcutaneous, and bony deformities. These patients appear more prone to develop autoantibodies and systemic features.

HISTOPATHOLOGY

The hallmark of scleroderma is fibrosis. During the early stages of scleroderma, obvious histologic changes of fibrosis may not be evident (2). However, vacuolization and destruction of blood vessel endothelial cells and basal lamina reduplication may be observed by electron microscopy.

With deep elliptical biopsies of early morphea lesions, the presence of a dense inflammatory dermal and subcutaneous infiltrate composed of lymphocytes (predominately CD4), macrophages, and plasma cells can be detected (34,35). Eosinophils and mast cells occur less frequently. Fibrosis follows the onset of the inflammatory infiltrate. As the scleroderma lesion matures, epidermal atrophy, entrapment of skin appendages, and disappearance of the inflammatory infiltrate occur. Collagen replaces the dermis and subcutaneous tissue.

LABORATORY STUDIES

In addition to antinuclear, anti-ssDNA antibodies and rheumatoid factor activity, as noted before, patients with localized scleroderma commonly demonstrate blood and tissue eosinophilia. The magnitude of blood eosinophilia correlates with disease activity and degree of skin involvement. For example, generally the highest level of eosinophils is detected in generalized morphea and linear scleroderma. In contradistinction, localized morphea have lower eosinophil counts (36,37). Eosinophilia is rare in progressive systemic sclerosis.

Hypergammaglobulinemia is detected in approximately 50% of patients with linear scleroderma and correlates with disease activity (36).

PATHOGENESIS

During the past 25 years, evidence has shown that scleroderma may be a T-cell–mediated disease resulting in stimulation of fibroblasts that subsequently produce various extracellular matrix proteins including type I, II, and VII collagens; glycosaminoglycans; and fibronectin [reviewed by Wigley and Povost [1] and Liu and Connolly [38]). The exact mechanism of how this putative T-cell–mediated autoimmune disease pertubates and fibroblast proliferation and overproduction of collagen and various other extracellular matrix proteins has been, and is, an area of active investigation.

In the 1970s, histologic and immunohistologic studies, initially by Fleischmajer and Nedwich (34), demonstrated that elliptical deep biopsies of early sclerodermatous lesions displayed the presence of an inflammatory cell infiltrate composed predominately of T cells, monocyte-macrophages, and an admixture of eosinophils in a perivascular distribution deep in the reticular dermis in close proximity to the subcutaneous tissue. Furthermore, the T cells were predominately $CD4^+$ (35).

In the early 1970s, LeRoy (39,40) demonstrated that the cultured fibroblasts from lesional skin in patients with scleroderma overproduced collagen and other extracellular matrix components. Furthermore, this abnormal overproduction of collagen was maintained *in vitro* for several passages. Additional studies indicated that fibroblasts in the reticular perivascular regions demonstrated increased collagen messenger RNA (mRNA) transcripts (41). It was also learned that conditioned medium from stimulated human peripheral mononuclear cells could induce normal fibroblasts to overproduce collagen and glycosaminoglycans (42,43).

Recent research has been focused attempting to understand the molecular mechanisms responsible for the initiation and maintenance of the scleroderma active fibroblasts. As noted before, it is a working hypothesis that the fibrosis that is the hallmark of scleroderma is induced by the T-lymphocytes and monocyte-macrophages at the dermal subcutaneous level of early sclerodermatous lesions (44). It should be noted that with established lesions, the inflammatory infiltrate is either markedly diminished or absent.

Other cells may also be capable of inducing fibroblast collagen production. For example, there is evidence indicating that activated vascular endothelial cells, perhaps representing vascular injury, are capable of up-regulating the expression of adhesion molecules leading to recruitment of inflammatory cells (45). Furthermore, coculture of normal fibroblasts and activated endothelial cells demonstrate that endothelial cells can elaborate factors capable of inducing fibroblasts to proliferate and produce increased matrix proteins (38,46).

It is also conceivable that mast cells, which are readily detected in connective tissue, may play a role. The production of histamine, heparin, and tryptase may serve to increase not only vasopermeability but also fibroblast matrix production (38,47,48). For example, in the tight skin–positive (Tsk^+) mouse model, disodium chromoglycolate prevents dermal fibrosis (49).

Cytokines and growth factors play key roles in fibroblast modulation. The cytokines and growth factors capable of enhancing or inhibiting fibroblast collagen synthesis are listed in Table 5.3.

TABLE 5.3. Factors in Fibroblast Modulation

Cytokines promoting fibroblast collagen synthesis:
Transforming growth factor-β, connective tissue growth factor, interleukin-4, interleukin-6 (oncostatin-m), insulin growth factor-1, endothelin-1
Cytokines suppressing fibroblast collagen synthesis:
Interferons-α, -β, -γ; interleukin-10; tumor necrosis factor-α

From Lui B, Connolly MK. The pathogenesis of cutaneous fibrosis. *Semin Cutan Med Surg* 1998;17:3–11, with permission.

Currently, evidence indicates transforming growth factor-β (TGF-β) composed of multiple isoforms (TGF-β 1, 2, and 3) may provide the early stimulus for fibroblast overproduction of collagen (38). In *in vivo* experiments in mice, TGF-β injected subcutaneously induces fibrosis and granuloma formation (50). It also induces proliferative responses in human dermal fibroblast via the up-regulation of platelet-derived growth factor-α (PDGF-α) receptors (51). In addition to up-regulating PDGF receptors, there is evidence that TGF-β induces transcriptional activation of collagen, fibronectin, and glycosaminoglycans genes in fibroblasts, resulting in overproduction (38).

Despite these impressive histochemical and *in situ* hybridization observations, data demonstrating elevated TGF-β levels in plasma of patients with localized as well as other forms of scleroderma have been inconstant (reviewed by Liu and Connolly [38]). In addition, inconsistent results regarding mRNA expression of TGF-β isoforms and the protein products of the isoforms have been observed. Data from cultured scleroderma fibroblasts indicate normal amounts of TGF-β proteins as well as receptors (52).

It should be noted, however, that despite these equivocal or negative findings, TGF-β is found in the early inflammatory lesions (blood vessel location). Thus, it may be capable of initiating fibrosis in fibroblasts.

Other factors may be responsible for maintaining the autonomous phenotype of the scleroderma fibroblast (38). One possible factor is connective tissue growth factor (CTGF), which is induced by TGF-β and is capable of stimulating collagen and other extracellular matrix protein synthesis by fibroblasts (53). Unlike TGF-β mRNA, which is detected during the inflammatory phase of scleroderma, CTGF mRNA is overexpressed in the fibrotic phase. Furthermore, CTGF injected subcutaneously into mice induces granulation tissue and fibrosis (54).

Additional data indicate that the lymphokines interleukin-1 (IL-1), IL-4, and IL-6 and the IL-6–related molecule oncostatin M are capable of stimulating human fibroblast *in vitro* to produce collagen and other matrix proteins (55–58). Furthermore, *in situ* hybridization has demonstrated increased mRNA levels in lesional skin as well as increased quantities of IL-4 and IL-6 proteins. Increased serum levels of IL-4 in patients with scleroderma have been reported (59).

Plasma endothelin-l is increased in patients with scleroderma (60). Furthermore, endothelins stimulate fibroblast proliferation and collagen synthesis *in vitro* and patients with scleroderma appear to produce increased quantities of endothelin (61).

Other studies indicate that insulin growth factor is capable of inducing increased collagen synthesis *in vitro* (62).

As noted before, PDGF-α, which can be up-regulated by TGF-β, has been detected in scleroderma lesions and has been shown to be capable of inducing fibroblast proliferation (63).

Tissue inhibitor of metalloproteinase-l (TIMP-1) may play a role in modulating scleroderma fibroblasts (38). TIMP-1 is capable of inducing proliferation of a scleroderma fibroblast. Anti–TIMP-1 antibody blocks this proliferating activity in scleroderma fibroblasts (64,65). In addition, TIMP-3 is induced by TGF-β and mRNA TIMP-3 inhibitor is elevated in scleroderma skin fibroblasts (65).

Cytokines, especially T-cell–derived interferon-γ (IFN-γ), are capable of suppressing fibroblast collagen and matrix protein synthesis. Also, IL-10 and tumor necrosis factor-α (TNF-α) suppress collagen synthesis (66,67).

In addition to cytokines and growth factors, other molecules may induce fibroblast collagen production. For example, oxygen in free radical formation, a product of ischemia and reperfusion, which theoretically can occur in scleroderma, may have an effect on fibroblastic activity (1,38). Superoxide free radical formation and nitric oxide are capable of inducing collagen synthesis by human fibroblasts (68,69).

In summary, although it has been over two decades since Fleischmajer's group demonstrated in early sclerodermatous lesions a lymphocytic monocytic macrophage infiltrate at the dermal subcutaneous level in early sclerodermatous lesions and LeRoy's studies demonstrating autonomous fibroblasts overproduction of collagen and other extra matrix proteins, the exact molecular mechanism(s) as to how activated mononuclear cells induce and maintain the scleroderma fibroblast phenotype is/are unknown.

ANIMAL MODELS FOR SCLERODERMA

In the Tsk mouse, mast cells appear to play a role in inducing fibrosis. Reportedly, mast cells play a role in graft versus host disease as well as interstitial pulmonary fibrosis (38). In the Tsk mouse, disodium chromoglycolate fed to the mouse throughout adult life prevents the development of dermal fibrosis. However, lymphocytes appear to have an important role in the pathogenesis of the Tsk mouse. In adoptive transfer experiments, it has been shown that progression of dermal fibrosis was markedly suppressed in Tsk^{+} $CD4^{-/-}$ mice (49). In the Tsk mouse model, these studies suggested a prominent role for CD4 lymphocytes in the development of skin fibrosis.

Bleomycin, which induces pulmonary fibrosis as a complication of therapy, is capable of inducing dermal fibrosis in severe combined immunodeficient (SCID) mice by subcutaneous injection. In addition, bleomycin is capable of inducing dermal sclerosis in the absence of mast cells in genetically mast cell–deficient WBB-6, F1-W/Wv mice. Furthermore, bleomycin induces skin fibrosis in SCID mice and directly induces up-regulation of TGF-β mRNA. These studies indicate that the bleomycin effect on fibroblasts does not involve lymphocytes (70).

Other studies indicate that bleomycin induces myofibroblasts to differentiate into fibroblasts, overproducing collagen. These studies demonstrate the expression of alpha smooth muscle actin (α-SMA) in the fibroblast in lesional skin as well as in the fibrosis lung in this mouse model (70). This significant increase in immunoreactive fibroblastic cells for α-SMA in lesional skin occurs in parallel with the induction of dermal sclerosis. Other studies demonstrate that with the concomitant treatment with anti–TGF-β antibody and bleomycin, the number of α-SMA–positive fibroblasts significantly decreases (approximately 50%) together with the reduction of dermal sclerosis. These studies suggest that bleomycin alters myofibroblasts into fibroblastic cells capable of producing increased quantities of dermal fibrosis and that this is mediated, at least in part, by TGF-β.

ROLE OF *BORRELIA BURGDORFERI* INFECTION IN THE PATHOGENESIS OF MORPHEA

Although for almost 20 years, it has been suggested that various forms of localized scleroderma may be induced by *Borrelia burgdorferi*, the exact role, if any, of a spirochetal infection remains controversial (71). A most recent study from Germany that used serologic as well as polymerase chain reaction (PCR) techniques demonstrated no evidence for *B. burgdorferi* in a group of 54 patients with morphea (72). Furthermore, it should be noted that each individual patient was evaluated for a history of tick bites and the clinical presence of erythema chronicum migrans. This study is important because it occurred in southern Germany, a geographic area with a high prevalence of tick-borne *B. burgdorferi* infections. Other investigators, on the basis of their positive studies, have proposed that morphea might be caused by certain subspecies of *B. burgdorferi* found exclusively in certain geographic areas.

This author, however, believes that the lack of positive sophisticated serologic tests, negative PCR findings, the absence of a history of tick bites, and morphologic evidence of erythema chronicum migrans provide definitive data establishing a lack of an etiologic role of a *B. burgdorferi* infection in the pathogenesis of localized scleroderma.

It should be noted that most of the positive reports of the association of cutaneous scleroderma with *B. burgdorferi* have come from Europe. In a large study from the United States, Tuffanelli (73) was unable to find an association.

SCLERODERMA-LIKE CUTANEOUS SYNDROMES

Eosinophilia-Myalgia Syndrome

This syndrome, characterized by myalgia, dermatitis, respiratory symptoms, paresthesias, edema, and muscle weakness appeared in epidemic form in the United States in 1989. Some patients developed generalized morphea-like lesions (12,4,38). Approximately 1,500 cases occurred (reviewed Mori et al. [74]). The cause was traced to the ingestion of products containing L-tryptophan, ostensibly from a single supplier. Extensive studies indicated a minute contamination of the implicated L-tryptophan (an L-tryptophan dimer 1,1-ethylidenebis L-tryptophan (Peak E). This Peak E has been shown to be capable of directly stimulating collagen production in dermal fibroblasts. This occurs by transcriptional activation of the collagen promoter (75,76).

Unfortunately, although the skin symptoms significantly improved over several years (with cessation of L-tryptophan usage), peripheral neuropathy and myopathy had a tendency to persist. In addition, progressive cognitive dysfunction has been noted (1). Furthermore, the age- and sex-adjusted mortality rates appears to be at least three times higher in these patients than in the general population or in asymptomatic individuals who have used L-tryptophan (74).

Unfortunately, isolated case reports still appear in the literature of the occurrence of eosinophilia-myalgia syndrome in individuals who have no history of L-tryptophan use (74). These studies suggest that other unidentified contaminants exist in our society capable of inducing this syndrome.

One such syndrome is the toxic oil syndrome reported in Spain in the late 1970s that was induced by adulterated cooking oil. Recently, an aniline contaminant has been detected in L-tryptophan preparations. This compound, 3-(phenylamino)-L-aniline, is metabolized in the liver to 3-(phenylamino)-1,2-propanediol (PAP). This PAP metabolite had been implicated in the Spanish toxic oil syndrome epidemic. These studies suggest that the eosinophilia-myalgia syndrome and the Spanish toxic oil syndrome may be etiologically related (74).

Role of Eosinophils in Fibrosis

Both eosinophilic myalgia syndrome and the Spanish toxic oil syndrome, in addition to demonstrating a striking cutaneous fibrosis, were associated with a very prominent eosinophilia. One putative component of eosinophils, major basic protein (MBP), may play a role as a fibrogenic cytokine. Recent studies indicate that MBP alone or synergistically with TGF-β can induce the production of IL-6 by normal fibroblasts. IL-6 enhances collagen production (74). Also, degranulation of eosinophils can induce quiescent fibroblast to transform into α-SMA–positive myofibroblast. As noted before, myofibroblasts produce fibrosis in the bleomycin mouse model.

Eosinophilic Fasciitis

This disease is characterized by prominent peripheral and tissue eosinophilia occurring in affected areas of the skin. The initial features of eosinophilic fasciitis may be quite similar to those of the eosinophilic myalgia syndrome (1,74). During the acute stage, patients have pronounced swelling and pitting of the extremities. On many occasions, this initial stage followed vigorous exercise. With progression, the tissue swelling dissipates and is followed by induration of the skin and the onset of morphea-like lesions (4). The morphea-like lesions occur in approximately 30% of patients. A peculiar "groove sign" occurs on the inner aspect of the upper arm caused by lack of fibrosis along blood vessels (Fig. 5.9). Unlike systemic sclerosis, Raynaud phenomenon, sclerodactyly, and facial involvement do not occur. Capillary nailfold abnormalities are not detected. However, joint contractures leading to immobility may occur. Eosinophilic fasciitis may also be complicated by carpal tunnel syndrome, peripheral neuropathy, and inflammatory arthritis (77–79). These patients may have hematologic abnormalities including aplastic anemia, hemolytic anemia, lymphoma, and B-cell lymphocytic leukemia (80–83).

The etiology of eosinophilic fasciitis is unknown. Eosinophilic fasciitis patients have been shown to produce elevated quantities of IFN-γ as well as IL-5 *in vitro* (IL-5 promotes eosinophilia). Local degranulation of eosinophils may be responsible for the fibrogenesis. In addition, mast cells are often detected and may also con-

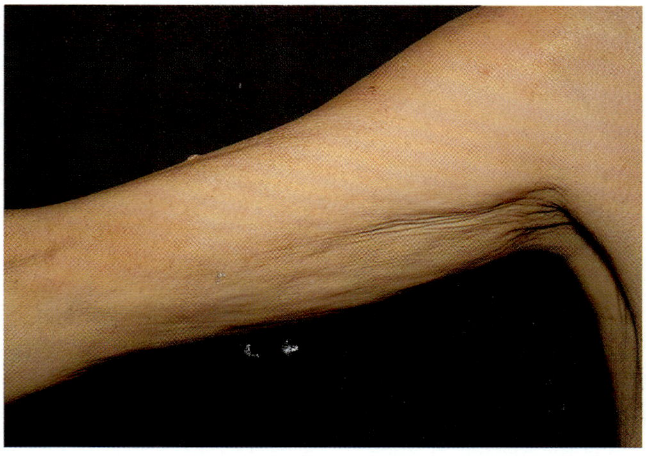

Figure 5.9. "Groove sign" demonstrating linear depression along blood vessels of upper arm of a patient with eosinophilic fasciitis.

tribute to fibrogenesis. It has been noted that fibroblasts from the fascia of eosinophilic fasciitis patients demonstrate increased collagen gene expression. In addition, these fascial fibroblasts demonstrate elevated CTGF and TGF-β 1 mRNA expression. These studies suggest an autocrine mediated stimulatory loop involving TGF-β and CTGF in the pathogenesis of the tissue fibrosis in eosinophilic fasciitis (74).

Scleredema

This is a striking chronic edematous disease most commonly seen in association with adult onset of diabetes producing induration of the neck, shoulder girdle, and upper extremities (1,2,4,84). It can occur acutely in association with an upper respiratory infection. Rarely, the face may be involved. Recent evidence indicates that scleredema may occur in association with an HIV infection (85). The cutaneous induration of scleredema is often self-limited, generally resolving within a 2-year period. Raynaud phenomenon, sclerodactyly, and abnormal cuticle nailfold capillary microscopy are absent. Biopsy of the affected area demonstrates amorphous material giving a positive stain with toluidine blue or colloidal iron. On occasions, a monoclonal gammopathy may be detected in adults with scleredema, and this gammopathy may proceed to the development of multiple myeloma (86).

Scleromyxedema

This disease exists in two forms: one in which sclerosis (scleromyxedema) is dominant; the other in which mucinosis (papular mucinosis) is characteristic (1,2,4). Scleromyxedema may mimic progressive systemic sclerosis (Fig. 5.10). However, Raynaud phenomenon, sclerodactyly, and cuticle nailfold capillary microscopic abnormalities are absent. Biopsies demonstrate amorphous material giving a positive reaction with colloidal iron, toluidine blue, or Alcian blue stains. Fibroblasts appear to be increased but inflammation is not prominent.

In general, scleromyxedema and papular mucinosis are associated with the presence of a monoclonal gammopathy, predominately IgG λ (87). Rarely myeloma has been described. On occasions, acute neurologic signs as well as encephalopathy have been described in association with scleromyxedema (88). Recently, a diffuse skin induration similar to scleromyxedema has been described in hemodialysis patients (89). This has also been referred to as vephrogenic fileosing demopahy. Biopsy of these patients demonstrate similar pathologic changes to those seen in scleromyxedema.

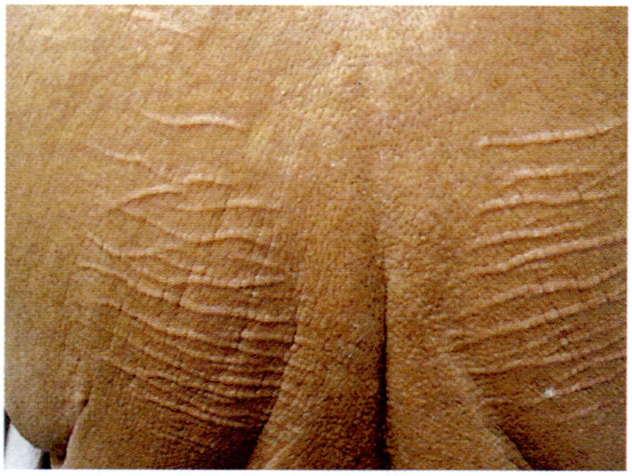

Figure 5.10. Widespread lesions of scleromyxedema displaying peculiar linear lesions on the lower back. Softening of these lesions occurred following PUVA therapy.

TREATMENT

Localized scleroderma may resolve without treatment. For a review of the treatment of scleroderma and localized scleroderma, see Table 5.4 and the article by Sapadia and Fleischmajer (90). Unfortunately, there are few controlled trials. For the most part, therapy has been empiric. In the past, topical as well as oral corticosteroids, antimalarials, and D-penicillamine have been used with varying degrees of reported success. Although previously, once enthusiastically used, a double-blind study showed D-penicillamine had little or no effect on systemic or localized scleroderma (91). Methotrexate in combination with intravenous pulse methylprednisolone has been successfully employed in children with localized scleroderma (92).

Most important, a plethora of reports have recently appeared in the literature that suggest phototherapy with or without psoralens may be effective in the treatment of patients with localized scleroderma. Topical applications of psoralens in the form of a gel as well as oral psoralens have been shown to be effective in the treatment of scleroderma (93–102).

The mechanism of action of ultraviolet (UV) light is an area of intense investigation (Fig. 5.11). There is evidence that UV-A is a potent stimulus for the cutaneous expression of Smad7 antagonist of the Smad signal transduction system. Smad7 binds to the cytoplasmic domain of the TGF-β receptor blocking TGF-β–induced responses, which in turn prevents extracellular matrix formation including collagen (103).

There is also recent evidence that UV light, A-1 (UV-A1, 340 to 400 nm) phototherapy is effective in clearing sclerotic plaques, even those of long duration. Investigations have demonstrated that UV-A1 induces interstitial collagenase (matrix metalloproteinase 1 [MMP-1]) (104).

These experiments indicate that UV light irradiation induces collagenase activity in fibroblasts of sclerotic plaques. This activity, plus the modulation of the TNF-β receptor and UV light's observed suppression of inflammatory infiltrates suggests that PUVA and UV-A1 may be potent therapeutic agents in diseases characterized by excessive collagen production which include all forms of cutaneous morphea (plaque morphea, guttate morphea, morphea profundus, bullous or vesicular morphea, linear morphea, generalized morphea, nodular (keloidal) morphea and atrophoderma of Passini and Pierini. From collaborations

TABLE 5.4. Treatment of Scleroderma

Therapy of localized scleroderma (morphea)
Corticosteroids (topical and intralesional)
Topical calcipotriene
PUVA
Linear scleroderma
Corticosteroids (intralesional for en coup de sabre)
Psoralen—UV-A baths
UV-A alone (340–400 nm)
PUVA, calcitrol
Oral calcitrol
Topical calcipotriene
Generalized morphea
PUVA
Psoralen—UV-A baths
UV-A alone (340–400 nm)
Oral calcitrol, topical calcipotriene
Methotrexate
Methotrexate plus corticosteroids

From Spadin AN, Fleischmajer R. Treatment of scleroderma. *Arch Dermatol* 2002;138:99–105, with permission.

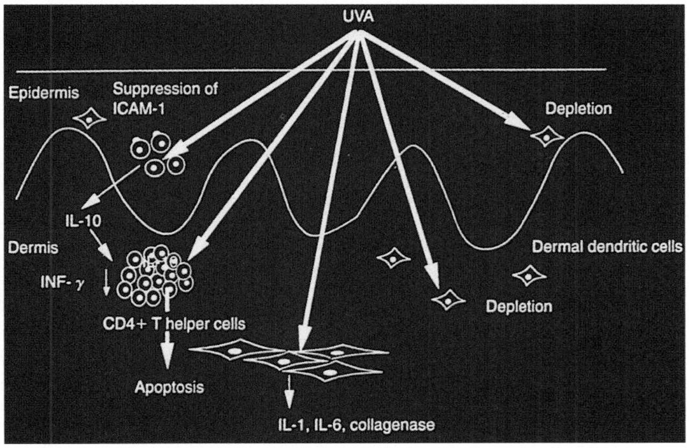

Figure 5.11. Possible mechanisms for therapeutic effects of UVA and PUVA on scleroderma. *1,* Suppressive effect on inflammatory infiltrates at dermal subcutaneous perivascular areas. *2,* Inhibition of collagen production by scleroderma fibroblasts. *3,* Induction of collagenase activity.

with Warwick Morison, Dr. Provost can personally attest to the effectiveness of PUVA therapy in the treatment of localized, generalized morphea and acrosclerotic scleroderma. They have also successfully treated scleredema of Buschke and have noted pronounced improvement in patients with scleromyxedema associated with an IgG lambda paraprotein.

Finally, there is some evidence to indicate that analogues of vitamin D [calcitrol (1α,25-dihydroxycholecalciferol) and calcipotriene] may have some benefit in the treatment of localized scleroderma (105–107). A recent study indicates that topical calcipotriol ointment plus low-dose UV-A1 is effective in treating childhood morphea (108). A double-blind, placebo-controlled study, however, of oral calcitrol for the treatment of localized scleroderma failed to show benefit as did a double-blind, placebo-controlled study of interlesional IFN-γ for the treatment of localized scleroderma (109,110).

REFERENCES

1. Wigley FM, Provost TT. Scleroderma. In: Provost TT, Flynn JA, eds. *Cutaneous medicine: cutaneous manifestations of systemic diseases.* Hamilton, Ontario, Canada: BC Decker, Inc. 2001:104–126.
2. Greenberg AS, Falanga V. Localized cutaneous sclerosis. In: Sontheimer RD, Provost TT, eds. *Cutaneous manifestations of rheumatic diseases.* Baltimore: Lippincott Williams & Wilkins, 1996:141–155.
3. Sontheimer RD, Callen JP, Camisa C, et al. Guidelines of care for scleroderma and sclerodermoid disorders. *J Amer Acad Dermatol* 1996;35:609–614.
4. Tuffanelli DL. Localized scleroderma. *Sem Cutan Med Surg* 1998;17:27–33.
5. Christiansen HB, Dorsey CS, O'Leary PAA, et al. Localized scleroderma: a clinical study of two hundred-thirty five cases. *Arch Dermatol* 1956;74: 629–639.
6. Yamani K, Ihn H, Kubo M, et al. Anti-U3snRNP in localized scleroderma. *Ann Rheum Dis* 1993;1157.
7. Ohtaki N, Mijamoto C, Orita M, et al. Concurrent morphea and neonatal lupus erythematosus in a boy born to a mother with SLE. *Br J Dermatol* 1986; 115:85–90.
8. Soma Y, Tamaki T, Kikuchi K, et al. Coexistence of morphea and systemic sclerosis. *Dermatology* 1993;186:103–105.

8a. Birdi N, Laxer RM, Thorner P, et al. Localized scleroderma progressing to systemic disease; case report and review of the literature. *Arthritis Rheum* 1993;36:410–415.

9. Wong SS, Holt PJ. Generalized morphea and primary biliary cirrhosis: a rare association and improvement with oxpentifylline. *Clin Exp Dermatol* 1992;17: 371–373.
10. De P, Lloyd J, Rashid AM, et al. Morphea presenting shortly after the onset of Schmidt's syndrome. *Clin Exp Dermatol* 2001;25:167–169.
11. Falanga V. Fibrosing syndromes of childhood. *Adv Dermatol* 1991;6:145–159.
12. Doyle JA, Connolly SM, Winkelmann RK. Cutaneous and subcutaneous inflammatory sclerosis syndromes. *Arch Dermatol* 1982;118:886–891.
13. Piette WW, Dorsey JK, Foucar E. Clinical and serologic expression of localized scleroderma and review of the literature. *J Am Acad Dermatol* 1985;13:342–350.
14. Synkowski DR, Lobitz WC, Provost TT. Bullous scleroderma. *Arch Dermatol* 1981;117:135–137.

14a. Kobayaski T, Willeberg A, Serup J, et al. Generalized morphea with blisters; a case report. *Acta Dermatol-Venereol* 1990;70:454– 456.

15. Mayorquin FJ, McCurley TL, Leveinier JE, et al. Progression of childhood linear scleroderma to fatal systemic sclerosis. *J Rheumatol* 1994;21:1955–1957.
16. Lehman TJ. The Parry-Romberg syndrome of progressive facial hemiatrophy and linear scleroderma en coup de sabre: mistaken diagnosis or overlapping conditions. *J Rheumatol* 1992;19:844–845.
17. Falanga V, Medsger TA Jr, Reichlin M, et al. Linear scleroderma: clinical spectrum, prognosis and laboratory abnormalities. *Ann Intern Med* 1986;104: 849–857.
18. Falanga V, Medsger TA Jr, Reichlin M. High titers of antibodies to single-stranded DNA in linear scleroderma. *Arch Dermatol* 1985;121: 345–347.
19. Jamane K, Ihn H, Kuboo M, et al. Anti-U1RNP antibodies in patients with localized scleroderma. *Arch Dermatol Research* 2001;293:455–459.
20. Arnett FC, Tan FK, Uziel Y, et al. Autoantibodies to the extracellular matrix microfibrillar protein Fibrillin-1 in patients with localized scleroderma. *Arthritis Rheum* 1999;42:2656–2659.
21. Fugimoto M, Kikuchi K, Tamaki T, et al. Distribution of anti-p80-coilin autoantibody in collagen diseases and various skin diseases. *Br J Dermatol* 1997;137:916–920.
22. Schainberg CG, Rodrigues-Periera RM, Cossermelli W. Linear scleroderma and systemic lupus erythematosus. *J Rheumatol* 1990; 17:1427–1428.
23. Baumgarten AK, Sukenik S, Horowitz J. Linear scleroderma, hemiatrophy and systemic lupus erythematosus. *J Rheumatol* 1989;16:1141–1143.
24. James WD, Berger TG, Butler DF, et al. Nodular (keloidal) scleroderma. *J Am Acad Dermatol* 1984;11:1111–1114.
25. Jablonska S, Szczepanski A. Atrophoderma Pasini-Pierini: is it an entity? *Dermatologia* 1962;125:226–242.
26. Kencka D, Blaszcyk M, Jablonska S. Atrophoderma Pasini-Pierini is a primary abortive morphea. *Dermatology* 1995;190:203–206.
27. Molta CT, Khan MA, Aponte CJ, et al. Familial occurrence of systemic sclerosis, rheumatoid arthritis and other immunological disorders; report of two kindreds with study of HLA antigens and review of the literature. *Clin Exp Rheumatol* 1989;7:229–236.
28. Arnett FC, Bias WB, McLean RH, et al. Connective tissue disease in southeast Georgia: a community based study of immunogenetic markers and autoantibodies. *J Rheumatol* 1990;17:1029–1035.
29. Curtis AC, Jansen TG. The prognosis of localized scleroderma. *Arch Derm* 1958;78:749–757.
30. Peterson LS, Nelson AM, Su WP, et al. The epidemiology of morphea (localized scleroderma) in Olmstead County 1960-1993. *J Rheumatol* 1997;24:73–80.

30a. Curtis AC, Jansen TG. The prognosis of localized scleroderma. *Arch Dermatol* 1958;78:749–757.

31. Winkelmann PK, Connolly SM, Doyle JA. Localized scleroderma and systemic disease. In: Kukita A, Seiji M, eds. *Proceedings of the XVI International Congress of Dermatology Tokyo, Japan* May 23-28 1982 Toyko: University of Tokyo Press, 1983.
32. Maricq HR. Capillary abnormalities, Raynaud's phenomenon and systemic sclerosis in patients with localized scleroderma. *Arch Dermatol* 1992;128: 630–632.
33. Moore EC, Cohen F, Farooki Z, et al. Focal scleroderma and severe cardiomyopathy; patient report and brief review. *Am J Dis Child* 1991;145:229–231.
34. Fleischmajer R, Nedwich A. Generalized morphea, I: histology of the dermis and subcutaneous tissue. *Arch Derm* 1972;106:509–514.
35. Aberer E, Klade H, Hobisch G. A clinical, histological and immunochemical comparison of acrodermatitis chronica atrophicans and morphea. *Am J Dermatopathol* 1991;13:334–341.
36. Falanga V, Medsger TA, Reichlin M, et al. Linear scleroderma; clinical spectrum, prognosis and laboratory abnormalities. *Ann Intern Med* 1986;104:849–857.
37. Falanga V, Medsger TA. Frequency, levels and significance of blood eosinophilia in systemic sclerosis, localized scleroderma and eosinophilia fasciitis. *J Am Acad Dermatol* 1987;17:648–656.
38. Liu B, Connolly MK. The pathogenesis of cutaneous fibrosis. *Semin Cutan Med Surg* 1998;17:3–11.
39. LeRoy EC. Connective tissue synthesis by scleroderma fibroblasts in cell culture. *J Exp Med* 1972;135:1351–1362.
40. LeRoy EC. Increased collagen synthesis by scleroderma skin fibroblasts *in vitro*: a possible defect in the regulation of activation of the scleroderma fibroblast. *J Clin Invest* 1974;54:880–889.
41. Peltonen J, Kahari L, Jaakkola S, et al. Evaluation of transforming growth factor β and type I procollagen gene expression in fibrotic skin disease by *in situ* hybridization. *J Invest Dermatol* 1991;94:365–371.
42. Johnson RL, Ziff M. Lymphokine stimulation of collagen accumulation. *J Clin Invest* 1976;58:240–252.
43. Worrall JG, Whiteside TL, Prince RK, et al. Persistence of scleroderma-like phenotype in normal fibroblasts after prolonged exposure to soluable mediators from mononuclear cells. *Arthritis Rheum* 1986;29:54–64.
44. Fleischmajer R, Perlish JS, Duncan M. Scleroderma: a model for fibrosis. *Arch Derm* 1983;119:955–962.
45. Kahaleh MB. The role of vascular of endothelium in the pathogenesis of connective tissue disease: endothelial injury, activation, participation and response. *Clin Exp Rheum* 1990;8:595–601.

46. Denton CP, Xu S, Black CM, et al. Scleroderma fibroblasts show increased responsiveness to endothelial cell derived IL-1 and bfgf. *J Invest Dermatol* 1997;108:269–274.
47. Gruber BL. Mast cells: accessory cells which potentiate fibrosis. *Int Rev Immunol* 1995;12:259–279.
48. Gruber BL, Kew RR, Jeloska A, et al. Human mast cells activate fibro-blasts: tryptase is a fibrogenic factor stimulating collagen messenger ribonucleic acid synthesis and fibroblast chemotaxis. *J Immunol* 1997;158:2310–2317.
49. Walker MA, Harley RA, LeRoy EC. Inhibition of fibrosis in the TSK mice by blocking mast cell degranulation. *J Rheumatol* 1987;14:299–301.
50. Roberts AB, Sporn MB, Assoian RK, et al. Transforming growth factor type beta: rapid induction of fibrosis and angiogenesis *in vivo* and stimulation of collagen formation in vitro. Proc Nat Acad Sci U S A 1986;83:4167–4171.
51. Jiminez SA, Hitraya E, Varga J. Pathogenesis of scleroderma: collagen. *Rheum Dis Clin North Am* 1996;22:647–674.
52. Needleman BW, Choi J, Burrows-Mezu A, et al. Secretion and binding of transforming growth factor-beta by scleroderma and normal dermal fibroblasts. *Arthritis Rheum* 1990;33:650–656.
53. Igarashi, A, Bradham DM, Okochi H, et al. Connective tissue growth factor. *J Dermatol* 1992;19:642–643.
54. Frazier K, Williams S, Kothapalli D, et al. Stimulation of fibroblast cell growth, matrix production and granulation formation by connective tissue factors. *J Invest Dermatol* 1996;107:408–411.
55. Gillery P, Ferutin C, Nicolas JF, et al. Interleukin-4 stimulates collagen gene expression in human fibroblast monolayer cultures: potential role in fibrosis. *FEBS Lett* 1992;302:231–234.
56. Duncan MR, Berman B. Stimulation of collagen and glycosaminoglycan production in cultured adult dermal fibroblasts by recombinant human interleukin-6. *J Invest Dermatol* 1991;97:686–692.
57. Duncan MR, Hasan A, Berman B. Oncostatin M stimulates collagen and glycosaminoglycan production by cultured normal fibroblasts. *J Invest Dermatol* 1995;104:128–133.
58. Kawaguchi Y, Harigai, Suzuki K, et al. Interleukin 1 receptor on fibroblasts from systemic sclerosis patients induces excessive functional responses to interleukin 1 beta. *Biochem Biophys Res Commun* 1993; 190:154–161.
59. Needleman BW, Wigley FM, Stai RW. Interleukin 1, interleukin 2, interleukin 4, interleukin 6, tumor necrosis factor alpha, and interferon-gamma levels in sera from patients with scleroderma. *Arthritis Rheum* 1992;35:67–72.
60. Morelli S, Ferri C, Poletlini E, et al. Plasma endothelin-1 levels, pulmonary hypertension and lung fibrosis in patients with systemic sclerosis. *Am J Med* 1995;99:255–260.
61. Dawes KE, Cambrey AD, Campa JS, et al. Changes in collagen metabolism in response to endothelin-1: evidence for fibroblast heterogeneity. *Int J Brochem Cell Biol* 1996;28:229–238.
62. Gillery P, Lepeue A, Marquart FX, et al. Insulin-like growth factor-1 (IGF-1) stimulates protein synthesis and collagen gene expression in monolayer and lattice cultures of fibroblasts. *J Cell Physiol* 1992;152:389–396.
63. Gay S, Jones RE Jr, Huang CQ, et al. Immunohistologic demonstration of platelet derived growth factor (PDGF) and sis-oncogene expression in scleroderma. *J Invest Dermatol* 1989;92:301–303.
64. Kikuchi K, Kubo M, Sato S, et al. Serum tissue inhibitor of metalloproteinases in patients with systemic sclerosis. *J Am Acad Dermatol* 1995;33:973–978.
65. Mattila L, Airola K, Ahonen M, et al. Activation of tissue inhibitor of metalloproteinases-3 (TIMP-3) mRNA expression in scleroderma skin fibroblasts. *J Invest Dermatol* 1998;110:416–421.
66. Duncan MR, Berman B. Persistence of reduced-collagen-producing phenotype in cultured scleroderma fibroblasts after short-term exposure to interferons. *J Clin Invest* 1987;79:1318–1324.
67. Reitamo S, Remity A, Tamai K, et al. Interleukin-10 modulates type I collagen and matrix metalloproteinase gene expression in cultured human skin fibroblasts. *J Clin Invest* 1994;94:2489–2492.
68. Silverstein JL, Steen VD, Medsger TA Jr, et al. Cutaneous hypoxia in patients with systemic sclerosis (scleroderma). *Arch Dermatol* 1998;124:1379–1382.
69. Shaffer MR, Efron PA, Thornton FJ, et al. Nitric oxide, an autocrine regulator of wound fibroblast synthetic junction. *J Immunol* 1997;158:2375–2381.
70. Yamamoto T, Nishika K. Animal model of sclerotic skin: increased expression of alpha smooth muscle actin in fibroblastic cells in bleomycin-induced scleroderma. *Clin Immunol* 2002;102:77–83.
71. Weide B, Waltz T, Garbe C. Is morphea caused by *Borrelia burgdorferi*? *Br J Dermatol* 2000;142:636–644.
72. Weide B, Schittek B, Klyscz T, et al. Morphea is neither associated with features of *Borrelia burgdorferi* infection, nor is this agent detectable in lesional skin by polymerase chain reaction. *Br J Dermatol* 2000;143:780–785.
73. Tuffanelli DL. Do some patients morphea and lichen sclerosis et atrophicus have a *Borellia* infection? *Am J Dermatophathol* 1987;9:371–373.
74. Mori Y, Kahari V-M, Varga J. Scleroderma-like cutaneous syndromes. *Curr Rheumatol Rep* 2002;4:113–122.
75. Takagi H, Ochoa MS, Zhou L, et al. Enhanced collagen synthesis and transcription by Peak E, a contaminant of L-tryptophan preparations associated with the eosinophilia-myalgia syndrome epidemic. *J Clin Invest* 1995;96: 2120–2125.
76. Hitraya EG, Jimenez SA, Ludwicka A, et al. Increased activity of A1 (I) procollagen promotor in skin fibroblasts from patients with chronic eosinophilia-myalgia syndrome. *Int J Biochem Cell Biol* 1977;29:135–141.
77. McGrory BJ, Schmidt IU, Wold LE, et al. Carpal tunnel syndrome associated with eosinophilic fasciitis. *Orthopedics* 1998;21:368–370.
78. Moriguchi M, Terai C, Kuroki S, et al. Eosinophilic fasciitis complicated with peripheral neuropathy. *Intern Med* 1998;37:417–420.
79. Garcia VP, deQuiros JF, Caminal L. Autoimmune hemolytic anemia associated with eosinophilic fasciitis. *J Rhematol* 1998;25:1864–1865.
80. Masouka H, Kikuchi K, Takahasi S, et al. Eosinophilic fasciitis associated with low-grade T-cell lymphoma. *Br J Dermatol* 1998;139:928–930.
81. Bonnotti B, Chauffer B, Caillot D, et al. Successful treatment with anti-thymocyte globulin and cyclosporin A of a severe aplastic anemia associated with an eosinophilic fasciitis. *Br J Rheumatol* 1998;37:1358–1359.
82. Farrell AM, Ross JS, Bunker CB. Eosinophilic fasciitis associated with autoimmune thyroid disease and myelodysplasia treated with pulsed methylprednisolone and antihistamines. *Br J Dermatol* 1999;140:1185–1187.
83. Naschitz JE, Misselevich I, Rosner I, et al. Lymph node-based malignant lymphoma and reactive lymphadenopathy in eosinophilic fasciitis. *Am J Med Sci* 1999;318:343–349.
84. Rho YW, Suhr KB, Lee JH, et al. A clinical observation of scleroderma adultorium and its relationship to diabetes. *J Dermatol* 1998;25:103–107.
85. Rongroletti F, Ghigliotti G, DeMarch R, et al. Cutaneous mucinosis and HIV infection. *Br J Dermatol* 1998;139:1077–1080.
86. Stables GI, Taylor PC, Highet AS. Scleroderma associated with para-proteinemia treated by extracorporeal photopheresis. *Br J Dermatol* 2000;142: 781–783.
87. Lister RK, Jolles S, Whittake S, et al. Scleromyxedema: response to high dose intravenous immunoglobulin (hdi-Vlg). *J Am Acad Dermatol* 2000;43:403–408.
88. Johkura K, Susuki K, Hasegawa O, et al. Encephalopathy in scleromyxedema. *Neurology* 1999;53:1138–1140.
89. Cowper SE, Robin HS, Steinberg SM, et al. Scleromyxedema-like cutaneous diseases in renal dialysis patients. *Lancet* 2000;356:1000–1001.
90. Sapadia AN, Fleischmajer R. Treatment of scleroderma. *Arch Dermatol* 2002; 138:99–105.
91. Clements PJ, Furst DE, Wong WK, et al. High dose versus low-dose D-penicillamine in early diffuse systemic sclerosis. *Arthritis Rheum* 1999;42: 1194–1203.
92. Uziel Y, Feldman BM, Krafchik BR, et al. Methotrexate and corticosteroid therapy for pediatric localized scleroderma. *J Pediatrics* 2000;136:91–95.
93. El-Mofty M, Zaher H, Bosseila M, et al. Low-dose broad band UVA in morphea using a new method for evaluation. *Photodermatol, Photoimmunol Photomed* 2000;16:43–49.
94. Steger JW, Matthews JH. UVA therapy for scleroderma. *J Am Acad Dermatol* 1999;40:787.
95. Camacho NR, Sanchez JE, Martin RF, et al. Medium dose UVA-1 phototherapy in localized scleroderma and its effect on CD 34–positive dendritic cells. *J Am Acad Dermatol* 2001;45:697–699.
96. deRie MA, Bos JD. Photochemotherapy for systemic and localized scleroderma. *J Arch Acad* 2000;43:725–726.
97. deRie MA, Bos JD. Photochemotherapy for systemic and localized scleroderma. *J Arch Acad* 2000;43:725–726.
98. Gruss CJ, vonKobyletzki G, Behrens-Williams C, et al. Effects of low-dose ultraviolet A-1 phototherapy on morphea. *Photodermatol, Photoimmunol Photomed* 2001;17:149–155.
99. Arangane Y, Kawada A, Maeda A, et al. Disseminated scleroderma of a Japanese patient successfully treated with bath PUVA photo-chemotherapy. *J Cutaneous Med Surg* 2001;135–139.
100. Oikarinen A, Knuutinen A. Ultraviolet A sun bed used for the treatment of scleroderma. *Acta Derm Venerol* 2001;81:432–433.
101. Grundmann-Kollmann M, Ochsendorf F, Zollner TM et al. PUVA-cream photochemotherapy for treatment of localized scleroderma. *J Am Acad Dermatol* 2000;43:675–678.
102. Morrison WL. Psoralen UVA therapy for linear and generalized morphea. *J Am Acad Dermatol* 1997;37:657–659.
103. Quan T, He T, Voorhees J, Fisher G. Ultraviolet irradiation blocks cellular responses to transforming growth factor-beta by down regulating its type II receptor and inducing Smad7. *J Biol Chem* 2001;276:26349–26356.
104. Gruss C, Reed JA, Altmeyer P, et al. Induction of interstitial collagenase (MMP-l) by UVA-l phototherapy in morphea fibroblasts. *Lancet* 1997;350: 1295–1296.
105. Eist EF, VanSuijiekom-Smit LW, Orange AP. Treatment of linear scleroderma with oral l,25 dihydroxyvitamin Ds (calcitrol) in seven children. *Pediatr Dermatol* 1999;16:53–58.
106. Huishol MM, Pavel S, Breedveld FA, et al. Oral calcitrol as a new therapeutic modality for generalized morphea. *Arch Dermatol* 1994; 130:1290–1293.
107. Cunningham BB, Landells DR, Langman C, et al. Topical calcipotriene for morphea/linear scleroderma. *J Am Acad Dermatol* 1998;39:211–215.
108. Kreuter A, Gambichler T, Avermaete A, et al. Combined treatment with calcipotriol ointment and low-dose ultraviolet A1 phototherapy in childhood morphea. *Pediatric Dermatol* 2001;18:241–245.
109. Hulshof MM, Bavinck JNB, Bergman W. Double-blind, placebo-controlled study of oral calcitrol for the treatment of localized and systemic sclerosis. *J am Acad Dermatol* 2000;43:1017–1023.
110. Hunzelmann N, Anders S, Fierlbeck G, et al. Double-blind, placebo-controlled study of intralesional interferon gamma for the treatment of localized scleroderma. *J Am Acad Dermatol* 1997;36:433–435.

CHAPTER 6

Mucocutaneous Manifestations of Sjögren Syndrome

Steven R. Flint, Rosemarie Watson, and Thomas T. Provost

DEFINITION

Sjögren syndrome is a chronic, progressive inflammatory, multi system rheumatologic disease, characterized by an exocrinopathy of the salivary and lacrimal glands. However, vaginal dryness also frequently occurs and may antedate by decades the diagnosis of Sjögren syndrome. The monograph by the Swedish ophthalmologist Heinrich Sjögren (1) (1933) described the association of lacrimal and salivary gland failure presenting as keratoconjunctivitis sicca and xerostomia with rheumatoid arthritis. Although Leber (1882) (2), Hadden (1888) (3), Mikulicz (1892) (4), and Gougerot (1926) (5) had all described the same condition with different emphases, the eponym is ascribed to Sjögren in recognition of his original thesis and his lifelong dedication to the investigation of the disorder [for a review, see (6)].

The designation of Mikulicz syndrome was historically used to identify any salivary gland swelling caused by a lymphocytic infiltration. Causes of such a histopathologic picture are varied and include lymphoreticular disease, granulomatous disease such as sarcoidosis, bacterial sialoadenitis, and sialosis; in addition, a group of patients with salivary gland lymphoid infiltrates, hypergammaglobulinemia, and autoantibodies were also classified as having Mikulicz disease. This latter group was shown to have the salivary gland pathologic features identical to Sjögren syndrome. Today, the term "Mikulicz disease" has fallen into disuse.

Sjögren syndrome is a heterogeneous condition and is classified as primary or secondary. Primary Sjögren syndrome is characterized as keratoconjunctivitis sicca with xerostomia in the absence of any definable connective tissue disease, although there may be other extraglandular features (Table 6.1). A lymphocyte-aggressive or pseudolymphoma subset with widespread lymphohistiocytic infiltrations and lymphadenopathy has been described by Strand and Talal (7). Most of these patients have primary Sjögren syndrome.

When the clinical triad of lacrimal and salivary gland failure in association with a definable connective tissue disease is seen, (most commonly rheumatoid arthritis, as in Sjögren original description), the term "secondary Sjögren syndrome" is used.

In the past, Sjögren syndrome has been estimated to affect between 0.1% and 3% of the U.S. population. It is second only to rheumatoid arthritis in frequency, affecting approximately 4 million people (in the United States). The wide variation in the reported incidence probably reflects a previous lack of consensus diagnostic criteria. No single test is diagnostic for the disorder. However, seven different diagnostic criteria recently have been proposed, each with different degrees of inclusion stringency. This has led to difficulties comparing and evaluating data in the scientific literature. A European community consensus was published in 1993 (8), and modified in 1996 (9) (see Appendix). All the authors of this chapter, on the basis of their clinical experiences, believe this to be the superior classification. It is also the opinion of the authors that Sjögren syndrome, because of its insidious onset and vague systemic symptoms, remains underdiagnosed.

Dry mouth is a common complaint. Table 6.2 lists the causes of dry mouth. Many medications can cause the symptom of xerostomia, which complicates the diagnosis (Table 6.3). This dryness can be induced by interfering with the neural control of salivation or by affecting the quality and composition of the saliva produced.

Sjögren syndrome is generally a disease of older patients (sixth to seventh decades) but has been infrequently described in children. There is no recognized racial predisposition, but there is a striking male-to-female ratio of 1:9. Male patients with Sjögren syndrome generally have a more benign disease than females, with fewer serologic abnormalities and extraglandular manifestations (10).

Morbidity is not only related to the declining function of exocrine glands, but in secondary Sjögren syndrome, there is the comorbidity and mortality of the underlying connective tissue disorder.

PATHOGENESIS

Immunogenetic Studies

Immunogenetic, autoantibody, and viral studies have provided information possibly related to the pathogenesis of Sjögren syndrome.

Relatives of patients with Sjögren syndrome have an increased frequency of autoimmune diseases and autoantibod-

TABLE 6.1. Extraglandular Manifestations of Sjögren Syndrome

Arthritis
Polymyositis
Raynaud phenomenon
Pulmonary disease
Interstitial
Necrotizing bronchoalveolitis
Chronic active hepatitis
Primary biliary cirrhosis
Renal disease
Interstitial
Glomerulonephritis
Thyroiditis
B-cell lymphomas
Vasculitis
Peripheral and central nervous system disease

ies (Table 6.4) (11,12). Amongst first-degree relatives, there are increased frequencies of antinuclear, anti–single-stranded DNA (anti-ssDNA), biologic false-positive test for syphilis (BFP-STS), and anti-Ro(SS-A) antibodies.

In addition to familial aggregation of autoantibodies and autoimmune diseases in Sjögren syndrome pedigrees, there is a close immunogenetic relationship between alleles in the major histocompatibility complex (MHC) and the expression of anti-Ro(SS-A) antibodies (13,14). Anti-Ro(SS-A) antibodies are frequently detected in patients with Sjögren syndrome (see later). There are two anti-Ro(SS-A) antibody response patterns: anti-Ro(SS-A) and anti-La(SS-B); anti-Ro(SS-A) alone (13). The anti-Ro(SS-A) and anti-La(SS-B) response is most commonly detected in Sjögren syndrome whereas the anti-Ro(SS-A) response in the absence of anti-La(SS-B) is more commonly detected in systemic lupus erythematosus (SLE). The anti-Ro(SS-A) and anti-La(SS-B) antibody response is associated with the serologically defined HLA-B8, DR3, DQw2, DRw52 haplotype (Table 6.5).

The anti-Ro(SS-A) antibody response, most frequently seen in SLE, is associated with the HLA-DR2, DQw1 haplotype. Heterozygosity (HLA-DQw1/DQw2 is associated with the highest anti-Ro(SS-A) antibody titers (15,16).

TABLE 6.2. Causes of Dry Mouth (Xerostomia)

Salivary gland disease
Sjögren syndrome
Radiotherapy
Hepatitis C infection
Human immunodeficiency virus infection
Graft versus host disease
Amyloidosis
Sarcoidosis
Hyperlipoproteinemia types IV and V
Lymphoma and early leukemia
Hemochromatosis
Cystic fibrosis
Ectodermal dysplasia
Psychogenic
Anxiety
Depression
Bulimia nervosa
Dehydration
Diabetes mellitus and diabetes insipidus
Severe hemorrhage, diarrhea, and vomiting
Drugs (see Table 6.3) and polypharmacy

TABLE 6.3. Drugs That Cause Dry Mouth

Drugs with anticholinergic activity (decreased volume)
Tricyclic antidepressants
Atropinics
Antihistamines
Major tranquilizers/neuroleptics
Antiemetics
Drugs with sympathomimetic activity (decreased volume and compositional changes)
Amphetamines
Decongestants
Appetite suppressants
Bronchodilators
Others (decreased volume and compositional changes)
Diuretics
Lithium
Retinoids
α blockers
β blockers
Angiotensin-converting enzyme inhibitors
Calcium channel blockers
Benzodiazepines
Morphine and derivatives
Antacid H_2 blockers
Disopyramide
Interleukin-2
Dideoxyinosine

Restriction-fragment length polymorphism has demonstrated alleles responsible for the highest anti-Ro(SS-A) and anti-La(SS-B) responses are associated with heterozygosity for HLA-DQw2.1/DQw6 (subtypes of HLA-DQw2 and DQw1, respectively) (17).

Nucleotide sequence studies of DQA1 and DQB1 chain alleles reveal 100% of anti-Ro(SS-A) antibody–positive patients with Sjögren syndrome or SLE possess a glutamine residue at position 34 of the outermost domain of the DQA1 chain and/or a leucine at position 26 of the outermost domain of the DQB1 chain. Additional studies have determined that a dosage effect of these alleles is present. For example, those patients with anti-Ro(SS-A) and anti-La(SS-B) antibodies generally have all four of their DQA1/DQB1 chains (one set on each haplotype) containing these amino acid residues. These data strongly suggest these amino acid residues localized to the floor of the antigen-binding cleft of the HLA-DQA1/DQB1 heterodimer may be important in binding the peptides responsible for the anti-Ro(SS-A) and anti-La(SS-B) antibody responses. (11,17).

These studies also indicate the HLA associations are not disease-specific but are associated with the anti-Ro(SS-A) and anti-La(SS-B) antibody responses. For example, if you subtract the anti-Ro(SS-A) antibody–positive patients (as determined by gel double diffusion) from a total cohort of patients with Sjögren syndrome or SLE, you remove the statistically significant associations of Sjögren syndrome with the HLA-DR3 phenotype and the HLA-DR2 and HLA-DR3 phenotypes with SLE (T.T.P. and Frank Arnett, personal observations 1985).

AUTOANTIBODY STUDIES

Gel double-diffusion studies indicate that between 40% and 45% of patients with Sjögren syndrome demonstrate anti-Ro(SS-A) precipitin antibodies (14,18). Approximately 15% to 20% demonstrate anti-La(SS-B) precipitin antibodies. Enzyme-linked immunosorbent assay (ELISA) techniques using the same sera demonstrated a 90% frequency of anti-Ro(SS-A) antibodies and a 70% frequency of anti-La(SS-B) antibodies.

TABLE 6.4. Autoimmune Diseases in Family Members of Probands with Primary and Secondary Sjögren Syndrome

Proband diagnosis				
Primary Sjögren syndrome	SLE	RA	UCTD	
Proband, no.	20	20	7	
Positive family history of autoimmune disease	18 (35)*	6 (30)	4 (20)	3 (43)
Autoimmune diagnosis of family members				
Sjögren syndrome	9 (12)	1 (5)	0	0
SLE	2 (5)	2 (10)	0	0
RA	7 (14)	3 (15)	2 (10)	2 (29)
Multiple sclerosis	0	0	0	0
Systemic sclerosis	1 (2)	0	0	0
Myasthenia gravis	0	0	0	0
Thyroid disease	7 (14)	1 (5)	1 (5)	2 (29)

*Numbers in parentheses represent percentage.
RA, rheumatoid arthritis; SLE, systemic lupus erythematosus; UCTD, undifferentiated connective tissue disease.
From Reveille JD, Wilson RW, Provost TT, et al. Primary Sjögren syndrome and other autoimmune diseases in families. *Ann Intern Med* 1984;101:748–756, with permission.

These studies indicate that the frequency of these antibodies in patients with Sjögren syndrome depends, at least in part, on the techniques used to measure the anti-Ro(SS-A) and anti-La(SS-B) responses.

Primary Sjögren syndrome is a very heterogeneous disease with respect to expression of anti-Ro(SS-A) and anti-La(SS-B) antibodies. In a study of 50 lip biopsy–proven patients with Sjögren syndrome referred by allergists, general internists, dermatologists, gynecologists, ophthalmologists, and rheumatologists, a 30% frequency of anti-Ro(SS-A) and a 15% frequency of anti-La(SS-B) antibodies were detected using both gel double-diffusion and ELISA techniques (19).

These studies indicate patient selection bias is important to consider when evaluating the frequency of antibody responses in patients with Sjögren syndrome. Those patients with Sjögren syndrome with extraglandular manifestations (i.e., arthritis, pulmonary disease, etc.) are generally anti-Ro(SS-A) antibody–positive and are most likely to be evaluated by a rheumatologist. In contradistinction, allergists, ophthalmologists, and gynecologists frequently evaluate patients with Sjögren syndrome with only mucous membrane dryness, having little if any, extraglandular manifestations of their disease. These patients are generally anti-Ro(SS-A) antibody–negative.

Dermatologists frequently see a population of patients with Sjögren syndrome with cutaneous vasculitis. These patients with Sjögren syndrome frequently are anti-Ro(SS-A) antibody–positive and have extraglandular manifestations including peripheral and central nervous system manifestations (Tables 6.6 and 6.7) (20).

TABLE 6.5. HLA-DR and DQ Specificities in Anti-Ro(SS-A) Whites with Primary Sjögren Syndrome[a]

	Anti-Ro + SS	Anti-Ro – SS	Controls
HLA	(*n* = 24)	(*n* = 13)	(*n* = 79)
DR3	67%[b,c]	23%[b]	20%[c]
DRw52a	75%[a]	38%	39%[a]
DQw2.1	67%[b,c]	23%[b]	20%[c]
DQw2.1/DQw6	29%[d]	0%	3%[d]

From Reveille JD, Arnett FC. The immunogenetics of Sjögren syndrome. *Rheum Dis Clin North Am* 1992;18:539–550, with permission.
[a] $p = 0.004$, RR = 4.6.
[b] $p = 0.03$, RR = 6.7.
[c] $p = 0.00005$, RR = 7.9.
[d] $p = 0.0002$, RR = 16.

Immunoblotting studies have demonstrated that the anti-Ro(SS-A) antibody response in Sjögren syndrome recognizes a 52-kDa Ro(SS-A) protein [reviewed in (13)]. In contradistinction, the anti-Ro(SS-A) antibody response in SLE recognizes a 60-kDa Ro(SS-A) protein. [The best evidence at present indicates the anti-Ro antibody response is directed at the 60-kDa macromolecule and that some of these antibodies (HLA-DR3 patients) cross-react with the 52-kDa macromolecule.] Mothers of infants with neonatal lupus possess anti-Ro(SS-A) antibodies that recognize the 52-kDa protein (they are also HLA-DR3–positive) (21,22).

Most recent studies indicate that anti 52-kDa anti-Ro(SS-A) antibodies bind to L-type cardiac calcium channels (21). It is theorized that these maternally derived antibodies pass across the placenta, bind to fetal cardiac calcium channels and induce an inflammatory response, the result of which is fibrotic replacement of the cardiac conduction system and the development of isolated congenital heart block [neonatal lupus erythematosus (NLE)] (22,23) (see Chapter 13).

The 52-kDa and 60-kDa nuclear and cytoplasmic proteins are associated with small RNAs known as hY1, hY3, hY4, and hY5 RNAs. Molecular cloning studies of the Ro(SS-A) autoantigens have determined that the 52-kDa and the 60-kDa are different proteins, sharing little, if any, sequence homology. The 60-kDa polypeptide has an RNA binding domain and a zinc finger motif. It is theorized the RNA binding motif binds the hY RNAs and the zinc finger motif may interact with the 52-kDa protein (13).

The 52-kDa protein possesses a zinc finger motif, as well as leucine zipper domains. It has been proposed because of the presence of the zinc finger motif and the leucine zipper domains, the 52-kDa protein may be involved in the regulation of gene expression (13).

Anti-Ro(SS-A) antibody–positive sera also react with a synthetic construct of the calcium binding protein, calreticulin (CR). The nature of this relationship is unknown. However, immunization studies in mice have demonstrated spreading of the immune response (intermolecular epitope spreading) from the Ro 52 to the Ro 60 to CR. These studies are interpreted to indicate that CR under certain circumstances must be associated *in vivo* with the Ro 52 and Ro 60 molecules (24).

Anti-La(SS-B) antibodies are directed against an RNA binding protein that transiently binds all RNA polymerase III tran-

TABLE 6.6. Association of Various Clinical Hematologic and Serologic Features in Sjögren Syndrome with Anti-Ro(SS-A) Antibodies

	Anti-Ro[+a] (n = 33)	Anti-Ro[−] (n = 42)	p Value
Clinical features			
Vasculitis	24	5	0.0005
Salivary gland enlargement	26	15	0.0005
Lymphadenopathy	19	4	0.0005
Purpura	12	1	0.0005
Hematologic features			
Anemia	19	6	0.0005
Leukopenia	14	3	0.01
Thrombocytopenia	7	1	0.025
Serologic features			
Hypergammaglobulinemia	21	8	0.025
RF	29	17	0.0005
ANA	23	10	0.0005
Cryoglobulinemia	7/13	0/22	0.001
Hypocomplementemia	11	2	0.005

ANA, antinuclear antibodies; RF, rheumatoid factor.
[a]Detected by gel double diffusion.
From Alexander et al. Ro (SS-A) and La (SS-B) antibodies in the clinical spectrum of Sjögren syndrome. *J Rheumatol* 1982;9:239, with permission.

scripts as well as precursors of RNA and 5s RNA. Studies by Gottesfeld et al. (25) and by Gottlieb and Steitz (26) indicate that *in vivo* transcription of RNA polymerase III genes is inhibited if the La(SS-B) protein is depleted with anti-La(SS-B) antibodies from the transcription extract. Furthermore, the few RNA transcripts produced in the La(SS-B)-depleted extract are truncated (loss of several uridylate residues at the 3′ end) (27). These data are interpreted as indicating the La(SS-B) protein is a transcription as well as a termination factor for all RNA polymerase III transcripts. Because the La(SS-B) protein and the hY5 Ro(SS-A) ribonuclear protein may be at least transiently complexed, it has been hypothesized, but not proven, that the Ro(SS-A) polypeptide may also be involved in RNA polymerase III transcription (28).

Most recent studies indicate that the sera of mothers of infants with NLE possess antibodies directed against a 75-kDa phosphoprotein and bind to a recombinant fusion protein encoded by α-fodrin complementary DNA (cDNA). In addition, anti–SS-A/Ro 52-kDa antibodies have been shown to block the cardiac 5-HT4 serotoninergic receptor. The role of these antibody specificities in the pathogenesis of Sjögren syndrome and other autoimmune diseases is an area of intense scientific investigations (29–31).

Cells undergoing apoptosis (programmed cell death) express a species of Ro(SS-A) and La(SS-B) macromolecules on the cell-surface membranes. Furthermore, keratinocytes cultured in the presence of 17β-estradiol or exposed to ultraviolet light express these "autoantigens" on their cell surface. These studies suggest that cells so pertubated are at risk for a possible immunologic-mediated cellular injury involving anti-Ro(SS-A) and anti-La(SS-B) antibodies (13). Theoretically, these apoptotic cells with their cell-surface expression of these putative "autoantigens" may also play a role in driving an autoimmune response to these antigens.

Epitope mapping of Ro(SS-A) and La(SS-B) peptides have thus far failed to establish a definite relationship of one or several epitopes with clinical features of disease expression [lupus erythematosus (LE) or Sjögren syndrome]. Tertiary protein structures (conformational) rather than linear protein sequences may be responsible for epitopes that correlate with disease expression (32).

Some SS patients possess antisalivary duct antibodies. These antibodies appear to be epiphenomenon induced by salivary duct damage. Recently antimuscarine receptor M3 antibodies have been detected in patients with Sjögren syndrome. These antibodies block muscarine receptor activity in rats (33). Although the exact role, if any, in Sjögren syndrome is unknown, their presence could help explain the general lack of correlation between the degree of salivary gland inflammation and salivary gland flow rates in Sjögren syndrome. Recently, the presence of this antibody also has been correlated with autonomic system dysfunction in a patient with Sjögren syndrome

TABLE 6.7. Neurologic Disorders Reported in Patients with Sjögren Syndrome

- Focal brain abnormalities
  - Motor and sensory nerve defects
    - Multiple sclerosis–like disease
  - Movement disorders
  - Cerebellar focal lesions
  - Brainstem focal lesions
    - Trigeminal neuropathy
    - Sensorineural hearing defect
  - Seizures
- Nonfocal brain abnormalities
  - Aseptic meningitis
  - Cognitive dysfunction
    - Alzheimer-like disease process
  - Psychiatric disorders
    - Hysteria and conversion reactions
    - Anxiety and depression
- Spinal cord disorders
  - Dorsal root ganglionitis
    - Subacute sensory neuronopathy
  - Transverse myelitis
  - Chronic progressive myelitis
  - Brown Sequard syndrome
  - Neurogenic bladder
- Autonomic nervous system involvement
- Peripheral nervous system involvement
  - Phrenic nerve involvement producing "shrinking lung syndrome"

presenting with gastrointestinal bloating and bladder irritability (34).

VIRAL STUDIES

Viral infection has been hypothesized to play a pathogenic role in Sjögren syndrome. Many latent forms of viruses are found in the salivary gland. All herpes viruses are possible candidates. For example, Epstein–Barr virus (EBV) DNA has been detected in salivary gland biopsies of patients with Sjögren syndrome. However, this is not a specific finding because EBV has been detected in the absence of clinical evidence of Sjögren syndrome (35) [reviewed in (25)].

Schofield and Harley (36) have presented evidence for sequence homology between the Ro (SS-A) macromolecule and the vesicular stomatitis virus capsid. Also, subsequent studies indicate anti-La(SS-B) antibodies precipitate a ribonuclear protein associated with EBV-encoded RNAs. These data suggest molecular mimicry perhaps between a viral infection such as EBV or another virus and the production of an anti-Ro(SS-A) and/or anti-La(SS-B) antibody response may be operative in Sjögren syndrome.

The possible role of retroviruses in the pathogenesis of Sjögren syndrome has received attention. Talal et al. (37) found that sera from some patients with Sjögren syndrome contain antibodies directed against the retroviral protein p24. Patients with human acquired immunodeficiency syndrome (AIDS) have been reported to have a syndrome termed "diffuse infiltrative lymphocytosis" (DILS) [reviewed in (38)]. This syndrome is characterized by bilateral parotid gland enlargement and xerostomia. Xerophthalmia and keratoconjunctivitis sicca occur less frequently. Anti-Ro(SS-A) and anti-La(SS-B) antibodies are absent. Furthermore, the salivary gland inflammatory infiltrate is composed predominantly of CD8 T cells, in contradistinction to the CD4 T cells detected in Sjögren syndrome. In addition, in DILS, HLA associations are markedly different from those found in Sjögren syndrome.

Recent studies suggest that at least 50% of patients infected with hepatitis C have salivary gland lymphohistiocytic infiltrates. However, few of these patients develop sicca symptoms or serologic abnormalities (39).

HISTOPATHOLOGY OF THE SALIVARY GLANDS

The cardinal histopathologic features of Sjögren syndrome affecting the major salivary glands are a patchy inflammatory infiltrate of $CD4^+$ lymphocytes, histiocytes, and plasma cells (Figs. 6.1 and 6.2). This is accompanied by acinar atrophy and fibrosis (40). In the early stages of the disease, the lymphocytic infiltration is focal and periductal (focal sialoadenitis), but as the disease advances, normal acini and ducts are replaced by the infiltrate to produce the benign lymphoepithelial lesion, also referred to as myoepithelial sialoadenitis (MESA) (41).

In early disease, ductal cells may proliferate, and in end-stage disease, islands of salivary epithelium are seen, which are called epimyoepithelial islands.

As a diagnostic procedure, a major salivary gland biopsy carries an unacceptable risk of fistula and scar formation and with parotid biopsy; there is the additional risk of facial nerve palsy. Major salivary gland biopsy, however, is indicated if there is a suspicion of lymphoma.

Minor salivary gland tissue, unlike that of major glands, is easily accessible, and biopsy carries less morbidity. A paramedian incision is performed midway between the corners and midline of the lip, and at least five lobules of gland are dissected from beneath clinically normal mucosa. The wound heals by primary intention. This procedure allows sufficient tissue for assessment and is the preferred technique (Figs. 6.3–6.5) (42). Labial nerve damage is a rare complication. There is good correlation between major salivary gland and labial salivary gland biopsy features (43). Epimyoepithelial islands, however, are very rarely seen in labial salivary gland biopsies.

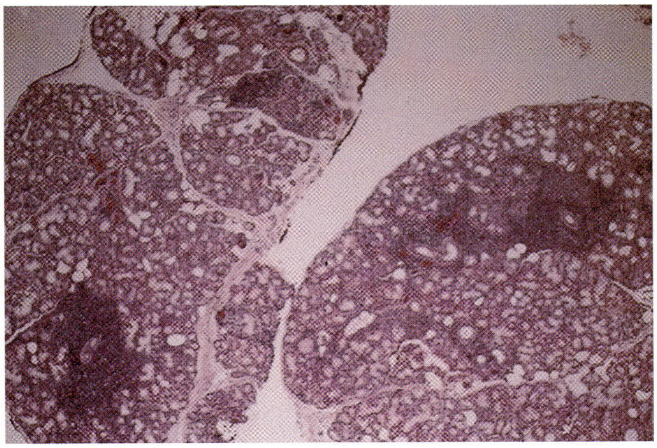

Figure 6.1. Focal aggregates (original magnification, ×100) of a lymphohistiocytic infiltrate invading the acinar and ductal portions of the minor salivary glands of a patient with Sjögren syndrome. Note the patchy nature of the infiltrate.

Quantitative grading of the distinctive periductal focal aggregates was introduced by Chisholm and Mason (43). A focus is defined as an aggregate of more than 50 mononuclear cells. They concluded that focus scores of more than one per 4-mm^2 area of gland were seen only in patients with connective tissue disease. High focal scores appear to be a particular feature of primary Sjögren syndrome. Focus scores above one are considered diagnostic by many authorities, if the biopsy is taken from an area with normal overlying mucosa. Nonspecific focal sialoadenitis may be seen underlying such mucosal disorders as lichen planus or traumatic lesions (42).

The labial gland biopsy is objective, and there is good reproducibility and interexaminer agreement. Most important, the procedure excludes other causes of xerostomia such as amyloidosis or sarcoidosis. However, false-negative labial gland biopsy has been found in patients with Sjögren syndrome who

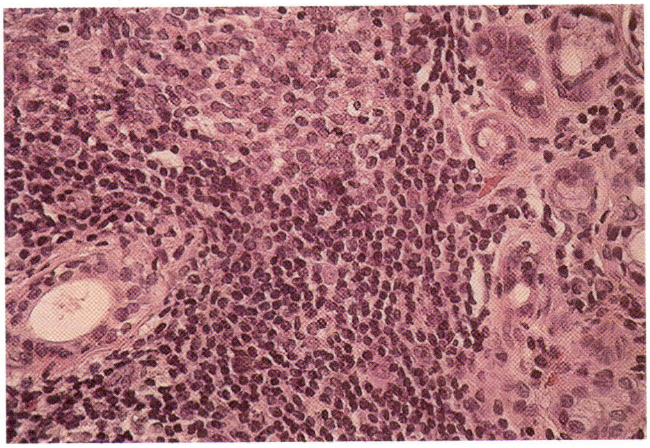

Figure 6.2. Lymphohistiocytic infiltrate (original magnification, ×300) in a minor salivary gland of a patient with Sjögren syndrome.

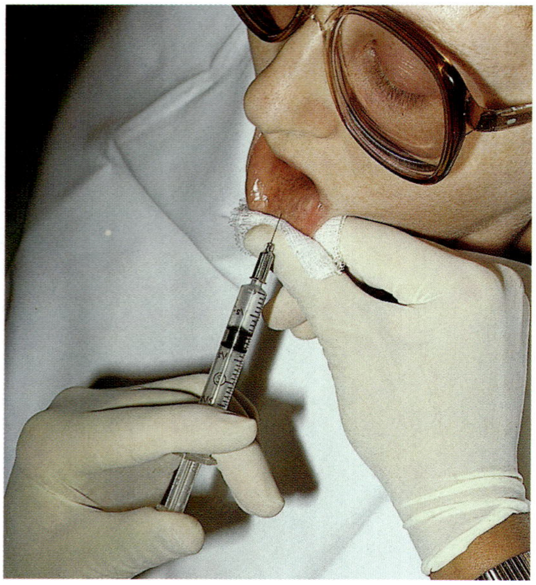

Figure 6.3. Injection of lower lip with lidocaine with epinephrine.

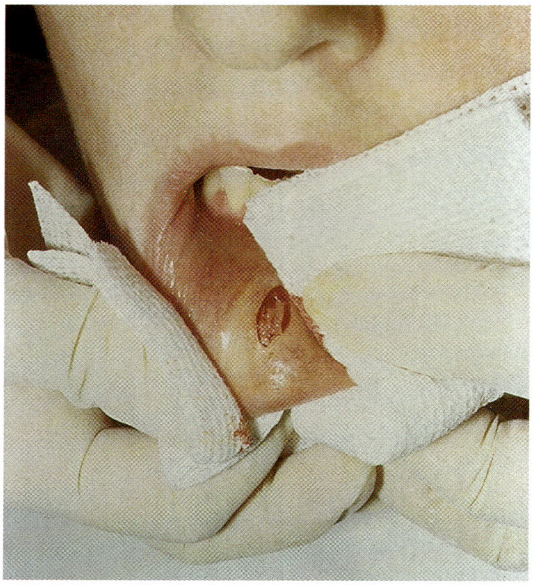

Figure 6.5. Exposure of minor salivary glands in lower lip.

were confidently diagnosed by other criteria. However, repeated biopsy may establish the diagnosis; a false-positive biopsy is rarely seen.

The histopathologic appearance of Sjögren syndrome of the labial gland, although distinctive, is not pathognomonic. Thus, a positive labial gland biopsy remains only part of the diagnostic criteria.

In the experience of one of the authors (T.T.P.) with several hundred biopsies, the minor salivary gland biopsy has proved problematic in some cases. Early in the disease, the inflammatory infiltrate is patchy (i.e., one gland may be totally involved and the other glands sampled not involved; thus, sampling error may occur). Furthermore, with extensive disease, the glands show fatty metamorphosis and fibrosis, two features not addressed in the current morphologic criteria.

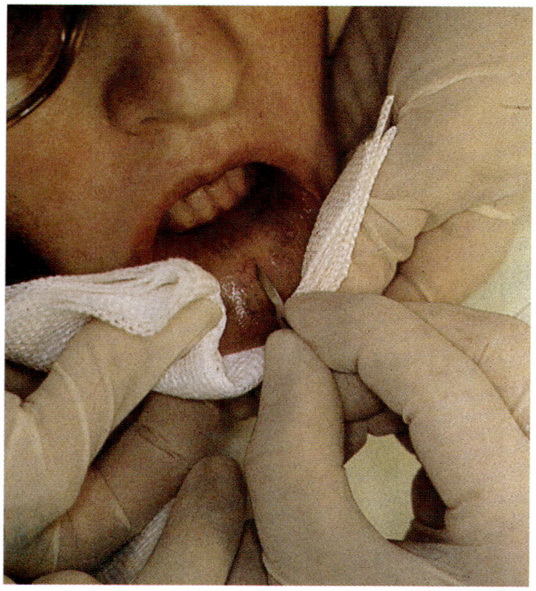

Figure 6.4. A 1-inch vertical paramedian incision of lower lip.

It should be noted that lymphohistiocytic infiltrates similar to those seen in the salivary gland biopsies occur in other organs (e.g., thyroid, liver, kidney, lung, etc.) and in all probability are responsible, at least in part, for the extraglandular manifestations of Sjögren syndrome.

ORAL MANIFESTATIONS

Oral complaints are often the presenting feature of Sjögren syndrome, usually manifesting as dry mouth. However, many patients with xerostomia do not complain of it. Frequently, they complain of oral soreness, burning mouth, dysphagia, or difficulties with eating dry food (the "cracker test") or with denture control and frequently use liquids to assist in swallowing food and talking (44). In severe cases, a characteristic clicking quality of the speech occurs due to the tongue sticking to the palate. The lips may be dry and cracked and, in women, the "lipstick-on-teeth" sign may be present (45).

Oral signs are characteristic; the mouth may appear frankly dry with glazed, erythematous, wrinkled mucosa in advanced cases, but in the early stages, there is simply an absence of normal salivary pooling on the floor of the mouth or frothy saliva along lines of mucosal contact (Fig. 6.6). Typically the examining mirror will adhere to the buccal mucosa. Massage of the major salivary glands will not elicit salivary flow. The tongue often looks dry and there may be erythema and depapillation (Fig. 6.7). In long-standing cases, the dorsum of the tongue takes on a lobulated appearance. Clearance of food debris is often reduced.

Complaints of abnormal or reduced taste may occur, and taste buds are not only decreased in number, which may be seen as a normal age change, but are also abnormal. Abnormalities of olfaction may also occur, which may compound disorders of taste.

The oral ecology changes. *Candida albicans* infection or carriage is virtually ubiquitous, and may manifest as sore

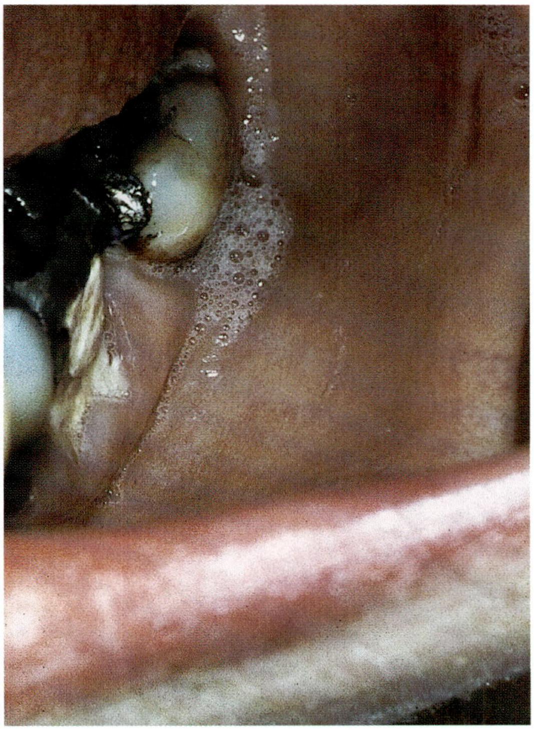

Figure 6.6. Frothy saliva at the line of mucosal contact—an early sign of xerostomia.

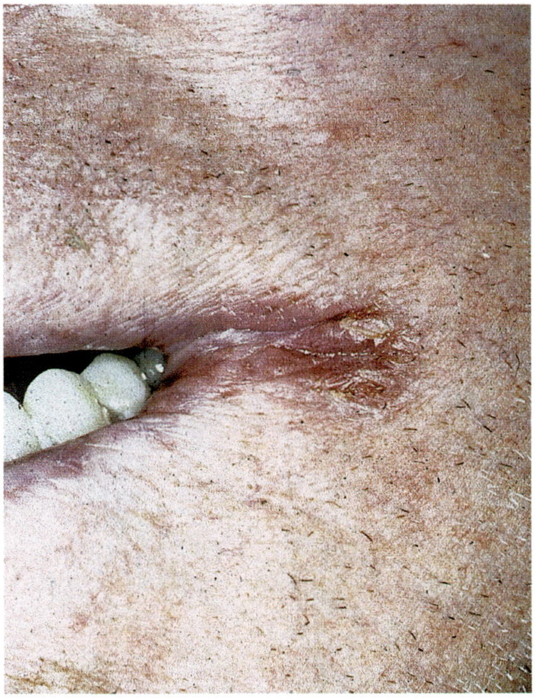

Figure 6.8. Angular cheilitis (perlèche) in a patient with Sjögren syndrome.

mouth, angular cheilitis (perlèche) (Fig. 6.8), or denture stomatitis. In addition, salivary pH is significantly reduced, as are numbers of commensals, such as *Streptococcus salivarius*, *Neisseria*, *Veillonella*, and *Micrococcus* species, while the numbers of pathogens such as *C. albicans* and *Staphylococcus* are increased. In the dentate, caries may become severe, characteristically affect the cervical and incisal surfaces, and are associated with heavy plaque deposits (Fig. 6.9). The dental caries may be particularly aggressive. Evidence for an increase in the susceptibility to periodontal disease or dental calculus is equivocal.

Painless swelling of the major salivary glands occurs in as many as one third of all patients with primary and secondary Sjögren syndrome at some stage of the disease but is rarely the presenting feature (Fig. 6.10). In the series of 171 cases by Whaley and Buchanan (46), one third had persistent enlargement. Within the primary Sjögren syndrome group, episodic salivary gland swelling may occur in 70%. Pseudolymphoma of the major glands is a particular feature, which may progress to lymphoma (47). Acute ascending bacterial sialoadenitis secondary to hyposecretion may be a presenting feature. Sjögren syndrome is the most common underlying condition in bacterial sialoadenitis in ambulant patients, and is generally caused by *Staphylococcus*, *Pneumococcus* or *Streptococcus* species.

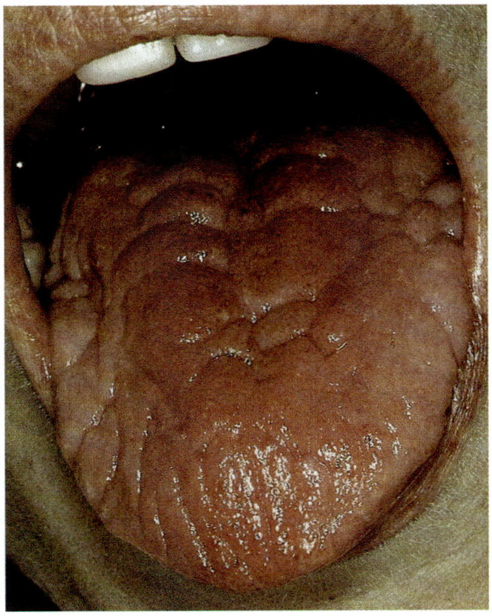

Figure 6.7. Lobulation of the tongue in long-standing xerostomia.

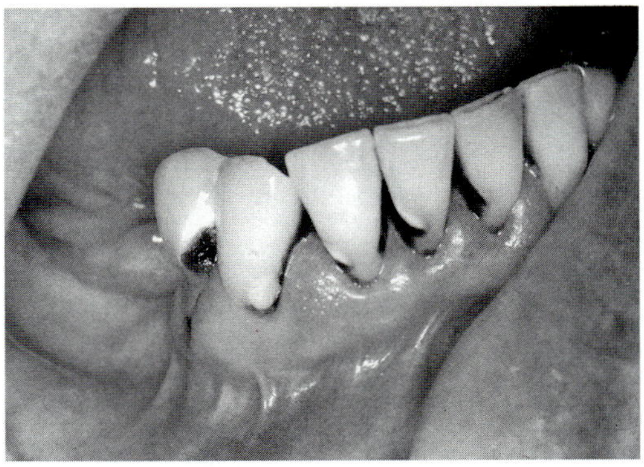

Figure 6.9. Cervical (neck) cavities in a patient with Sjögren syndrome.

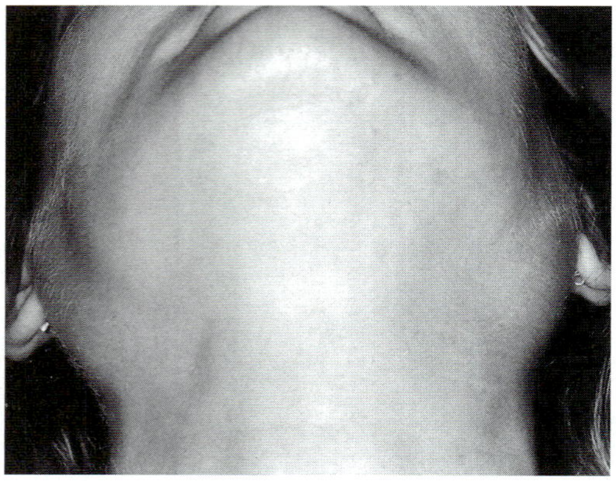

Figure 6.10. Bilateral parotid swelling in a patient with Sjögren syndrome.

EVALUATION OF SALIVARY GLAND FUNCTION AND CHANGES IN SJÖGREN SYNDROME

The previously described clinical signs give subjective assessment of salivary gland function. However, objective tests are available. The simplest method for assessment of whole salivary flow rate (sialometry) is to ask the patient to spit into a weighed container every minute for up to 15 minutes. The patient should be resting and instructed to have not eaten or put anything in the mouth for the previous 90 minutes. Resting and stimulated salivary flow can be measured. For stimulated flow rates, the patient chews (45 chews per minute) a rubber band or paraffin wax. Whole stimulated saliva is collected every minute for 5 minutes. In general, there is agreement that unstimulated (basal) whole salivary flow rates below 0.1 to 0.2 mL per minute and stimulated whole flow rates below 0.7 mL per minute are the lower limits for normal flow rates. In the Saxon test, preweighed gauze is chewed for 2 minutes and saliva collected. The gauze is then weighed again. These simple tests are reliable for the demonstration of salivary hypofunction in adults.

Individual major gland flow rates can be investigated using specialized equipment. The simplest gland to investigate is the parotid. A Lashley, Carlsson–Crittenden (Fig. 6.11), or Curby

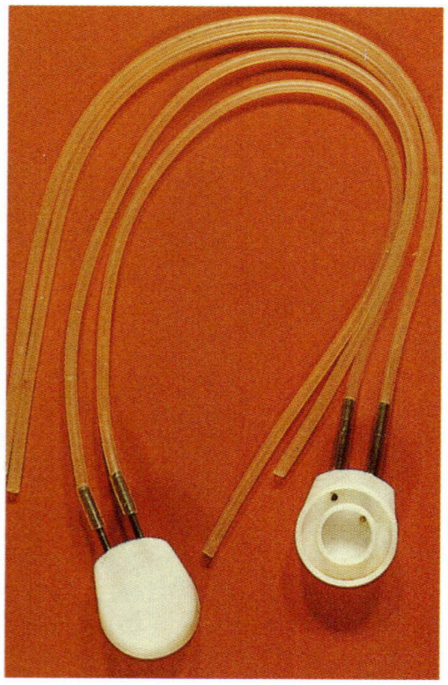

Figure 6.11. The Carlsson–Crittenden cup for parotid sialometry.

cup is placed over the orifice of Stenson duct and gentle suction applied to the outer ring. Saliva produced by the gland will flow down the central ring and can be collected in an attached tube. The parotid gland can be stimulated by the application of 2% citric acid to the tongue. The submandibular and sublingual gland flow rates can be measured using a Truelove apparatus or by cannulating the Wharton duct. Normal standardized unstimulated flow rates are 0.03 to 0.05 mL per minute per gland for parotid, 0.06 mL per minute per gland for submandibular, and more than 0.5 mL per minute per gland for both stimulated major glands. Salivary flow from the minor salivary glands is difficult to measure. Various devices and techniques from simple filter-paper absorption to specific commercial products have been used.

Qualitative changes in the saliva itself (sialochemistry) have been investigated, but the results are disappointing. Salivary levels and activity of enzymes and inflammatory mediators such as kallikrenin, lactoferrin, salivary isoamylase, β_2-microglobulin, serum immunoglobulins, and secretory IgA have not proved to be reliably discriminatory.

Sialography involves the hydrostatic retrograde injection of a radioopaque dye into a Wharton or Stenson duct and imaging with extraoral radiography to visualize the duct architecture. The typical sign seen in Sjögren syndrome is punctate sialectasis, but it is not pathognomonic.

Computed tomography (CT) and, particularly, nuclear resonance imaging are useful for the detection of salivary gland enlargements and masses (48). A "salt and pepper" appearance on CT is suggestive of Sjögren syndrome (49). Scintigraphy is a reliable, functional test. Intravenously injected ^{99m}Tc–sodium pertechnetate is preferentially taken up by the salivary glands (50). Imaging is by a gamma camera and the rate of clearance of the radionuclide correlates with flow rates. Ultrasonography may be useful, particularly if there are cystic lesions as may be seen in HIV-related salivary gland disease (51). Single-photon emission computed tomography shows promise as an investigative technique in the diagnosis of Sjögren syndrome, but is not widely available (52).

TREATMENT OF ORAL MANIFESTATIONS

Currently, there is no treatment that has been proven to arrest progression of lacrimosalivary gland failure in the disease, although there have been a few longitudinal studies. The rate of progression of the disease is variable, but irreversible. The mainstay of treatment, therefore, is symptomatic and aimed at prevention of the oral diseases that are a consequence of the xerostomia.

There are a number of liquid salivary substitutes available based on carmellose sodium or mucins. Other preparations are sugar-free, acidic sialogogues in the form of troches (pastilles) or tablets. In severe xerostomia, however, there may be insufficient saliva to dissolve them. Pilocarpine and cevimeline are cholinergic agonists that increase salivary flow. Excessive sweating is the dose-limiting side effect, although cevimeline may have more specific cholinergic agonist activity for the M3 muscarinic salivary receptor.

Prevention of dental caries is of paramount importance and patients should see their dentists for regular prophylaxis and early treatment of dental caries, which can be rampant in this group of patients. Whenever possible, fluoride-containing filling materials should be used, and this should be supplemented by regular use of fluoride mouth rinses.

Oral candidiasis is a regular complication of xerostomia and can be managed by periodic use of systemic (fluconazole) and topical (clotrimazole troches, nystatin, oral suspension, etc.) antifungal agents, along with antiseptic mouth rinses, such as chlorhexidine. Brown extrinsic staining of the tongue and teeth is a complication of long-term use of chlorhexidine mouthwashes.

Oral candidiasis occurs more frequently in patients with Sjögren syndrome with dentures. Scouring of the mucosal surface of the denture with nystatin powder using a toothbrush is very helpful.

Systemic treatment with ambroxol, hydroxychloroquine, retinols, and intramuscular nandroline has also been reported. One of the authors (T.T.P.) has noted increased mucous membrane moisture in some patients with Sjögren syndrome treated for several years with hydroxychloroquine (200 mg twice daily).

Unfortunately, in patients with secondary Sjögren syndrome taking immunosuppressive drugs for the underlying connective tissue disease, there appears to be little effect of the drugs on progression of the lacrimosalivary component of the syndrome.

OCULAR SJÖGREN SYNDROME

The major symptom of ocular involvement in Sjögren syndrome is dryness secondary to a chronic, progressive inflammatory destruction of the lacrimal glands [reviewed in (53)]. A foreign-body sensation due to repeated blinking and rubbing of the eyes (which produces minor corneal abrasions) may be the first manifestation. Blurring of vision due to drying of the cornea is a common complaint but photophobia is rare and raises the suspicion of uveitis. Severe dryness can produce a deep aching pain in the eyes. The eye symptoms tend to worsen during the day in contrast to blepharitis (worse in the morning), which is often confused with sicca syndrome. The irritation associated with blepharitis is due to accumulation of bacterial infection products overnight. Blepharitis may also be exacerbated by preservatives in ocular lubricants.

The evaluation of ocular dryness is problematic. The most commonly used test is the Schirmer test (Fig. 6.12). However, blepharitis, contact lenses, viral infections, irradiation, and drugs may also induce dryness. The list of drugs causing dry

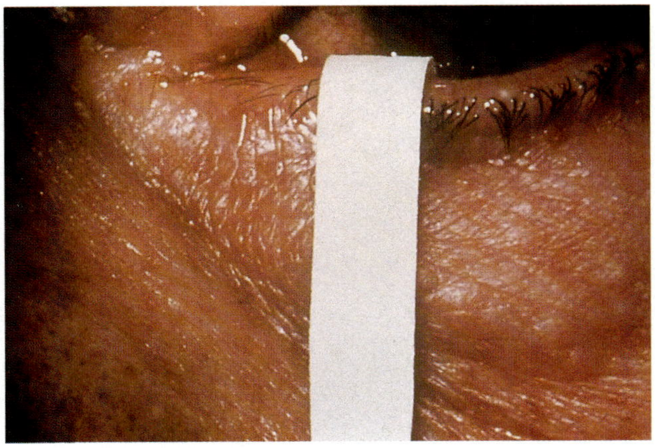

Figure 6.12. Schirmer test. In a patient with Sjögren syndrome, a filter-paper wick is placed under the lower eyelid after application of a local anesthesia. After 5 minutes, the distance that the tears have migrated along the filter paper is measured. Healthy individuals have more than 5-mm migration. In this patient, there are virtually no tears to migrate.

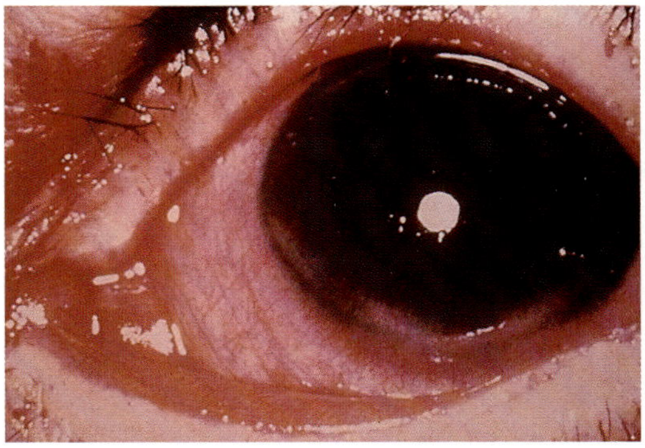

Figure 6.13. Rose bengal dye test. Note filiform staining of the cornea in this patient with Sjögren syndrome with severe dryness (sicca).

eyes is similar to those causing dry mouth (Table 6.3). The most common drugs causing dry eyes seen by ophthalmologists include antidepressants, antihistamines, retinoids, beta-blockers, and birth control pills. Unlike ocular dryness in Sjögren syndrome, these forms of ocular dryness generally respond to the instillation of artificial tears two to four times a day. In marked contradistinction, patients with Sjögren syndrome characteristically must apply artificial tears hourly, or even more frequently (53).

The signs of ocular Sjögren syndrome are varied. Conjunctival injection is common. The cornea loses its luster and the light reflex may be distorted rather than sharp and crisp. Small filiform defects may occur in the inferior portion of the cornea adjacent to the conjunctiva. The supravital rose bengal dye is useful in detecting these defects (Fig. 6.13). This dye is limited by a significant stinging sensation that may last for 20 minutes. Lissamine green dye, which has no associated stinging sensation, can be used as an alternative. An additional sign of ocular involvement in Sjögren syndrome is a decrease in the aqueous component of the tears, resulting in an increased mucin and oil production. Patients with ocular Sjögren syndrome can sometimes pull long strings of mucin from their eyes. Because of the severe dryness, large areas of epithelium may slough off. These cells tend to roll up and adhere to the corneal surfaces, producing filaments.

TREATMENT OF OCULAR MANIFESTATIONS

The mainstay of treatment of ocular Sjögren syndrome is artificial tears. These are available as nonviscous and more viscous preparations. A variety of preservative-free products is now available. It is generally advised to use preservative-free products if the lubricants are needed more than four times daily. Trial and error will determine individual preference for viscous or less viscous products. In addition, lubricant ointments are important adjuncts in the treatment of ocular Sjögren syndrome. These lubricants are applied at night.

In the authors' experience, bedroom humidifiers are beneficial for patients with ocular, as well as oral, Sjögren syndrome symptomatology. In addition, wearing underwater goggles containing water-soaked soft cotton at night is an effective means of humidifying dry eyes.

Punctal occlusion of the lacrimal nasal duct to preserve normal tear film is also a common therapeutic approach. A temporary punctal occlusion is performed with silicone plugs and if beneficial, a permanent ductal occlusion is accomplished by electrocautery following local anesthesia. Topical cyclosporine may have some promise in keratoconjunctivitis sicca; clinical trials are now in progress.

OTHER MUCOUS MEMBRANE INVOLVEMENT

Although the mucous membranes of the eyes and mouth are most commonly affected in Sjögren syndrome, it should not be forgotten that severe sinus and nasal xerosis frequently occurs in these patients. Many such patients have recurrent nonallergic rhinitis and sinusitis. In fact, a number of these patients with Sjögren syndrome initially seek evaluation from allergists because of recurrent rhinitis and sinusitis. These patients are usually negative for routine allergy skin testing. Increasing the ambient humidity with a humidifier, especially in the bedroom, or using large leafy plants (which must be constantly watered) in the house to create a greenhouse effect, are effective means of treating this annoying complication of Sjögren syndrome.

Vaginal dryness is a very common complication of Sjögren syndrome, and is much more frequently present than has been previously appreciated (54). Frequently, the presence of vaginal dryness may be detected only by direct questioning of the patient. The hyposecretion in the vaginal area is associated with chronic low-grade bacterial infections. Dyspareunia is common. Candidal vaginitis is also a common complication and can be successfully treated using a vaginal moisturizer together with nystatin vaginal suppositories at night.

EXTRAGLANDULAR MANIFESTATIONS

Sjögren syndrome is a systemic disease (7,14,46). The extraglandular manifestations are presented in Table 6.1. It should be noted that in general, patients with Sjögren syndrome with extraglandular manifestations are generally, but not always, anti-La(SS-B) and/or anti-Ro(SS-A) antibody–positive. Table 6.6 presents the association of various clinical, hematologic, and serologic features in patients with Sjögren syndrome demonstrating anti-Ro(SS-A) antibodies.

The following is a brief discussion of the extraglandular manifestations of Sjögren syndrome. Obviously some extraglandular features fall outside the realm of dermatology. (For more thorough discussion, please consult internal medicine, neurologic, or rheumatologic textbooks.)

Arthritis

Approximately 30% to 60% of patients with Sjögren syndrome have arthritis indistinguishable from rheumatoid arthritis. In many instances, the arthritis antedates by years the diagnosis of SS.

Rheumatoid factor (RF) is commonly detected in patients with Sjögren syndrome. The anti-Ro(SS-A) antibody cross-reacts with an epitope on the $F(ab')_2$ fragment of IgG, which probably explains at least in part the high frequency of RF activity in patients with Sjögren syndrome (55).

Polymyositis

Polymyositis is seen in 5% to 10% of patients with Sjögren syndrome (56). Muscle enzymes are generally only mildly elevated. Muscle biopsies demonstrate a perivascular mononuclear inflammatory infiltrate (Fig 6.14A,B).

Raynaud's Phenomenon

Raynaud's phenomenon is commonly detected in patients with Sjögren syndrome. The frequency is 20% to 40%. There also appears to be an increased frequency of carpal tunnel syndrome in patients with Sjögren syndrome, although the exact frequency is unknown.

Pulmonary Disease

Upper airways xerosis is common in Sjögren syndrome. It may be complicated by bacterial sinusitis. Interstitial lung disease is an uncommon feature of Sjögren syndrome (57,58). Bronchial lavage techniques indicate that approximately 50% of patients with Sjögren syndrome demonstrate increase quantities of alveolar inflammatory cells; however, these patients are generally asymptomatic. Necrotizing bronchial alveolitis is a very uncommon complication in Sjögren syndrome (Fig. 6.15).

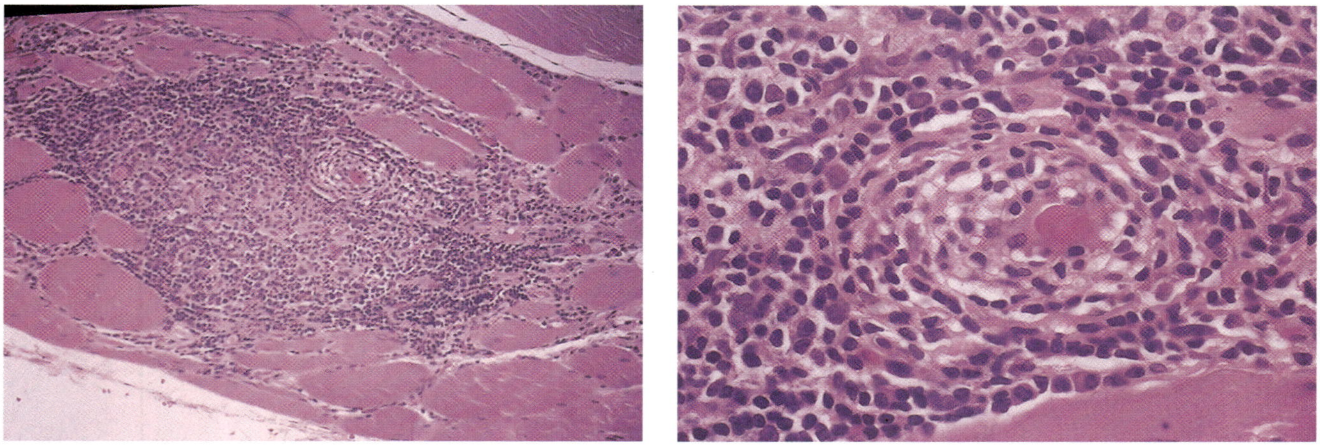

A B

Figure 6.14. A: Pathologic features of a muscle biopsy of a patient with Sjögren syndrome who had severe muscle weakness. Note perivascular lymphohistiocytic infiltrate (original magnification, ×100). **B:** Prominent perivascular infiltrate in same patient as depicted in **A** (original magnification, ×300).

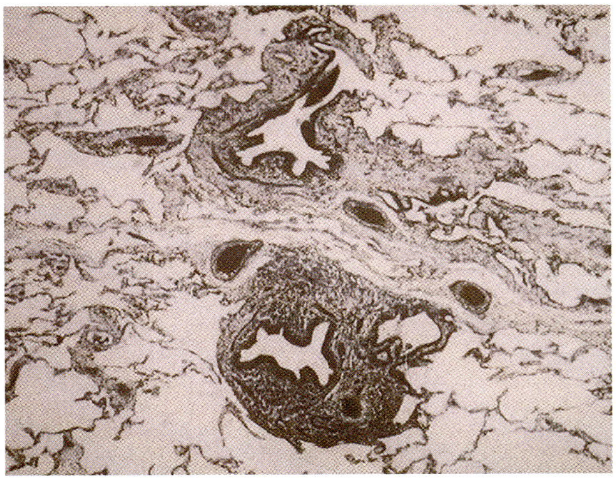

Figure 6.15. Pathogenic features of an anti-Ro(SS-A)–positive female patient with Sjögren syndrome initially presenting with urticaria-like vasculitic lesions and dyspnea. Note lymphohistiocytic infiltrate around terminal bronchi (necrotizing bronchial alveolitis). Pulmonary studies revealed an obstructive pattern (original magnification, ×40).

Chronic Active Hepatitis

Approximately 10% of patients with Sjögren syndrome produce anti–smooth muscle antibodies indicative of an immunologic insult, which can be associated with chronic active hepatitis and cryptogenic cirrhosis. In general, liver enzyme abnormalities are modest (56).

Primary Biliary Cirrhosis

There is an increased frequency of Sjögren syndrome in patients with primary biliary cirrhosis (59). The frequency has been reported as high as 70%. Anti-Ro(SS-A) antibodies have been reported in as many as 20% of patients with primary biliary cirrhosis.

Gastrointestional Manifestations

On occasion, various parts of the gastrointestinal tract may demonstrate a lymphohistiocytic infiltrate of the lamina propria (stomach, intestines) (60). At times, this may be symptomatic (i.e., diarrhea). Celiac disease has recently been reported in 14% of 34 patients with Sjögren syndrome (61).

Renal Disease

Glomerulonephritis may occur in Sjögren syndrome but is unusual (58). It is thought to result from immune complexes. More common is renal involvement in Sjögren syndrome, with a lymphohistiocytic inflammatory interstitial nephritis involving predominantly the distal tubules. This produces renal tubal acidosis and has been reported to occur in 20% of some Sjögren syndrome cohorts (58). Much less frequently, the interstitial inflammation may involve the more proximal renal tubules and induce aminoaciduria, calcuria, glucosuria, and so forth.

Thyroiditis

As many as 30% of patients with Sjögren syndrome develop evidence of Hashimoto thyroiditis associated with serum antimicrosomal and antithyroglobulin antibodies (58).

There is also some evidence to suggest subclinical pancreatic involvement as detected by secretin and pancreozymin tests. However, there is no evidence of increased frequency of diabetes mellitus.

B-cell Lymphomas

There is a 30- to 40-fold increased risk of lymphoma in patients with Sjögren syndrome (62,63). Most of the lymphomas are extranodal. Cutaneous and salivary glands are common sites of occurrence. The lymphomas are generally marginal cell or marginal cell derived. Translocation of the proto-oncogene bcl-2 t(14;18) is frequently detected. Cutaneous amyloid nodules have been detected adjacent to cutaneous lymphoma infiltrates (T.T.P., personal observation).

In addition to lymphomas, other hematologic abnormalities are also detected including leukopenia, lymphopenia, and thrombocytopenia. Antibodies directed against these three hematopoietic cells have been found.

It is interesting to note that platelets express cell-surface Ro(SS-A) macromolecules. In one of the author's experience (T.T.P.), 10% of patients with idiopathic thrombocytopenic purpura, possessed anti-Ro(SS-A) antibodies. In addition, it should be noted that thrombocytopenia can be a feature, and at times the sole feature, of neonatal lupus syndrome in infants born of anti-Ro(SS-A) antibody–positive mothers (64).

CENTRAL NERVOUS SYSTEM

Occasionally, neurologic disorders may be the presenting feature of Sjögren syndrome (65–76). Table 6.7 lists the spectrum of neurologic disease. Studies strongly suggest that a small-vessel inflammatory vasculopathy involving the vasa nervorum of the peripheral nerves (Fig. 6.16), as well as small blood vessels in

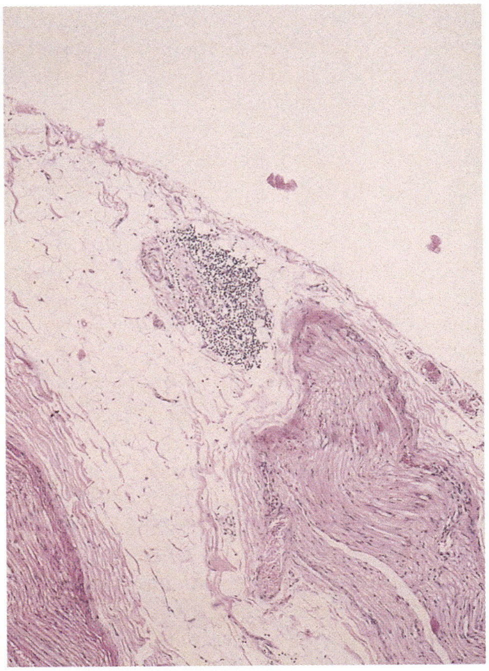

Figure 6.16. Peripheral nerve biopsy (sural nerve) demonstrating mononuclear vasculopathy of vasa nervorum (original magnification, ×40).

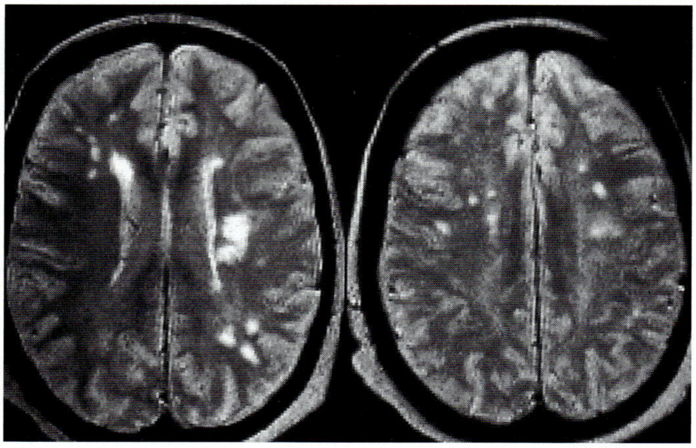

Figure 6.17. Magnetic resonance imaging of the bra n of an anti-Ro(SS-A) antibody–positive patient with Sjögren syndrome demonstrating infraction in right subcortical white matter as well as multiple enhanced T2-weighted images in the paraventricular white matter. Findings on enhanced T2-weighted images are thought to represent a vascular insult.

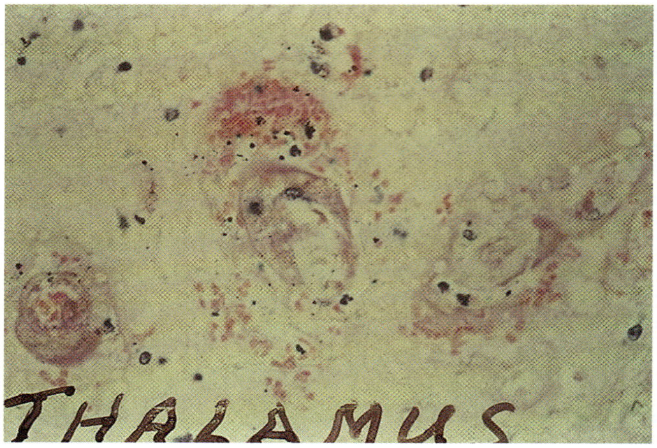

Figure 6.18. Brain autopsy findings in an anti-Ro(SS-A) antibody–positive patient with Sjögren syndrome with a history of recurrent palpable and nonpalpable purpura of the lower extremities for many years. This specimen demonstrates a smudging necrosis of the blood vessel walls associated with diapedesis of red blood cells and in other areas hemosiderin deposition indicative of a previous vascular insult.

the brain as detected by nuclear magnetic resonance images in the periventricular white matter (Fig. 6.17) and autopsy (Fig. 6.18) are probably responsible for the diverse clinical findings.

CUTANEOUS MANIFESTATIONS

The cutaneous manifestations associated with Sjögren syndrome are listed in Table 6.8.

Xerosis

Dryness of the skin (xerosis) is a common complaint in patients with Sjögren syndrome. For example, in their classic paper, Bloch et al. (56) reported 33 (53%) of 62 patients with this complaint. Xerosis is frequently accompanied by pruritus. Hyperpigmentation may be seen in areas of skin subjected to repeated scratching, and on occasion, the features of neurodermatitis may occur. Dry scalp may result in loss of luster to the hair. On occasion, patients also complain of severe dryness of the external ear canal with impaction of dried cerumen.

The pathogenesis of xerosis in Sjögren syndrome is unknown. The sebaceous glands are the major source of lubrication of the skin, with the sweat glands contributing a secondary component. In a few patients, a lymphohistiocytic infiltrate of the eccrine sweat glands has been demonstrated (77).

Recent studies of patients with primary Sjögren syndrome show disturbance of both the sympathetic and parasympathetic arms of the autonomic nervous system. Mandl et al. (78) documented a significant increase in the vasoconstrictor (VAC) index in patients with Sjögren syndrome compared with controls. The VAC index is a measurement of finger-skin blood flow, which is a sensitive test for detection of sympathetic dysfunction. Kovacs et al. (79) reported that patients with Sjögren syndrome have a reduced response to intracutaneous carbachol injection, indicating cholinergic dysfunction. The cause is unclear and maybe due to an immunologic or inflammatory mechanism. Mandl et al. suggest that a disturbance in neurotransmission at a receptor or postreceptor level and subsequent autonomic dysfunction may contribute to the exocrine inefficiency. Further studies are needed in this area to determine if sebaceous gland dysfunction is also playing a role in this distressing complaint (80).

With intense pruritus, the diagnosis of dermatitis herpetiformis should be considered in these patients. One of us (R.W.) has observed this condition occasionally in patients with Sjögren syndrome. This is not surprising in view of the high incidence (14%) of celiac disease recently reported in 34 patients with primary Sjögren syndrome and the common genetic background (HLA-DR3) in both Sjögren syndrome and dermatitis herpetiformis (61).

Vasculopathy

Cutaneous vasculitis occurs in Sjögren syndrome and although the exact frequency is unknown, it appears to occur more commonly in patients with Sjögren syndrome demonstrating anti-Ro(SS-A) antibodies (81). Our studies at a tertiary medical center (Johns Hopkins) detected evidence of cutaneous vasculitis in approximately 25% of 92 patients with Sjögren syndrome.

Patients may present with palpable and nonpalpable purpura or urticaria-like lesions located predominately over the lower extremities (Fig. 6.19). In addition to anti-Ro(SS-A) antibodies, RF and hypergammaglobulinemia are frequently seen. The clinical features are identical to Waldenström hypergammaglobulinemia. Indeed, Strauss (82) and Kyle et al. (83) have

TABLE 6.8. Cutaneous Manifestations of Sjögren Syndrome

Xerosis
Palpable and nonpalpable purpura
Urticaria-like vasculitic lesions
Erythema multiforme–like, erythema perstans, and erythema nodosum–like lesions
Cutaneous lymphoma
Nodular amyloidosis
Sweet syndrome
Annular erythematous lesions (donut lesion) described predominantly in Japanese patients

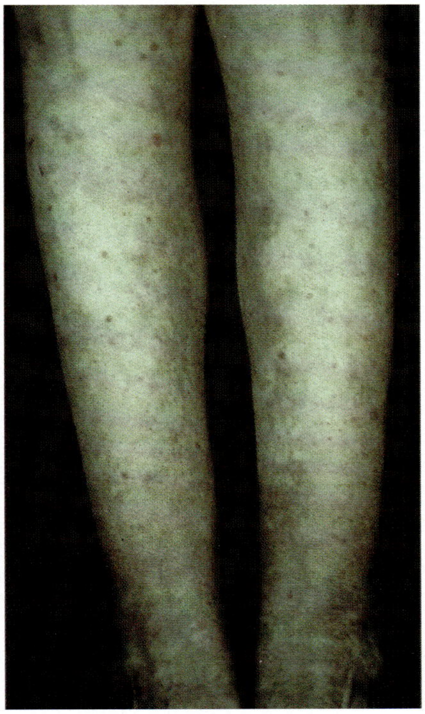

Figure 6.19. Palpable and nonpalpable purpura of the lower extremities. Recent lesions are characterized by erythematous papules and hemosiderin "tattooing" of the skin indicative of previous vasculitic lesions. Biopsy of acute lesions demonstrated a leukocytoclastic angiitis. Patient was anti-Ro(SS-A) antibody–positive and had longstanding Sjögren syndrome with the recent onset of cutaneous lupus lesions.

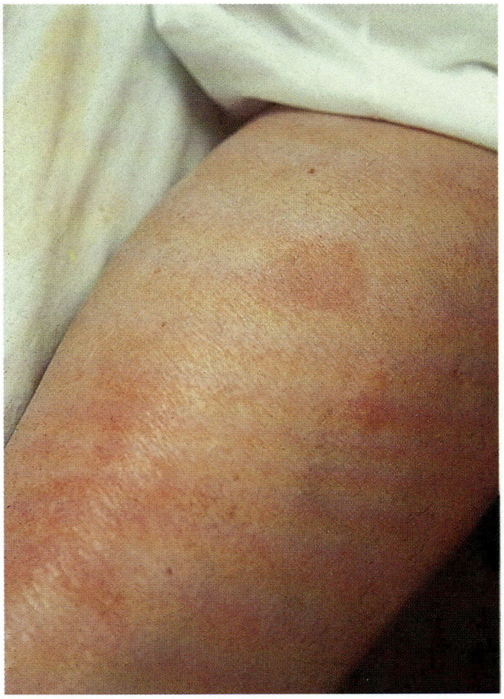

Figure 6.20. Urticaria-like lesions in a patient with Sjögren syndrome. The patient was anti-Ro(SS-A)–positive and had necrotizing bronchial alveolitis. Her lung biopsy is shown in Fig. 6.15. Biopsy demonstrated a leukocytoclastic vasculitis.

noted the frequent diagnosis of Sjögren syndrome among such patients. Purpuric lesions may be associated with ulcerations. Purpura frequently occurs in waves of activity (showers) often aggravated by increased activity or prolonged weight bearing.

In addition to the purpuric lesions on the lower extremities, patients with Sjögren syndrome may also demonstrate urticaria-like lesions (Fig. 6.20) (84,85). These urticaria-like lesions are characterized by persistent erythematous, edematous plaques. Petechiae may or may not be present in these plaques. Frequently, light touch to these lesions produces an annoying painful sensation (hyperpathia). Unlike the urticarial lesions associated with IgE-mediated allergic responses, these lesions persist for days rather than hours and may be accompanied by residual hyperpigmentation.

On biopsy, the palpable and nonpalpable purpuric lesions of the lower extremities and the urticaria-like lesions most commonly demonstrate a leukocytoclastic vasculitis involving small blood vessels high in the papillary portion of the dermis (Fig. 6.21) (85). Occasionally, mononuclear inflammatory vasculopathy in which mononuclear cells invade the blood vessel wall can be detected (Fig. 6.22). Our studies indicate that the mononuclear inflammatory infiltrate is *not* the late phase of a leukocytoclastic angiitis because repeated biopsies in these patients have shown a persistence of the mononuclear cells. The leukocytoclastic vasculitis is associated with evidence of seroreactivity [anti-Ro(SS-A) antibodies rheumatoid factor activity, etc.] (85). In contradistinction, the mononuclear vasculopathy is associated with seronegativity (Table 6.9). Cryoglobulins may occur in patients with Sjögren syndrome with leukocytoclastic vasculitis.

More recently, antineutrophil cytoplasmic antibodies (ACNA) were reported in 11% (9 of 82) of patients with primary Sjögren syndrome (86). Forty-four percent of patients positive for these antibodies had cutaneous vasculitis. Seven patients had p-ANCA and two patients had an atypical ANCA. Antibodies to c-ANCA were not seen. The meaning of these findings is unknown.

Over the years, we have determined that it is not possible to predict which histopathologic pattern (leukocytoclastic or mononuclear vasculopathy) is present by examining the clinical morphologic features of the palpable and nonpalpable purpura and the urticaria-like vasculitic lesions.

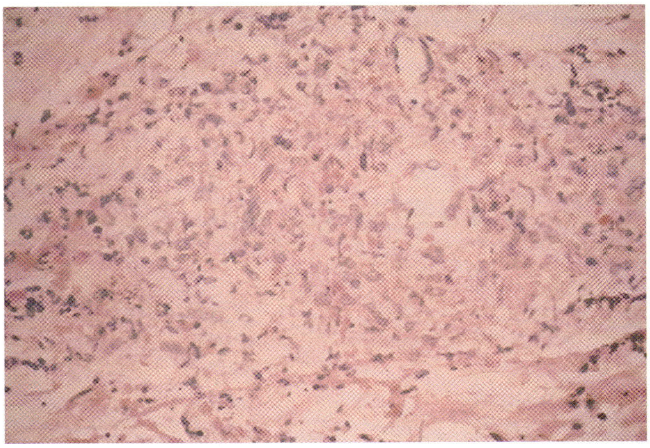

Figure 6.21. Leukocytoclastic vasculitis in a biopsy of a patient with anti-Ro(SS-A)–positive Sjögren syndrome.

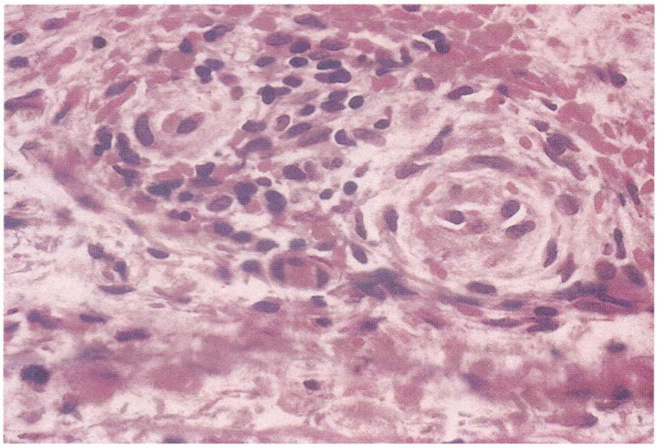

Figure 6.22. Mononuclear vasculopathy in biopsy of a patient with Sjögren syndrome. In general, the mononuclear vasculopathy occurs in serologically negative patients.

Although the palpable and nonpalpable purpuric lesions of the lower extremities and the urticaria-like vasculitic lesions are the most common manifestations of vasculitis in Sjögren syndrome, the vasculitis may present as petechiae, digital ulcers, erythema multiforme–like lesions, erythema perstans, nodular vasculitis, and, at times, nonspecific erythematous macules (84,85).

Donut-like Cutaneous Lesions

Japanese investigators have described raised, erythematous, plaquelike lesions with central clearing in their patients with Sjögren syndrome (Fig. 6.23A,B). These lesions are clinically, but not histologically, reminiscent of Sweet syndrome. Pathologically, the lesions are characterized by a perivascular mononuclear infiltrate. Some interface dermatitis is detected in approximately 30% of patients. T cells ($CD4^+$) are the dominant cells in the inflammatory infiltrate. These lesions are associated with the almost-universal presence of the HLA-DRw52 phenotype. The HLA-DR3 phenotype is rare in Oriental patients. These patients frequently have prominent clinical features of Sjögren syndrome and possess anti-Ro(SS-A) and anti-La(SS-B) antibodies (87–93).

Some American investigators have questioned whether these Japanese patients really have LE in addition to Sjögren syndrome. However, after personally examining a number of these Japanese patients, the senior author (T.T.P.) determined that he had not seen these plaquelike, "donut," erythematous lesions in over 200 anti-Ro(SS-A) antibody–positive American patients (white and black) with SLE and Sjögren syndrome. Recently, however, other investigators have described the annular erythema of Sjögren syndrome in a white woman (93). Studies on these lesions by our group indicate heavy mucin deposition may be present (Thomas Horn and T.T.P., personal observations 1994). Because mucin is very hydroscopic, this finding could conceivably explain, at least in part, the edematous nature of these lesions.

On unusual occasions, Sweet syndrome has been described in patients with Sjögren syndrome (94,95). These lesions are erythematous, edematous plaques demonstrating a diffuse neutrophilic dermal infiltration.

Cutaneous Lupus and Sjögren Syndrome Overlap

Patients with a combination of Lupus Erythematosus and Sjögren syndrome are generally in the sixth decade of life and are anti-Ro(SS-A) antibody–positive.

The most common type of lupus lesion seen in these patients is subacute cutaneous lupus erythematosus (SCLE) (Figs. 6.24 and 6.25) (96,97). Unlike anti-Ro(SS-A)–positive patients with isolated SCLE, overlap patients have a more guarded prognosis. Their disease process is complicated by pulmonary, neurologic, and renal diseases. In our experience, each of these complications occurs in approximately 33% of patients. Cutaneous vasculitis may occur and thyroiditis is frequent.

In addition to the Sjögren syndrome/LE overlap syndrome, it has also been recognized that anti-Ro(SS-A) antibody–positive patients with Sjögren syndrome may, on occasion, give birth to children with the classic neonatal lupus syndrome (99). Furthermore, some anti-Ro(SS-A) antibody–positive mothers, who are asymptomatic at the time they give birth to infants with the neonatal lupus syndrome, will eventually develop clinical features of Sjögren syndrome or Sjögren syndrome/LE overlap (99).

These two observations indicate that the clinical distinction between anti-Ro(SS-A) antibody–positive female patients with Sjögren syndrome and those with LE may not be as sharp as once believed. HLA studies indicate that a large proportion of anti-Ro(SS-A) antibody–positive female patients described under the rubric of primary Sjögren syndrome, SCLE, mothers of neonatal lupus infants, and the Sjögren syndrome/LE overlap syndrome share an increased frequency of the HLA phenotypes B8, DR3, DQ2, and DRw52. The reason for the phenotypic different clinical expressions of these patients is unknown (100). As noted before, studies by Reveille and Arnett have demonstrated that all anti-Ro(SS-A) antibody–positive patients demonstrate specific amino acid substitutions (glutamine at position 34 of the outermost domain of HLA-DQA1 alleles and leucine at position 26 of the DQB1 alleles). In addition to the establishment of a similar immunogenetic background between

TABLE 6.9. Serologic Correlation with Histopathologic Type of Vascular Disease in Sjögren Syndrome

	ANA	Hyperglob	RF	Anti-Ro	Anti-La
Leukocytoclastic angiitis (%) $n = 27$	21 (78)	14 (52)	18 (67)	20 (74)	12 (44)
Mononuclear vasculopathy (%) $n = 18$	7 (39)	2 (11)	3 (17)	2 (11)	2 (11)
p Value	0.02	0.01	0.002	0.0006	0.036

ANA, antinuclear antibody; hyperglob, hypergammaglobulinemia; RF, rheumatoid factor.
From Molina R, Provost TT, Alexander EL. Two histopathologic prototypes of inflammatory vascular disease in Sjögren syndrome: differential association with seroreactivity to rheumatoid factor and antibodies to Ro (SS-A) and with hypocomplementemia. *Arthritis Rheum* 1985;28:1251, with permission.

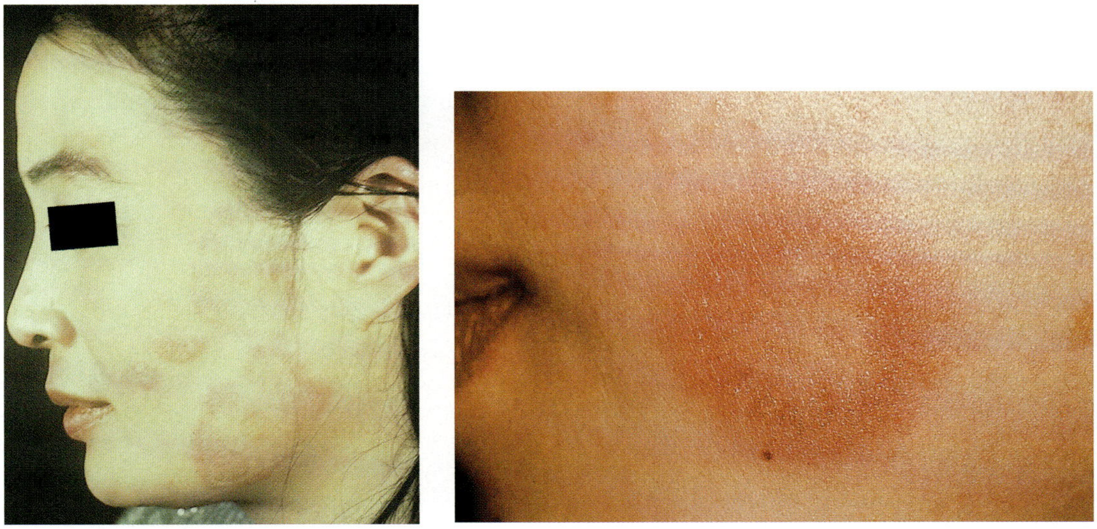

A B

Figure 6.23. A: Donut-like erythematous plaque lesion with central clearing in this anti-Ro(SS-A) antibody–positive patient. (From Tekiski Nishikawa, M.D., Keo University, Tokyo, with permission.) **B:** Close up of "donut-like" lesion in an anti-Ro(SS-A) antibody–positive Japanese female patient. (From Tekishi Nishikawa, M.D., Keo University, Tokyo, with permission.)

these anti-Ro(SS-A) antibody–positive female patients, these studies also demonstrate that the anti-Ro (SS-A) antibody response is under strict control by alleles localized to the MHC. Furthermore as noted above, the anti-Ro(SS-A) antibody response in HLA-DR3 patients frequently possess anti-Ro(SS-A) antibodies that cross react with the 52-kDa macromolecule and bind cardiac L-chain calcium channels.

The interrelationship between various phenotypic presentations of anti-Ro(SS-A)–antibody positive HLA-DR3–positive females and the neonatal lupus syndrome is presented in Fig. 6.26 (see Chapters 2 and 13).

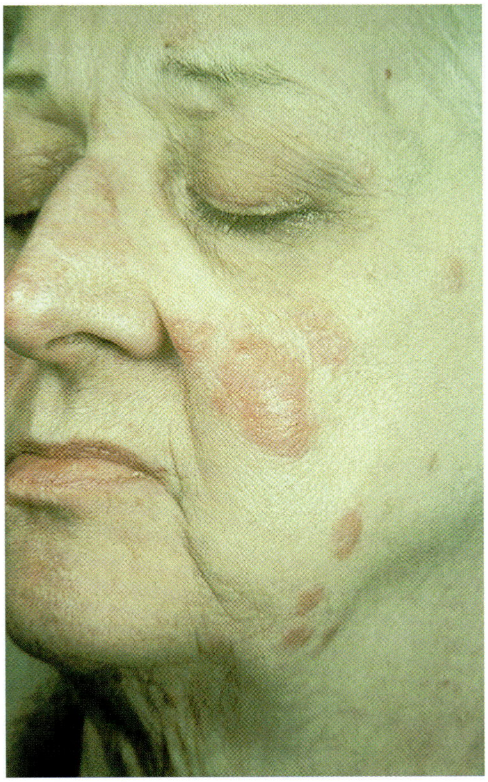

Figure 6.24. Patient with anti-Ro(SS-A) antibody–positive Sjögren syndrome with recent onset of erythematous-like facial lesions. These lesions demonstrated interface dermatitis compatible with lupus erythematosus. The patient suddenly died and autopsy demonstrated a diffuse central nervous system vasculopathy. Her brain autopsy findings are presented in Fig. 6.22. She also had lower extremity vasculitic lesions, which are depicted in Fig. 6.16.

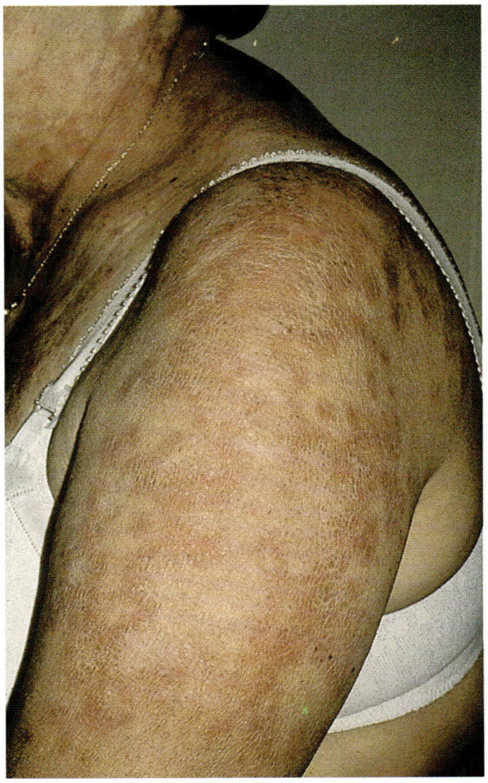

Figure 6.25. Widespread annular polycyclic lesions of subacute cutaneous lupus erythematosus in a 60-year-old patient with Sjögren syndrome and anti-Ro(SS-A) antibodies.

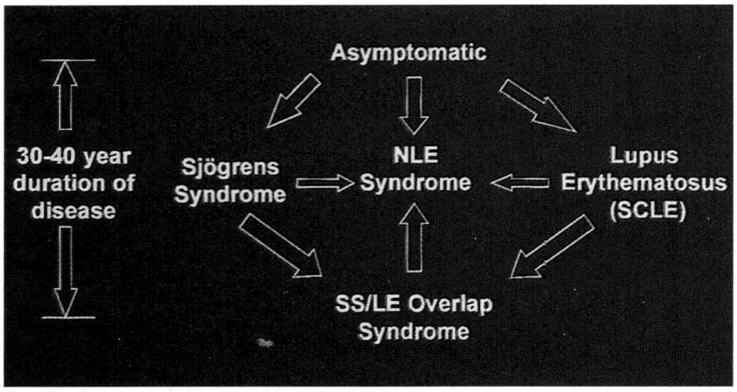

Figure 6.26. Depiction of close interrelationship of phenotypically different anti-Ro(SS-A) antibody, HLA-DR3–positive females. These patients may be initially asymptomatic and with time phenotypically differentiate toward lupus erythematosus (subacute cutaneous lupus erythematosus) or Sjögren syndrome. Some of these patients develop features of both Sjögren syndrome and lupus erythematosus. If their disease process occurs during the childbearing years, they are at risk to give birth to a child with the neonatal lupus syndrome.

Treatment of Cutaneous Disease

The treatment of dry skin involves daily baths with oily bath additive, soap substitutes, and liberal emollients. Vasculitis localized to the skin may be managed with dapsone, colchicine, or a brief course of oral corticosteroids. Systemic vasculitis carries a more guarded prognosis and requires more aggressive treatment with systemic corticosteroids and immunosuppressive agents (i.e., azathioprine or cyclophosphamide). The cutaneous features of Sjögren syndrome/LE overlap syndrome are usually controlled by photo protection, antimalarials, or dapsone.

SUMMARY

Sjögren syndrome is a complex, multisystem disease that may present in many different ways depending which organs or body systems are predominantly affected (101). Consequently, patients with Sjögren syndrome may attend many medical and surgical departments with no definitive diagnosis. Delay in diagnosis may be due to the following:

1. Patients may not recognize mucosal dryness as abnormal due to its insidious onset and thus not report this symptom to their physicians.
2. Patients may only have one mucous membrane affected for years and may not connect it with their current symptomatology.
3. Many doctors tend to associate the systemic symptomatology and serology with LE rather than Sjögren syndrome.

Long-term follow up of patients with Sjögren syndrome is required to minimize the damaging effects of mucosal dryness. The presence of small-vessel cutaneous vasculitic lesions in a subset of patients with Sjögren syndrome may reflect an associated systemic vasculitis, which often manifests as chronic, repetitive peripheral and central nervous system involvement. Early diagnosis and investigation to determine subtle systemic disease are important. Our studies suggest that these lesions are inflammatory and that early intervention with immunosuppression and/or steroid therapy may prove beneficial.

APPENDIX

California Criteria for Diagnosis of Sjögren Syndrome: Primary Sjögren Syndrome[1]

SYMPTOMS AND OBJECTIVE SIGNS OF OCULAR DRYNESS

1. Schirmer test less than 8 mm of wetting per 5 minutes, and
2. Positive rose bengal staining of cornea or conjunctiva to demonstrate keratoconjunctivitis sicca.

SYMPTOMS AND OBJECTIVE SIGNS OF DRY MOUTH

1. Decreased parotid flow rate using Lashley cups or other methods
2. Abnormal findings from biopsy of minor salivary gland (focus score of more than two based on average of four evaluable lobules).

SEROLOGIC EVIDENCE OF SYSTEMIC AUTOIMMUNITY

1. Elevated rheumatoid factor more than 1:320, or
2. Elevated antinuclear antibody more than 1:320, or
3. Presence of anti-SS-A(Ro) or anti-La(SS-B) antibodies.

SECONDARY SJÖGREN SYNDROME

Characteristic signs and symptoms of Sjögren syndrome (described before), plus clinical features sufficient to allow a diagnosis of rheumatoid arthritis, systemic lupus erythematosus, polymyositis, scleroderma, or biliary cirrhosis.

EXCLUSIONS

Sarcoidosis, preexistent lymphoma, human immunodeficiency virus, hepatitis virus B or C, primary fibromyalgia, and other known causes of autonomic neuropathy, keratitis sicca, or salivary gland enlargement

"Definite" Sjögren syndrome requires objective evidence of dryness of the eyes/mouth and autoimmunity, including a characteristic minor salivary gland biopsy (criteria IA, IB, and IC). "Probable" Sjögren syndrome does not require a minor salivary gland biopsy but can be diagnosed by demonstrating decreased salivary function (criteria IA, B-1, and IC).

European Criteria for Diagnosis of Sjögren Syndrome[2]

OCULAR SYMPTOMS

Positive response to question of daily dry eyes for 3 months, or
Sand or gravel feeling in eyes, or
Need for tears substitutes more than three times a day

ORAL SYMPTOMS

Positive response to question of daily dry mouth for more than 3 months, or
Recurrent or persistent swollen glands, or
Frequent drinking of fluids to aid swallowing of food

[1]From Fox RI, Robinson CA, Curd JG, et al. Sjögren syndrome: proposed criteria for classification. *Arthritis Rheum* 1986;29:577–585, with permission.

[2]Vitali C, Bombardieri S, Moutsopoulos HM, et al. Preliminary criteria for the classification of Sjögren's syndrome: results of a prospective concerted action supported by the European Community. *Arthritis Rheum* 1993;36:340–347, with permission.

OCULAR SIGNS

Positive test results from either a Schirmer test (≤ 5 mm in 5 minutes), or
a Rose Bengal score (≥ 4 according to van Bijsterveld scoring system).

HISTOPATHOLOGY

A focus of ≥1 on a minor salivary biopsy (focus = aggregations of 50 or more mononuclear cells per 4 mm^2 of glandular tissue)
Objective evidence of salivary gland involvement
Positive test results by salivary scintigraphy, parotid simulation, or unstimulated salivary flow (≥ 1.5 mL in 15 minutes)

Autoantibodies

Presence of anti-Ro(SS-A), anti-La(SS-B), or antinuclear antibodies or rheumatoid factor

Sjögren syndrome is diagnosed if four or more criteria are present.

Information Sources for Patients with Sjögren Syndrome

Carsons S, ed: *The New Sjögren's Syndrome Handbook.* Oxford, Oxford University Press, 1998.

Additional patient information is available from the National Sjögren's Syndrome Association; 3201 W. Evans Dr., Phoenix, AZ 85023; tel.: (800) 395-6772; or the Sjögren's Foundation, Inc., 382 Main St., Port Washington, NY 11050; tel: (516) 767-2866.

WEBSITES FOR SJÖGREN SYNDROME ASSOCIATIONS

Brazil: http://www.lagrima-brasil.org.br/
Columbia: http://www.reumacib.org.co/
Japan: http://www.fujita-hu.ac.jp/ktorikai/sjs.html
The Netherlands: http://www.spin.nl/nvsp0301.htm
Sweden: http://www.sjögrensyndrom.se/
United Kingdom: http://ourworld.compuserve.com/homepages/bssassociation/
United States: http://www.sjögrens.org

REFERENCES

1. Sjögren H. Zur Kenntnis der Keratoconjunctivitis sicca (Keratitis Filiformis bei hypofurktion der Tranendrusen). *Acta Opthal* 1933;11:1.
2. Leber, Ueber die Entstenhurg der Netzhautablosung. *Ber Versamnl Ophthal Ges Stuttg* 1882;14:165.
3. Hadden WB. On "dry mouth," or suppression of the salivary and buccal secretions. *Trans Clin Soc Lond* 1888;21:176.
4. Mikulicz JH. *Uber eine eigenartige symmetrische Erkankung der Tranen – und Mundspeicheldrusen.* Beitr Chir. Fortschr. Gewidmet: Theodor Billroth. Stuttgart, 1892:610–630.
5. Gougerot H. Inuffisance progressive et atrophie des glans salivaries et muqueuses de la bouche, des glands salivaries et muqueuses de la bouche, des conjonctives (et porfoes des mugueuses, nasale laryngee, vulvarre) secheresse de la bouche, des conjenctive etc. *Bull Med* 1926;40:360.
6. Talal N. Sjögren's syndrome: historical overview and clinical spectrum of disease. *Rheum Dis Clin North Am* 1992;18:507.
7. Strand V, Talal N. Advances in the diagnosis and concept of Sjögren's syndrome, autoimmune exocrinopathy. *Bull Rheum Dis* 1980;30:1046–1052.
8. Vitali C, Bombardieri S, Moutsopuolos HM, et al. Preliminary criteria for the classification of Sjögren's syndrome: results of a prospective concerted action supported by the European community. *Arthritis Rheum* 1993;36:340–347.
9. Vitali C, Bombardieri S, Moutsopuolos HM, et al. Assessment of the European classification criteria for Sjögren's syndrome in a series of clinically defined cases: results of a prospective multicentre study. *Ann Rheum Dis* 1996;55:116–21.
10. Molina R, Provost TT, Arnett FC, et al. Primary Sjögren's syndrome in men: clinical serologic and immunogenetic features. *Am J Med* 1986;80:23.
11. Reveille J, Arnett FC. The immunogenetics of Sjöogren's syndrome. *Rheum Dis Clin North Am* 1992;18:539–550.
12. Reveille J, Wilson RW, Provost TT, et al. Primary Sjögren's syndrome and other autoimmune diseases in families: prevalence and immunogenetic studies in six kindreds. *Ann Intern Med* 1984;101:748—756.
13. Chan EKL, Andrade Lec. Antinuclear antibodies in Sjögren's syndrome. *Rheum Dis Clin North Am* 1992;18:551.
14. Alexander EL, Arnett FC, Provost TT, et al. Ro (SS-A) and La (SS-B) antibodies in the clinical spectrum of Sjögren's syndrome. *J Rheumatol* 1982;9:239.
15. Harley JB, Reichlen M, Arnett FC, et al. Gene interaction at HLA DQ enhances autoantibody production on primary Sjögren's syndrome. *Science* 1986;232:1145.
16. Hamilton RG, Harley JB, Bias WB, et al. Two Ro (SS-A) autoantibody responses in systemic lupus erythematosus. Correlation of HLA DR/DQ specificities with quantitative expression of Ro (SS-A) auto antibody. *Arthritis Rheum* 1988;31:496.
17. Reveille JD, Macleod MJ, Whittington K, et al. Specific amino acid residues in the second hypervariable region of HLA-DQA1 and DQB1 chain genes promote the Ro (SS-A)/La (SS-B) auto antibody responses. *J Immunol* 1991;146: 3871–3876.
18. Harley JB, Alexander EL, Bias WB, et al. Anti Ro/SS-A and anti La/SS-B in patients with Sjögren's syndrome. *Arthritis Rheum* 1986;29:196.
19. Provost TT, Levin LS, Watson MM, et al. Detection of anti Ro (SS-A) antibodies by gel double diffusion and a sandwich ELISA in systemic lupus erythematosus and subacute cutaneous lupus erythematosus and Sjögren's syndrome. *J Autoimmun* 1991;4887.
20. Alexander EL, Provost TT, Stevens MB, et al. Neurologic complications of primary Sjögren's syndrome. *Medicine* 1982;61:245.
21. Boutjdir M, Chen L, Zhag ZH, et al. Arrhythrogenicity of IgG and anti 52kD SSA/Ro affinity purified antibodies from mothers of children with congenital heart block. *Circ Res* 1997;80:354.
22. Buyon JE, Winchester RJ, Slade SG, et al. Identification of mothers at risk for congenital heart block and other neonatal lupus syndromes in their children. *Arthritis Rheum* 1993; 36:1263.
23. Julkunen H, Kaaja R, Wallgren E, et al. Isolated congenital heart block: fetal and infant outcome and familial incidence of heart block. *Obstet Gynecol* 1993; 82:11.
24. Kinoshita G, Keech CI, Sontheimer RD, et al. Spreading of the immune response from 52-kDa and 60kDa Ro to calreticulin in experimental autoimmunity. *Lupus* 1998;7:7.
25. Gottesfeld JM, Andrews DL, Hoch SO, et al. Association of an RNA polymerase III transcription factor with a ribonuclear protein complex recognized by autoimmune sera. *Nucleic Acid Res* 1984;12:3185–3200.
26. Gottlieb E, Steitz JA. The RNA binding protein La influences both the accuracy and the efficiency of RNA polymerase III transcription *in vitro. EMBO J* 1989;8:841.
27. Gottlieb E, Steitz JA. Function of mammalian La protein: evidence for its action in transcription termination by RNA polymerase III. *EMBO J* 1989;8:851.
28. Boire G, Craft J. Human Ro ribonuclear protein particles: characterization of mature structure and stable association with La polypeptide. *J Clin Invest* 1990;85:1182.
29. Wang D, Buyon JP, Zhu W, et al. Defining a novel 75kDa phosphoprotein associated with SS-A/Ro and identification of distinct human auto antibodies. *J Clin Invest* 1999;104:1265.
30. Miyagawa S, Yanagi K, Yoshioka A, et al. Neonatal lupus erythematosus: maternal IgG antibodies bind to a recombinant-terminal fusion protein encoded by human alpha fodrin CDNA. *J Invest Dermatol* 1998;116:1189.
31. Eftekhari P, Salle L, Lezoualc'h F, et al. Anti SS-A/Ro 52 auto antibodies blocking the cardiac 5-HT4 serotininergic receptor could explain neonatal lupus congenital heart block. *Eur J Immunol* 2000;308:1782
32. Boire G, Lopex-Longo FS, Lapointe S, et al. Sera from patients with autoimmune disease recognize confirmational determinants on the 60kD Ro/SSA protein. *Arthritis Rheum* 1991;34:722.
33. Bacman S, Sterin-Borda L, Camusso JJ, et al. Circulating antibodies against rat parotid gland: muscarinic receptors in primary Sjögren's syndrome. *Clin Exp Immunol* 1996;104:454–459.
34. Waterman A, Gordon TP, Rischmueller M, et al. Muscarinic receptor antibodies in Sjögren's syndrome. *Arthritis Rheum* 2000;43:1647–1654.
35. Venables PJW, Rigby SP. Viruses in the etiopathogenesis of Sjögren's syndrome. *J Rheumatol* 1997;24:3.
36. Schofield RH, Harley J. Autoantigenicity of Ro (SS-A) antigen is related to a nucleocapsid protein of vesicular stomatitis virus. *PNAS* 1991;81:3343.
37. Talal N, Dauphinee MJ, Dang T, et al. Detection of serum antibodies to retroviral proteins in patients with primary Sjögren's syndrome (autoimmune exocrinopathy). *Arthritis Rheum* 1990;33:774.
38. Itescu S, Winchester R. Diffuse infiltrative lymphocytosis syndrome: a disorder occurring in human immune deficiency virus-1 infection that may present as a sicca syndrome. *Rheum Dis Clin North Am* 1992;18:683.
39. Manus MP, Rambesch EJ. Autoimmunity and extrahepatic manifestations of hepatitis C virus infection. *J Hepatol* 1999;31[Suppl 1]:39.
40. Mason DK, Chisholdm DM. *Salivary glands in health and disease.* London: WB Saunders, 1975:38–41, 194–200.

41. Godwin JT. Benign lymphoepithelial lesions of the parotid gland (adenolymphoma, chronic inflammation, lymphoepithelioma, lymphocytic tumor, Mikulicz disease): report of eleven cases. *Cancer* 1952;5:1089–1096.
42. Daniels TE. Labial salivary gland biopsy in Sjögren's syndrome: assessment as a diagnostic criterion in 362 suspected cases. *Arthritis Rheum* 1984;27: 147–156.
43. Chisholm DM, Mason DK. Labial salivary gland biopsy in Sjögren's syndrome. *J Clin Pathol* 1968;21:656–660.
44. Chen MS, Daly TE. Xerostomia and complete denture retention. *Oral Health* 1980;70:27–29.
45. Ruiz-Arguelle GJ. The "lipstick-on-teeth" sign in Sjögren's syndrome. *N Engl J Med* 1986;315:1030–1031.
46. Whaley K, Buchanan WW. Sjögren's syndrome and associated diseases. In: Parker CW, ed. *Clinical immunology.* Philadelphia: WB Saunders, 1980:637.
47. Sutcliffe J, Inanc C, Speight PM, et al. Predictors of lymphoma development in primary Sjögren's syndrome. *Semin Arthritis Rheum* 1998;28:80–87.
48. March DE, Rao V, Zwillenberg D. Computed tomography of salivary glands in Sjögren's syndrome. *Arch Otolaryngol Head Neck Surg* 1989;105–106.
49. Takashima S, Takeuchi N, Morimoto S, et al. MR imaging of Sjögren's syndrome: correlation with sialography and pathology. *J Comput Assist Tomogr* 1991;15:393–400.
50. Kohn WG, Ship JA, Atkinson JC, et al. Salivary gland 99mTc scintigraphy: a grading scale and correlation with major salivary flow rates. *J Oral Pathol Med* 1991;21:70–74.
51. Kawamura H, Taniguchi N, Itoh K, et al. Salivary gland echography in patients with Sjögren's syndrome. *Arthritis Rheum* 1990;30:505–510.
52. Nakamura T, Oshiumi Y, Yonestsu K, et al. Salivary SPECT and factor analysis in Sjögren's syndrome. *Acta Radiol* 1991;32:406–410.
53. Friedlanender MH. Ocular manifestations of Sjögren's syndrome: keratoconjunctivitis sicca. *Rheum Dis Clin North Am* 1992;18:591.
54. Marchesoni D, Mazzauega B, DeSandre P, et al. Gynaecological aspects of primary Sjögren's syndrome. *Eur J Obstet Gynecol Reprod Biol* 1995;63:49–53.
55. Manula MJ, Fox OF, Yamagata, et al. The Ro (SS-A) autoantigen as an immunogen: some anti Ro (SS-A) antibody binds IgG. *J Exp Med* 1986;86: 1889–1901.
56. Bloch KJ, Buchanan WW, Wohl MJ, et al. Sjögren's syndrome: a clinical, pathological and serologic study of 62 cases. *Medicine* 1965;44:187.
57. Boulware DW, Hedgpeth MT. Lupus pneumonitis and anti Ro (SS-A) antibodies. *J Rheumatol* 1989;16:479–481.
58. Simmons-O'Brien E, Chen S, Watson R, et al. One hundred anti-Ro (SS-A) antibody positive patients: a 10-year follow up. *Medicine* 1995;74:109–130.
59. Penner E, Reichlin M. Primary biliary cirrhosis associated with Sjögren's syndrome: evidence for circulating and tissue deposited Ro/Anti Ro immune complexes. *Arthritis Rheum* 1982;25:1250.
60. Sobhani I, Brousse N, Vissuzaine C, et al. A diffuse T lymphocytic gastrointestinal mucosal infiltration associated with Sjögren's syndrome resulting in a watery diarrhea syndrome and responsive to immunosuppressive therapy. *Am J Gastroenterol* 1998;93:2584–2586.
61. Iltanen S, Collins P, Korfela M, et al. Celiac disease and markers of celiac disease latency in patients with primary Sjögren's syndrome. *Am J Gastroenterol* 1999;94:1042–1046.
62. Kassan SS, Thomas Tl, Moutsopoulos HM, et al. Increased risk of lymphoma in sicca syndrome. *Ann Intern Med* 1978;89:888.
63. Royer B, Cazals-Hatem D, Sibilia J, et al. Lymphomas in patients with Sjögren's syndrome are marginal zone–B cell neoplasms, arise in diverse extranodal and nodal sites, and are not associated with viruses. *Blood* 1997; 90:766.
64. Watson R, Kang JE, May M, et al. Thrombocytopenia in the neonatal lupus syndrome. *Arch Dermatol* 1988;124:560–563.
65. Alexander E. Central nervous system disease in Sjögren's syndrome. *Rheum Dis Clin North Am* 1992;18:637.
66. Alexander EL, Provost TT, Stevens MB, et al. Neurologic complications of primary Sjögren's syndrome. *Medicine* 1982;61:245.
67. Alexander EL, Alexander GE. Aseptic meningitis in primary Sjögren's syndrome. *Neurology* 1982;33:593.
68. Alexander EL, Provost TT. Sjögren's syndrome: association of cutaneous vasculitis with nervous system disease. *Arch Dermatol* 1987;123:801.
69. Alexander EL, Beall S, Gordon B, et al. Magnetic resonance imaging (MRI) in primary Sjögren's syndrome with central nervous system disease: new clues to pathogenesis. *Arthritis Rheum* 1986;29:S63.
70. Alexander EL, Craft C, Provost TT, et al. Necrotizing arteritis and spinal subarachnoid hemorrhage in Sjögren's syndrome. *Ann Neurol* 1986;11:632.
71. Alexander EL, Provost TT, Stevens MB, et al. Sjögren's syndrome: central nervous system manifestations. *Neurology* 1981;31:1391.
72. Alexander EL, Provost TT, Stevens MB, et al. Neurologic complications of primary Sjögren's syndrome. *Medicine* 1982;61:247.
73. Alexander EL, Beall S, Gordon B, et al. Magnetic resonance imaging of cerebral lesions in patients with Sjögren's syndrome. *Ann Intern Med* 1988;108: 815.
74. Alexander EL, Malinow K, Lejewski JE, et al. Primary Sjögren's syndrome with central nervous system dysfunction mimicking multiple sclerosis. *Ann Intern Med* 1986;104:323.
75. DeLaMonte SM, Hutchins GM, Gupta PK. Polymorphous meningitis with atypical mononuclear cells in Sjögren's syndrome. *Ann Neurol* 1983;14:455.
76. Lafitte C. Neurological manifestations in Sjögren's syndrome. *Arch Neurol* 2000;57:411–413.
77. Whaley K, Williamson J, Chisholm DM, et al. Sjögren's syndrome, I: sicca components. *Q J Med* 1973;166:279.
78. Mandl T, Bornhyr SV, Casterfors J, et al. Sympathetic dysfunction in patients with primary Sjögren's syndrome. *J Rheumatol* 2001;28:296–301.
79. Kovacs L, Totok T, Bari F, et al. Impaired microvascular response to cholinergic stimuli in primary Sjögren's syndrome. *Ann Rheum Dis* 2000;59:48–53.
80. Sais G, Admella C, Fantova MJ, et al. Lymphocytic autoimmune hidradenitis cutaneous vasculitis and primary Sjögren's syndrome. *Br J Dermatol* 1998;139: 1073.
81. Alexander EL, Arnett FC, Provost TT, et al. Sjögren's syndrome: association of anti-Ro (SS-A) antibodies with vasculitis, hematologic abnormalities, and serologic hyperreactivity. *Ann Intern Med* 1983;98:155.
82. Strauss WG. Purpura hypergammaglobulinemia of Waldenstrom. *N Engl J Med* 1959;260:857.
83. Kyle RA, Gleich GJ, Bayed ED. Benign hypergammaglobulinaemic purpura of Waldenstrom. *Medicine* 1971;50:113.
84. Behrman HT, Leek K. Sjögren's syndrome. *Arch Dermatol Syphil* 1950;61:63.
85. Alexander EL, Provost TT. Cutaneous manifestations of primary Sjögren's syndrome: a reflection of vasculitis in association with anti-Ro (SS-A) antibodies. *J Invest Dermatol* 1991;32:406–410.
86. Font J, Ramos-Casals M, Cervera R, et al. Anti neutrophil cytoplasmic antibodies in primary Sjögren's syndrome: prevalence and clinical significance. *Br J Rheumatol* 1998;37:1287–1291.
87. Teramoto N, Katayama I, Arai H, et al. Annular erythema: possible association with Sjögren's syndrome. *J Am Acad Dermatol* 1989;20:596.
88. Katayama I, Asai T, Nishioka K, et al. Annular erythema associated with primary Sjögren's syndrome: analysis of T cell subsets in cutaneous infiltrates. *J Am Acad Dermatol* 1989;21:1218.
89. Katayama I, Teramato N, Arai H, et al. Annular erythema: a comparative study of Sjögren's syndrome with subacute cutaneous lupus erythematosus. *Int J Dermatol* 1991;30:365.
90. Nishikawa T, Provost TT. Differences in clinical, serologic and immunogenetic features of white versus Oriental anti- SSA/Ro positive patients [editorial]. *J Am Acad Dermatol* 1991;25:6563.
91. Ruzicka T, Faes J, Arai H, et al. Annular erythema associated with Sjögren's syndrome: a variant of systemic lupus erythematosus. *J Am Acad Dermatol* 1991;25:557.
92. Kawakami T, Saito. The relationship between facial annular erythema and anti-SS-A/Ro antibodies in three East Asian women. *Br J Dermatol* 1999;140: 136–1470.
93. Harmowitz JE, McCauliffe DP, Seykora J, et al. Annular erythema of Sjögren's syndrome in a white woman. *J Am Acad Dermatol* 2000;42:1069–1072.
94. Prystowsky SD, Fye KH, Goitte KD, et al. Acute febrile neutrophilic dermatoses associated with Sjögren's syndrome. *Arch Dermatol* 1978;114:1234.
95. Levenstein MM, Fisher BK, Fisher LL, et al. Simultaneous occurrence of subacute cutaneous lupus erythematosus and Sweet's syndrome: a marker of Sjögren's syndrome? *Int J Dermatol* 1991;30:640.
96. Provost TT, Alexander E, Talal N, et al. The relationship between anti-Ro (SS-A) antibody positive Sjögren's syndrome and anti-Ro (SS-A) antibody positive lupus erythematosus. *Arch Dermatol* 1988;124:63.
97. Steinberg AD, Talal N. The co-existence of Sjögren's syndrome and systemic lupus erythematosus. *Ann Intern Med* 1971;74:55.
99. Provost TT, Watson R, Simmons-O'Brien E. Anti-Ro (SS-A) antibody positive Sjögren's/lupus erythematosus overlap syndrome. *Lupus* 1997;6:105–115.
99. Watson RM, Lane AT, Barnett NK, et al. Neonatal lupus erythematosus: a clinical, serological, and immunogenetic study with review of the literature. *Medicine* 1984;63:362.
100. Provost TT, Watson R. Anti-Ro (SS-A) HLA-DR3 positive women: the interrelationship between some ANA negative, SS, SCLE, and NLE mothers in SS/LE overlap female patients. *J Invest Dermatol* 1993;100:14S.
101. Talal N. What is Sjögren's syndrome and why is it important? *J Rheumatol* 2000;27[suppl 61]:1–3.

CHAPTER 7

Rheumatoid Arthritis

Carlin B. Hollar and Joseph L. Jorizzo

Rheumatoid arthritis (RA) is a multisystem, autoimmune connective tissue disease. It was first described by Soranus in the second century and first called "rheumatoid arthritis" in 1876 by Garrod (1). The hallmark of the disease is a progressive, commonly symmetric, polyarthritis that can result in destruction of joint function and premature morbidity and mortality. Extraarticular manifestations are seen, often in more aggressive forms of the disease (2). Multiple organs may be affected including the skin, heart, and lungs, among others. The rheumatoid nodule is the most common and well-known dermatologic lesion in RA, but a variety of cutaneous manifestations can be seen.

Approximately 1% of the adult population is affected with RA (3). Women are affected two to three times more commonly than men. Onset is usually in the fourth and fifth decades. Most patients follow a chronic course characterized by exacerbations and remissions. Five percent have a very aggressive, "malignant" form with multiple extraarticular manifestations (4). Eighty percent are disabled after 20 years. Life expectancy is decreased by 3 to 18 years (5).

Evidence suggests that RA is a multifactorial autoimmune process. Studies on twins suggest that both environmental and genetic factors play a role (5). Any of a variety of insults to the joints may initiate an inflammatory process in a genetically predisposed patient. Associations between RA and certain subtypes of HLA-DR1 and HLA-DR4 have been established (6,7). Inflammation is initiated when major histocompatibility complex (MHC) class II molecules present antigens to $CD4^+$ T cells, activating them. These activated T cells, in turn, stimulate monocytes, macrophages, and fibroblasts to release inflammatory cytokines such as interleukin-1 (IL-1), IL-6 and tumor necrosis factor-α (TNF-α) (8). Activated T cells also stimulate B cells to produce immunoglobulins. There is a disruption in the normal balance between adequate inflammatory response required for healing and excessive inflammatory response that results in destruction.

Rheumatoid factor is an IgM (or IgA) autoantibody directed against the Fc portion of IgG. It is present in as many as 80% of patients with RA and often in those with the more aggressive forms of the disease (9). Its presence suggests a role for immune complexes in this disease process. The lack of rheumatoid factor in some affected patients does not eliminate the possibility of immune complex disease, but suggests the presence of other autoantibodies. Some autoantibodies currently under investigation include: antikeratin antibody (AKA), antiperinuclear factor (APF), and anti-RA33 antibody (10). Like many autoimmune diseases, cellular and humoral immunities play a role in disease pathogenesis.

RA often begins with general constitutional symptoms such as fatigue, anorexia, vague musculoskeletal complaints, and generalized weakness. It may be weeks or months before the characteristic synovitis presents. The American College of Rheumatology has set guidelines for the diagnosis of RA (Table 7.1) (11). Synovial inflammation, which affects joints, tendons, and bursae, usually results in warmth but not erythema of the affected area. There is significant pain associated with stretching of the joint capsule. There is characteristic involvement of the proximal interphalangeal joints and metacarpophalangeal joints with sparing of the distal interphalangeal joints. The developing pattern of joint involvement is very suggestive of the diagnosis. Chronic inflammation may result in late structural deformities that are clinically obvious. The "swan neck" deformity results from hyperextension of the proximal interphalangeal (PIP) joint and compensatory flexion of the distal interphalangeal (DIP) joint leading to radial deviation of the hand with ulnar deviation of the digits. Flexion contracture of the PIP joint and extension of the DIP joint is referred to as the "boutonniere" deformity. Similar structural deformities can occur in the feet.

TREATMENT OF RHEUMATOID ARTHRITIS

The exact cause of RA is unknown and initial treatments have been general antiinflammatory medications. There is no single therapy that is the treatment of choice. Many drugs are used, frequently in combination. Analgesics and antiinflammatory agents such as acetaminophen, which relieves pain somewhat, and nonsteroidal antiinflammatory drugs (NSAIDs), which reduce inflammation, help symptomatically, but do not alter the underlying disease course. Selective COX-2–inhibitor NSAIDs, such as celecoxib and rofecoxib, have a reduced incidence of nephrotoxicity and gastrointestinal side effects and are therefore better tolerated by patients. These types of treatments have been considered "first line" in pyramidal treatment protocols in the past. However, more is now known about the importance of aggressive therapy to alter the disease

TABLE 7.1. 1987 American College of Rheumatology Revised Criteria for the Classification of Rheumatoid Arthritis (Modified)

Criterion	Definition
Morning stiffness	Morning stiffness in and around the joints, lasting at least 1 h before maximal improvement
Arthritis of three or more joint areas	At least three joint areas simultaneously afflicted with soft-tissue swelling or joint fluid observed by a physician. The 14 possible areas are (right or left): PIP, MCP, wrists, elbow, knee, ankle, and MTP joints
Arthritis of hand joints	At least one area swollen in a wrist, MCP, or PIP joint
Symmetric arthritis	Simultaneous involvement of the same joint areas on both sides of the body (bilateral involvement of PIP, MCP, or MTP acceptable without perfect symmetry)
Rheumatoid nodules	Subcutaneous nodules over bony prominences or extensor surfaces or in juxtaarticular regions (observed by a physician)
Serum rheumatoid factor	Abnormal amount of serum rheumatoid factor by any method for which the result has been positive in less than 5% of control subjects
Radiographic changes	Erosions or unequivocal bony decalcification localized in or most marked adjacent to the involved joints

MCP, metacarpophalangeal; MTP, metatarsophalangeal; PIP, proximal interphalangeal.
From Winchester R, Dwyer E, Rose S. The genetic basis of rheumatoid arthritis. *Rheum Dis Clin North Am* 1992;18:761–783, with permission

course in the early years, with the goal of preventing permanent joint damage.

Disease-modifying antirheumatic drugs (DMARDs), previously considered "second line," are now used early in the disease process. DMARDs reduce acute-phase reactants, decrease inflammation, prevent joint damage, and produce overall disease modification (4). These DMARDs include methotrexate, antimalarials, sulfasalazine, azathioprine, cyclosporine, penicillamine, and leflunomide. Systemic glucocorticoids are potent antiinflammatory agents and have been used, but have a significantly toxic side-effect profile, especially when used over long periods.

Newer additions to the antirheumatic armamentarium are considered biologic response modifiers and many act directly on cytokines. The most well-known and now commercially available members of this category are the anti-TNFα agents, etanercept and infliximab. Etanercept (Enbrel; Wyeth, Philadelphia, PA) is a recombinant human TNF dimeric receptor fusion protein consisting of the ligand-binding portion of the human 75-kDa TNF receptor linked to the Fc portion of human IgG1. This treatment is given as a subcutaneous injection twice per week. Infliximab (Remicade; Schering-Plough, Kenilworth, NJ) is a chimeric (mouse/human) IgG1 monoclonal antibody to TNF-α. It is given intravenously every 6 to 8 weeks. Both etanercept and infliximab block the interaction between TNF-α and its receptors, rendering TNF-α biologically inactive. Both have been shown to significantly decrease the synovitis and retard the progression of cartilage destruction (12). Other biologic response modifiers are currently under investigation, including anti–IL-6 and anti–IL-1 agents.

CUTANEOUS MANIFESTATIONS

In addition to the debilitating joint destruction, disease of numerous other organ systems contributes to the morbidity and mortality in patients with RA. A discussion of all extraarticular manifestations is beyond the scope of this chapter. Dermatologic manifestations range from the well-recognized rheumatoid nodule, to manifestations of cutaneous vasculitis, to associated processes such as pyoderma gangrenosum and autoimmune bullous diseases.

Rheumatoid Nodules

Rheumatoid nodules are the classic cutaneous manifestation of RA. They are not diagnostic for this disease and can be seen in other processes, especially other connective tissue diseases. The lesions occur in 20% to 30% of patients with seropositive RA (13). Rheumatoid nodules are extremely relevant clinically as they correlate with more severe arthritis, higher levels of rheumatoid factor, and with an increased incidence of rheumatoid vasculitis (9). Clinically, they are firm, dome-shaped, skin-colored papules within the subcutaneous tissue and they are mobile and nontender (Fig. 7.1). They are most often located over pressure points such as the extensor surface of the forearms, the Achilles tendons, and the olecranons. However, any subcutaneous site can be affected. Visceral involvement has also been noted with nodules occurring at sites including the lungs, heart, larynx, and serosal surfaces (9,14–16).

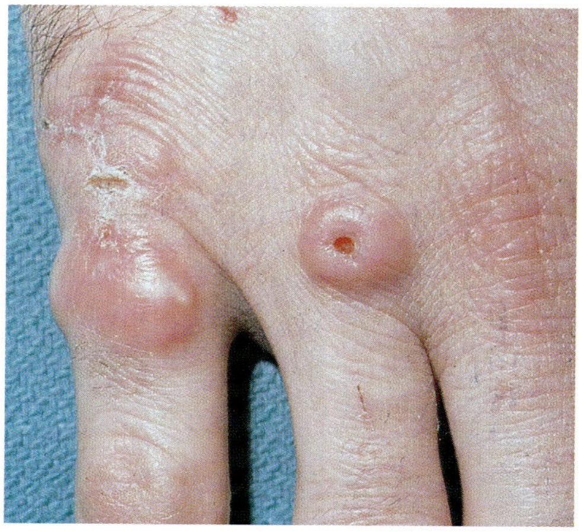

Figure 7.1. Rheumatoid nodules. Subcutaneous, firm, dome-shaped, skin-colored nodules, which usually appear on extensor surface.

Histopathologically, the rheumatoid nodules manifest three characteristic zones. The central zone contains necrotic connective tissue fibers. The middle zone shows palisading granulomas, which are the most striking histopathologic feature of the rheumatoid nodule. The granulomas are surrounded by a third zone of fibrotic tissue reaction containing fibroblasts, plasma cells, and lymphocytes. In 1953, Sokoloff et al. (17) proposed a link between the vasculitis often seen in patients with RA and this palisading granulomatous reaction. Subsequently, many later authors have agreed (18). The presence of rheumatoid factor within rheumatoid nodules suggests the possibility of immune complex–mediated vasculitis as the initiating event in rheumatoid nodule development (18).

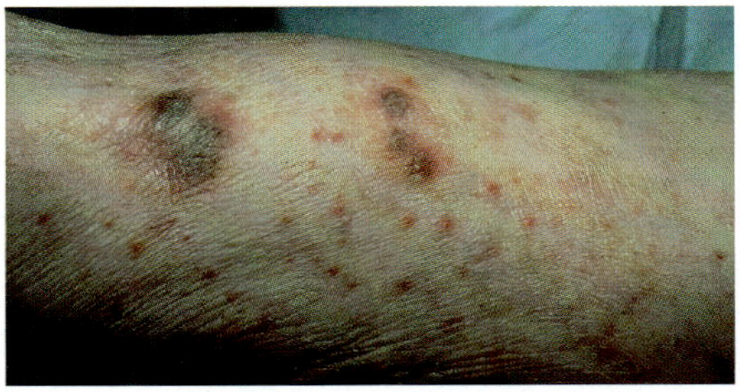

Figure 7.2 Small-vessel necrotizing vasculitis. Palpable purpura, the classic manifestation of small-vessel vasculitis.

Other Palisaded Dermatoses

Patients with RA may have other dermatoses with similar histopathologic findings as the rheumatoid nodule. Rheumatoid papules are erythematous to violaceous papules, occurring most often on the digits of patients with RA. They are clinically similar to granuloma annulare and histopathologically, they are similar to rheumatoid nodules except that the necrobiotic granuloma is located in the superficial dermis, instead of the subcutaneous tissue. Similarly, a strong association between active RA and lesions similar to necrobiosis lipoidica diabeticorum has been noted (19). These lesions, often located on the lower extremities of patients with high-titer rheumatoid factor again represent palisaded granulomas with central degenerated collagen and neutrophilic debris. This is now known as superficial ulcerating rheumatoid necrobiosis (18). Chu et al. (18) suggest a similar etiology for all of these palisaded granulomas in patients with RA: an immune complex–mediated leukocytoclastic vasculitis, leading to degeneration of collagen, resulting in a granulomatous reaction pattern (18).

CUTANEOUS VASCULITIS

Cutaneous vasculitis, a complication seen in approximately 5% to 15% of patients with RA, is associated with positive, often high-titer, rheumatoid factor; advanced erosive disease; and increased patient morbidity and mortality (20). The clinical implication is that the primary joint inflammatory process is poorly controlled. Manifestations are often precipitated by abrupt discontinuation of systemic therapy with resultant rebound circulating immune complex disease. Cutaneous vasculitis can be classified by the size of the largest vessel involved and by the presence or absence of systemic involvement. The severity of the vasculitis cannot be defined by the cutaneous examination alone; a thorough evaluation searching for systemic involvement is essential. Rheumatoid vasculitis can be conceptualized as a spectrum of disease in cutaneous vessels, ranging from severe with multisystem larger vessel vasculitis, to moderate with cutaneous small-vessel and possibly systemic small-vessel vasculitis, and mild with Bywaters lesions only.

Severe rheumatoid vasculitis results from a systemic arteritis of small to medium arteries. Histologically, this is a leukocytoclastic vasculitis with endothelial swelling, polymorphonuclear leukocyte invasion of vessel walls with necrosis, leukocytoclasis, and extravasation of red blood cells. Peripheral neuropathy presenting as mononeuritis, mononeuritis multiplex, or distal symmetric neuropathy may be the first sign (21). Neuropathy is thought to result from vasculitis of the vaso nervorum. Gangrene of the digits, nailfold thromboses and infarcts, and deep cutaneous ulcers can also be seen. Less common manifestations of this larger vessel vasculitis include ischemic bowel disease, cerebral vasculitis, pulmonary vasculitis, and vasculitic glomerulonephritis (21).

Moderate rheumatoid vasculitis results from limited small-vessel vasculitis involving the postcapillary venules. Histopathologically it is also a leukocytoclastic vasculitis. Patients most often present with cutaneous lesions, most characteristically, palpable purpura, on dependent sites (Fig 7.2). Cutaneous small-vessel vasculitis can be seen in many disease states and can be caused by infection, drugs, foreign protein, or immune complexes (autoimmune diseases). Moderate rheumatoid vasculitis is believed to be an immune complex–mediated vasculitis in patients with high-titer rheumatoid factor that represents IgM (or IgA)/IgG immune complexes. Systemic signs and symptoms likely result from immune complex deposition in multiple organs.

Mild rheumatoid vasculitis describes cutaneous manifestations of RA that occur in the absence of systemic vasculitis, and includes nailfold telangiectasias with thromboses, minute digital ulcerations, digital petechiae, livedo reticularis, and digital pulp papules also known as Bywaters lesions (9). Bywaters lesions are purpuric papules that primarily affect the pulp of the distal digits (Fig. 7.3). Histopathologic examination of these lesions again reveals leukocytoclastic vasculitis. Bywaters lesions differ from rheumatoid nodules in that no palisading granulomatous response is found in histologic specimens (22).

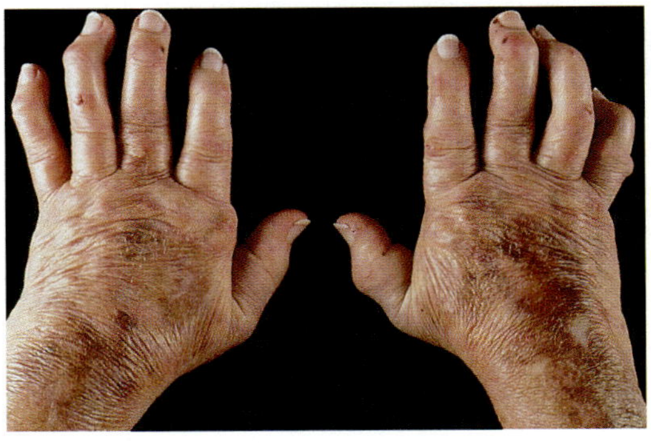

Figure 7.3. Bywaters lesions. Distal digital purpuric papules.

NEUTROPHILIC DERMATOSES

Several neutrophilic dermatoses occur in patients with RA. These include pyoderma gangrenosum, rheumatoid neutrophilic dermatosis, acute febrile neutrophilic dermatosis (Sweet's syndrome), erythema elevatum diutinum, subcorneal pustular dermatitis (Sneddon–Wilkinson's disease) and neutrophilic lobular panniculitis. Sweet's syndrome is a reactive dermatologic disease also associated with other systemic autoimmune diseases, infections, and myelodysplastic malignancies. Its association with RA has been well described (23). Erythema elevatum diutinum, thought to be a chronic plaque form of leukocytoclastic vasculitis, has been noted in patients with severe RA (9,24). Pustular panniculitis in patients with RA has most recently been termed "neutrophilic lobular panniculitis" (25).

Pyoderma Gangrenosum

Pyoderma gangrenosum (PG) is a condition characterized by acute, necrotizing, rapidly expanding cutaneous ulcers (Fig. 7.4). These ulcers may occur on any cutaneous site, yet they most commonly occur on the lower extremities and abdomen. Lesions begin as erythematous papulopustules. They quickly expand to become fluctuant, painful ulcerations with dusky, undermined borders. When lesions heal, they demonstrate a characteristic atrophic "papyraceous" scar. PG can be seen in association with multiple systemic diseases such as Crohn disease, ulcerative colitis, RA, and malignancies, especially hematologic malignancies (26). In patients with RA, the lesions have often been confused with venous stasis ulcers, necrobiosis lipoidica diabeticorum, and bacterial pyoderma. No histologic pattern is pathognomonic for pyoderma gangrenosum and it is ultimately a clinical diagnosis of exclusion. However, histopathologic examination often reveals neutrophils in the dermis with signs of endothelial swelling and deposits of immunoglobulins and/or complement factors in dermal blood (27). (This may be an important finding or an epiphenomenon.) Some authors believe that early lesions represent a neutrophilic vascular reaction (28).

Rheumatoid Neutrophilic Dermatosis

Rheumatoid neutrophilic dermatosis is a rare cutaneous manifestation seen in patients with severe RA. All but one patient reported in the English literature has had a positive rheumatoid factor and all have had severe disease (29). This presents as chronic, erythematous, "urticaria-like" plaques and papules over the extensor surfaces of the extremities and the trunk (29). The lesions are usually nontender, nonscaling, and nonmigratory. They may persist for weeks to months, and ulceration may occur. Histopathologically, a dense neutrophilic infiltrate is seen throughout the dermis without an associated vasculitis (29). It may be difficult to distinguish rheumatoid neutrophilic dermatosis from acute febrile neutrophilic dermatosis (Sweet disease), which also occurs in patients with RA.

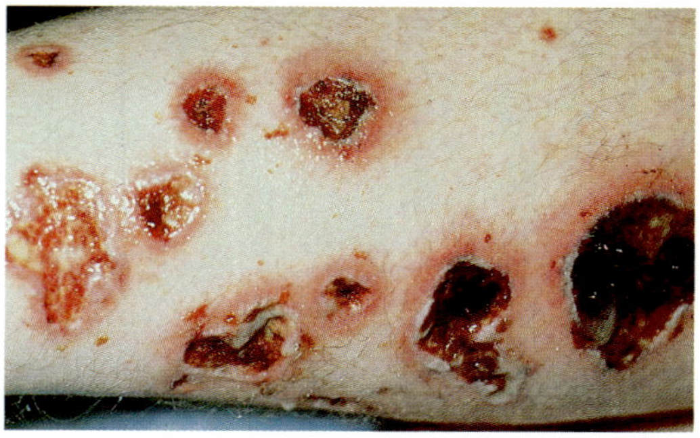

Figure 7.4. Pyoderma gangrenosum. Note undermined border.

LEG ULCERS

Cutaneous ulceration, primarily of the lower extremities, is frequently found in patients with chronic, debilitating disease. Lower extremity ulceration in patients with RA may be due to an associated disease process such as rheumatoid vasculitis or pyoderma gangrenosum, as discussed before. Symmetric lower extremity ulcerations in patients with RA, resembling necrobiosis lipoidica diabeticorum, have been called superficial ulcerating rheumatoid necrobiosis (19). These are now classified with other palisading dermatoses in these patients, as described before. More common causes of lower extremity ulceration should also be considered, such as venous stasis ulcers and "pressure sores." The presence of lower extremity ulcers, granulocytopenia, and splenomegaly in a patient with RA is diagnostic for Felty syndrome.

Felty's Syndrome

Felty's syndrome is the occurrence of RA and granulocytopenia, splenomegaly, and refractory leg ulcers (Fig 7.5). It occurs in less than 1% of all patients with RA (30). Leg ulcers are a common feature of the syndrome and although the pathogenesis has not been well established, it is thought that abnormal immune function may play a role. Patients with Felty's syndrome also develop recurrent, therapy-resistant, cutaneous bacterial infections (30).

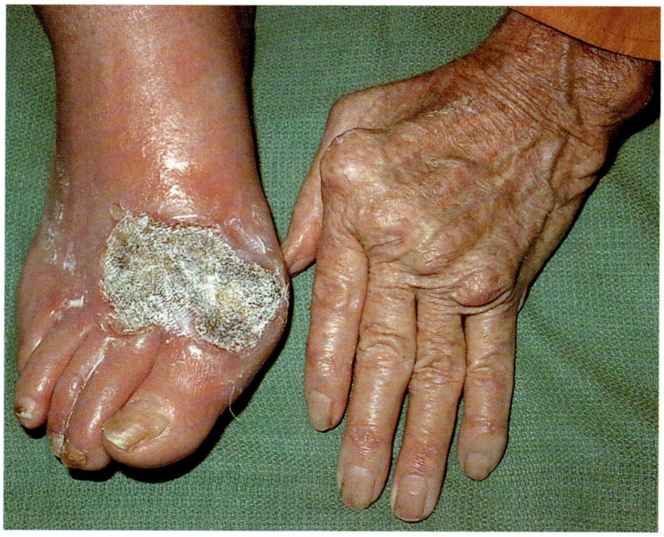

Figure 7.5. Felty's syndrome. Rheumatoid arthritis, granulocytopenia, splenomegaly, and lower extremity ulcers.

CUTANEOUS ATROPHY WITH STELLATE SCARRING

Patients with RA occasionally present with livedo reticularis, a reticulated vasodilatory response that occurs predominantly on the trunk and on entire extremities. The lesions are nonpalpable and often quite subtle (Fig 7.6). The reticulated pattern results from the occlusion of distal vessels that supply the upper skin with a compensatory vasodilation of surrounding vessels. Ulceration and scarring are common. Patients with RA may also have livedoid vasculopathy. Also known as atrophie blanche, these initially purpuric lesions on the lower extremities can progress to infarctive ulcerations and stellate scaring. Their confusion with livedo reticularis has been reviewed (31).

OTHER CONDITIONS OF NOTED INTEREST

Autoimmune bullous diseases have been reported in patients with RA. The most commonly noted association has been with bullous pemphigoid (32). Case reports and series have also been reported regarding patients with RA with cicatricial pemphigoid, pemphigus vulgaris and foliaceous, and dermatitis herpetiformis (9). Patients with lupus erythematosus who develop bullae have been shown to have antibodies to type VII collagen, as with epidermolysis bullosa acquisita (33). Perhaps this may be the case in patients with RA, as well. Epidermolysis bullosa acquisita has been described in patients with RA. There are also reports in the literature of patients with RA with lichen sclerosis et atrophicus, mucinous nodules, and porphyria cutanea tarda (34–36). Yellow nail syndrome, red lunulae, longitudinal ridging of the nails, palmar erythema, and erythromelalgia have also been noted. Patients with RA have a generalized thinning of the skin.

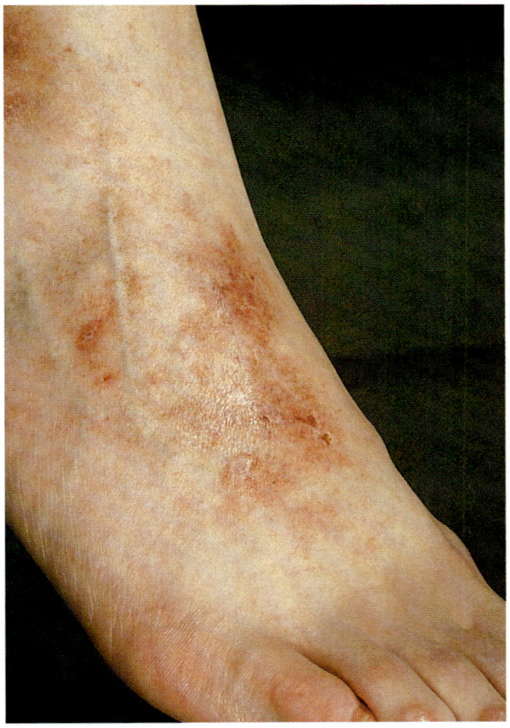

Figure 7.6. Livedo reticularis or atrophie blanche.

It is also important to remember the possibility of cutaneous reactions to medicines used to treat RA. Reaction-pattern dermatoses such as erythema nodosum, urticaria, or erythema multiforme may be seen in patients with RA. These may result as a reaction to the primary disease process or to the medications used to treat it. Overlap syndromes can occur between RA and other connective tissue diseases. In these cases, the patient may present with cutaneous manifestations of the associated connective tissue disease.

REFERENCES

1. Harris ED. Clinical features of rheumatoid arthritis. In Ruddy S, Harris ED Jr, Sledge CB, et al, eds. *Kelley's textbook of rheumatology,* 6th ed. Philadelphia: WB Saunders, 2000:967–1000.
2. Turesson C, Jacobsson L, Bergstrom U. Extra-articular rheumatoid arthritis: prevalence and mortality. *Rheumatology* 1999;38:668–674.
3. Lawrence RC, Helmick CG, Arnett FC, et al. Estimates of the prevalence of arthritis and selected musculoskeletal disorders in the United States. *Arthritis Rheum* 1998;41:778–799.
4. Seymour HE, Worsley A, Smith JM, et al. Anti-TNF agents for rheumatoid arthritis. *Br J Clin Pharmacol* 2001;51:201–208.
5. Maini RN, Zvaifler N. Rheumatoid arthritis and other synovial disorders. In: Klippel JH, Dieppe PA, eds. *Rheumatology,* 2nd ed. Philadelphia: Mosby, 1998: 5.1–5.3.
6. Winchester R, Dwyer E, Rose S. The genetic basis of rheumatoid arthritis. *Rheum Dis Clin North Am* 1992;18:761–783.
7. Ollier W, Thomson W. Population genetics of rheumatoid arthritis. *Rheum Dis Clin North Am* 1992;18:741–759.
8. McInnes IB. Rheumatoid arthritis: from bench to bedside. *Rheum Dis Clin North Am* 2001;27:373–387.
9. Jorizzo JL, Daniels JC. Dermatologic conditions reported in patients with rheumatoid arthritis. *J Am Acad Dermatol* 1983;8:439–457.
10. Meyer O, Combe B, Elias A, et al. Autoantibodies predicting the outcome of rheumatoid arthritis: evaluation in two subsets of patients according to severity of radiographic damage. *Ann Rheum Dis* 1997;56:682–685.
11. Arnett FC, Edworthy SM, Bloch DA, et al. The American Rheumatism Association 1987 revised criteria for the classification of rheumatoid arthritis. *Arthritis Rheum* 1988;31:315–324.
12. Kalden, JR. How do the biologics fit into the current DMARD armamentarium? *J Rheumatol* 2001;62[Suppl]:27–35.
13. Toshiyuki Y, Ohkubo H, Nishioka K. Skin manifestations associated with rheumatoid arthritis. *J Dermatol* 1995;22:324–329.
14. Laloux L, Chevalier X, Maitre B, et al. Unusual onset of rheumatoid arthritis with diffuse pulmonary nodulosis: a diagnostic problem. *J Rheumatol* 1999;26: 920–922.
15. Woo P, Mendelsohn J, Humphrey D. Rheumatoid nodules of the larynx. *Otolaryngol Head Neck Surg* 1995;113:147–150.
16. Abbas A, Byrd BF III. Right-sided heart failure due to right ventricular cavity obliteration by rheumatoid nodules. *Am J Cardiol* 2000;86:711–712.
17. Sokoloff L, McCluskey RT, Bunim JJ. Vascularity of the early subcutaneous nodule of rheumatoid arthritis. *AMA Arch Pathol* 1953;55:475–495.
18. Chu P, Connolly MK, LeBoit PE. The histopathologic spectrum of palisaded neutrophilic granulomatous dermatitis in patients with collagen vascular disease. *Arch Dermatol* 1994:130:1278–1283.
19. Jorizzo JL, Alansky AJ, Stanley RJ. Superficial ulcerating necrobiosis in rheumatoid arthritis: a variant of the necrobiosis lipoidica-rheumatoid nodule spectrum. *Arch Dermatol* 1982;118:255–259.
20. Voskuyl AE, Wsinderman AH, Westedt ML, et al. Factors associated with the development of vasculitis in rheumatoid arthritis: results of a case-control study. *Ann Rheum Dis* 1996;55:190–192.
21. Danning CL, Illei GG, Boumpas DT. Vasculitis associated with primary rheumatologic diseases. *Curr Opin Rheumatol* 1998;10:58–65.
22. Craig SD, Jorizzo JL, White WL, et al. Cutaneous signs of rheumatic disease: acral purpuric papules in a patient with clinical rheumatoid arthritis. *Arthritis Rheum* 1994;37:957–959.
23. Gay-Crosier F, Dayer JM, Chavaz P, et al. Rheumatoid neutrophilic dermatitis/Sweet's syndrome in a patient with seronegative rheumatoid arthritis. *Dermatology* 2000;201:185–187.
24. Balbir-Furman A, Schapira D, Bergman R, et al. Erythema elevatum diutinum—a rare cause of nodulosis in a patient with rheumatoid arthritis. *J Rheumatol* 2000;27:2291–2293.
25. Tran TA, Dupree M, Carlson A. Neutrophilic lobular (pustular) panniculitis associated with rheumatoid arthritis. *Am J Dermatopathol* 1999;21:247–252.

26. Bennett ML, Jackson JM, Jorizzo JL, et al. Pyoderma gangrenosum: a comparison of typical and atypical forms with an emphasis on time to remission—case review of 86 patients from 2 institutions. *Medicine* 2000;79:37–46.
27. von den Driesch P. Pyoderma gangrenosum: a report of 44 cases with follow-up. *Br J Dermatol* 1997;137:1000–1005.
28. Jorizzo JL, Solomon AR, Zanolli MD, et al. Neutrophilic vascular reactions. *J Am Acad Dermatol* 1988;19:983–1005.
29. Brown TS, Fearneyhough PK, Burruss JB, et al. Rheumatoid neutrophilic dermatitis in a woman with seronegative rheumatoid arthritis. *J Am Acad Dermatol* 2001;45:596–600.
30. Rosenstein ED, Kramer N. Felty's and pseudo-Felty's syndromes. *Semin Arthritis Rheum* 1991:21:129–142.
31. Milstone LM, Braverman IM. PURPLE (oops! Atrophie blanche) revisited. *Arch Dermatol* 1998:134:1634.
32. Taylor G, Venning V, Wojnarowska F, et al. Bullous pemphigoid and autoimmunity. *J Am Acad Dermatol* 1993;29:181–184.
33. Chan LS, Lapiere JC, Chen M, et al. Bullous systemic lupus erythematosus with autoantibodies recognizing multiple skin basement membrane components, bullous pemphigoid antigen 1, laminin-5, laminin-6, and type VII collagen. *Arch Dermatol* 1999;135:569–573.
34. Albornoz MA, Greenblatt JM, Myers AR. The development of rheumatoid arthritis in a patient with lichen sclerosus et atrophicus [letter]. *Int J Dermatol* 1999;38:238–239.
35. Nihei Y. Cutaneous mucinous nodules associated with proliferating synovitis of rheumatoid arthritis. *J Dermatol* 1999;26:229–235.
36. Chalem P, Ghnassia AM, Nordmann Y, et al. Porphyria cutanea tarda affecting a rheumatoid arthritis patient treated with methotrexate: association or coincidence? *Rheumatology* 1999;38:453–456.

CHAPTER 8

Primary Systemic Vasculitis

Warren W. Piette

PRIMARY SYSTEMIC VASCULITIS: GENERAL CONSIDERATIONS

Classification of Vasculitis with Historic Perspective

Vasculitis is most simply defined as a syndrome of vessel-directed inflammatory injury, regardless of the size of the vessel or type of inflammation (1–4). Traditionally, cutaneous syndromes are not considered vasculitic despite lesions of palpable purpura when the vessel-directed inflammation is composed primarily of mononuclear cells [e.g., pityriasis lichenoides et varioliformis acuta (PLEVA), erythema multiforme] (5). Conversely, vasculitis has been ascribed to some syndromes that often show little inflammation (e.g., livedoid vasculitis) but prominent intravascular fibrin. More important, syndromes of straightforward cutaneous microvascular occlusion are all too often considered as variants of vasculitis in discussions or reviews of vasculitic syndromes.

The evolution of currently recognized syndromes began in 1837. Many classifications for vasculitis have been proposed, focusing mostly on systemic vasculitides that may or may not involve the skin (1–4,6–12). Despite these classifications, terms such as "hypersensitivity vasculitis," "polyarteritis nodosa" (PAN), or "Henoch–Schönlein purpura" (HSP) do not have universally accepted definitions. Zeek (6) originally used the term "hypersensitivity vasculitis" to refer to patients with disseminated necrotizing lesions affecting small arteries and often the glomeruli. The term "hypersensitivity vasculitis" has since been used for conditions in which skin involvement dominates the clinical picture and in which evidence of serious visceral involvement is rare; some criteria exclude this diagnosis if any extracutaneous involvement is found (12–14). The term "polyarteritis" has been used in naming at least five clinically distinct syndromes, some of which are followed primarily by pediatricians, others by rheumatologists, and still others by dermatologists. Each group of physicians may be unfamiliar with syndromes outside their usual patient population. In addition, no current working classification adequately addresses the palette of vasculitic syndromes that may affect the skin, with or without systemic involvement. Two of the more recent classifications include the American College of Rheumatology (ACR) and the Chapel Hill Consensus Group classifications (CHCG) (10,12,13). There is a low rate of concordance for diagnosis when cases are classified by both the ACR and CHCG classification schemes (15). This may relate in part to differences in intent for the designing the two classifications. Classifying a disease is different from defining the essential elements underlying conditions such as Wegner's granulomatosis (WG) and Giant cell arteritis (GCA). Unlike the ACR classification, the CHCG did not aim to provide surrogate clinical or laboratory correlates for such essential elements. Table 8.1 compares the ACR and CHCG classifications, lists an alternative classification that attempts to address some of the problems with these classifications as they relate to vasculitis in the skin, and lists the usual presentation of these vasculitides in the skin.

A major difficulty with all classification systems is that primary vasculitic syndromes are primary only by exclusion. Vasculitis associated with rheumatoid arthritis, systemic lupus erythematosus (SLE), and similar rheumatic diseases have been included within the term "rheumatic vasculitis." A variety of medications, infections, and underlying diseases can also lead to secondary vasculitides. Vasculitic lesions in patients with secondary vasculitis are in most instances clinically identical to lesions caused by the "primary" vasculitides involving the same size vessels (8,16). Obviously, the prognosis and treatment of a vasculitic syndrome might be significantly altered by the finding of an underlying condition such as inflammatory bowel disease, malignancy, or a treatable infection. For example, HSP syndrome triggered by a particular medication might have the same acute risks for extracutaneous involvement and severe cutaneous disease as an idiopathic syndrome of predominant IgA vasculitis. However, the long-term prognosis, including the risk of renal insufficiency, would be very different, assuming the patient never again received the offending medication. Another overlap with respect to primary and secondary vasculitic syndromes is the role of hepatitis viruses in certain vasculitides. Hepatitis B infection has been associated with cutaneous vasculitis, glomerulonephritis, cryoglobulinemic vasculitis, and PAN, and hepatitis C is now thought to account for most cases of mixed essential cryoglobulinemia. Despite this, classifications of primary systemic vasculitides include mixed essential cryoglobulinemia and PAN as primary syndromes, without distinguishing between idiopathic and viral-associated syndromes.

Epidemiology

Vasculitic syndromes are uncommon but not rare. The incidence rates of primary systemic vasculitides were 115 and more than 439 per million adult population in two European countries. Secondary systemic vasculitis in one of these countries was estimated at 26.5 per million (17). Prospective population-

TABLE 8.1. Vasculitis Classifications

ACR Criteria	CHCC		Comments	Proposed Classification: by Major Pathogenic or Identifying Feature	Usual Cutaneous Presentation
Hypersensitivity vasculitis. 3 of 5 criteria: age at disease onset >16 y; medication at disease onset; palpable purpura; maculopapular rash; biopsy including arteriole and venule, with granulocytes in peri- or extravascular location.	Cutaneous leukocytoclastic angiitis	Isolated cutaneous leukocytoclastic angiitis without systemic vasculitis or glomerulonephritis	ACR: Uses age and medication as criteria for classification; maculopapular rash is nonspecific descriptor. CHCC; No requirement for immune complex, no allowance for even minor extracutaneous involvement.	IgG/IgM immune complex, small-vessel leukocytoclastic vasculitis *Exclude* cryoglobulinemia, rheumatic vasculitides *Distinguish* between idiopathic and syndromes secondary to drug, infection, or malignancy	Palpable purpura on legs, with density of lesions increasing toward most dependent area of legs. Sometimes have a serum sickness–like presentation, with urticaria, fever, arthralgias. Lesions in SBE most often localized on upper extremities, may be cryoglobulin and RF +.
Henoch–Schönlein purpura. 2 of 4 criteria: palpable purpura; age ≤20 at disease onset; bowel angina; wall granulocytes on biopsy of arterioles or venules	Henoch–Schönlein purpura (HSP)	IgA-dominant immune deposits affecting small vessels, typically involves skin, gut, and glomeruli; associated with arthralgia or arthritis	ACR: Uses age and bowel angina as criteria, which bias toward diagnosis in children. Does not require presence of IgA, and syndrome in adults can be mimicked by many other vasculitides. CHCC: Does not exclude IgA-rich variants of cryoglobulinemia or rheumatic vasculitis.	IgA immune complex (HSP) small-vessel leukocytoclastic vasculitis *Exclude* cryoglobulinemia and rheumatic vasculitides, esp. lupus. *Distinguish* between idiopathic and syndromes secondary to drug, infection, or malignancy.	Palpable purpura on legs, with density of lesions increasing toward most dependent area of legs. May also show retiform palpable purpura, which is more specific. Extracutaneous findings more common than with IgG/IgM complexes. Long-term renal sequelae do not depend on presence of full HSP syndrome. Adults more frequently have limited syndrome, but still have greater risk of recurrent disease, cutaneous necrosis, and extracutaneous disease compared with IgG/IgM-associated disease.
—	—	—	—	Urticarial Vasculitis Normocomplementemic Hypocomplementemic HUVS (see text) Distinguish between idiopathic, food, drug, infection, and lupus-related disease.	Urticaria/angioedema-like lesions last longer than 24 h, usually show leukocytoclastic vasculitis. HUVS has C1q antibody, renal, pulmonary disease. May occur with lupus.
Mixed cryoglobulinemic vasculitis: not addressed in original ACR criteria	Essential cryoglobulinemic vasculitis	Vasculitis with cryoglobulin immune deposits in small vessels; associated with serum cryoglobulins, skin and glomeruli often involved, may manifest as nephritis or pulmonary–renal vasculitic syndrome	—	—	—
Polyarteritis subsets Infantile PAN/Kawasaki disease—not listed in ACR vasculitis criteria. ACR primer suggests using Japanese Kawasaki Research Committee criteria adopted by CDC case definition.	Kawasaki disease	Arteritis involving large, medium, and small arteries, and associated with mucocutaneous lymph node syndrome; coronary arteries are often involved; aorta and veins may be involved; usually occurs in children	— —	Infantile PAN CHCC properly describes involvement; Japanese Kawasaki Research Committee guidelines as adopted by CDC are best diagnostic criteria.	Skin lesions in this syndrome are . not vasculitic. Mucocutaneous findings in criteria: polymorphous rash; injection of conjunctiva, oral or pharyngeal mucosa; erythema, fissuring of lips; strawberry tongue; erythema or edema of hands/feet; membranous desquamation of fingertips.

PAN requires 3 of 10 criteria: Wt loss ≥4 kg; livedo reticularis; testicular pain or tenderness; myalgias, weakness, leg tenderness; mono- or polyneuropathy; diastolic BP >90; Elevated BUN or creatinine level; HBV; arteriographic abnormality (defined); biopsy of small or medium artery containing PMN	PAN	Necrotizing inflammation of medium or small arteries without glomerulonephritis or vasculitis in arterioles, capillaries, or venules	ACR: HBV is one of criteria. Definition would include benign cutaneous PAN subsets CHCC: Does not distinguish HBV and non-HBV syndromes.	CHCC classification. Suggest that HBV status be appended to diagnosis, because of potential to affect therapy and prognosis.	There are no vessels in the skin of the size that are affected by this syndrome. There are two cutaneous findings that have been reported: palpation of arterial aneurysm (i.e., radial artery at wrist), and digital necrosis due to digital artery lesions.
No ACR category for benign cutaneous PAN	No CHCC category for benign cutaneous PAN		Benign cutaneous PAN involves smaller vessels than classical PAN, but in size range of MPA. However, benign cutaneous PAN should be ANCA-negative and extracutaneous findings are limited to those listed in last column	Benign cutaneous PAN involves arterioles, capillaries, or venules, ANCA-negative. Occasional cases are HCV associated, and this should be appended to diagnosis.	Localized livedo reticularis, tender nodules or ulcers, usually on legs. May have fever, myalgia, myositis, arthritis, arthralgias, especially legs. ANCA-negative.
—	—	—	As above.	Childhood BCPAN. Same as adult form, except HCV association not reported. ANCA-negative.	Findings same or similar to adult form, but extracutaneous findings perhaps more common. Neonatal cases reported in infants born to affected mother.
No ACR category to distinguish microscopic polyangiitis.	Microscopic polyangiitis	Necrotizing vasculitis. With few or no immune deposits affecting small vessels; may also involve small and medium arteries; necrotizing glomerulonephritis very common, pulmonary capillaritis often occurs	—	Microscopic polyangiitis: CHCC classification. Expect ANCA positivity.	Palpable purpura or retiform palpable purpura lesions that are not distributed in a gravity-dependent fashion.
Wenger granulomatosis 2 of 4 criteria: nasal or oral inflammation; abnormal chest radiograph; urinary sediment (RBC casts or >5 RBC/HPF); granulomatous inflammation on biopsy	Wegener granulomatosis	Granulomatous inflammation involving the respiratory tract, and necrotizing vasculitis affecting small to medium vessels; necrotizing glomerulonephritis is common	—	Wegener granulomatosis. CHCC classification describes involvement, ACR criteria useful in diagnosis. ANCA positive in most cases, but less so in limited cases.	Palpable purpura or retiform palpable purpura lesions which are not distributed in a gravity dependent fashion. Skin lesions show leukocytoclastic vasculitis without granuloma.
Churg–Strauss syndrome 4 of 6 criteria: asthma; eosinophilia (>10% WBC); mono- or polyneuropathy; pulmonary infiltrates, nonfixed; paranasal sinus abnormality; extravascular eosinophils	Churg–Strauss syndrome	Eosinophil-rich and granulomatous inflammation of respiratory tract and necrotizing vasculitis affecting small to medium vessels and associated with asthma and blood eosinophils	—	Churg–Strauss syndrome. CHCC classification describes involvement, ACR criteria useful in diagnosis.	Palpable purpura 45%, maculopapular rash 40%, subcutaneous nodules 20%.

(continued)

TABLE 8.1. *(continued)*

ACR Criteria	CHCC		Comments	Proposed Classification: by Major Pathogenic or Identifying Feature	Usual Cutaneous Presentation
Giant cell arteritis 3 of 5 criteria: age at disease onset >50 y; new headache; temporal artery abnormality; elevated erythrocyte sedimentation rate; abnormal artery biopsy	Giant cell (temporal) arteritis	Granulomatous arteritis of the aorta and its major branches, with a predilection for the extracranial branches of the carotid artery; often involves the temporal artery, usually occurs in patients older than 50 y and often is associated with polymyalgia rheumatica	—	Giant cell arteritis. CHCC classification describes involvement, ACR criteria useful in diagnosis.	Rarely involves skin. Visible or palpable temporal arteries or scalp tenderness most common. Gangrene of scalp or tongue rare.
Takayasu arteritis 3 of 6 criteria: age at disease onset ≤40 y; claudication of extremities; decreased brachial artery pulse; BP difference >10 mm; bruit over subclavian arteries or aorta; arteriogram abnormality	Takayasu arteritis	Granulomatous inflammation of the aorta and its major branches; usually occurs in patients younger than 50 y	Skin involvement rare	CHCC describes involvement; ACR useful for diagnosis	Erythema nodosum–like lesions, pyoderma gangrenosum–like lesions, panniculitis-like lesions, purpura, necrotic or ulcerated nodules

ACR, American College of Rheumatology; CHCC, Chapel Hill Consensus Group Classification; SBE, subacute bacterial endocarditis; HUVS, hypocomplementemic urticarial vasculitis syndrome; PAN, polyarteritis nodosa; CDC, Centers for Disease Control and Prevention; BUN, blood urea nitrogen; HBV, hepatitis B virus; PMN, polymorphonuclear leukocyte; ANCA, antineutrophil cytoplasmic antibodies; HCV, hepatitis C virus; RBC, red blood cell; HPF, high-power field; WBC, white blood cell; BP, blood pressure.

TABLE 8.2. Comparative Incidence of Vasculitis Presenting to Rheumatologists and Dermatologists

Disease	Presenting to Rheumatologist *N* = 1,000	Presenting to Dermatologist *N* = 101
Polyarteritis nodosa	12%	7%
Churg–Strauss	2%	2%
Wegener granulomatosis	8.5%	3%
Hypersensitivity vasculitis	9%	38%
		16% Idiopathic
		13% Drug-associated
		9% Infection-associated
Henoch–Schönlein	8.5%	4%
Giant cell (temporal) arteritis	21%	—
Takayasu	6%	—
Kawasaki, rheumatic vasculitides	21%	21% rheumatic, no Kawasaki
Other (urticarial, cryoglobulin, etc.)	13%	27%
		10% Urticaria, angioedema
		9% Malignancy-associated
		3% Cryoglobulinemia
		3% Granuloma faciale
		2% Hypergammaglobulinemic purpura

based estimates of incidence and prevalence are few, but such studies should eliminate referral bias and provide an accurate population based denominator. One such study from England found an annual incidence of primary systemic vasculitis of 19.8 per million, with a point prevalence of 144.5 per million (18). Improvement in diagnostic tools may greatly affect epidemiologic data. For example, the reported annual incidence of WG and microscopic polyangiitis in Leicester, United Kingdom, increased from 1.5 per million population to 6.1 per million after antineutrophil cytoplasmic antibodies (ANCA) testing became readily available (17).

Two studies may offer some insight into the incidence of subsets of vasculitis derived from large series of patients. Table 8.2 compares cases over a 5-year period by rheumatologists from 48 centers in the United States, Canada, and Mexico with cases seen by dermatologists at a major referral center (10). Since cutaneous vasculitis is rare in Takayasu arteritis and temporal arteritis, and not seen in Kawasaki disease, these three diagnostic categories should be rare in a dermatologic series. Patients with cutaneous lesions associated with symptomatic systemic disease might be expected to present more often to a rheumatologic practice. Conversely, patients with syndromes that predominantly affect the skin and seldom induce prominent systemic findings would be expected to comprise a much higher percentage of a dermatologic practice. Despite this, the frequencies of WG and Churg–Strauss are not too dissimilar between the two studies and practice types. Also, although the percentage figures for polyarteritis are reasonably close for each group, the population of patients with polyarteritis seen by rheumatologists is likely to be enriched for patients with classic PAN and microscopic polyangiitis, whereas it is likely that the dermatologic group contains mostly patients with benign cutaneous PAN and a few patients presenting with microscopic polyangiitis.

General Cutaneous Morphologic Considerations

Different syndromes of inflammatory injury of cutaneous blood vessels often have very similar morphologic presentations (19). Idiopathic small-vessel vasculitis may present as palpable purpura with a central necrotic pustule, indistinguishable from lesions of septic vasculitis with an immune complex component as seen in gonococcemia. The history and physical findings typically differ in these two settings, however, and the correct diagnosis can often be suspected before a single laboratory test is drawn or biopsy taken. The PLEVA syndrome may also produce lesions of palpable purpura with a necrotic center, but this syndrome is one of primarily mononuclear cell–mediated vessel injury, with a distinctive clinical history and cutaneous distribution, and usual absence of extracutaneous findings.

The morphology at the bedside can suggest simple hemorrhage, inflammatory hemorrhage, or hemorrhage secondary to occlusion or ischemia of the microvasculature. Unfortunately, discussions of vasculitis frequently mix syndromes of inflammatory hemorrhage with syndromes of noninflammatory (bland) occlusion. Beginning the process of distinguishing these syndromes at the bedside is critical to appropriate and efficient evaluation of patients with lesions of purpura and vasculitis (19).

Vasculitic lesions in the skin may present as urticarial papules, palpable purpura, nodules, or ulcers (1,8,11,19–21). The most characteristic presentation is that of palpable purpura (Fig. 8.1). Early lesions of small-vessel vasculitis contain

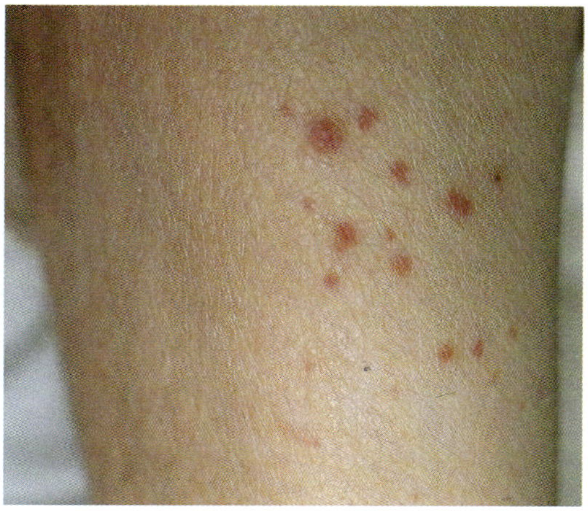

Figure 8.1. Lesion of classic palpable purpura. This lesion should partially blanch.

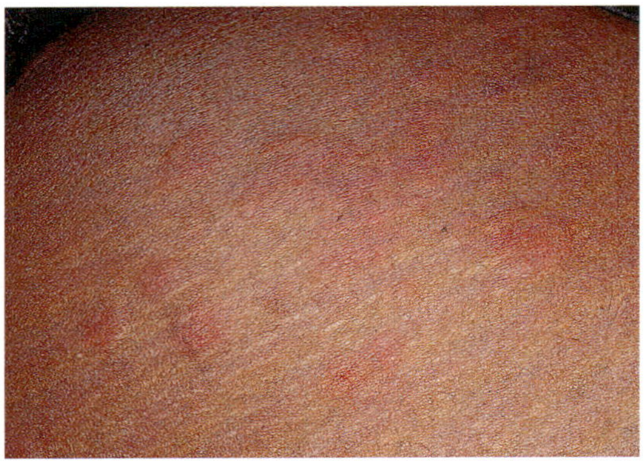

Figure 8.2. Lesions of urticarial vasculitis may have minimal to no purpuric component.

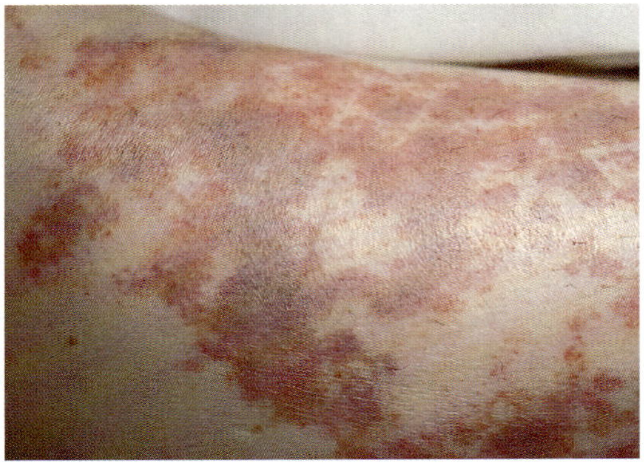

Figure 8.4. Noninflammatory (bland) retiform purpura lesions in a patient with disseminated intravascular coagulation. Biopsy shows microvascular occlusion.

a blanchable component of erythema and a nonblanchable residual component of visible hemorrhage (19). Occasionally, small-vessel vasculitis may present as urticarial lesions, which may or may not have a component of visible hemorrhage. This is the characteristic presentation of urticarial vasculitis (Fig. 8.2). A target or "bulls-eye" lesion consists of a central vesicular, purpuric, or superficial necrotic change, surrounded by a zone of normal-to-slightly pale skin (thought to be secondary to edematous pallor), and surrounded in turn by a zone of completely blanchable erythema (Fig. 8.3). Target lesions strongly suggest the diagnosis of erythema multiforme. This is not a leukocytoclastic vasculitis, but instead a mononuclear cell inflammatory process that may have a component of vessel-directed injury. It can cause not only target lesions, but variants can produce lesions of typical palpable purpura (usually secondary to drug reactions). Both the distribution of lesions (acral and mucosal) and the histology are helpful in recognizing the nontargeted presentation of purpuric erythema multiforme. Inflammatory hemorrhage may be induced by or localized by physical trauma (Köebner or isomorphic phenomenon), leading to linear or geometric patterns of palpable purpura (22).

Syndromes of bland (noninflammatory) microvascular occlusion may also present with palpable purpura. Examples of such syndromes include intravascular gelling of cryoglobulins or cryofibrinogens, microthrombosis occurring in some patients with inherited or acquired protein C or protein S deficiency, purpura fulminans, coumarin necrosis, disseminated intravascular coagulation, antiphospholipid antibody syndrome (lupus anticoagulant), platelet plugging in heparin necrosis or myeloproliferative disease, or embolic occlusion due to cholesterol–arteriosclerotic emboli (11,19). Because these syndromes begin as bland occlusion or thrombosis, an initial erythema is usually lacking (19). However, increased vascular permeability favors local protein-rich edema formation producing palpable lesions, and vessel ischemia or necrosis results in perivascular hemorrhage and intravascular clot propagation. Because these processes extend intravascularly and perivascularly, they frequently show a retiform (reticulate, livedoid, netlike) or branching pattern (Fig. 8.4). Occasionally, only a nonretiform eschar will signal this process (Fig. 8.5).

Whereas inflammation with erythema typically precedes hemorrhage in vasculitic syndromes, early lesions of noninflammatory occlusion most often show little or no erythema. Erythema in inflammatory lesions typically fades over hours to days as the inflammation subsides, accentuating the residual hemorrhage. In contrast, erythema in noninflammatory microvascular occlusion usually develops later, as a response to ischemic injury or necrosis. In this setting, erythema is a sign of a wound healing response. The difference in evolution over time between inflammatory vessel injury and noninflammatory occlusion highlights the importance of determining the age of lesions clinically, since late lesions of bland occlusion with necrosis and a wound healing response may resemble early lesions of inflammatory hemorrhage, both clinically and histologically. A late lesion of inflammatory hemorrhage, which has lost its erythematous component, would also have transitioned histologically from a leukocytoclastic to a chronic nonspecific inflammatory infiltrate (23–25). Absence of erythema is not an invariable finding with cuta-

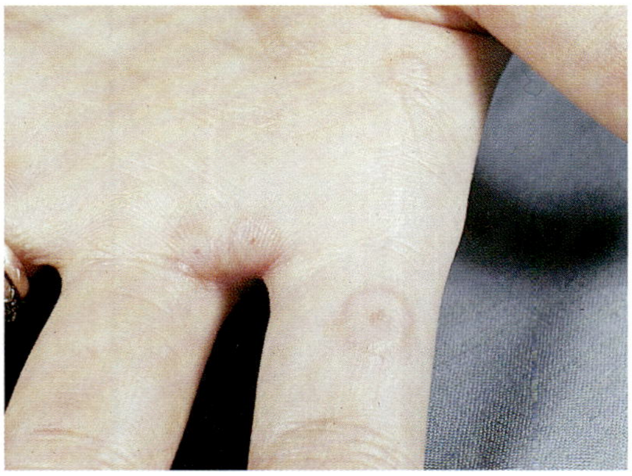

Figure 8.3. Typical target lesion of erythema multiforme.

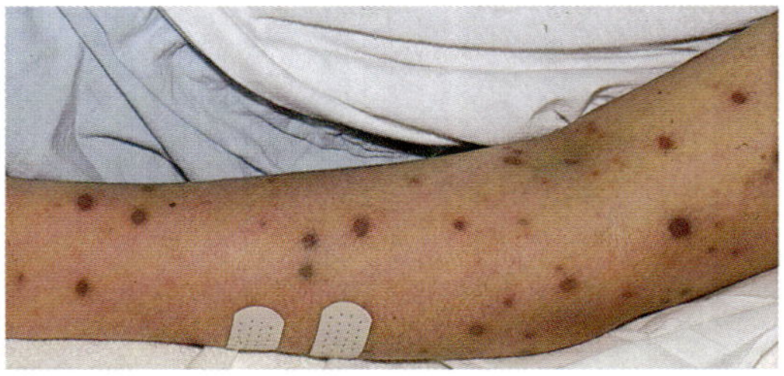

Figure 8.5. Round papules of noninflammatory eschar in an immunosuppressed patient with *Acremonium* sepsis. Biopsy shows fungal elements in and invading through the vessel wall, with surrounding thrombosis.

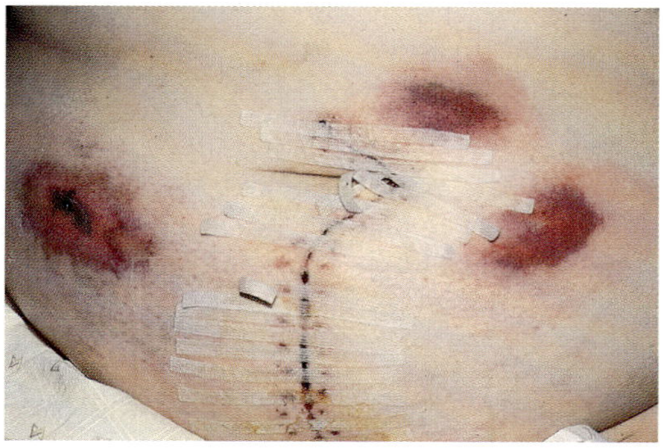

Figure 8.6. Heparin necrosis showing erythema surrounding an area of retiform hemorrhage. Biopsy shows bland occlusion of dermal vessels.

neous occlusion syndromes, however. For example, coumadin or heparin necrosis may frequently show prominent early erythema surrounding the infarctive sites (Fig. 8.6). This erythema may be secondary to initial ischemic injury in the subdermal fat.

Occasionally, lesions show both prominent early erythema and retiform morphology. Syndromes involving small dermal vessels exclusively and manifesting as this inflammatory retiform morphology are usually IgA vasculitis, although IgA vasculitis most often presents as classic palpable purpura only (Fig. 8.7) (26). A similar morphology of inflammatory retiform purpura can occur in vasculitic syndromes that involve a range of vessel sizes in the dermis and sometimes in the fat, as in WG, some polyarteritis subsets, and mixed cryoglobulinemia (Fig. 8.8).

The presence of nodules, large areas of inflammatory necrosis, or larger ulcerations imply injury to vessels usually larger than those found in the dermis (1,8,11,19–21) (Fig. 8.9). The largest cutaneous vessels supplying skin are the small arterioles and venules in the adipose tissue, although these vessels are smaller than the vessels involved in classic PAN syndromes. This means that skin lesions of vasculitis are exclusively small-vessel lesions, although a range of vessel sizes may be involved, and the larger vessels within this size range are frequently termed "medium-sized." The term "small-vessel vasculitis" typically refers to syndromes that primarily affect the dermal vessels, whereas syndromes of mixed-size vessel involvement may also involve the slightly larger vessels in the fat. Inflammatory nodules of vasculitis in deep dermis or fat do not always produce hemorrhage visible at the dermal surface; therefore, the absence of purpura clinically does not exclude

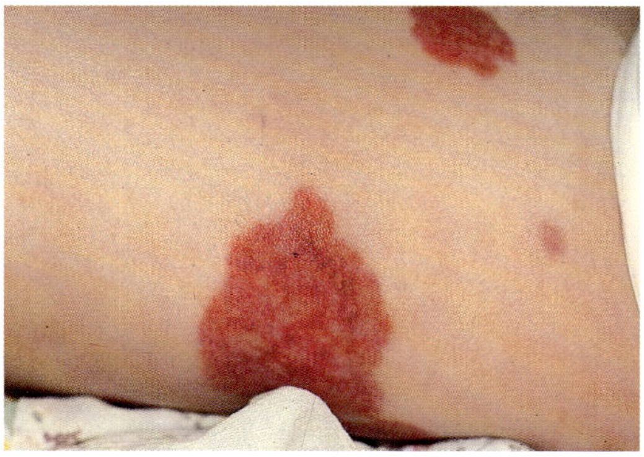

Figure 8.7. Inflammatory retiform purpura in IgA vasculitis.

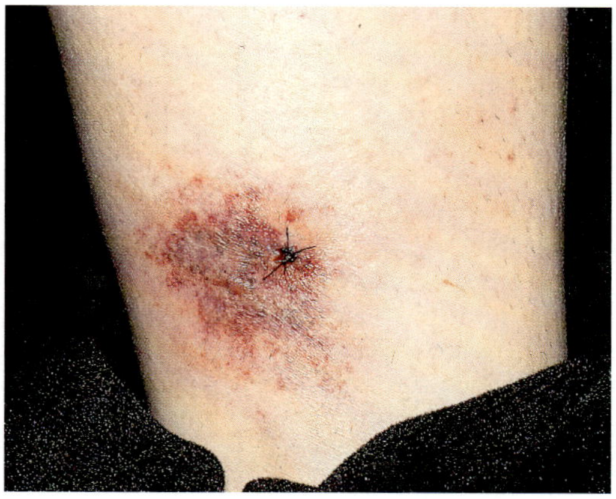

Figure 8.8. Inflammatory retiform purpura in Wegener granulomatosis.

vasculitis. However, other syndromes such as the panniculitides are much more commonly the cause of nonpurpuric inflammatory nodules in the fat.

Pathogenesis of Vasculitis

IMMUNE COMPLEX–TRIGGERED DISEASE

Deposition of circulating immune complexes with subsequent vessel damage has emerged as the major immunopathologic event associated with many of the vasculitic syndromes, especially those producing exclusively small-vessel leukocytoclastic vasculitis. Implicated antigens include proteins (e.g., serum sickness), medications, foods and food additives, infections (e.g., hepatitis B and C, subacute bacterial endocarditis), endogenous antigens (e.g., DNA, rheumatoid factor binding to IgG), presumed tumor antigens in malignancy, and even antigens in fumes from photocopy paper (11,27–30).

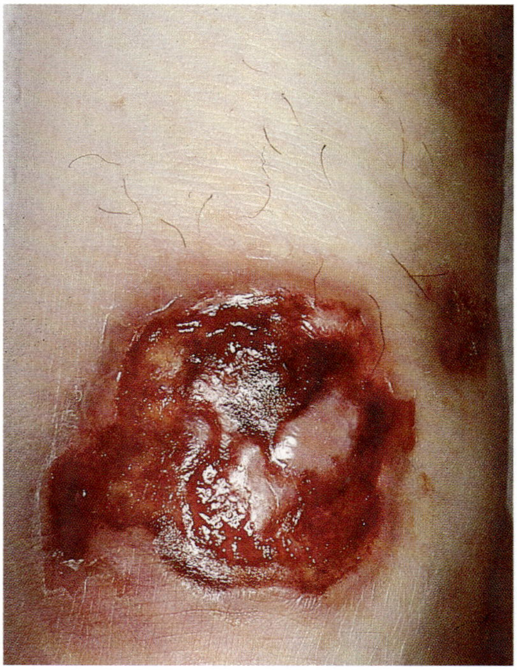

Figure 8.9. Cutaneous ulcer resembling pyoderma gangrenosum on the anterior aspect of the ankle of a patient with Wegener granulomatosis.

The mechanism of tissue damage in immune complex vasculitis is inferred from experimental models and clinical studies in serum sickness syndromes or Arthus reactions (23,31–38). The conventional pathogenesis begins with the formation of soluble immune complexes in antigen excess conditions, which then precipitate or are trapped in blood vessel walls in areas of increased vascular permeability, such as those secondary to inflammation. This increased permeability is attributed to release of vasoactive amines from mast cells under the influence of specific IgE or from platelets. Complement activation follows, and activated complement components (especially C5a) act in part as chemoattractants. Neutrophils infiltrate the vessel wall at the site of immune complex deposition and directly damage the vessel wall. This damage may result in hemorrhage at the site of attack, or in fibrinoid degeneration with compromise of the vascular lumen and downstream ischemic damage to the vessel wall with hemorrhage. The size, charge, and other physical properties of immune complexes, the turbulence of blood flow, the hydrostatic pressure within vessels, the response of the endothelium to injury, and the regional and microenvironmental differences in the properties and reactivities of endothelial cells, as well as previous vascular injury are important variables in the elicitation and subsequent modulation of vasculitis syndromes. Lymphocytes may also play a role through release of cytokines, or through the effects of natural killer or lymphokine-activated killer T-cell activity (33). More recent work has begun to question this immune complex trapping theory, with some evidence suggesting that immune complexes bind through Fc receptors to inflammatory cells with modulation of a local inflammatory response independent of trapped or precipitated complexes (39). Evidence also suggests that the interaction of cytokine production and specific and sequential adhesion molecule expression on endothelial cells and inflammatory cells is central to the induction of cutaneous lesions of leukocytoclastic vasculitis (36–38,40).

OTHER POTENTIAL MECHANISMS

Many other factors affecting the development of vasculitis include genetic predisposition, immunoregulatory mechanisms, cytokine and chemokine effects, the effectiveness of the reticuloendothelial system in clearing immune complexes from the circulation, and the endothelial elaboration of inflammatory mediators and endothelial–platelet and endothelial–leukocyte adhesive interactions (33,34,36–38,40–42).

Lymphocytes may be the prime effectors of injury in some small-vessel vasculitis. Other mechanisms of vasculitis are likely, and may include antibody-mediated endothelial cytotoxicity, delayed hypersensitivity or other cell-mediated forms of inflammation (especially in vascular reactions of transplant rejection syndromes), or the interplay of endothelial cells and antibody-activated neutrophils (38).

Antineutrophil Cytoplasmic Antibodies and Vasculitis. In 1982, Davies et al. (43) described eight patients with arthralgias, myalgias, and focal, segmental crescentic glomerulonephritis without glomerular immune deposits (44). Half of these patients also had dyspnea or hemoptysis. Their sera contained an autoantibody that stained the cytoplasm of neutrophils on indirect immunofluorescent assay. In 1984, Hall et al. (45) suggested that these ANCA might represent a diagnostic test for systemic vasculitis. One year later, van der Woude et al. (46) linked ANCA to WG, an association soon confirmed by others (44). By 1989, a large study from the United States and Europe reported that 90% of patients with active systemic WG were ANCA-positive (47). Patients with active limited WG had a 65% to 70% incidence of ANCA positivity, and patients with WG in remission had a 35% incidence of ANCA positivity. Subsequently, ANCA positivity was reported in PAN, primarily the microscopic PAN subset, and in Churg–Strauss syndrome (44).

In 1988, a second form of ANCA (termed "p-ANCA," for perinuclear) was reported by Jennette and Falk (48) in a group of patients with pauci-immune crescentic glomerulonephritis. This ANCA bound specifically to neutrophil myeloperoxidase, and was the first proof that ANCA activity was directed against lysosomal enzymes of neutrophils and monocytes. A third ANCA pattern, designated atypical ANCA, was reported in 1992 (44,49).

The localization of ANCA staining in formalin-fixed neutrophils is always cytoplasmic, indicating that cytoplasmic antigens are the targets. However, ANCA staining used ethanol- or acetone-fixed neutrophils allows translocation of some of the antigens, accounting for the perinuclear pattern of staining seen in both the p-ANCA and the "very perinuclear" pattern seen with the atypical ANCA (44,50). The antigens that are the target of c-ANCA are proteinase 3 (85% to 90%), and cationic antimicrobial protein 57 and other antigens (10% to 15%). p-ANCA usually binds to myeloperoxidase (90%) and uncommonly to cathepsin G, elastase, lactoferrin, and other granule enzymes (10%). The antigen specificity for patients with ANCA-positive vasculitis varies by syndrome (Tables 8.3 and 8.4).

ANCA testing is done both by immunofluorescence (IIF) and by enzyme-linked immunosorbent assay (ELISA) methods, and each method has its role. An international consensus statement on ANCA testing recognizes four ANCA patterns by IIF staining: c-ANCA, c-ANCA (atypical), p-ANCA, and atypical ANCA (see Table 8.4) (50).

TABLE 8.3. Vasculitis and Nephritis Associations of Antineutrophil Cytoplasmic Antibodies (ANCA)

Disease	Anti-PR-3[a] (%)	Anti-MPO[a] (%)	Other Antigen (%)	Negative ANCA (%)
Wegener granulomatosis	80–85	10	5–10	—
Microscopic polyangiitis	45	45	5–10	—
Churg–Strauss syndrome	10	70	—	20
Classic polyarteritis nodosa	10	20	—	70
Overlap vasculitis	40	20	40	—
Pauci-immune-crescentic glomerulonephritis	30	65	5	

From Goeken JA. Antineutrophil cytoplasmic and anti-endothelial cell antibodies: new mechanisms for vasculitis. *Curr Opin Dermatol* 1995;2:75–82, with permission.
[a]Anti-PR-3 is a C-ANCA pattern; anti-MPO is a P-ANCA pattern.

TABLE 8.4. Immunofluorescence ANCA Patterns, Antigen Specificities, and Disease Associations (see also Table 7.3)[a]

There are four ANCA patterns distinguished by IIF testing, with subsets determined by ELISA antigen specificity:

C-ANCA: classic granular cytoplasmic fluorescence with central or interlobular accentuation.
C-ANCA occur in at least 70% of patients with active generalized WG, less frequently in patients with limited (nonrenal) disease, and in 30% of patients with MPA. Almost all of these are PR3-ANCA.

C-ANCA (atypical): diffuse flat cytoplasmic fluorescence without interlobular accentuation.
C-ANCA (atypical) accounts for about half the cytoplasmic fluorescence patterns on routine ANCA screening. In this pattern the corresponding antigen is not the expected PR3 with C-ANCA, but instead is MPO, bactericidal/permeability-increasing protein, or unknown (majority).
C-ANCA (atypical) has no clinical significance.

P-ANCA: pattern shows perinuclear fluorescence, with or without nuclear extension and includes granulocyte-specific ANA staining.
P-ANCA with MPO specificity occur in 50%–80% of patients with active MPA (including renal only) and up to 25% of patients with WG.
P-ANCA (usually non-MPO specificity) occur in 50%–70% of patients with ulcerative colitis, 20%–40% of patients with Crohn disease, 80% of patients with chronic active hepatitis, 25%–35% of patients with rheumatoid arthritis, and about 20% of patients with systemic lupus erythematosus[c], and in other autoimmune diseases. In these patients, ANCA levels are often low and of uncertain clinical significance.
Most neutrophil fluorescence patterns detected on routine laboratory screening are not found in patients with primary small-vessel vasculitides[c]. The most common IIF pattern is a P-ANCA that lacks the nuclear fluorescence seen in most MPO-related ANCA.

Atypical ANCA: distinct from C-ANCA (atypical), includes all other neutrophil-specific or monocyte-specific IIF reactivity, and most commonly stains both cytoplasmic and perinuclear areas.
Antigen specificities for P-ANCA and atypical ANCA (formerly U-ANCA) include α-enolase, catalase, high-mobility-group nonhistone chromosomal proteins, actin, cathepsin G, elastase, lactoferrin, lysozyme, and other unknown targets.
Atypical ANCA occur in patients with inflammatory bowel disease, rheumatoid arthritis, and some types of drug-induced vasculitis. All forms of P-ANCA and atypical ANCA fluorescence occur only with ethanol- and acetone-fixed neutrophils; formalin-fixed cells stained with the same sera would give C-ANCA–type staining.

ANCA, antineutrophil cytoplasmic antibodies; ELISA, enzyme-linked immunosorbent assay; WG, Wegener granulomatosis; IIF, immunofluorescence; ANA, antinuclear antibody.

In WG and MPA, ANCA levels usually decline with treatment, but increase in about 50% of patients with relapse[c]. IIF testing should be performed on all patients suspected of having WG or MPA, since 10% of WG or MPA patients will be positive only on IIF, and negative on ELISA.[c] Most patients with active WG have C-ANCA with PR3 specificity, varying from 60% in patients with localized disease to 96% in patients with generalized disease[b]. However, up to 25% of patients with active generalized WG have been reported to have P-ANCA staining with MPO specificity.[c]

About 60% of patients with MPA or pauciimmune segmental necrotizing glomerulonephritis have P-ANCA with MPO specificity, and 30% have C-ANCA with PR3 specificity. ANCA are less common in patients with Churg–Strauss syndrome, and the patterns and specificities resemble those found in MPA.[c]

[a]From Hagen E, Daha M, Hermans J, et al. The diagnostic value of standardized assays for ANCA in idiopathic systemic vasculitis: results of an international collaborative study. *Kidney Int* 1998;53:743–753, with permission.

[b]From Mohan N, Kerr G. Diagnosis of vasculitis. *Best Pract Research Clin Rheumatol* 2001;15:203–223, with permission.

[c]From Savige J, Gillis D, Benson E, et al. International consensus statement on testing and reporting of antineutrophil cytoplasmic antibodies (ANCA). *Am J Clin Pathol* 1999;111:507–513, with permission.

Disease Associations of Antineutrophil Cytoplasmic Antibodies. Many different diseases have been associated with positive ANCA testing (see Tables 8.3 and 8.4)(44,49–55). The c-ANCA pattern predominates in WG, but is not specific.

In patients with new-onset WG, microscopic polyangiitis, and idiopathic pauci-immune necrotizing glomerulonephritis, a prospective study found a sensitivity of 85% for IIF, and 81% for ELISA (54). The specificity of c-ANCA (IIF) was 95%, but that of p-ANCA (IIF) was only 81%. Using IIF and ELISA together improved the specificity of both assays to 99%, but decreased the sensitivity to 67% to 82%, depending on the diagnosis (54,55).

For diagnostic purposes, IIF is an appropriate screening test for ANCA, but a positive IIF test should always be confirmed by an antigen-specific ELISA at least for anti-PR3 and anti-MPO (55). A p-ANCA (IIF) without an ELISA has a low specificity for systemic vasculitis.

Pathogenic Role for Antineutrophil Cytoplasmic Antibodies. Whether ANCA contribute to the development of vasculitis, or are merely a marker of systemic vasculitis is not clear, but a plausible scenario for their role is becoming increasingly likely (56). Infection has long been implicated in the onset or exacerbation of WG. A possible pathogenic role begins with infection-related leukocyte stimulation with cytokine release, including interleukin-1 and tumor necrosis factor-α (TNF-α). During periods of active vasculitis, elevated levels of TNF can be detected in serum and at sites of vasculitis. Activation of neutrophils and monocytes by these cytokines induces lysosomal movement toward the cell membrane, making ANCA antigens, especially PR3 or MPO, accessible to circulating antibodies. Experimentally, on binding to the leukocyte cell membrane, the ANCA antibody can induce a respiratory burst and degranulation. If this occurs *in vivo*, endothelial damage would be an expected consequence. Binding of primed neutrophils to endothelium occurs via α_2 integrins and up-regulated intercellular adhesion molecule-1 (ICAM-1) and vascular cell adhesion molecule-1 (VCAM-1). Primed neutrophils interacting with ANCA become fully activated, undergo respiratory burst activity, and the free radicals and enzymes released lead to endothelial cell death and vascular injury. This model has been partly confirmed in a mouse model (57).

PR3-ANCAs can also act by interfering with the interaction between PR3 and its natural inhibitor, α_1-antitrypsin, prolonging the enzymatic activity of PR3 and possibly increasing vascular injury (58). Similarly, MPO-ANCAs may interfere with binding of MPO with its natural inhibitor, ceruloplasmin.

Antiendothelial Cell Antibodies. Antiendothelial cell antibodies have been reported in many different diseases, including WG, microscopic PAN, Kawasaki disease, Takayasu arteritis, SLE, dermatomyositis, systemic sclerosis, Behçet disease, HLA-matched graft rejection, IgA nephropathy, hemolytic-uremic syndrome, thrombotic thrombocytopenic purpura, and preeclampsia (38,59). Some antiendothelial cell antibodies recognize cytokine-inducible molecules (e.g., in Kawasaki disease), whereas others recognize constitutive endothelial cell antigens (e.g., in WG and microscopic polyangiitis) (38). Because antiendothelial cells have been reported in such a wide spectrum of diseases, it is unclear when their presence is pathogenic.

General Therapeutic Considerations

Therapy for small-vessel leukocytoclastic vasculitis should first be directed toward any identified precipitating factor or underlying disease. For example, if vasculitis is drug-induced, withdrawal of the offending agent may be the only therapy required. In the occasional case where food antigens are a possible cause, alteration in diet may be helpful, both in diagnosis and in therapy (60). Appropriate therapy for a streptococcus-associated vasculitis would be the use of antibiotics to treat the infection or carrier state.

Unfortunately, many cases of vasculitis have no clear cause. Most forms of idiopathic small-vessel limited leukocytoclastic vasculitis are self-limited, resolving in 2 to 3 weeks. In such cases, therapy should be directed toward relief of symptoms. Reduction of activity and leg elevation or compression stockings may be all that are indicated. Antihistamines may be useful in patients with pruritus and occasionally helpful in patients with urticarial vasculitis. Nonsteroidal antiinflammatory agents are useful for relief of arthralgias or myalgias, but are seldom helpful in preventing or treating new lesions. Reportedly, antimalarial drugs are helpful in some cases of cutaneous vasculitis, primarily in livedoid vasculitis or some subsets of lupus vasculitis, but do not seem to be effective in most cases of idiopathic small-vessel leukocytoclastic vasculitis.

Dapsone, a drug used by dermatologists primarily for the treatment of dermatitis herpetiformis, is also used for the treatment of leprosy and its vasculitic complications. It is also useful in idiopathic small-vessel leukocytoclastic vasculitis, and is probably the drug of choice in erythema elevatum diutinum. Dapsone is used in dosages of 25 to 200 mg per day orally. As several weeks of therapy may be required to judge its effectiveness in an individual patient with vasculitis, other therapies may be more appropriate for patients in whom rapid relief of symptoms or interruption of lesion formation is needed. Dapsone has several significant side effects, including hemolysis, and rarely, agranulocytosis or neuropathy (61,62). Hemolysis is an expected and dose-related complication in all patients, but it is especially severe in patients with glucose-6-phosphate dehydrogenase deficiency. Occasionally, patients with minimal-to-modest hemolysis not ordinarily requiring discontinuation of the drug will have a disproportionate production of methemoglobin. Patients with increasing fatigability, decreasing exercise tolerance, or other symptoms that might be due to decreased oxygen-carrying capacity of the blood should have their methemoglobin level checked. Laboratory monitoring of patients on dapsone therapy should include complete blood count (CBC), liver enzymes, blood urea nitrogen (BUN) level, and creatinine level at the initiation of therapy. Recommendations for further monitoring vary, but a reasonable approach is checking a CBC weekly or biweekly during the first month of therapy, monthly for 2 to 3 months, and CBC and liver enzyme screen every 3 to 4 months thereafter. Granulocyte colony-stimulating factor was used to shorten the recovery time for dapsone-induced agranulocytosis in one patient (62).

Colchicine should probably be a first-line agent in the treatment of symptomatic idiopathic cutaneous leukocytoclastic vasculitis (63–65). In addition to treating cutaneous lesions, it may also be effective in treating arthritis in these patients. Its mechanism of action is unknown. Begun at 0.6 mg once or twice daily, it can be increased to three times a day in some patients; the major limitation on dose increases is gastrointestinal side effects. When effective, benefit is usually evident within 2 weeks of initiation. Its incidence of serious side effects when given orally is rare, although intravenous colchicine has been implicated as a cause of aplastic anemia. Once control has been achieved, control can often be maintained on a slow taper, and the drug can be stopped after 2 weeks of clinical resolution. The recurrence of lesions usually responds to the reinstitution of therapy. Colchicine is not appropriate for primary use in patients with serious systemic disease.

The role of oral corticosteroids in treating idiopathic small-vessel vasculitis is controversial, with conflicting reports of efficacy in this and other vasculitic syndromes. Certainly, in skin-limited or skin-predominant vasculitic syndromes, steroids are seldom indicated. However, even in patients with skin-limited disease, progression of vasculitic lesions to plaques, vesicles, or nodules, often with ulceration, may warrant corticosteroids. In addition, many patients may achieve symptomatic relief from arthritis only with corticosteroid use. A short course of corticosteroid therapy when lesser therapies have failed, or would be expected to act too slowly, may be useful in such settings (66). However, there are no reports of a controlled trial to support a long-term benefit from corticosteroids in isolated small-vessel leukocytoclastic vasculitis, thus steroids should not be used routinely for the management of vasculitis.

In patients in whom the potential short-term benefits appear to outweigh the well-known risks of corticosteroid therapy, an initial oral single daily dose of 40 to 60 mg is usually sufficient to control symptoms and lesion formation. The dose should be discontinued by tapering over a 2- to 3-week period. Alternate therapies should be considered for patients who do not respond to this therapy or in patients whose disease recurs on tapering.

Azathioprine may be effective treatment for small-vessel vasculitis (67,68). When colchicine or dapsone therapy has failed or is not tolerated, and chronic cutaneous vasculitis is being controlled primarily with corticosteroids, azathioprine should be considered as adjunctive therapy early in the course, just as steroid-sparing agents are used in many rheumatic syndromes. When effective, azathioprine may eventually allow the discontinuation of corticosteroids in patients with chronic small-vessel leukocytoclastic vasculitis. The effective dose for cutaneous vasculitis is probably between 50 and 150 mg per day. It is a relatively safe drug when used appropriately, although careful monitoring is important. Once a stable dose is achieved, monitoring of hematologic and hepatic screens is warranted at least every 3 to 4 months. Pancreatitis can occur, and some patients develop gastric intolerance or a febrile reaction that may preclude its use.

Corticosteroid therapy is much more routinely given as treatment for patients with the more aggressive (and usually larger vessel) vasculitic syndromes. Prednisone is the usual agent, given as 1 mg/kg per day orally, occasionally in divided doses every 6 hours in fulminant cases (69). The decision to taper to an alternate-day regimen or to discontinue corticosteroid therapy is based on clinical response.

In many instances, corticosteroid therapy is insufficient. This is especially true in patients with WG, where the addition of cyclophosphamide therapy was a major advance in improving prognosis and has become the treatment of choice as either daily oral or cyclic intravenous pulse therapy (70–74). The usual oral regimen is 1 to 2 mg/kg per day of oral cyclophosphamide. The dose is adjusted to maintain the total leukocyte count above 3,000/mm^3 and the neutrophil count above 1,000 to 1,500/mm^3, assessed weekly (70). In patients with fulminant disease, intravenous cyclophosphamide may be given at a dose of 4 mg/kg daily for 3 days, changing to the lower dosage daily oral regimen after the third day. Patients should be treated for 1 year after achieving remission, and then the cyclophosphamide should be stopped and the patient followed carefully for evidence of relapse. Cyclophosphamide therapy is not without significant risk. Complications include hemorrhagic cystitis, bone marrow suppression, opportunistic infections, gonadal dysfunction and possibly sterility, and rarely, bladder carcinoma, leukemia, or lymphoma (70,74).

The newest area of therapy in vasculitis relates to the use of biologic therapies. Etanercept is a recombinant fusion protein consisting of two TNF receptors linked to the Fc portion of human IgG1. Randomized trials of this agent are in progress, following promising results in a small number of patients with therapy-resistant WG when given as 25 mg subcutaneously twice weekly (75). Infliximab is an anti–TNF-α antibody reported to induce prompt symptomatic responses in patients with treatment-refractory systemic vasculitides, including WG, rheumatic vasculitis, and cryoglobulinemia (76).

Rituximab is a human/mouse chimeric monoclonal antibody that reacts with CD20 antigen on B-lymphocytes and induces complement- and antibody-dependent cellular cytotoxicity. Its use has been associated with partial to complete remissions in type II mixed cryoglobulinemia (77). Intravenous immunoglobulin has been used successfully to treat leukocytoclastic vasculitis (78). The use of interferon-α is discussed in the cryoglobulinemia section. Many other potential avenues of biologic intervention may be of use in treating vasculitis (75).

SPECIFIC VASCULITIC SYNDROMES

Leukocytoclastic Small-Vessel Vasculitis

Syndromes of small-vessel leukocytoclastic vasculitis tend to cause palpable purpura, to involve vessels the size of those in the dermis, and to share pathologic features. The three syndromes most closely associated with these clinical findings include cutaneous leukocytoclastic vasculitis (and its variants), HSP, and essential mixed cryoglobulinemia. The remaining major vasculitides most characteristically involve medium-to-large vessels, although they may also involve the small dermal vessels. These syndromes will be discussed by diagnostic category.

IGG/IGM IMMUNE COMPLEX SMALL-VESSEL LEUKOCYTOCLASTIC VASCULITIS (CUTANEOUS LEUKOCYTOCLASTIC VASCULITIS, HYPERSENSITIVITY VASCULITIS)

Small-vessel leukocytoclastic vasculitis is a common disease, affecting the sexes with approximately equal frequency and occurring at all ages (3,4,35). Multiple names have been applied to this syndrome, most commonly hypersensitivity vasculitis, allergic vasculitis, cutaneous–systemic vasculitis, or small-vessel necrotizing vasculitis. In the initial description of hypersensitivity angiitis by Zeek, all patients died within a few weeks of onset (79). Certainly, many of her original cases would not be among the same group of patients to whom most authors assign the term "hypersensitivity vasculitis" today. Most patients with IgG/IgM immune complex vasculitis (hypersensitivity vasculitis) do well on minimal therapy today. The classification of vasculitis proposed by the CHCG clarifies and simplifies the assignment of diagnostic categories to patients with cutaneous vasculitides. This classification substitutes the term "cutaneous leukocytoclastic angiitis" for hypersensitivity vasculitis and limits its use to patients with *no* evidence of extracutaneous vasculitic disease (13). It would also reclassify as microscopic PAN most other cases that have traditionally been considered hypersensitivity vasculitis or cutaneous–systemic small-vessel vasculitis. This is clearly a significant departure from current practice. In light of this, an argument can be made that the CHCG classification criteria for cutaneous leukocytoclastic vasculitis are too narrow.

Relationship Between Cutaneous and Systemic Features of Disease. Some patients with systemic involvement secondary to a small-vessel leukocytoclastic vasculitis may have no cutaneous involvement. Likewise, many patients with a cutaneous leukocytoclastic vasculitis may have no clinical evidence of extracutaneous vasculitis. However, it is common for patients with cutaneous leukocytoclastic vasculitis limited to small dermal vessels to have at least some extracutaneous findings, most commonly arthralgias or arthritis, fever, myalgia, renal or gut involvement (1,7,79,80).

As with Zeek's cases, some patients in frequently cited earlier studies of small-vessel cutaneous leukocytoclastic vasculitis might today be reclassified as complete or incomplete syndromes of HSP, microscopic PAN, small-vessel limited WG, and perhaps even rheumatic vasculitis (1,7,79,80). Inclusion of such cases would obviously affect the reported incidence of extracutaneous involvement in hypersensitivity vasculitis. Still, the current consensus seems to be that small dermal vessel leukocytoclastic vasculitis is often skin-limited, but may include extracutaneous involvement in a pattern similar to that of HSP (4,11,81–84).

For example, in a survey by Liss and Wolverton of 58 patients with hypersensitivity vasculitis, 13 patients were shown by rechallenge to have vasculitis secondary to a drug. The frequency of extracutaneous involvement in 44 of these patients included renal (43%), arthralgias (32%), fever (20%), myalgias (11%), liver (9%), lung (9%), gastrointestinal (5%), cardiac (2%), and central nervous system (2%). Haber et al. (85) found similar frequencies of internal involvement.

The ACR criteria for vasculitis raise two different issues. These criteria include hypersensitivity vasculitis, but rely primarily on histologic criteria to distinguish this syndrome (11,86). Patients who present with skin lesions limited to the small-vessel component of PAN or granulomatous vasculitides might fit ACR criteria for cutaneous hypersensitivity vasculitis (11). Patients with neutrophilic dermatoses with prominent perivascular neutrophilic infiltrates without histologic criteria for vasculitis might also be misclassified with hypersensitivity vasculitis using ACR criteria.

The second and perhaps more important problem is that patients were initially classified as having hypersensitivity vasculitis or Henoch–Schönlein purpura, partly by age of onset, and subsequently age criteria were determined to be important criteria for distinguishing between these two syndromes (11,87). If the patient is greater than 16 years of age, the criteria is biased against HSP. If the patient is 16 years of age or older, the criteria is biased toward a diagnosis of HSP.

Cutaneous Manifestations. Cutaneous small-vessel leukocytoclastic vasculitis primarily affects the postcapillary venules of dermal vessels, and manifests in the skin most classically as palpable purpura 3 to 10 mm in diameter. Lesions are often asymptomatic, but may burn, itch, or be tender (11). Individual lesions of small dermal vessel leukocytoclastic vasculitis evolve over a period of hours from erythematous macules to erythematous papules (which may have an urticarial appearance), and usually become purpuric (1,11,20,21). Such lesions at the peak of development typically have both a blanchable (erythematous) component and a nonblanchable (hemorrhagic) component, and partial blanching of such lesions is expected. These lesions are usually round or oval (Figs. 8.1 and 8.10). Occasionally, the central area may form pustules or hemorrhagic vesicles, and may necrose and ulcerate if the inflammation is severe enough.

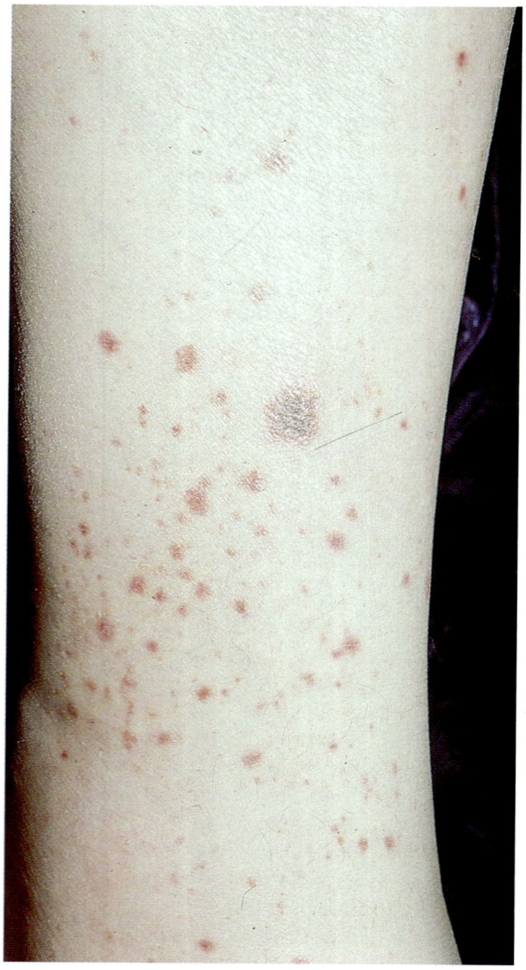

Figure 8.10. Typical distribution of palpable purpura in cutaneous small-vessel leukocytoclastic vasculitis.

Once the initial injury phase is complete, the erythema gradually fades and the edema subsides, leaving a residual purpuric macule or papule. Postinflammatory hyperpigmentation is a common finding. If sufficient dermal necrosis has occurred, a persistent palpability and erythema may develop, correlating with a wound healing response. Other less common presentations include vesicles, bullae, subcutaneous nodules, or ulcerations (1,82).

Lesions of small-vessel leukocytoclastic vasculitis typically arise in crops, persist for less than a month, and spontaneously subside (1,11). Scarring is unusual, although it occurs after ulcer development. Lesions are most common in dependent areas: typically the lower legs and ankles, or posterior legs, back, and buttocks in bedridden patients. In severe cases, lesions can be extensive, although they are still more densely distributed in dependent areas, and usually spare intertriginous areas. Lesions may also occur at sites of trauma due to köebnerization, or under tight-fitting clothing (22).

Pathology and Immunopathology. Traditional criteria for hypersensitivity vasculitis include the histopathologic findings of leukocytoclastic vasculitis, affecting primarily postcapillary venules. These findings include a neutrophil-rich infiltrate, nuclear dust from degeneration of neutrophil nuclei (leukocytoclasis), and fibrinoid necrosis. It is clear, however, that the timing of the biopsy has an important effect on the histologic appearance of the infiltrate and the immunoreactants found in the vessel wall. Studies on experimentally induced immune complex deposition in guinea pigs and later in humans have shown early deposition of immune complexes and complement components, but disappearance (clearance) of these immune complexes as the neutrophilic infiltrate increases. By 24 hours after the lesional stimulus, immunoreactants have largely disappeared from vasculitic lesions (23,32,88). Serial biopsies in patients with histamine-induced leukocytoclastic vasculitis have shown an increase in the degree of inflammatory infiltrate, hemorrhage, nuclear dust, and fibrin deposition over a 24-hour period following the injection of histamine into the normal-appearing skin of patients with an active vasculitis (23). Serial biopsies of spontaneous lesions in patients with leukocytoclastic vasculitis have validated these findings, and have also shown that biopsies taken of lesions 48 hours old or older show a marked decrease in neutrophilic infiltrate and an increase in mononuclear cell infiltrate (25). The variability of histologic and IIF findings in immune complex–mediated vasculitis and the possibility of other forms of small-vessel, nonleukocytoclastic vasculitis or inflammatory hemorrhage, as has been reported in Sjögren syndrome, PLEVA, or erythema multiforme, make appropriate selection of a lesion for biopsy critical (24,25,89,90). Secondary vasculitic change is also a frequent finding in biopsies taken from the edge of nonvasculitic cutaneous ulcers; therefore, histologic findings alone cannot be taken as evidence of a primary leukocytoclastic vasculitis.

The sensitivity of direct IIF in immune complex vasculitis appears to be between 60% and 80% (91). In light of the previous discussion, this sensitivity is dependent on the timing of the biopsy in the evolution of the lesion; those biopsies showing the most solid evidence of leukocytoclastic vasculitis are the least likely to have any remaining specific IIF findings. Ideally, biopsies should be taken of lesions that are less than 18 hours old (91).

The specificity of immune complex deposition is also a problem. For example, immunoglobulin and complement deposition may be seen in vessel walls in several nonvasculitic settings: in sun-damaged skin, at the margin of nonvasculitic ulcers, in lesions of dermatitis, and possibly in a variety of other inflammatory but nonvasculitic settings (91–97). Despite this, a granular staining pattern of immune deposits in and directly around the vessel wall suggests a diagnosis of immune complex vasculitis. Deposition of IgM is the least specific finding, whereas the deposition of IgG or IgA is somewhat more likely to suggest a pathogenic role for the immunoreactants.

Laboratory Manifestations. Aside from biopsy findings, laboratory abnormalities in leukocytoclastic vasculitis are nonspecific. The most common abnormal finding is an elevated erythrocyte sedimentation rate, followed by leukocytosis, eosinophilia, or anemia (3,82). Cryoglobulins, rheumatoid factor, antinuclear antibodies, and decrease in complement levels are seen less commonly, and their incidence often depends on the presence of associated diseases such as rheumatoid arthritis or systemic lupus. Evidence of extracutaneous involvement may also be found; abnormal urinalysis, elevated creatinine or BUN, or abnormal liver enzyme levels are the most common. A routine blood count and differential, a urinalysis, and screening panel for renal or liver abnormalities may be indicated in all patients; certainly patients with bowel symptoms or significant extracutaneous disease should also be screened for occult gastrointestinal bleeding. However, judicious use of laboratory tests is warranted, and further testing should depend on the history and physical findings and the duration of symptoms or recurrence of lesions. It is not clear whether a full panel of cryoglobulins, rheumatoid factor, antinuclear antibody (ANA), ANCA, serum complement, total hemolytic complement, chest radiograph, hepatitis screen, circulating immune complex screen, malignancy workup, or other tests are indicated or even appropriate in an individual with a single brief episode of mild cutaneous leukocytoclastic vasculitis with mild arthralgias, no history of previous similar episodes or extracutaneous symptoms, and otherwise unremarkable physical findings.

Differential Diagnosis. Having firmly established a diagnosis of small-vessel cutaneous leukocytoclastic vasculitis, the next step is to determine its likely etiology and the presence of extracutaneous disease. The classification of the vasculitis will bear directly on the likelihood of finding current or future extracutaneous development. Patients with an isolated episode of apparently skin-limited cutaneous vasculitis with or without arthralgias should receive minimal laboratory screening as outlined before, but careful counseling and follow-up. The persistence of cutaneous vasculitis beyond 3 weeks, the development of extensive cutaneous disease, the presence of associated extracutaneous symptoms or findings, the history of multiple chronic extracutaneous symptoms preceding the episode of vasculitis, or the finding of physical or laboratory evidence of extracutaneous involvement should prompt a more extensive initial laboratory evaluation. Likewise, recurrence of even minimal cutaneous vasculitis after the initial resolution of lesions should prompt a detailed evaluation.

The possibility of a food or drug reaction; an infection; an underlying connective tissue disease or malignancy; a chronic inflammatory disease such as Crohn disease, ulcerative colitis, or primary biliary cirrhosis; or a congenital complement component deficiency triggering the vasculitis must be kept in mind. Infections implicated in triggering acute episodes of vasculitis are many, but hepatitis B and C, subacute bacterial endocarditis, and bowel-related bacteremia in bowel bypass (stasis) syndrome are thought to be important causes of identifiable persistent antigenemia and chronic vasculitic syndromes. Malignancies associated with leukocytoclastic vasculitis are usually lymphoreticular or hematopoietic in origin (11,98–101). Solid tumors have rarely been reported in association with vasculitis, but the nature of the association is unclear. In 71% of reported cases of vasculitis associated with solid-tumor malignancy, however, manifestations of vasculitis appeared before or concurrent with recognition or relapse of the tumor (102).

It should also be noted that syndromes such as PAN, WG, allergic granulomatosis of Churg–Strauss, and lupus and rheumatoid vasculitis may all present with vasculitis limited to small vessels and isolated pathologic findings of leukocytoclastic vasculitis. Therefore, the presence of isolated small dermal vessel disease cannot be used at presentation to rule out these possibilities. Again, the disease course, the development of lesions implying larger vessel involvement, or the presence of recurrent disease or significant extracutaneous disease makes these diagnoses more likely.

Bronchiectasis has been associated with recurrent episodes of cutaneous and systemic small-vessel vasculitis in a small number of patients (103–106). Patients with bronchiectasis have been shown to have a high incidence of circulating immune complexes. The vasculitic episodes seemed to correlate with exacerbation of underlying chronic bronchitis (105). When IgA is prominent in the immunoreactants and serum IgA is predominantly elevated, these patients would seem to fit in the IgA vasculitis category. Prominent gastrointestinal findings were present in one such patient (105).

In a study of 82 patients with cutaneous leukocytoclastic vasculitis, 44 patients had apparently idiopathic vasculitides, whereas the remaining vasculitides were thought to be due to food or drugs (nine cases), infection/drug (three cases), infection (eight cases), connective tissue disease (17 cases), and Crohn disease (one case) (82). Of the 82 patients, 21 were self-referred and most had no systemic symptoms and infrequent laboratory abnormalities. In the physician-referred group of 61 patients, over half had one or more symptoms and laboratory abnormalities. Forty-two of these patients showed one or more of the systemic disease manifestations. The musculoskeletal system was most commonly involved (43%, usually arthralgias), whereas renal (15%) and pulmonary (8%) were the next two systems most frequently involved.

Previous studies of primarily small-vessel vasculitis that may have included some patients with lupus, rheumatoid arthritis, PAN, and perhaps other vasculitic syndromes have noted the following associations: idiopathic (39% to 61%), drugs (0% to 59%), infections (0% to 30.5%), collagen vascular disease (0% to 17%), and malignancy (0% to 6.5%) (7,79,83,107). The incidence of extracutaneous findings in some series, again with the caveat that some patients might be reclassified under current criteria, was joints (50%), kidneys (38% to 60%), lungs (20% to 30%), and gastrointestinal tract (15% to 22%) (7,79,108).

Management of Skin Lesions and Prognosis. The prognosis in individual patients obviously depends on the extent and severity of cutaneous disease and on the presence and severity of extracutaneous findings. The prognosis in most patients with uncomplicated small dermal vessel leukocytoclastic vasculitis is very good. Most of the severe disease, deaths, or chronic organ dysfunction are likely due to other vasculitic syndromes. Therapy has been discussed previously.

Cutaneous Small-Vessel Leukocytoclastic Vasculitis: Variants. There are a number of syndromes of small-vessel vasculitis syndromes that are often included in the spectrum of small-vessel leukocytoclastic vasculitis but for which either there is a known etiology or a clinical presentation distinctive enough to warrant their separation.

Drug-induced. Only a small fraction of drug reactions takes the form of vasculitis (109–111). Drug-induced vasculitis is most often reported as small-vessel lymphocytic and monocytic inflammatory injury, rather than as leukocytoclastic vasculitis (112,113). Agents most often associated with vasculitis include allopurinol, penicillin, aminopenicillins, sulfonamides, thiazides, pyrazolones, hydantoins, and propylthiouracil. ANA and ANCA may be produced with propylthiouracil, as well as a distinctive vasculitis involving the face and ear lobes, with erythema and later purpura. Serum preparations and vaccines are the expected cause of serum sickness, while serum sickness-like reactions are most often due to β-blockers, streptokinase, or β-lactam antibiotics (111). In a recent study of published cases of drug-induced vasculitis, the most commonly associated medications in descending order were propylthiouracil, hydralazine, colony-stimulating factors, allopurinol, cefaclor, minocycline, D-penicillamine, phenytoin, isotretinoin, and methotrexate (114). Vasculitic skin lesions have been reported with each of these medications. ANCA positivity was reported with propylthiouracil, hydralazine, allopurinol, minocycline, penicillamine, and phenytoin. In most cases, vasculitis resolved following discontinuation of the drug.

Serum Sickness and Serum Sickness–like Reactions. In 1905, von Pirquet and Schick described serum sickness in children treated with horse serum containing diphtheria antitoxin. More recently, serum sickness has been noted in patients treated with horse antithymocyte globulins or human diploid-cell rabies vaccine (115–117). Serum sickness or serum sickness–like reactions are characterized by the occurrence of fever, rash, polyarthralgias, and lymphadenopathy 7 to 14 days after primary exposure and 2 to 4 days after secondary exposure to a heterologous protein such as intravenous antithymocyte globulin or streptokinase (classic serum sickness), or a drug such as penicillin or sulfa (serum sickness–like reaction) (115,116,118).

Serum sickness or serum sickness–like reactions usually spare mucosa, but are associated with a morbilliform eruption, and sometimes with urticaria, fever, and arthralgias. More than 90% of cases are drug-induced; fewer than 5% are fatal (111). Vasculitis is uncommon; occasional patients will have typical cutaneous vasculitis, which may rarely progress to a systemic vasculitis. Serum sickness may have distinctive skin findings (115,116). Typically, erythema first occurs on the sides of the fingers, toes, and hands, followed by a morbilliform eruption in two thirds of patients, sometimes with urticaria. Urticaria is seldom seen alone. About half the cases have visceral involvement. Rash, fever, constitutional symptoms, arthralgia, and arthritis are the most frequent clinical findings. Serum C3 and C4 are markedly decreased (115,116). The urticaria–arthritis syndrome of hepatitis B may present as serum sickness–like reaction, or with lesions more typical of urticarial vasculitis (28).

Urticarial Vasculitis. Urticarial vasculitis is a relatively newly recognized subset of vasculitis, first reported as a syndrome of urticarial lesions, synovitis, hypocomplementemia, occasionally glomerulonephritis or abdominal pain, and histologic findings of leukocytoclastic vasculitis (119). In 1982, chronic obstructive pulmonary disease was added to the list of associated complications seen with hypocomplementemic vasculitis (120). The syndrome of urticarial vasculitis has continued to broaden. Many patients do not have hypocomplementemia, and histology of leukocytoclastic vasculitis is not required for diagnosis (121–123). The urticaria–arthritis syndrome of hepatitis B infection is often a form of urticarial vasculitis rather than urticaria, secondary to hepatitis B antigen–antibody complexes (28).

Lesions of urticarial vasculitis are likely to be painful or burning, to persist for longer than 24 hours, to show some evidence of purpura clinically, and to show more prominent perivascular infiltrates, most classically with evidence of leukocytoclastic vasculitis and at least microscopic hemorrhage (see Fig. 8.2) (122). In contrast, lesions of urticaria are pruritic, short lasting (< 24 hours), not purpuric, and characterized histologically by the presence of little or no perivascular infiltrate and no evidence of vasculitis. Other skin manifestations in this syndrome include angioedema, macular erythema, livedo reticularis, cutaneous nodules, and bullae (123,124). Approximately 70% of patients are women.

In a study of 72 patients with urticarial vasculitis, only about a third of patients had elevated erythrocyte sedimentation rates or a depressed CH_{50}, a fourth had decreased C3 levels, and fewer than 10% had a depressed C4. Patients with nephritis in this series had abnormal urinary sediments. Patients with hypocomplementemia were more likely to have purpuric lesions, arthralgias, abdominal pain, chronic obstructive pulmonary disease, a neutrophilic dermal infiltrate, and positive vascular IIF when compared to patients who were normocomplementemic (122). Urticarial vasculitis may be caused by or associated with medications, foods, viral diseases, serum sickness, serum sickness–like reactions, physical urticarias, connective tissue diseases, or monoclonal gammopathies (124,125). Urticaria in patients with collagen vascular disease is more likely to be urticarial vasculitis with leukocytoclastic change, and the lesions of urticarial vasculitis often correlate with systemic disease activity (126–128). Urticarial vasculitis occurs in 5% to 10% of patients with SLE, and may rarely be a presenting sign (123). Conversely, one large study reports that SLE was associated with 54% of patients with hypocomplementemic vasculitis, but only 3% of the normocomplementemic group (129). In this same study, all hypocomplementemic patients were female, compared with equal distribution by gender in the normocomplementemic group. Therapy with a variety of agents is occasionally successful; the most frequently administered therapies showing some degree of success include antihistamines, nonsteroidal antiinflammatory drugs, antimalarials, and most often, corticosteroids (122,129,130).

Wiesnieski et al. (123) have proposed separating urticarial vasculitis into normocomplementemic urticarial vasculitis, hypocomplementemic urticarial vasculitis, and a new group termed "hypocomplementemic urticarial vasculitis syndrome" (HUVS) (123). The last subset of patients is distinguished by both a more severe clinical syndrome and by the presence of an IgG antibody to the C1q component of complement (C1q precipitin) (123,129). The patients with HUVS typically have urticarial vasculitis and often angioedema and eye inflammation, arthritis or arthralgia, frequent but usually mild renal disease, obstructive pulmonary disease (often severe), serum complement activation with hypocomplementemia, and the C1q precipitin. Although 28% to 47% of patients with SLE may have an IgG antibody to C1q, and 50% of the patients with HUVS have had a positive ANA test, clinical and serologic findings distinguish these two groups. Angioedema, eye inflammation, and obstructive pulmonary disease are common in HUVS but rare in SLE. Anti–double-stranded DNA and anti–extractable nuclear antigen antibodies are not seen in HUVS. Severe renal disease is common in lupus but rare in HUVS (104). Despite the severe and often fatal pulmonary disease in HUVS, the serum α_1-antitrypsin levels are normal in these patients. Colchicine, nonsteroidal antiinflammatory drugs, danazol, tricyclic antidepressants including doxepin, and histamine-1 (H_1) and H_2 blockers have all been ineffective in treating patients with

HUVS. Prednisone taken in oral doses of 30 to 60 mg daily has suppressed or decreased the urticarial vasculitis in most patients, and dapsone or hydroxychloroquine has been helpful as adjunctive therapy in some. Treatment of the pulmonary disease is difficult; cigarette smoking seems to be a strong risk factor in the progression of pulmonary disease in at least some of these patients.

Pustular Vasculitis. Certain neutrophilic dermatoses such as Sweet syndrome, pyoderma gangrenosum, the pustular vasculitis category that is idiopathic or associated with intestinal bypass syndrome (bowel stasis, dermatitis–arthritis), or Behçet disease can mimic or be mimicked by leukocytoclastic vasculitis (131–135). Lesions with prominent perivascular neutrophilic infiltrates without evidence of vessel wall destruction may develop in these patients. Patients may also have associated fevers, myalgias, polyarthralgias, or arthritis.

Infection-Related Vasculitis. Many infections can trigger a syndrome of leukocytoclastic vasculitis. Recognized infectious triggers include group A streptococcus, *Staphylococcus aureus* or *Streptomyces albus*, hepatitis (A, B, and C), influenza, cytomegalovirus, infectious mononucleosis, otitis media, chronic meningococcemia, gonococcemia, human immunodeficiency virus (HIV) infection, subacute bacterial endocarditis, infected shunts, and *Mycobacterium leprae* (11,124,136,137). Bacteremia can trigger a true septic vasculitis with both viable organisms and leukocytoclasis in lesions or can serve as an antigen for a more chronic immune complex vasculitis (137–139).

Erythema Elevatum Diutinum. A variant of small-vessel vasculitis localized to the skin, erythema elevatum diutinum, was reported in 1894 by Radcliffe-Crocker and Williams (140). It is an uncommon syndrome of chronic small-vessel leukocytoclastic vasculitis, usually attributed to antecedent streptococcal infection, and may be increased in incidence in HIV-infected patients (141–143). It is reviewed in Chapter 10.

LEUKOCYTOCLASTIC SMALL-VESSEL VASCULITIS: HENOCH–SCHÖNLEIN PURPURA

HSP is characterized by palpable purpura, arthralgia, gastrointestinal signs and symptoms, and glomerulonephritis. It has a remarkable tendency to resolve and recur several times over a period of weeks or months, usually ending in spontaneous resolution. A small percentage of patients progress to chronic disease.

HSP has been considered a subset of hypersensitivity vasculitis in most classification systems. It has been classified as a distinct entity in the ACR and the CHCG proposals (11,13,144). The ACR classification is biased against this diagnosis in adults because age is considered a major diagnostic criterion for HSP. It may be more common in adults than currently recognized if predominance of IgA immunoreactants in idiopathic cutaneous small-vessel vasculitis is included in the HSP spectrum, whether or not there are extracutaneous findings of HSP (26). IgA-predominant immune complexes associated with vasculitis may be increased in patients with lupus, cryoglobulinemia, or IgA gammopathies, so that special attention should be paid to excluding these diseases, in addition to underlying drugs or infections, before diagnosing idiopathic IgA vasculitis.

Epidemiology. Two large pediatric series of HSP, both published in 1960, shared a number of key findings: an increased incidence in boys (1.6 to 1.8:1.0), a peak incidence between 2 and 5 years of age, and a history of a recent upper respiratory infection (66% to 75%) (145,146). More recent studies have found a background incidence of HSP in children under age 15 years of approximately two to 10 cases per 10,000 children per year, and a mean age of 6 years (147–151). Approximately 75% of children are younger than 8 years, and 90% are younger than 10 years (151). Most epidemiologic studies have been performed in Europe and the Middle East. In childhood, boys are more frequently affected (60%) than are girls (40%) (145,151, 152).

Upper respiratory infections frequently precede HSP (148, 149,151). Group A β-hemolytic streptococcus has been the most frequently identified pathogen in children with HSP, but infection with these bacteria, or any other organism, has not yet been directly linked to the pathogenesis of HSP.

The incidence of HSP in adults is about one tenth that of children, about 1.3 to 1.4 cases per 100,000 adults per year (151,153,154). The mean age of onset is around 50 years of age, with men and women affected with equal frequency (151,155). Preceding infection is less common in adults than in children.

Medications are more often associated with HSP in adults than in children, undoubtedly, in part, because medication use is much more frequent in adults (114,151,155). Other associations include food sensitivity, pregnancy, familial Mediterranean fever, cryoglobulinemia, and some cancers (lymphoma, colonic, bronchial, prostatic) (156). More loosely implicated triggers include toxins (thiram) and insect bites. A single report suggests that trauma may precipitate HSP-like disease, and that in one family this tendency might be familial (157).

Familial Clustering and Inherited Factors in IgA Vasculitis. Identical 7-year-old twin boys each had a proven adenovirus infection at the same time (158). A few days later, one child developed florid HSP, with severe gastrointestinal symptoms, transient joint symptoms, and an acute nephritic syndrome that progressed to nephrotic syndrome and renal insufficiency. A renal biopsy showed severe proliferative glomerulonephritis with crescents and marked deposition of IgA, IgG, C3, and fibrin in the mesangium as well as subepithelial deposits in the glomeruli. The second twin developed hematuria and abdominal pain but no rash. A renal biopsy showed mesangial proliferative glomerulonephritis with mesangial deposits of IgA, and to a lesser extent IgG and C3. His subsequent clinical course was characteristic of Berger disease (IgA nephropathy).

A second family study of IgA nephropathy found one adult member with HSP (159). She had recurrent purpuric rashes accompanied by severe renal involvement, and ultimately died in renal failure from cerebral hemorrhage. Her serum IgA was twice normal, and a renal biopsy later in her course demonstrated predominantly IgA complexes in the mesangium. Including the proband, four family members had IgA nephropathy, and six of seven family members had significantly elevated serum IgA levels. Both of these family studies suggest a linkage of HSP and Berger nephropathy.

Inherited defects in complement, particularly within the alternate pathway of complement activation, have also been implicated as a predisposing factor for HSP. Complete deficiency of C2 has been associated with HSP in three cases (160–162). Some authors found a significant increase in complete deficiencies of either the C4A or C4B complement isotype in children and adults who had HSP or IgA nephropathy in Kentucky (163,164). Properdin deficiency has been associated with IgA nephropathy (165). Additional studies have found C4B deficiency in pediatric patients with IgA nephropathy (166,167). Somewhat larger studies of adult and pediatric patients could not confirm this finding, but there may be worldwide regional variations in this finding (168).

Etiologic Factors/Pathogenesis. Differences in the definition of HSP complicate the evaluation of the literature pertinent to cutaneous vasculitis, particularly since the description of this syndrome antedated the availability of IIF studies. Some authors regard HSP as an appropriate term for any syndrome of leukocytoclastic vasculitis that is associated with arthritis or arthralgias, fever, abdominal pain, and renal disease with hematuria or proteinuria, regardless of or, in the absence of, direct IIF studies of lesional skin. Other authors regard the significant presence of IgA deposition in the affected vessels as important in the definition of HSP regardless of the presence or absence of extracutaneous findings (13,26,35,156,169–171).

IgA Complexes, Skin and Kidney. One of the more frequent findings noted when circulating or deposited immune complexes have been studied is the predominance of IgA immune complexes in HSP. Childhood HSP is less likely to be confused with other vasculitides that are more frequently seen in adults. In light of this, multiple studies of HSP syndromes exclusively or predominantly in children have shown evidence of either IgA deposition in lesional vessel walls, elevated serum IgA immune complex levels, or elevated levels of IgA-bearing peripheral blood lymphocytes (169–175).

In HSP, the membrane attack complex of complement localizes in the kidneys with deposits of IgA rather than IgG or IgM. This attack complex is also found in skin lesions and less commonly in uninvolved areas of skin, implicating IgA-mediated triggering of the membrane attack complex formation (176,177). Other studies have demonstrated C3, properdin, and factor B in the skin and kidneys without evidence of earlier complement components, suggesting that complement is activated by the alternate pathway in HSP (178–180). HSP can occur in patients with complete C2 deficiency, and therefore in the absence of complement activation through the classic pathway, suggesting that the alternative pathway of complement activation is central to the pathogenesis (162). Although IgA is thought to activate complement via the alternative pathway, there is surprisingly little experimental evidence to support this. The strongest evidence comes from experiments by Hiemstra et al. (181) suggesting that polymeric IgA is capable of activating the alternative pathway of complement.

Links Between IgA Nephropathy in HSP and Berger nephropathy. The tentative link between HSP and Berger/IgA nephropathy began with the report by Baart de la Faille-Kuyper et al. (178) in 1973 of four patients with both HSP and nephropathy, who had vessel wall deposits of IgA in purpuric lesions and IgA deposits in their renal mesangium. IgA antibodies or complexes are found in dermal capillaries in both syndromes, as well as increases in serum polymeric IgA and IgA-bearing blood leukocytes (172,182–188). IgA nephropathy is the most common form of glomerulonephritis in the world, accounting for up to 10% of patients treated for end-stage renal disease (189). It is most common in young adults, especially males, and is characterized clinically by recurrent episodes of gross or microscopic hematuria. Such episodes are often associated with minor flulike illnesses or vigorous exercise. The disease recurs in kidney transplant recipients, and disappears from kidneys if an affected kidney is inadvertently transplanted to someone without Berger disease (190).

Prominent mesangial deposits of IgA are required for the diagnosis. Serum IgA levels are increased in about 50% of cases, and biopsy of normal skin often reveals perivascular deposits of IgA, C3, and fibrin. Patients with IgA nephropathy may develop some of the clinical features of HSP, such as arthralgias, abdominal pain, or skin lesions, or may rarely develop into a classic HSP syndrome (185). Conversely, the elevation of IgA-bearing peripheral blood lymphocytes in children with HSP returned to normal after the acute symptoms of HSP had subsided in those patients without nephritis, but were elevated for more than 12 months in those children who developed nephritis, despite disappearance of the purpuric eruption (174). IgA rheumatoid factors are reported in approximately half of patients with either syndrome, and evidence suggests a renal antigen common to both diseases (191–193). HSP nephritis (but not HSP) and IgA nephropathy are both associated with HLA-Bw35 (194–196). Reports suggest a familial clustering of IgA nephropathy (197–201). The frequency of end-stage renal disease is 13% to 20% 10 years after diagnosis, and 25% to 34% 20 years after diagnosis (202).

IgA antibody can exist in a monomeric or a dimeric form, and can belong to one of two subclasses, IgA1 or IgA2. In patients with IgA nephropathy, excess amounts of IgA are produced in the bone marrow and in mucosal sites, such as the tonsils (203,204). Patients with Berger nephropathy, alcoholic cirrhosis, and HSP have elevated dimeric IgA in their serum, unlike the monomeric IgA typical of serum (156,190,205). The serum IgA also differs in other ways in these patients: it is more negatively charged, and has an abnormal carbohydrate content that is deficient in galactose, sialic acid, or both (151,206). The IgA eluted from glomeruli and in circulating complexes shows these changes as well, and belongs exclusively to the IgA1 (bone marrow–derived) subclass, and not to the IgA2 subclass (151,190,205). The reasons for this selective production by bone marrow of abnormal IgA, and why it selectively binds to glomeruli are not clear (151,190).

Cutaneous Manifestations. A palpable petechial or purpuric rash, sometimes associated with contiguous erythematous plaques, is characteristic (26,145,152,155). Especially in children, the rash is frequently urticarial at onset, then fades and is replaced by purpuric macular or papular lesions that can

TABLE 8.5. Distribution of Specific Findings in Pediatric Henoch–Schönlein Purpura by Age (Study of 131 Children)

Findings	Incidence <2 Yr Old	Incidence >2 Yr Old
Gastrointestinal symptoms in 2/3, 4 with intussusception	29%	75%
Hematuria in 40% (60% microscopic, 40% gross)	23%	43%
Average duration of syndrome	2 wk	>4 wk
Recurrences	<25%	Nearly 50%
Localized cutaneous edema in two-thirds (usually scalp, periorbital area, hands, or feet)	Twice as common in those <3 y old; not seen in patients 8 y or older	
Joint symptoms in two-thirds, usually ankles or feet	No difference in joint symptoms by age	

From Allen M, Diamond LK, Howel DA. Anaphylactoid purpura n children. *Am J Dis Child* 1960;99:833–854, with permission.

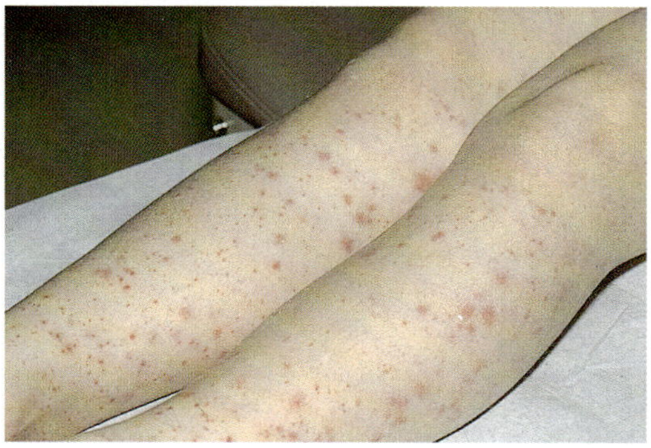

Figure 8.11. Lesion of classic palpable purpura in a patient with IgA vasculitis.

become confluent (145). In addition to urticarial lesions, erythema multiforme–like lesions are also frequent in childhood HSP. The distribution is roughly symmetric and favors the lower limbs but may involve the thighs and buttocks. The upper limbs or abdomen are occasionally affected. In the study by Allen et al. (145), localized edema in childhood was common, occurring in two thirds of children in one large series, with scalp, periorbital area, hands, and feet as the most common sites. Facial or scalp edema was often painful. Edema was much more common in younger patients, and was not seen in children older than 8 years (Table 8.5).

The distribution of lesions in adults is similar to that seen in pediatric patients. However, in adults it is more common for purpura to appear without any preceding lesion. In the series of Cream et al. (155), localized edema occurred in approximately half the adult patients, but usually in dependent areas. Blistered, necrotic, or ulcerated lesions, uncommon in children, developed in 16% of the adults in this series. In HSP, symptoms tend to persist, and recurrences are common in children older than 2 years of age and in adults (see Table 8.5) (26,145,152,155).

In addition to urticarial lesions, erythema multiforme–like lesions, and classic palpable purpura lesions typical of small-vessel inflammatory hemorrhage, a more distinctive morphology can be seen in IgA-predominant small-vessel leukocytoclastic vasculitis (Fig. 8.11) are seen.This morphology consists of superficial plaques of palpable purpura, erythema (demonstrated by partial blanching on pressure), purpura (demonstrated by persistence of some blood color on pressure), and retiform (netlike) patterning of lesional margins or of more intense areas of hemorrhage or necrosis within the lesions (Figs. 8.7 and 8.12) (26). There is a tendency toward bridging of adjacent lesions. This morphology can occasionally be seen in cutaneous lesions of vasculitis syndromes, which involve a mixture of vessel sizes, such as WG, but should be distinguished from the nonerythematous retiform purpura of microocclusive (bland occlusion, thrombotic) syndromes (see discussion of morphology) (19).

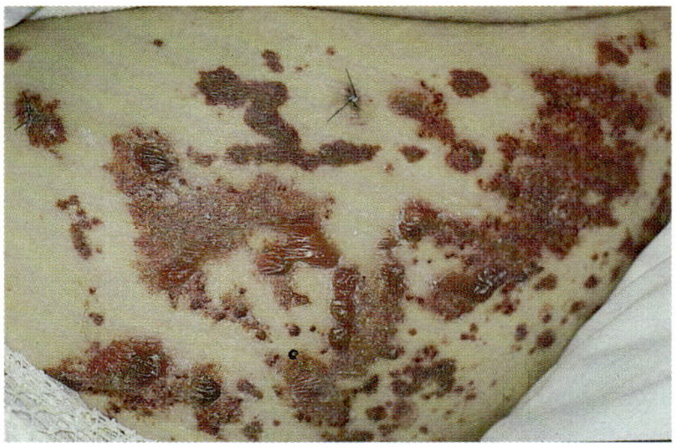

Figure 8.12. Inflammatory retiform purpura in IgA vasculitis. The erythema has faded, but retiform necrotic vesicles and residual dermal hemorrhage remain.

Acute Hemorrhagic Edema. Probably first described by Snow in 1913, the recognition of the syndrome of acute hemorrhagic edema (AHE) is credited to Finkelstein and Seidlmayer in 1938 to 1939. Europeans have recognized AHE of the infant (postinfectious cockade purpura, Finkelstein disease, Seidlmayer syndrome) as a benign disorder of children, 5 to 24 months of age (207–211). This condition is a form of cutaneous leukocytoclastic vasculitis, often preceded by upper respiratory tract infection or drug ingestion. There is an increased incidence in the winter (207,209). This syndrome is characterized by the symmetric distribution of large purpuric plaques over the extremities and face. These lesions may begin as painful petechiae or ecchymoses, which become edematous and later targeted or cockaded (209). The trunk and mucous membranes are typically spared. Localized edema may accompany or precede the purpuric lesions. Involvement of extracutaneous sites is unusual, although fever or generalized edema may occur. The usual course is one of spontaneous resolution over a 1- to 3-week period (207,209).

Given the remarkable similarity of the symptom complex of HSP in children under 2 years of age (see Table 8.5) to the presentation of AHE, and the transient presence of relevant immune complexes in lesions of leukocytoclastic vasculitis, it seems reasonable to consider that at least a portion of patients in the AHE group fit within the spectrum of IgA-associated HSP in children under 2 years of age. Many consider AHE simply to be a variant of HSP, but the low incidence of lesional IgA deposits in some reports of AHE leaves some room for dispute (209,210,212–215). It is possible that the low incidence of finding IgA deposits in patients with AHE is related to the maturation pattern of infant antibody production. Serum IgA levels are 1% of adult level at birth, and do not reach adult levels until adolescence. By 12 and 24 months of age, when AHE is most common, serum IgA levels are 19% and 25% of adult levels, respectively (216). This might result in decreased detection of IgA deposits on lesional biopsy in young infants and perhaps an inflammatory response less damaging to vessels.

Relationship Between Cutaneous and Systemic Features of Disease. In the series by Cream et al. (155) of adult HSP patients, over 80% developed systemic involvement, and in most, the skin was the first organ affected, although symptoms and signs of internal involvement could precede the rash by as long as 28 days.

The incidence of signs and symptoms in the 131 children studied by Allen et al. (145) included 100% incidence of rash (required), fever in 75%, arthritis or arthralgia in 68%, abdominal pain in 53%, guaiac-positive stools in 49%, melena in 38%, and hematemesis in 11%. However, patients younger than 2 years of age tended to have a different constellation of cutaneous and extracutaneous findings than did patients older than 2 years (see Table 8.5).

JOINTS. Joint involvement consists of an arthralgia of variable intensity, often diffuse and migratory; signs of inflammation are unreliable (152). The arthralgia affects mainly the ankles (40%), the knees (30%), and the elbows or wrists (25%), and usually affects more than one joint. The incidence of joint involvement may be higher in adults than in children, and may occur in as many as 50% to 90% of patients (152,215). Of course, if the diagnosis of HSP is determined by syndrome constellation rather than by predominant immunoreactant, by definition nearly all patients would be expected to have arthritis or arthralgias.

A complicating factor in the evaluation of patients with IgA vasculitis and arthralgias or renal disease is the possible association of inflammatory bowel disease or seronegative spondyloarthropathies with IgA nephropathy and, rarely, IgA vasculitis. Included in the seronegative spondyloarthropathies are ankylosing spondylitis, psoriatic arthritis, Reiter syndrome, and the arthritis of inflammatory bowel disease. The coexistence of inflammatory bowel disease and ankylosing spondylitis is well known: 4% of patients with ankylosing spondylitis have inflammatory bowel disease, whereas 6% (range, 1% to 25%) of patients with inflammatory bowel disease have ankylosing spondylitis (217,218). Each of the seronegative spondyloarthropathies has been associated with IgA nephropathy. Two patients with inflammatory bowel disease and ankylosing spondylitis have been reported with both IgA nephropathy and IgA vasculitis (217).

GASTROINTESTINAL. Gastrointestinal involvement occurs in 50% to 70% of patients, but again, the incidence of gut involvement is affected by the diagnostic criteria for HSP. Colicky abdominal pain is most common; bloody diarrhea or melena is frequently reported in children. Intussusception is rare, occurring in 2.5% to 5%, and can mimic acute abdominal perforation (152,219). Actual perforation is more rare but quite serious, and rarer still is duodenojejunal stenosis. Malabsorption, exudative enteropathy, hemorrhagic pancreatitis, hydrops of the gallbladder, and pseudomembranous colitis may also occur as very rare complications.

RENAL. There are three types of renal involvement. The most common is that of acute glomerulonephritis present at the same time that joint, gut, or cutaneous findings are active, and this usually resolves with treatment or time in concert with resolution of other syndrome features. A much less common form is acute crescentic glomerulonephritis, seen primarily in children, which is rapidly progressive and treatment-resistant. The third type is the most indolent, IgA mesangial nephropathy.

Nephritis occurs in 50% to 80% of adults, but only 20% to 40% of children (151). In the series of 224 children with HSP reported by Sterky and Thilén, 22% had renal findings, and in follow-up of 176 of these patients, 28% had abnormal urinary findings (Table 8.6) (146). In an occasional case, the nephropathy can precede the extrarenal manifestations by months or even years (185,220,221). In patients with HSP, renal involvement usually occurs within 3 months of presentation (152,222). Gross or microscopic hematuria, with or without proteinuria, is the usual presentation.

TABLE 8.6. Renal Involvement in Children with Henoch–Schönlein Purpura

Renal involvement in 22%
Boys:girls, 3:1
Renal involvement:
Resolved by 3 mo in 50%
Resolved by 1 y in 84%
Persisted >2 y in 11% of those who had renal involvement
In total, of 154 children followed for >2 y, 7 (4.5%) still had renal involvement on follow-up
2.5% of 119 children without renal involvement at presentation later developed findings

From Sterky G, Thilén A. A study on the onset and prognosis of acute vascular purpura (the Schönlein-Henoch syndrome) in children. *Acta Paediatr* 1960;49: 217–229, with permission.

In earlier studies, rates of renal failure in children with HSP nephropathy ranged from 13.5% to 24% (220,223). In more recent studies of patients with HSP nephropathy, 1% to 5% of children develop end-stage renal disease, versus 10% to 20% in adults (151,215,224–227). HSP-related renal disease accounts for roughly 10% (3% to 15%) of children entering into end-stage renal failure programs (156,215). About 7% of all childhood glomerular nephropathies are due to HSP (136,220). Recent studies in children with severe HSP nephritis have suggested that addition of azathioprine or cyclophosphamide might be of some benefit in inducing complete or partial remissions (215,228,229).

In follow-up of a cohort of 26 boys and 26 girls with HSP into adult life, children with severe HSP purpura and glomerulonephritis were much more likely to have renal impairment as adults (35%), compared with children with mild or no renal symptoms at onset (7%) (230). Relative risk was 5 for men and 2 for women. Despite this lower risk for renal impairment, 70% of 23 pregnancies were complicated by hypertension, proteinuria, or both, a finding documented in other long-term studies (231). In adults over age 20, of more than 6,000 patients reported to the United Kingdom MRC Glomerulonephritis Registry between January 1976 and July 1986, only 47 cases (72% male) were cases of HSP nephritis (232). Follow-up data (mean, 37 months) were available in 43 of these patients: 33% were well, 27% had abnormal urinary sediment and/or hypertension, 11% had chronic renal impairment, 9% had end-stage renal failure, and 16% were dead (232). Other long-term follow-up studies have similarly found that hypertension or renal insufficiency is more frequent than in the general population (231). Hypertension occasionally develops in the absence of urinary abnormalities (233).

Results of transplantation for renal failure due to HSP nephropathy are variable, but the risk of rejection or graft failure due to recurrent disease may be significant, with four of 12 children with HSP nephropathy in one study developing renal failure after transplantation (234).

Liver disease may also be linked to IgA nephropathy. Van de Wiel et al. (235) reported that 68% of 34 patients with cirrhosis had IgA deposits in their skin, but no evidence of vasculitis. In addition to circulating IgA complexes in patients with cirrhosis, a variety of glomerular lesions have been reported from series of patients with cirrhosis, including mesangial IgA deposits. Although such deposits do not lead to renal dysfunction, at least one case has been reported that seems to link IgA complexes in cirrhosis with HSP. In that case, a rapidly progressive glomerulonephritis requiring long-term dialysis was followed by an episode of IgA cutaneous vasculitis (236).

OTHER EXTRACUTANEOUS FINDINGS IN HENOCH–SCHÖNLEIN PURPURA. Unusual presentations or sites of involvement include subcutaneous or muscular hemorrhage, ocular involvement, paroditis, intestinal infarction and perforation, esophageal involvement, hepatomegaly, asthma, hemoptysis, myocarditis, scrotal or testicular involvement, testicular swelling mimicking torsion, adrenal necrosis with Addison disease, pancreatitis, and neurologic findings such as seizures, hemiparesis, or subarachnoid hemorrhage (145,156,237,238).

Pathology and Immunopathology. The histology of HSP is that of a small-vessel leukocytoclastic vasculitis. Increasingly, the presence of IgA as the predominant immunoreactant is considered fundamental to the diagnosis of this syndrome. The histology and immunopathology of the renal disease are identical to those of Berger disease or IgA nephropathy (239).

An interesting finding from a study in 15 cases of pediatric vasculitis (mostly IgA vasculitis) is that perivascular dermal dendrocytes (factor XIIIa–positive dendritic cells) were the target of apoptotic destruction in every patient (240). It will be helpful to know if adult patients with IgA vasculitis show this perivascular dendrocytoclasis and to compare this group to factor XIIIa staining in IgG- or IgM-predominant small-vessel vasculitis.

Laboratory Manifestations. The usual nonspecific laboratory abnormalities typical of many patients with small-vessel leukocytoclastic vasculitis may be seen in HSP. In the typical case, the only tests to be monitored routinely are urinalysis, renal function, and perhaps stool testing for occult blood. Since IgA deposition is central to the diagnosis, biopsy for IIF is important, particularly in adults where the incidence of other small-vessel vasculitides is higher. Serum IgA levels may increase, and have recently been shown to be IgA1 (241). The finding of IgA as the predominant immunoreactant is not limited to idiopathic HSP, however. Patients with SLE, IgA monoclonal gammopathies, or multiple myeloma may develop syndromes of small-vessel vasculitis with similar prominent IgA deposition (W.W.P., personal observation).

Differential Diagnosis. In adults, differentiation of HSP from other vasculitic syndromes may be impossible in the absence of IIF microscopy (170). In children, SLE may rarely mimic this syndrome. Abdominal signs and symptoms of PAN or appendicitis may mimic those of HSP.

One of the more unusual concerns in the differential diagnosis of HSP is child abuse (242). In fact, HSP is one of the more dramatic syndromes of hemorrhage, which includes other vasculitides, and bleeding and clotting diatheses, which have been misdiagnosed as child abuse. Interestingly, trauma has rarely been cited as an inciting factor for HSP, both in individual cases and in families (157). Moreover, the gastrointestinal involvement in HSP may occasionally be severe and chronic enough to affect the vitamin K stores, and may result in purpura and hemorrhage related to vitamin K depletion independent of the more specific vasculitic lesions of HSP (243).

In children with the classic clinical findings of HSP, a biopsy is not necessarily indicated for diagnosis. However, in adults, particularly in patients with chronic, recurrent, or progressive disease, or with extracutaneous findings beyond mild arthralgias, a biopsy to attempt to confirm IgA deposition is prudent. In addition, in these patients with more active disease, consideration of other vasculitides is warranted, particularly if the biopsy does not show IgA deposition. Testing for systemic lupus, cryoglobulinemia, monoclonal gammopathy, rheumatoid factor, or ANCA may be indicated depending on the chronicity and severity of findings and the constellation of clinical disease present.

Management of Skin Lesions and Prognosis. Treatment of HSP should be guided by the clinical findings. Treatment includes identifying and eliminating possible causes such as infection or drugs. An underlying gammopathy might require cytotoxic therapy. Corticosteroids have been recommended in severe cases and have been used successfully to treat intestinal obstruction complicating this syndrome (156). Dapsone has been used effectively, and colchicine may prove effective in treating even very active cutaneous disease or arthralgias (244). Interestingly, in at least two patients with systemic lupus (and therefore would not be considered HSP) who have had florid extracutaneous involvement by lupus and an active cutaneous IgA vasculitis with inflammatory retiform morphology, the systemic disease has responded to high-dose corticosteroid therapy given for renal involvement, but the cutaneous vasculitis continued to worsen until colchicine at 0.6 mg orally twice daily was added (W.W.P., personal observation). The use of colchicine in IgA monoclonal gammopathy with vasculitis has not been tested.

A treatment of unproven efficacy and uncertain mechanism of action is the use of factor XIII concentrate in the treatment of recalcitrant HSP in adults (245–247). There are several reports of patients with HSP appearing to respond to infusions of factor XIII concentrate. There are several problems with interpreting these results. Despite the finding of factor XIIIa–positive perivascular dendritic cell apoptosis in one series of HSP, there is no clear-cut mechanism for factor XIII in the pathogenesis of HSP. As a clotting factor, factor XIII acts primarily to induce long-term stabilization of a clot by increasing the cross-linking between the molecular components of a clot. Levels of factor XIII reported in HSP are not low enough to approach the levels of congenital deficiency associated with a bleeding diathesis. Improvement following factor XIII infusion has occurred whether or not the factor XIII levels remained low or returned partially to normal. It is highly unlikely, if factor XIII administration has an effect in HSP, that the mechanism is mediated by elevation of only moderately low levels of factor XIII (25% to 30%) to a level near 70%.

In HSP, renal involvement typically determines prognosis, although severe gastrointestinal involvement and pulmonary involvement may be fatal (156). The prognosis of persistent HSP nephropathy appears similar to that of idiopathic IgA nephropathy, although HSP nephropathy may be more likely to remit spontaneously. In idiopathic IgA nephropathy, there is no clearly effective treatment. Factors such as greater age, male gender, hypertension, persistent proteinuria, impaired renal function at diagnosis, or glomerulosclerosis or interstitial fibrosis on renal biopsy are associated with more rapid progression in Berger disease.

As in most other forms of glomerulonephritis, severe proteinuria, impairment of renal function, and arterial hypertension predict a poor outcome, as may absence of the typical symptoms of recurrent macroscopic hematuria (202,206, 248–250). The potential therapies in IgA nephropathy have been reviewed (248). Therapy with fish oil n-3 fatty acids may slow progression of the IgA nephropathy (248,250). It appears that control of hypertension, preferably with an angiotensin-converting enzyme inhibitor, is the most effective measure known to influence the progression of idiopathic IgA nephropathy (202,206,248). Recognition and treatment of hypertension are likely to be similarly important in patients with HSP nephropathy.

LEUKOCYTOCLASTIC VASCULITIS: CRYOGLOBULINEMIC VASCULITIS, ESSENTIAL MIXED CRYOGLOBULINEMIA

Cryoglobulins are immunoglobulins that precipitate spontaneously on exposure to temperatures below 37°C, and are divided into three types based on their composition (251). A type I cryoglobulin is an isolated monoclonal immunoglobulin, most often IgM. Types II and III cryoglobulins are mixed cryoglobulins. Type II defines an immune complex of monoclonal immunoglobulin with rheumatoid factor activity binding to its antigen, the Fc portion of polyclonal IgG. The monoclonal component is again most often IgM, although it can be IgG or IgA. Type III cryoglobulins are mixed polyclonal complexes, composed of one or more classes of polyclonal immunoglobulins binding most often to IgG, but occasionally to nonimmunoglobulin molecules.

Cutaneous Manifestations. Cutaneous manifestations have been reported to occur in 67% to 100% of patients with cryoglobulinemia, and are often a presenting complaint (136, 251–253). Inflammatory, erythematous-to-purpuric macules or papules are expected findings. Raynaud disease is common. Other findings include leg ulcers (especially malleolar), petechiae, erythema multiforme–like lesions, livedo reticularis, cutaneous infarction or digital gangrene, urticaria and urticaria-like lesions, oral and nasal mucosal lesions, acrocyanosis, and erythrocyanosis.

Vasculitis has been reported as an infrequent finding in patients with type I cryoglobulinemia (88,254). A more frequent finding in type I disease may be noninflammatory hyaline thrombosis (253). Typically, reviews of the essential cryoglobulinemia syndromes do not segregate histology or cutaneous morphology by age of lesion. As mentioned previously, this has an important bearing on the interpretation of the pathophysiology of the lesion: early occlusion with subsequent necrosis, secondary inflammation, and secondary leukocytoclastic vasculitis versus early inflammation with erythema, induration and primary leukocytoclastic vasculitis followed by a mononuclear cell infiltrate and resolution. Studies such as these are extremely difficult to accomplish, especially in retrospect. Additionally, referral to major reporting centers often occurs later in the course of illness, and seclusion to a warm environment occurs naturally as a result of admission. Thus, it is often difficult to biopsy an early lesion.

One of the larger studies divided 59 patients into type I, II, or III (253). Despite histologic findings of vasculitis ranging from 33% for type I to 50% in patients with type II or III, and inflammatory lesions clinically in 92% to 100% of these patients, 71% of cutaneous infarctive lesions were seen in the type I patients. One interpretation of these findings is that they are consistent with occlusive infarction producing most skin lesion development in type I disease, and that vasculitic histology may be secondary to infarction in at least some of the type I lesions.

There is limited evidence that some type I cryoglobulin complexes may activate neutrophils after cryogelling (255). Thus, it is possible that type I cryoglobulins might induce a leukocytoclastic vasculitis, but this same study showed that the nonchilled, and therefore soluble, monoclonal cryoprotein did not activate neutrophils. This would suggest that cryogelling and microocclusion should occur first, and since ischemia or necrosis of the endothelium would likely follow microocclusion, leukocytoclasis *in vivo* would be likely to follow ischemic injury with necrosis as a secondary change.

Morphology can be very important in understanding the etiology of lesions in cryoprotein syndromes. Vessel injury due to cryofibrinogens or to monoclonal cryoglobulins (type I) causes vessel injury primarily by gelling in the cold and occluding vessels through cryoprotein gelling. Therefore, noninflammatory retiform (thrombotic) purpura is the expected morphology, and these conditions tend to cause acral lesions because those are the areas of the body that are most cold. Rarely, cryofibrinogens or cold agglutinins can cause similar lesions (256).

Because refrigeration of plasma or serum is at temperatures far below those normally expected in even acral-exposed winter skin, cryoprecipitation in the laboratory does not always translate into clinically relevant intravascular gelling with vessel occlusion. In fact, mixed cryoglobulins (type II and type III), despite cryoprecipitation in the laboratory, more typically produce an immune complex–mediated vasculitis involving small- and often medium-sized vessels. With immune complex disease (type II or III), the typical morphology is classic palpable purpura in dependent areas. Occasionally, when slightly larger vessels are involved, the skin lesions may have an inflammatory retiform morphology with erythema and induration, usually prominent in proportion to any accompanying necrosis (19).

Relationship Between Cutaneous and Systemic Features of Disease. Types II and III cryoglobulinemia are often associated with underlying collagen vascular diseases or acute and chronic infection (257). Essential cryoglobulinemia is the diagnosis given to the one third of patients with type II or III cryoglobulins who do not have an associated disorder. The category of essential mixed cryoglobulinemia is continually shrinking due to new tools to look for hepatitis B and C. Prior to the recognition of chronic hepatitis C as a significant underlying factor, from 28% to 57% of cases of mixed cryoglobulinemia were classified as idiopathic (258). Nearly all patients with mixed cryoglobulinemia have cryoprecipitate with rheumatoid factor activity (259). The prevalence of mixed cryoglobulinemia is higher in Southern Europe than in Northern Europe or North America, and this is related to the prevalence of hepatitis C infection in those geographic regions. In a study of 190 Italian patients referred to rheumatologists for mixed cryoglobulinemia, the mean age of patients was 50 years, the disease duration was 12 years, and females outnumbered males three to one (30). Purpura (91%), weakness (90%), and arthralgias (80%) were the three most common clinical features. The incidence of sicca syndrome, renal involvement (membranoproliferative glomerulonephritis), Raynaud phenomenon, and peripheral neuropathy ranged from 33% to 39% for each finding. Hepatitis C virus (HCV) RNA (88%) and anti-HCV antibodies (92%) were very common, anti–hepatitis B virus (HBV) antibodies (42%) were common, and HbsAg (4%) was rare.

Clinical features of cryoglobulinemia result primarily from vasculitis or occlusion of small vessels. Large-vessel involvement with aneurysm formation is rare (260). Dependent palpable purpura and arthritis or arthralgias are the most common presenting symptoms, but renal disease is also common. Gastrointestinal, peripheral and central nervous system, or pulmonary involvement is less frequent (251,252,259,261). Some patients may develop HSP-like abdominal symptoms (136). Gelling of cryoglobulins (monoclonal or mixed) may occur secondary to extreme osmotic shifts or changes in protein concentration and hematocrit as might be seen in transit through the renal circulation, but the extent to which this gelling is responsible for the renal disease is unclear (251).

Systemic disease is frequent and includes peripheral neuropathy, arthralgias, renal disease (proteinuria, azotemia, and/or hypertension), hepatic dysfunction, hepatosplenomegaly, intestinal vasculitis, and coronary vasculitis (251,262, 263). Associated diseases include autoimmune diseases such as SLE, Sjögren syndrome, and Behçet syndrome; lymphoproliferative diseases such as multiple myeloma, Waldenström macroglobulinemia, lymphoma, and chronic lymphocytic leukemia; and infections such as hepatitis, infectious mononucleosis, cytomegalovirus, subacute bacterial endocarditis, and toxoplasmosis (253,257).

Pathology, Immunopathology, and Laboratory Manifestations. Cryoglobulins are immunoglobulins that reversibly precipitate or gel on exposure to cold (251,264). Their detection and analysis are fundamental to the diagnosis of a cryoglobulinemia syndrome. The simplest screen involves drawing a serum (clot) and plasma sample, and maintaining it at 37°C until separation is complete. These tubes are then placed at 4°C for several days, to induce gelling of any cryoprotein. Monoclonal cryoglobulins (type I) are usually the earliest to gel, whereas mixed cryoglobulins (especially type III) may take several days to gel. Precipitation in both the serum and plasma tube suggests the presence of cryoglobulinemia. Precipitation in only the plasma tube suggests cryofibrinogenemia. A larger cryocrit in the serum tube compared to the plasma tube suggests the presence of both cryoglobulin and cryofibrinogen. Rewarming to 37°C with disappearance of the cryogel confirms cryogelling as opposed to nonspecific-protein precipitation. This screening method will not detect the presence of cold agglutinins, nor is it a sensitive method for detecting small quantities of cryoprotein.

Once a cryoglobulin is isolated, immunoelectrophoresis or immunofixation can be used to analyze its composition. Approximately 25% of cryoglobulins are type I monoclonal immunoglobulins (251,264). In order of frequency, they are IgM, IgG, IgA, or light chains. Type II cryoglobulins contain a monoclonal and a polyclonal element, and comprise approximately 25% of cryoglobulins. The monoclonal immunoglobulin always has rheumatoid factor activity, and is usually an IgM but can be an IgG or IgA rheumatoid factor. Unfortunately, current commercial assays detect only IgM rheumatoid factor. The antigen bound by the monoclonal rheumatoid factor is the Fc portion of polyclonal IgG, comprising the second component of type II cryoglobulins. The most common cryoglobulin in clinical practice is type III, accounting for about 50% of cryoglobulins, and nearly all of these are composed of polyclonal IgM rheumatoid factor binding to polyclonal IgG.

IIF studies of skin biopsy specimens usually reveal deposits in vessels of the same immunoglobulin components found in the patient's serum cryoglobulin (264). The spectrum of histologic findings on skin biopsy of vascular lesions includes vasculitis, inflammatory and noninflammatory purpura, noninflammatory (bland) hyaline thrombosis, and postinflammatory sequelae (253). Most studies have suggested a low incidence of vasculitis in type I cryoglobulinemia, emphasizing noninflammatory hyaline thrombosis as the more common cutaneous finding in this subset (88,251,254,265). Vasculitis has been reported as approximately equal in incidence to hyaline occlusion as a histopathologic finding in the skin (253). Whether this histologic picture is a result of late biopsy of a bland infarctive lesion or represents, in fact, a leukocytoclastic vasculitis triggered during cryoprecipitation, will require careful prospective study. Although type II and type III behave as cryoglobulins in the test tube, they more often induce clinical disease as immune complexes, and the expected histology is predominantly that of leukocytoclastic vasculitis rather than hyaline thrombosis.

Hepatitis and Cryoglobulinemia. It seems likely, based on accumulating evidence, that viral hepatitis is a significant cause of otherwise apparently idiopathic mixed cryoglobulinemia. Hepatitis A has been associated with cryoglobulinemia and cutaneous vasculitis, although the association is rare and may be secondary to the extremely low incidence of chronic infection associated with the hepatitis A virus (266–268). Hepatitis B has been implicated as an important underlying disease in mixed cryoglobulinemia (269,270). However, hepatitis C has emerged as a major cause of essential mixed cryoglobulinemia. In fact, up to 90% of patients with essential mixed cryoglobulinemia appear to have HCV RNA in their serum (271–273). Immune response to the virus elicits a response to the Fc portion of immunoglobulin with most elicited antibody having the Wa idiotype, presumably due to a cross-reactive idiotype on HCV and immunoglobulin (28). These viral and rheumatoid factor complexes precipitate on exposure to cold. In one study of 59 consecutive patients with chronic hepatitis C, rheumatoid factor was found in 71% and a serum cryoglobulin in 36% (274). Numerous studies find low levels of mixed cryoglobulins in greater than 50% of HCV-infected individuals, but also find only a small minority of these patients develop a mixed cryoglobulinemia syndrome (30).

In a study involving 115 consecutive patients with unselected mixed cryoglobulinemia, 45% had well-defined underlying diseases, whereas 55% were considered initially to have essential mixed cryoglobulinemia (275). Antibodies to HCV were found in 41% of the 115 patients, with an incidence of 27% in those with underlying disease and 52% of those thought initially to have essential or idiopathic disease. Among the 63 patients with essential mixed cryoglobulinemia, the 33 patients with anti-HCV antibodies were compared to the 30 patients who were antibody-negative. Antibody-positive patients had more frequent cutaneous involvement (Raynaud phenomenon, purpura, livedo, distal ulcers, or gangrenous changes) and higher serum cryoglobulin levels than the antibody-negative group of patients with essential mixed cryoglobulinemia.

A second study examined prospectively clinical, biochemical, and immunologic abnormalities in a series of 61 consecutive patients with chronic hepatitis C, compared to those in 61 patients with chronic hepatitis B, and to a control group of 61 age- and sex-matched subjects without markers of HCV and HBV infections (276). Cryoglobulinemia was found in 36% of the patients with HCV, four of whom had dermatologic and/or neurologic manifestations of vasculitis, and rheumatoid factor was present in 70%. Serum antitissue antibodies were detected in 41% of cases, mostly antinuclear and anti–smooth muscle antibodies. Salivary gland lesions were found in 49% of the patients, sometimes associated with lymphocytic sialoadenitis resembling that of Sjögren syndrome, but without Ro(SS-A) antibodies or features of sicca syndrome. The prevalences of cryoglobulinemia, rheumatoid factor, and antitissue antibodies were significantly higher than those in the control group and in patients with chronic hepatitis B. Lichen planus was present in 5% of the patients.

Differential Diagnosis. The differential diagnosis of essential mixed cryoglobulinemia includes those vasculitides that involve small or small- and medium-sized vessels, both in the skin and in other organs. At times, nearly all vasculitides that can affect these vessels, including HSP, PAN, WG, or the rheumatic vasculitides, may present with a constellation of findings suggestive of essential mixed cryoglobulinemia. Of course, diseases such as SLE or Sjögren syndrome may be the reason for high-titer mixed cryoglobulinemia (277). Further confusing the clinical picture, low-titer cryoglobulinemia may accompany some of the remaining vasculitides. Hypocomplementemia is found in 90% of patients with cryoglobulinemic vasculitis, with fluctuating C3 levels and usually low to very low C4 (278). This is an aid in distinguishing cryoglobulinemic vasculitis from ANCA-positive vasculitides, which can present with overlapping clinical features.

It is increasingly evident that chronic hepatitis secondary to the hepatitis A, B, and especially C viruses account for a major percentage of the previously idiopathic or essential mixed cryoglobulinemia group. In patients in whom noninflammatory infarctive or retiform lesions predominant, or whose histology suggests significant bland occlusion, a type I cryoglobulinemia, cryofibrinogenemia, cold agglutinin disease, or other microvascular occlusive syndrome should be considered. Clonal lymphoproliferative diseases such as multiple myeloma or lymphoma should be suspected in type I or II cryoglobulinemia, but it is also clear that hepatitis C can induce a type II syndrome. The diagnosis of essential mixed cryoglobulinemia is suggested by the clinical syndrome, supported by the presence of a type II or type III cryoglobulin, and confirmed by the exclusion of similar vasculitis syndromes and known associated diseases.

Management of Skin Lesions and Prognosis. Many patients do not require treatment. Of course, patients with cold-exacerbated disease should be protected from the cold. Cryoglobulinemic glomerulonephritis is almost exclusively associated with type II, rather than type III, mixed cryoglobulinemia (278). Bacteria-related cryoglobulinemic vasculitis (e.g., with infectious endocarditis) requires antibiotic therapy. Severe symptoms or renal involvement may respond to corticosteroid and immunosuppressant therapy, and in patients with underlying lymphoproliferative disease, the use of cytotoxic drugs may be of benefit (252,279). Plasmapheresis may be temporarily beneficial (280). Prednisone and immunosuppressive agents are not of proven efficacy, but can be indicated when manifestations with a poor prognosis are present (251,263). Boom et al. (281) described a patient with long-standing severe leukocytoclastic cutaneous vasculitis and type II cryoglobulinemia who failed to respond to therapy with immunosuppressive drugs, plasmapheresis, and colchicine. Therapy with high-dose γ-globulin intravenously for 5 days resulted in disappearance of vasculitis lesions within 3 weeks. Cryoglobulins, circulating immune complexes, and IgM paraprotein dropped and complement levels rose. There were no serious side effects and the patient remained in remission for at least 16 months.

Therapy of Hepatitis C in Patients with Cryoglobulinemia. Findings from several studies suggest that some patients with hepatitis C and mixed cryoglobulinemia may have a beneficial clinical response of their vasculitic symptoms to therapy with interferon-α (282–287). The introduction of interferon–ribavirin combination therapy has markedly improved clinical outcomes in hepatitis C–infected individuals, but the current sustained virologic response rate with this therapy is still only 40% (288). The standard combination regimen is 3 million units of interferon-α given subcutaneously three times weekly, and ribavirin 1,000 (patients < 75kg) or 1,200 mg (patients ≥ 75kg) orally. However, harmful immune-mediated side effects may occur, such as induction or worsening of peripheral sensory-motor neuropathy (30). Because of the low rate of response to interferon alone, the high rate of relapse following this therapy, and the risk of autoimmune complications, alternative regimens are usually considered.

Immunosuppressive agents are used to treat symptomatic patients with non–HCV-associated mixed cryoglobulinemia, HCV-associated cases in which antiviral therapy fails, and HCV-associated cases with acute exacerbations or rapidly progressive illness (30,278). Interferon therapy should probably not be started in HCV-associated cryoglobulinemic vasculitis until rapidly progressive symptoms are stabilized, despite the possibility that immunosuppression may enhance viral replication. Low-antigen-content diet, corticosteroids, plasma exchange, and other immunosuppressive agents, especially cyclophosphamide, may be considered in such cases (30). Oral cyclophosphamide at a dose of 50 to 100 mg per day for 2 to 6 weeks during tapering of plasmapheresis may prevent rebound of cryocrit levels after discontinuation of plasma exchange. Once a patient's symptoms are controlled, interferon and ribavirin can be used in an attempt to control the infection (289).

Polyarteritis Nodosa: Classic Polyarteritis Nodosa, Microscopic Polyangiitis, and Benign Cutaneous Polyarteritis Nodosa

The syndromes of PAN are a natural bridge from small-vessel vasculitis to the medium-sized vessel vasculitides because the histology is usually leukocytoclastic, and the vessels involved are frequently small and cutaneous, as in the microscopic polyangiitis group, or may be limited to medium-sized vessels as in classic PAN.

The classification of PAN has been at least as problematic as that of hypersensitivity vasculitis. Braverman (1), among others, has maintained that there are at least three clinical syndromes of PAN based on cutaneous findings: (a) vessel involvement limited to medium-sized vessels with both acute and chronic histologic changes; (b) vessel involvement of both small- and medium-sized vessels, usually with an acute necrotizing vasculitis histology; and (c) a possible subset of benign cutaneous PAN. Nevertheless, for many years studies of PAN have been reported without distinction between patients in the first two categories. In recent years, the diagnosis of microscopic polyarteritis has become increasingly more important. The CHCG separates PAN syndromes into classic PAN and microscopic polyangiitis, but does not recognize a benign cutaneous subset (12). Classic PAN is restricted to disease in which there is arteritis primarily in medium-sized arteries with no capillary or venular involvement, including no glomerulonephritis or alveolar capillaritis (37). Microscopic polyangiitis includes syndromes of pauci-immune (i.e., few or no immune deposits) small-vessel leukocytoclastic vasculitis, with or without occasional involvement of medium-sized arteries. The lack of immune deposits distinguishes microscopic polyangiitis from immune complex vasculitis such as mixed cryoglobulinemia or HSP. The term "polyangiitis" was selected in lieu of "polyarteritis" because many patients with microscopic polyangiitis do not have arterial vasculitis, but do have lesions in arterioles, venules, and capillaries. Similar vascular findings are seen in WG and Churg–Strauss syndrome, but the former is distinguished by the addition of granulomatous inflammation and the latter by the presence of asthma and eosinophilia (37). Likewise, most patients formerly classified as having polyangiitis overlap syndrome would fall into the microscopic polyangiitis category (12). Benign cutaneous PAN, an important syndrome in the dermatologic literature, will be discussed later.

Determining the incidence and prevalence of the PAN syndromes is difficult because, until recently, most series have not distinguished between variants. PAN appears to be an uncommon, but not rare, disease. Mean age at onset of systemic PAN is 48 to 50 years, with a male predominance (290,291).

CUTANEOUS MANIFESTATIONS

There are differences in cutaneous presentations between the subsets of polyarteritis due to differences in the sizes of the involved vessels.

Classic Polyarteritis Nodosa. Classic PAN involving only the skin is a rare occurrence (1). The only reliable cutaneous signs of classic PAN seem to be the following: ulceration resulting from infarction, peripheral gangrene of fingers and toes, ecchymoses resulting from the rupture of aneurysms and weakened walls of necrotic arteries, and subcutaneous nodules that are no larger than 5 to 10 mm and that follow the course of the arteries (1). The nodules represent aneurysmal dilatation of underlying arteries and may be pulsatile.

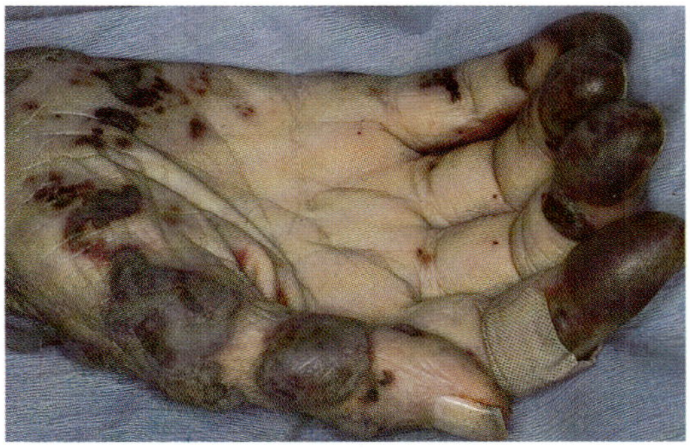

Figure 8.13. Microscopic polyangiitis. Purpuric plaques in a patient with glomerulonephritis, multisystem disease, and high-titer p-ANCA (perinuclear antineutrophil cytoplasmic antibodies), who died from sepsis following vasculitic bowel infarction.

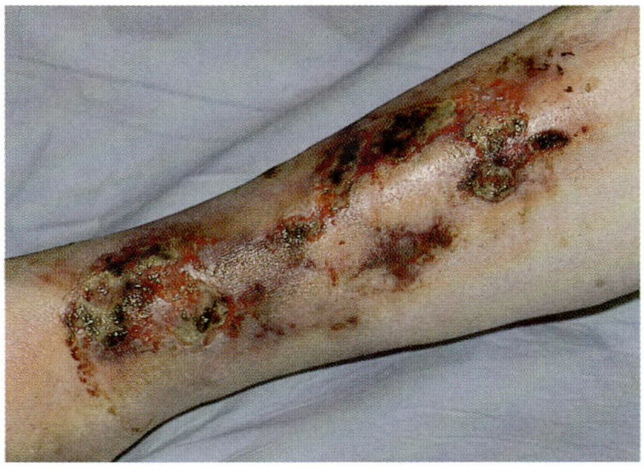

Figure 8.14. "Benign cutaneous" polyarteritis nodosa. Patient with 1-year history of progressive ulceration of tender nodules with surrounding livedo reticularis and areas of inflammatory retiform hemorrhage. Fever and myalgias are present but the patient is antineutrophil cytoplasmic antibodies–negative. Healing was achieved with pulse and daily corticosteroid therapy.

Microscopic Polyangiitis. As defined by the CHCG, both classic PAN and microscopic polyangiitis can affect arteries in the skin causing nodules, but only microscopic polyangiitis can also affect vessels smaller than arteries and cause purpura (13). Of course, involvement of the arterioles in the fat can lead to cutaneous nodule formation as well, and is the usual etiology of cutaneous nodules in microscopic polyangiitis. The skin is involved in about 30% to 40% of patients (290–293). Cutaneous manifestations include palpable purpura, splinter hemorrhages, and cutaneous ulcers (especially on the legs) (Fig. 8.13) (291–294). Livedo reticularis and tender subcutaneous nodules have not been reported in microscopic polyangiitis (290). However, until recently, most studies of cutaneous manifestations of PAN have failed to separate microscopic polyangiitis. In at least two studies, several patients classified as having benign cutaneous PAN because of tender cutaneous nodules, livedo reticularis, or characteristic cutaneous histology, would seem on the basis of lung and/or renal involvement to fit into the microscopic polyangiitis category instead (294,295). ANCA studies were not available in these patients. Until this is clarified, the presence or absence of tender nodules or livedo reticularis should probably not be considered unique to the benign cutaneous PAN category of patients.

Benign Cutaneous Polyarteritis Nodosa. A more limited form of PAN has also been described. Called benign cutaneous polyarteritis (periarteritis) nodosa, this vasculitis primarily involves arterioles located in the deep reticular dermis and upper subcutaneous fat (294,296). Cutaneous findings in benign cutaneous PAN can be similar to those of microscopic polyangiitis, but tender subcutaneous nodules are more frequently associated with the benign cutaneous form (Fig. 8.14) (296).

Except for infantile PAN (Kawasaki disease), which presents in a very different fashion, syndromes of polyarteritis, including benign cutaneous PAN, are rare in children (297,298). Of children reported, nearly all have had tender cutaneous nodules as part of their clinical presentation, and several have had digital cyanosis (297–299).

Interestingly, there appears to be a syndrome of cutaneous vasculitis in newborns of mothers with cutaneous PAN. This association in three cases suggests that a circulating factor may cross the placenta and may play a role in the genesis of this syndrome (298). In the patient of Stone et al. (298), digital cyanosis was followed by infarction of a toe, a finding that is otherwise extremely rare in benign cutaneous PAN. The mother of the proband in this report has had a second child, who also developed a neonatal benign cutaneous PAN syndrome (M. Seabury-Stone, personal communication). The affected children and their mother are ANCA-negative. Two additional children reported with benign cutaneous PAN were also ANCA-negative (299).

Relationship Between Cutaneous and Systemic Features of Disease. Most larger series of patients with PAN were published without regard to classic or microscopic subsets. Most patients present with fever, malaise, myalgias, and arthralgias (291,292,300,301). Many are also found to have hypertension, peripheral neuritis, and liver dysfunction. Pulmonary arteries are not involved in classic PAN, and bronchial artery involvement is uncommon. By definition, patients with glomerular or pulmonary alveolar capillary involvement could not be included as classic PAN in the CHCG classification, and would instead be grouped into microscopic polyangiitis (12).

The findings of a study of 64 patients with PAN are listed in Table 8.7 (2,302). Patients from the study of Leib et al. (302) were included in the summary of 507 patients by Cupps and Fauci (2), but are worth considering separately because patients with skin-limited disease were excluded from their 64-patient series.

Polyarteritis can be associated with methamphetamine abuse, allergic hyposensitization, drug reactions, rheumatoid arthritis, SLE, mixed cryoglobulinemia, familial Mediterranean

TABLE 8.7. Clinical Findings in Patients with Systemic Polyarteritis Nodosa Syndromes

Clinical Finding	Leib et al.[a] (%)	Cupps and Fauci[b] (%)
Fever	36	71
Musculoskeletal	73	64
Hypertension	55	54
Peripheral neuropathy	72 (includes CNS)	51
GI/liver	42	44
Skin	28	43
Cardiovascular	30	36
CNS	(see neuropathy)	23

CNS, central nervous system; GI, gastrointestinal.
[a]From Lieb ES, Restivo C, Paulus HE. Immunosuppressive and corticosteroid therapy of polyarteritis nodosa. *Am J Med* 1979;67(6):941–947.
[b]From Cupps TR, Fauci AS. The vasculitides. In Smith LH Jr, ed. *Major problems in internal medicine*. Vol. XXI. Philadelphia: WB Saunders, 1981.

fever, chronic hepatitis B antigenemia, as well as following B-streptococcal infections, acute postinfectious serous otitis, trichinosis, HIV infection, and possibly Parvovirus B19 infection (1,136,299,303–307). PAN in many of these settings has tended to involve small and large vessels; therefore, at least some patients with these associations would fit best in the microscopic polyangiitis category.

Patients with hairy cell leukemia appear to have an increased risk of developing a vasculitis, usually PAN (308–310). PAN has also been associated with a variety of other lymphoreticular malignancies (11). The etiology of these associations is unknown.

Most estimates of the hepatitis B–associated PAN range from 10% to 30% of patients, although an incidence of up to 54% hepatitis B antigen positivity has been reported in one series of 55 patients (136,311). In general, no clinical features have been identified that discriminate PAN patients with or without hepatitis B antigenemia. However, one recent study has suggested that orchitis may be more common and pulmonary disease less common in the hepatitis B–associated PAN subset (312).

Microscopic Polyangiitis. In patients with microscopic polyangiitis, sore throat and seasonal exacerbations are common (291,292). Renal disease is the most common clinical feature, especially glomerulonephritis, and 30% of patients have pulmonary involvement (269,291,292). Less common findings include abdominal pain, peripheral neuropathy, arthritis, oral and ocular involvement, hearing loss, epistaxis, and pericarditis or arrhythmia (see Fig. 8.13) (290).

Benign Cutaneous Polyarteritis Nodosa, Including Childhood Forms. Benign cutaneous PAN is distinguished by the lack of severe systemic disease (see Fig. 8.14) (11,313,314). Although cutaneous PAN is thought to be a localized vasculitic process, systemic features such as fever, neuropathy, myalgias, arthralgias, and arthritis are frequent (272–274,294,296,299). These findings are also seen in children with this syndrome (297–299). In addition, some patients have associated systemic diseases including inflammatory bowel disease (both Crohn and ulcerative colitis), hepatitis B infection, or paraproteinemia (294,315–317). Both systemic and cutaneous PANs are known to occur after upper respiratory infections, including streptococcal infections (299). In addition rheumatic heart disease, known sequelae of streptococcal infection may coexist with PAN (299).

An interesting finding that supports benign cutaneous PAN as a distinct PAN subset is an apparent association with inflammatory bowel disease, especially Crohn disease (316,318). There have been 11 cases with this association, and in most instances the Crohn disease preceded the development of the cutaneous (and apparently skin-limited) PAN. In at least one of the cases, the intestinal signs and symptoms of Crohn disease were used initially in reasonable but ultimately incorrect support of the diagnosis of systemic PAN. Sulfasalazine therapy may improve both PAN and bowel disease. Resection of diseased bowel may sometimes be followed by remission of the skin disease.

PATHOLOGY AND IMMUNOPATHOLOGY

In the acute stages of disease, polymorphonuclear neutrophils infiltrate all layers of the vessel wall and perivascular areas, leading to intimal proliferation and degeneration of the vessel wall. Mononuclear cells infiltrate the area as the lesions progress to the subacute and chronic stages. Fibrinoid necrosis of the vessels ensues with compromise of the lumen, thrombosis, infarction of the tissues supplied by the involved vessel, and in some cases hemorrhage. As the lesions heal, there is collagen deposition, which may lead to further occlusion of the vessel lumen. Aneurysmal dilatations up to 1 cm in size along the involved arteries are characteristic of classic PAN. Granulomas and substantial eosinophilia with eosinophilic tissue infiltrations are not characteristically found, and suggest allergic angiitis and granulomatosis. Because the vessels in the skin, including subcutaneous tissue, are smaller than those involved in classic PAN, a diagnosis of classic PAN is not possible from the skin biopsy findings alone (1,319).

Microscopic polyangiitis is a systemic vasculitis affecting small vessels of arteriolar or capillary size, associated with focal and segmental necrotizing glomerular nephritis (290, 291). The cutaneous histology of microscopic polyangiitis is that of leukocytoclastic vasculitis. Microscopic polyangiitis involves the small arterioles of the reticular dermis more often than other syndromes of cutaneous leukocytoclastic vasculitis, which usually involve only the postcapillary superficial dermal venules. Moreover, microscopic polyangiitis seems to spare the subcutaneous arterioles typically seen in benign cutaneous PAN (290).

Microscopic polyangiitis, WG, and Churg–Strauss vasculitis are all ANCA-positive syndromes and can cause dermal leukocytoclastic vasculitis. By immunohistologic examination, all three have minimal or no immune deposits (pauci-immune vasculitis) (13). WG and Churg–Strauss syndrome can also cause focal cutaneous and subcutaneous granulomatous inflammation manifested clinically as skin nodules. The presence of necrotizing granulomatous inflammation in the upper or lower respiratory tract (and sometimes skin) is indicative of WG, whereas the presence of asthma and eosinophilia is indicative of Churg–Strauss syndrome. In the absence of any of these specific features, microscopic polyangiitis becomes the diagnosis (13).

In a series of patients with benign cutaneous PAN, Diaz-Perez and Winkelmann (320) found in all cases a necrotizing arteritis involving the small- and medium-sized arteries in the panniculus and occasionally in the lower dermis. The small vessels of the middle and upper dermis showed only a nonspecific lymphocytic perivascular infiltrate (320). In addition, although some have argued that involvement of the vessels in deep reticular dermis and fat is more typical of benign cutaneous PAN than of cutaneous lesions of microscopic polyangiitis, this histologic distinction is probably not reliable (294). Biopsy findings in childhood benign cutaneous PAN are similar to those in adults (297–299).

LABORATORY MANIFESTATIONS

In over 75% of patients, the leukocyte count is elevated with a predominance of neutrophils (136). Eosinophilia is seen only rarely and when present at high levels, suggests the diagnosis of Churg–Strauss granulomatosis. The anemia of chronic disease may be seen, and an elevated erythrocyte sedimentation rate is usually present. Hypocomplementemia, positive rheumatoid factor, and circulating immune complexes are common findings. Other common laboratory findings reflect the particular organ involved. Hypergammaglobulinemia may be present, and 10% to 30% of patients have a positive test for HBsAg (136).

In a series selected for microscopic polyangiitis, most patients had an elevated erythrocyte sedimentation rate, a normochromic normocytic anemia, leukocytosis, and an elevated C-reactive protein (290). Rheumatoid factor was detected in fewer than 50% of patients, and ANA was usually negative, as was serologic evidence of hepatitis B infection.

The incidence of ANCA positivity in patients with classic PAN is low, regardless of whether the PAN is idiopathic or hepatitis B–associated (see Table 8.3) (44,290,321). In another series, ANCA positivity in 44 patients with classic PAN defined by CHCG criteria was 2% c-ANCA and 16% p-ANCA (MPO) (321). Of patients who were hepatitis B–positive, only two (9%) 22 were p-ANCA (MPO)–positive, and none had c-ANCA.

In contrast, microscopic polyangiitis is ANCA positive in nearly 100% of cases, split between p-ANCA and c-ANCA patterns (see Tables 8.3 and 8.4) (44,50). Patients with p-ANCA are much more likely to have microscopic polyangiitis than WG (12). WG is nearly 100% ANCA-positive, but in 80% to 85% of cases, the pattern is c-ANCA and the antigen specificity is PR3. In contrast, Churg–Strauss syndrome is ANCA-positive in 80% of cases, but usually with a p-ANCA pattern and MPO specificity. Results of ANCA testing in benign cutaneous PAN are very limited, but at least some patients with this syndrome are ANCA-negative (298,299) (see Fig. 8.14).

DIFFERENTIAL DIAGNOSIS

The diagnosis of PAN is based on the clinical presentation, the laboratory findings (especially ANCA positivity, pattern, and antigen specificity), and usually on the demonstration of characteristic findings of vasculitis on biopsy material of involved organs. WG, allergic granulomatosis of Churg–Strauss, or small-vessel vasculitides with necrotizing glomerular nephritis must be excluded as causes before the diagnosis of microscopic polyangiitis can be made (290,291). The association of the PAN syndromes with a variety of underlying conditions (as noted before) must be considered in evaluating patients at presentation. In the absence of easily accessible tissue for biopsy, the angiographic demonstration of involved vessels, particularly in the form of aneurysms of small- and medium-sized arteries in the renal, hepatic, and visceral vasculature, may be sufficient to make the diagnosis in the appropriate clinical setting. Aneurysms of vessels are not pathognomonic of classic PAN, and aneurysms need not always be present. Such aneurysms can also be seen in collagen vascular disease, WG, atrial myxoma, subacute bacterial endocarditis, and Kawasaki disease (136). Biopsy of symptomatic organs such as nodular skin lesions, painful testes, or muscle provides the highest diagnostic yields, whereas blind biopsy of asymptomatic organs is frequently negative.

The diagnosis of benign cutaneous PAN is one of exclusion. Nodules, which are characteristic of benign cutaneous PAN, are rare in classic PAN and less common in microscopic polyangiitis (291,300). The nodules of benign cutaneous PAN are usually painful and may ulcerate, and livedo reticularis often surrounds the nodules in a starburst pattern (320).

All forms of PAN (other than Kawasaki disease) are rare in childhood (297–299). Juvenile rheumatoid arthritis has been cited as an important differential consideration due to its presentation with cyclic high fevers, arthralgias, arthritis, and rash (297). However, the evanescent macular to finely papular or urticarial truncal eruption of juvenile rheumatoid arthritis is very different from the usual cutaneous manifestations of the PAN subsets. The possible association of underlying infection, especially streptococcal, is important to consider in pediatric patients (299).

MANAGEMENT OF SKIN LESIONS AND PROGNOSIS

The prognosis of untreated systemic PAN is extremely poor, with a 5-year survival rate of 10% to 13% (302). Renal failure, bowel infarction or perforation, or cardiovascular complications are the usual cause of death. Severe hypertension frequently hastens deterioration and complicates management. In patients with microscopic polyangiitis, death is usually from pulmonary hemorrhage or renal failure (291).

Patients with immediately life-threatening PAN or factors associated with a poor prognosis should be treated with cyclophosphamide and corticosteroid, using the WG protocol. Favorable therapeutic results have been reported in systemic PAN with the combination of prednisone 1 mg/kg per day and cyclophosphamide 2 mg/kg per day. This regimen has achieved up to a 90% long-term remission rate even following the discontinuation of therapy. However, in five large series reported from 1967 to 1995, the 5-year survival rate has remained constant, ranging between 55% and 63% (322). These figures suggest that the addition of other immunosuppressive agents to corticosteroid therapy may have had a minimal effect on the 5-year survival rate, but a large enough study directed at this issue has not been completed. Certainly, corticosteroid monotherapy improves the 5-year survival rate in PAN, and the question of whether cytotoxic agents improve remission or survival rates has been somewhat clouded because many studies include patients with Churg–Strauss in their analysis (73). Careful attention to the treatment of hypertension can lessen the acute and late morbidity and mortality associated with renal, cardiac, and central nervous system complications of PAN. Patients with cutaneous PAN who are ANCA-negative are at lower risk for having or subsequently developing small-vessel vasculitis in the skin or other organs (13).

In microscopic polyangiitis specifically, therapy with corticosteroids, cyclophosphamide, and azathioprine resulted in an improvement of the 5-year survival rate to 65% by 1985 (291). There have been no prospective studies that have specifically examined the treatment of microscopic polyangiitis alone (73). The rate of remission, relapse, and treatment resistance was studied in 97 ANCA-positive patients with either microscopic polyangiitis or necrotizing and crescentic glomerulonephritis treated with corticosteroids with or without cyclophosphamide (323). Both disease groups responded similarly to therapy, with a 56% remission rate with corticosteroids alone and 85% with the addition of cyclophosphamide. The cyclophosphamide-treated group had three-times lower risk of relapse than did the group treated with corticosteroids alone. Relapses occurred in 29% of patients, and generally responded to retreatment. Patients with life-threatening disease at the time of presentation may die before induction therapy can be completed, emphasizing the need for early diagnosis and treatment.

Long-term remissions have been reported in PAN associated with HBV antigenemia using the antiviral agent vidarabine in combination with plasma exchange with and without corticosteroids (312). A study of interferon-α2b and plasma exchange therapy in hepatitis B–associated PAN has reported effective clearing of vasculitis in six of six patients (324). Intravenous immunoglobulin therapy has been used to clear PAN-like vasculitis in two patients with chronic Parvovirus B19 infections (307). The therapy of choice for vasculitis in HIV-infected individuals is far from clear (305).

Treatment of hairy cell leukemia–associated PAN with prednisone or cyclophosphamide has been variably successful; therapy may worsen the cytopenias associated with the leukemia (308–310,325). Treatment with interferon-α has been successful in one case, while avoiding the cytopenic complications (325).

The prognosis for patients with benign cutaneous PAN is good, but a chronic course is common (11). Patients with predominantly cutaneous disease do not require aggressive therapy beyond that needed to control symptoms. Regular follow-up is advised. It is not appropriate to rely only on the presence of tender subcutaneous nodules with surrounding livedo reticularis in assigning a patient to this category. Based on negative ANCA testing in at least some patients who fit the benign cutaneous PAN profile, ANCA testing may be useful in distinguishing patients with relatively skin-limited disease, and in predicting a good prognosis for patients with similar cutaneous findings but a course ultimately more typical of microscopic polyangiitis. Future studies are needed to address this issue.

The use of nonsteroidal antiinflammatory agents or corticosteroids has resulted in clinical improvement in most children with benign cutaneous PAN (297–299). Antibiotic therapy, including prophylaxis, was also used in the treatment of some of these patients (299).

Granulomatous Vasculitis: Wegener Granulomatosis

WG is a diagnosis restricted to patients with granulomatous inflammation by the CHCG criteria (12). Patients with exclusively nongranulomatous small-vessel vasculitis involving the upper or lower respiratory tract (e.g., alveolar capillaritis) would fall into the category of microscopic polyangiitis.

Classic WG is characterized by the triad of necrotizing granulomas of the upper or lower respiratory tracts, focal glomerulonephritis, and varying degrees of systemic vasculitis. Limited WG involves only the respiratory tract.

The pathogenesis of this disease is not known. Immune complex disease is not the likely cause of WG, although circulating and deposited immune complexes are occasional findings. Delayed hypersensitivity reaction is a possible mechanism, but again there is insufficient evidence to support this mechanism as primary. As discussed before, there is a possible role of ANCA in the pathogenesis of WG and perhaps other vasculitides, but this remains a hypothesis under active investigation.

WG is an uncommon disease. In a recent series of 158 patients from the United States, the incidence was equal by sex, but extremely rare in black patients (2%) compared with white (97%) (326). The mean age of onset was 41 years, with a range of 9 to 78 years. Although approximately 15% of patients are younger than 19 years of age, only rarely does the disease occur before adolescence (326). In a recent series of 265 patients from the United Kingdom, the mean age was 50 years, with a range of 10 to 83 years, and a slight male to female predominance (55% to 45%, respectively) (327).

CUTANEOUS MANIFESTATIONS

In several larger series emphasizing systemic disease, specific cutaneous disease was present at diagnosis in 20% to 25% of patients with WG, occurred usually in 14% to 66% of patients sometime during the course of the disease, but was the presenting sign in only 8.6% to 25% (326–329). Two similar studies emphasizing cutaneous findings in 40 and 75 patients found a 45% to 47% overall incidence of skin or mucosal disease, respectively, and in 10% to 11%, respectively, of all patients these were the presenting findings (330,331). The difference in the incidence of cutaneous findings depends in part on the percentage of patients with generalized or chronic disease versus limited or early WG. Patients with limited disease comprised 70% of 244 patients and had only a 4.4% incidence of cutaneous disease, whereas the remaining 30% of patients with generalized disease had a 40% incidence of skin findings (328). The ratio of patients with generalized versus limited disease in this study seemed much lower than in the other studies cited, presumably accounting for the lower incidence of skin disease. The most commonly involved site is the leg, but lesions are also frequent on the trunk, upper extremities, face, and neck (328,330,332).

Purpuric lesions (sometimes necrotic or ecchymotic) are the most frequently encountered cutaneous lesions. Necrotic papules of the limbs are somewhat more suggestive of WG than of other vasculitides (331). Common lesional morphology includes palpable purpura, petechiae, ecchymoses, papules, hemorrhagic bullae, necrotic papules, ulcers, or subcutaneous nodules (see Fig. 8.8) (330–335). Ulcers may have a morphology and behavior resembling pyoderma gangrenosum (328,331,335–337) (see Fig. 8.9). Like pyoderma gangrenosum, they may follow trauma, such as intramuscular injection, or may evolve from painful pustules or nodules, although the rolled and undermined margin of pyoderma gangrenosum may be lacking. In one large series, 27% of patients with cutaneous findings had such ulcers (328).

Less common or uncommon manifestations include pustules, macules, petechiae, crusted plaques, vesicles, livedo reticularis, cysts, scars, ecchymoses, acral cyanosis, annular infarcts of fingers and toes, nonhealing surgical scars, auricular chondritis, palpebral xanthoma, necrosis of the penis, nailfold infarcts, and splinter hemorrhages of the fingernails (328,330–332,335). Saddle nose deformity is strongly suggestive of WG, but is rarely seen. The presentation of WG may mimic bowel disease, and perianal ulcers may be seen, usually associated with severe intestinal involvement (331).

The incidence of oral lesions has ranged from 10% to 50% in three series of patients with WG (331). The incidence of mucosal lesions at presentation has ranged from 5% to 6% (71,330). Mucosal lesions are usually ulcers. The oral ulcers of WG persist, unlike aphthae, which tend to remit and recur (331). Hyperplastic gingivitis (strawberry gums), manifesting as granular red-to-purple gingiva with petechiae, sometimes with loss of dentition, may be underrecognized (331). Gingival hyperplasia with petechiae is considered by some to be pathognomonic of WG (330). Genital ulcers are uncommon.

Relationship Between Cutaneous and Systemic Features of Disease. Patients with WG often present with nonspecific signs and symptoms of a systemic illness such as fever, malaise, weight loss, arthralgias, and myalgias. Upper airways disease manifested by sinus pain, purulent nasal discharge, epistaxis, nasal mucosal ulceration, and otitis media are common. Most patients also present with pulmonary disease. Renal disease is frequent and can be severe.

Of 35 patients with dermatologic lesions, eight had cutaneous lesions at presentation (331). These presenting lesions coexisted with extracutaneous lesions in seven and preceded them by 2 months in only one patient who presented with purpura. In the remaining 24 patients, extracutaneous lesions came first, and in three of these patients, the skin findings occurred only during relapse.

In a series of 40 patients with WG, Patten and Tomecki (330) were unable to find any prognostic links to cutaneous findings. However, Daoud et al. (328) noted that in their series of 244 patients, the overall risk of developing renal disease was 33.4%, whereas the subset of patients with cutaneous lesions had an 80% chance of developing kidney involvement during their disease course. In the series of Francès et al. (331), dermatologic manifestations were associated with a higher frequency of articular and renal involvement (68% vs. 25% and 80% vs. 47%, respectively). In this series, skin or mucosal lesions (except for xanthoma) indicated active systemic disease in all patients.

Eye involvement ranges from a mild conjunctivitis to eye pain, dacryocystitis, episcleritis, scleritis, granulomatous sclerouveitis, ciliary vessel vasculitis, visual loss, and retroorbital mass lesions leading to proptosis (333).

In the series of 265 cases from the United Kingdom followed from 1975 to 1985, WG was confined to the lung or upper respiratory tract in 22%, and renal disease occurred in 58% (327). The interval between the onset of symptoms and presentation was a mean of 7 months (median, 15 months; range, less than 1 to 132 months), and the interval between presentation and diagnosis was a mean of 6.5 months (median 20.9 months; range, less than 1 to 188 months), for a total mean interval of 13.5 months from the onset of symptoms to diagnosis. This is similar to the mean interval of 15 months reported in the United States report of 158 patients (333). The incidence of organ involvement as reported from these two large series is outlined in Table 8.8.

Pulmonary involvement may be manifested as asymptomatic infiltrates or may be clinically expressed as cough, hemoptysis, dyspnea, and chest discomfort. Subglottic from active disease or scarring may result in severe airway obstruction.

Renal disease generally dominates the clinical picture and, if left untreated, accounts directly or indirectly for most of the mortality (327,333). Although it may smolder in some cases as a mild glomerulitis with proteinuria, hematuria, and red blood cell casts, it is clear that once clinically detectable renal functional impairment occurs, rapidly progressive renal failure usually ensues unless appropriate treatment is instituted (333).

While the disease is active, most patients have nonspecific symptoms and signs such as malaise, weakness, arthralgias, anorexia, and weight loss. Fever may indicate activity of the underlying disease but more often reflects secondary infection, usually of the upper airway.

PATHOLOGY AND IMMUNOPATHOLOGY

The histologic hallmarks of WG are necrotizing vasculitis of small arteries and veins together with granuloma formation, which may be either intravascular or extravascular. Leukocytoclastic vasculitis is the most common cutaneous pathologic pattern in WG, accounting for 63%, 80%, and 82% of the histology of biopsied cutaneous lesions in three recent series (328,330, 331). In these same series, extravascular granuloma was seen in 6%, 10%, and 13%; granulomatous vasculitis occurred in none, 12.5%, and 17% of biopsied cutaneous lesions (mucosal biopsies excluded). Nongranulomatous biopsies correlated with purpuric lesions, and granulomatous biopsies with nonpurpuric lesions (328,330,331,334). Small dermal vessels were involved in 16 (57%) of 28 biopsies, slightly larger "medium-sized" cutaneous vessels in two (7%) of 28, and a mixture of vessel sizes in 10 (36%) of 28 (331). Direct IIF tests of purpuric skin lesions were done in seven patients; four of these were immunoglobulin-positive in blood vessels. The palisading granuloma seen in WG is characterized by focal necrobiosis, with a peripheral palisade of histiocytes and giant cells and is similar to that seen in Churg–Strauss syndrome. However, a polymorphonuclear infiltrate surrounding the necrosis is a frequent finding in WG, whereas tissue eosinophilia more typical of Churg–Strauss syndrome is usually absent (331,334,338).

Although cutaneous findings in WG can be helpful in confirming the diagnosis or a disease relapse when taken in context with the clinical picture, the pathologic features of lesions are not specific to WG alone. Necrotizing vasculitis can be observed in most primary and secondary vasculitides. Cutaneous extravascular necrotizing granuloma may occur in up to 50% of cases of Churg–Strauss syndrome, and this finding is occasionally seen in other syndromes such as PAN, SLE, rheumatoid arthritis, and lymphoproliferative diseases (339–341).

Gingival hyperplasia usually correlates with extravascular granuloma or granulomatous vasculitis on biopsy (331). Upper airway lesions, particularly those in the sinuses and nasopharynx, typically reveal inflammation, necrosis, and granuloma formation with or without vasculitis. Lung involvement typically appears as multiple, bilateral, nodular cavitary infiltrates, which on biopsy, almost invariably reveal the typical necrotizing granulomatous vasculitis. In its earliest form, renal involvement is characterized by a focal and segmental glomerulitis, which may evolve into a rapidly progressive crescentic glomerulonephritis. Granuloma formation is only rarely seen on renal biopsy.

Anderson et al. (327) found that histologic confirmation was most frequently obtained by examination of nasal biopsy specimens, and that multiple biopsies were often required. Focal proliferative glomerulonephritis is usually present on renal biopsies; granulomatous glomerulonephritis is uncommon (327,333).

LABORATORY MANIFESTATIONS

Frequent laboratory findings during active disease include an elevated erythrocyte sedimentation rate, elevated C-reactive protein level, mild anemia (usually normocytic, normochromic), leukocytosis (usually polymorphonuclear, occasionally with eosinophilia), mild hypergammaglobulinemia (particularly of the IgA class), thrombocytosis, elevated BUN and creatinine levels, and active urinary sediment (327,333). Rheumatoid factor may be positive in 25% of patients, and 40%

TABLE 8.8. Clinical Findings in Wegener Granulomatosis

	Hoffman[a] (N = 158)		
Finding or Organ Involved	Presentation	Overall	Anderson[b] (N = 256) Presentation
Fever	23%	50%	—
Musculoskeletal	32%	67%	20% Joints
Upper airway or ear	73%	92%	75% Airway 7% Ear
Lung	45%	85%	63%
Kidney	18%	77%	60%
Eye	15%	52%	14%
Skin	13%	46%	25%
Other organ	Rare	15% Nerve 8% CNS 6% Pericarditis	14% Node 4% Other

CNS, central nervous system.
[a]From Hoffman GS, Kerr GS, Leavitt RY, et al. Wegener's granulomatosis: an analysis of 158 patients. *Ann Intern Med* 1992;116:488–498.
[b]From Anderson G, Coles ET, Crane M, et al. Wegener's granuloma. A series of 265 British cases seen between 1975 and 1985. A report by a sub-committee of the British Thoracic Society Research Committee. *Q J Med* 1992;83:427–438.

may have circulating immune complexes (291). ANA testing was positive in 27% of 133 patients tested (327). Hypocomplementemia is not seen.

In one large series, c-ANCA testing was positive in 88% of patients with active WG and 43% of patients in remission; 5% of patients were p-ANCA–positive (see Table 8.4) (333). These figures are similar to those reported in patients with specific cutaneous findings, with c-ANCA positive in 83% of patients at least once during their disease (328). ANCA testing was positive in 94% of patients if done at the time of active skin lesions, but in only 47% of patients after successful treatment (328).

DIFFERENTIAL DIAGNOSIS

The diagnosis of WG is a clinicopathologic one made by the demonstration of necrotizing granulomatous vasculitis on biopsy of appropriate tissue in a patient with the clinical findings of upper and lower respiratory tract disease together with evidence of glomerulonephritis. Biopsies of upper or lower airway lesions offer the highest yield, with lung tissue more often yielding granulomatous vasculitis. Cutaneous lesions usually offer the most accessible lesions for biopsy, although the granulomatous components of WG are usually absent in skin biopsy.

WG needs to be differentiated from the other vasculitides, particularly allergic angiitis and allergic granulomatosis of Churg–Strauss, and from Goodpasture syndrome, tumors of the upper airway or lung, and infectious or noninfectious granulomatous disease. The presence of c-ANCA proves extremely helpful in the differentiation from most of the preceding nonvasculitic diseases. Destructive midline facial lesions (idiopathic midline destructive disease or idiopathic midline granuloma) is a rare syndrome now known to be mostly secondary to T cell/natural killer cell lymphomas, but occasionally mimicked by WG or by cocaine abuse (342,343). Such upper airway neoplasms may erode through the skin of the face, a feature very rarely seen in WG. Several of the cocaine-associated syndromes were ANCA-positive (343).

Lymphomatoid granulomatosis is another important disease to differentiate from WG; in fact, in early studies, its histology was included as a subset of Wegener vasculitis. Lymphomatoid granulomatosis is characterized by lung, skin, central nervous system, and kidney involvement in which atypical lymphocytoid and plasmacytoid cells infiltrate tissue in an angioinvasive manner. Approximately 50% of patients develop a true malignant lymphoma.

The ACR criteria for WG were developed before the wide availability of ANCA testing. Four criteria were established that separated WG from other vasculitides: abnormal urinary sediment (red cell casts or more than five red blood cells per high-power field), abnormal findings of chest radiograph (nodules, cavities, or fixed infiltrate), oral ulcers or nasal discharge, and granulomatous inflammation on biopsy. The presence of two or more of these four criteria was associated with a sensitivity of 88% and a specificity of 92% (344).

ANCA testing is an increasingly important component of establishing the diagnosis of WG. A positive ANCA is expected in most patients with active disease, usually with c-ANCA staining (44). Although ANCA positivity alone cannot confirm the diagnosis of WG because of its presence in other vasculitides, it is strongly supportive of the diagnosis. Likewise, the diagnosis of WG should be questioned in a patient with active systemic disease and a negative ANCA.

Many patients with cutaneous lesions of WG will develop only palpable purpura with simple leukocytoclastic vasculitis on biopsy. The misdiagnosis of some other vasculitic syndrome could easily result unless the frequent occurrence of small-vessel limited disease in the skin is recognized as a common finding in cutaneous WG. Pyoderma gangrenosum is a differential concern in those patients presenting with pyoderma gangrenosum–like ulcers in WG. Another area of potential misdiagnosis based on cutaneous lesions is the overlap in clinical presentation with perianal ulcers in both Crohn disease and WG. This differential can be further confused by the high frequency of positive ANCA testing in both disorders, although the ANCA pattern in Crohn is atypical, whereas that in WG is usually c-ANCA–positive (44,331).

Another atypical presentation of WG mimics giant cell arteritis. Of 345 patients with WG, five initially had features of giant cell arteritis, with biopsy-proven giant cell arteritis of temporal artery. All five were older than 60, had elevated erythrocyte sedimentation rates, and had either jaw claudication, sudden loss of vision, severe headaches with or without diplopia, or polymyalgia rheumatica at the time of initial examination. All five subsequently had pulmonary and renal lesions characteristic of WG, with typical histologic features or a positive ANCA (345).

At least one instance of a drug reaction mimicking WG has been reported (346). This was a case of α-methyldopa–induced systemic vasculitis accompanied by hepatic injury, and systemic granulomatous disease with fever, myalgias, fatigue, night sweats, and later arthritis beginning 11 days after α-methyldopa. A random nasal biopsy demonstrated necrotizing granulomatous inflammation. The syndrome persisted for 6 weeks after discontinuation of the drug, and then remitted spontaneously.

MANAGEMENT OF SKIN LESIONS, SYSTEMIC THERAPY, AND PROGNOSIS

Cutaneous manifestations respond well to cyclophosphamide therapy (331). The survival rate of patients with and without cutaneous findings differed significantly at 5 years in one series: 66% of those with skin lesions versus 87% of those without (331). However, the survival of those without cutaneous lesions seemed to drop abruptly at 10 years, and 10-year survival was near 60% for both groups (331). Gingival hypertrophy may have a good partial response to antibiotic therapy.

WG was formerly universally fatal, usually within a few months after the onset of clinically apparent renal disease. Disease affecting the upper or lower respiratory tract alone without constitutional findings has been treated with prednisolone alone or with sulfamethosoxazole–trimethoprim (74). In patients with systemic disease, corticosteroid therapy often improves symptoms, but fails to affect disease progression or survival in most patients. The combination of cyclophosphamide (2mg/kg per day oral) and oral corticosteroid (1mg/kg per day) is the treatment of choice for induction of remission in WG (73,74,333). Methotrexate and corticosteroid therapy has been successful in some patients with multifocal disease without threatened organ function, but cyclophosphamide should always be used in severely affected patients (74). Pulse cyclophosphamide therapy, while effective in inducing remission, does not seem to produce as good a long-term result as the daily oral regimen (73,74,333). Once remission is achieved, tapering doses or switching to safer drugs to maintain remission is recommended (73,74). Methotrexate or azathioprine is typically used for remission maintenance.

Corticosteroids should be administered together with cyclophosphamide (73,333). This can be given as prednisone, 1 mg/kg per day for the first month of therapy as a daily regimen, with gradual conversion to an alternate-day schedule followed by tapering and discontinuation after approximately 6 months. With this regimen, the prognosis is good, with marked improvement in 91% of patients and complete remission in 75%

(333). A number of patients who developed irreversible renal failure but who achieved subsequent remission on appropriate therapy have undergone successful renal transplantation.

In the National Institutes of Health (NIH) experience, long-term follow-up of patients has revealed that approximately 50% of remissions are later associated with one or more relapses (333). Reinduction of remission is usually achieved. However, 86% of patients ultimately had some degree of morbidity from irreversible features of their disease, such as varying degrees of renal insufficiency, hearing loss, tracheal stenosis, saddle nose deformity, and chronically impaired sinus function (333). The morbidity or mortality of other patients results from the toxicities of therapy. Death was considered to result from complications of treatment with cytotoxic drugs or prednisolone in 6% of patients in the large series of Anderson et al. (327). Aggressively tapering corticosteroid therapy using the regimen mentioned earlier minimizes the corticosteroid toxicity. However, cyclophosphamide-related toxicities are more frequent and severe. Cystitis to varying degrees occurred in 43% of the patients of Hoffman et al. (333) (NIH), bladder cancer in 3%, and myelodysplasia in 2%. Two patients developed lymphoma after 1.5 and 8.6 years of cyclophosphamide therapy (333).

Some patients cannot tolerate cyclophosphamide therapy, usually due to severe neutropenia at low doses of the drug, severe cystitis, or bladder cancer. Azathioprine, in doses of 1 to 2 mg/kg per day, in combination with prednisone, has proven effective in some patients, particularly in maintaining remission in those in whom remission was induced by cyclophosphamide (327,333). Although patients have improved while taking trimethoprim–sulfamethoxazole, this therapy remains unproven (73, 347–349).

Granulomatous Vasculitis: Allergic Granulomatosis of Churg and Strauss

In 1951, Churg and Strauss (350) reported 13 cases of severe asthma, fever, and hypereosinophilia with histologic findings of vascular and extravascular granulomas and necrotizing vasculitis.

In a subsequent series of 30 patients, all patients had bronchial asthma, peripheral eosinophilia, and systemic vasculitis that differed from PAN (351). In addition, in contrast to PAN, renal disease was rare. The clinical evolution of Churg–Strauss syndrome seemed to follow the pattern of allergic rhinitis, followed by asthma, then eosinophilia, tissue infiltration by eosinophils, and finally a vasculitis (352). There was a slight-to-moderate male predominance, with a mean age of onset for allergic rhinitis of 25 to 28 years, asthma of 33 to 35 years, and vasculitis of 38 years (352).

In 1983, Finan and Winkelmann (340) demonstrated the presence of cutaneous extravascular necrotizing granulomas in conditions other than Churg–Strauss syndrome. Moreover, in 1984 Lanham et al. (352) emphasized the histologic variability of the Churg–Strauss syndrome, with patients frequently lacking one or more of the "diagnostic" histopathologic features: tissue infiltration by eosinophils, necrotizing vasculitis, and extravascular granulomas. Proposed criteria included asthma, peak peripheral blood eosinophil count above 1,500/mm^3, and systemic vasculitis involving two or more extrapulmonary organs.

Proposed ACR criteria for Churg–Strauss syndrome include asthma, eosinophilia above 10%, mono- or polyneuropathy, nonfixed pulmonary infiltrates, abnormalities of the paranasal sinuses, and extravascular eosinophils present on biopsy (353). The presence of four or more of these six criteria yielded a diagnostic sensitivity of 85% and specificity of 99.7%. Using ACR criteria, a series of 20 patients was reported with a mean age at disease onset of 50 years (range, 16 to 74 years), and a 65% predominance of males (353).

CHCG criteria for this syndrome include the presence of eosinophil-rich and granulomatous inflammation involving the respiratory tract and necrotizing vasculitis affecting small- to medium-sized vessels, in association with asthma and eosinophilia (13). The presence of eosinophil-rich infiltrates is not by itself a discriminating feature since this can be seen in other vasculitides (12). These criteria are similar to those used by Lanham et al. (352) in their large review.

Leukotriene antagonists are a group of drugs useful in the treatment of asthma, often allowing reduction of prednisone requirements in severe asthma patients (354). It has been associated with the development of Churg–Strauss syndrome, but it is unclear whether it induces this syndrome, or whether it simply uncovers other features of the syndrome that were being suppressed by the higher dose of prednisone.

CUTANEOUS MANIFESTATIONS

Skin involvement is an important feature of Churg–Strauss syndrome. Cutaneous manifestations in Churg–Strauss syndrome are more frequent than in PAN, but resemble the type and frequency of involvement of the skin in hypereosinophilic syndrome (352). In the ACR group of 20 patients, the incidence of cutaneous findings included palpable purpura in 45%, maculopapular rash in 40%, and subcutaneous nodules in 20% (353). In general, lesions can be divided into three categories: erythematous macules or papules resembling erythema multiforme, hemorrhagic lesions from petechiae to ecchymoses, and cutaneous and subcutaneous nodules (Fig. 8.15) (338).

In the review of Lanham et al. (352), patient entry was defined by the presence of asthma, systemic vasculitis, and eosinophilia. Several of these patients had been previously

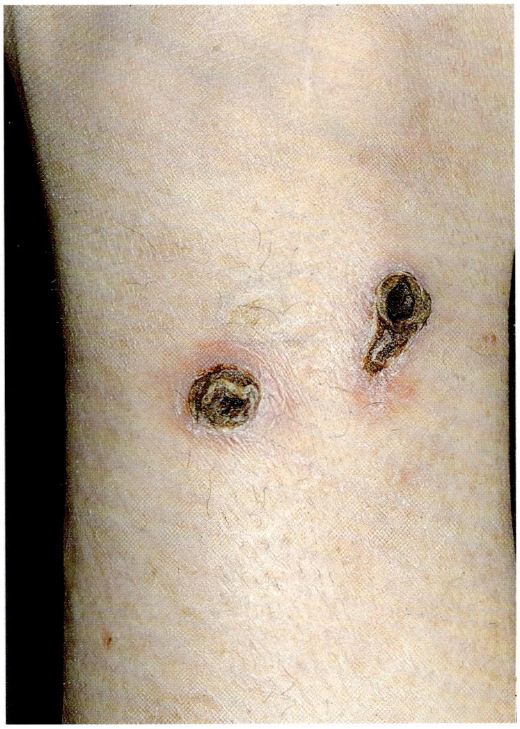

Figure 8.15. Ulcerating nodules below the knee of a patient with allergic granulomatosis of Churg and Strauss.

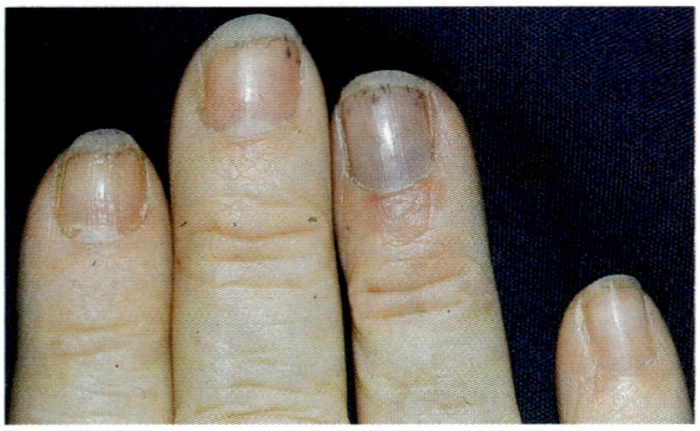

Figure 8.16. Splinter hemorrhages in a patient with allergic granulomatosis of Churg and Strauss (same patient as in Fig. 8.15).

reported under other diagnoses; the seeming rarity of Churg–Strauss syndrome may depend as much on classification as on incidence (311,352). Within this group of 154 patients, 70% developed cutaneous lesions. Purpura developed in 48%, most often on the extremities, erythema/urticaria in 35%, and subcutaneous nodules in 30%. The nodules were the most distinctive skin lesions of Churg–Strauss syndrome. Often tender, occasionally "pea-sized and stony hard," they occurred particularly on the scalp, symmetrically on the extremities, and rarely on the sacrum or buttocks (339). They are the most persistent, resolving with scarring within 2 to 3 months (338). Also occasionally reported in this syndrome are vesicles or papulovesicles (occasionally purpuric), cutaneous infarction, including nailfold infarction-splinter hemorrhage (Fig. 8.16), ulceration of nodules, nonpitting facial edema, and livedo reticularis (339). One patient developed an erythema multiforme–like erythematous eruption of the shoulders and buttocks.

Relationship Between Cutaneous and Systemic Features of Disease. Because of the high incidence of skin lesions in patients with Churg–Strauss syndrome, it is likely that cutaneous findings will develop during the course of a patient's illness. Asthma is unusual in PAN or in WG, but expected in Churg–Strauss syndrome (352). Apart from the characteristic pulmonary findings, the multisystem involvement in this disease is quite similar to that of classic PAN, except that renal disease is less common and usually less severe in Churg–Strauss syndrome.

As reported by Lanham et al. (352), upper or lower airway involvement included asthma in 100%, allergic rhinitis in 70%, pulmonary infiltrates in 72%, and Löffler prodrome in 40%. The nervous system was the next most frequently affected system, with peripheral neuropathy in 66% and a 27% incidence of central nervous system disease, followed by arthritis/arthralgia in 51%, and myalgia in 41%. Cardiac failure developed in 47%, pericarditis in 32%, and hypertension in 29%. Abdominal pain occurred frequently (59%), sometimes with diarrhea or bleeding. Although mild-to-moderate renal disease was found in 49%, only 9% developed renal failure.

PATHOLOGY AND IMMUNOPATHOLOGY

The three major types of histologic changes in Churg–Strauss syndrome are eosinophilic infiltration, granuloma formation, and necrotizing vasculitis (338). Histologically, the vascular and extravascular granulomas are composed of necrotic eosinophilic exudates, severe fibrinoid degeneration of collagen, and prominent epithelioid and giant cells (350). Eosinophilic tissue infiltration proceeds to eosinophil death, scattering of granules, and nuclear fragmentation. Fibrinoid swelling and eosinophilia of collagen follows, with eventual fiber destruction. Macrophages palisade around this central necrotic core, and Langhans or foreign-body giant cells appear (350,352). Involvement of small vessels is characteristic, but medium-sized vessels may also be involved. Arterial vessels are usually preferentially involved (338). In the Masi et al. (353) (ACR) series, granulomas were found in or near arteries, arterioles, or venules in 10% to 20% of cases; none in relation to veins. Vessels may show simply perivascular cuffing by eosinophils or a necrotizing vasculitis similar to PAN.

Necrotizing extravascular granulomatosis was reported in 22 (73%) of the series of Chumbley et al. (351), and fibrinoid necrosis of vessel walls in 12 (40%). The necrotizing vasculitis in Churg–Strauss syndrome may be indistinguishable from that in PAN or hypersensitivity vasculitis (311). Biopsy of the nodular lesions frequently reveals granulomas, whereas the other skin lesions more often show vasculitis (339,350). Granulomas may be particularly difficult to find by tissue biopsy, and are absent at autopsy in a considerable number of cases (352).

The Churg–Strauss granuloma is certainly not a specific histologic finding, although its presence is certainly suggestive of the diagnosis (340). Finan and Winkelmann (340) reviewed 27 cases with the findings of extravascular necrotizing (Churg–Strauss) granuloma, and found that only seven (26%) had allergic granulomatosis of Churg and Strauss. Including these seven cases, 14 (52%) had some form of systemic vasculitis; the additional seven cases included three of WG, one PAN, and three unclassified. Of the remaining 13 cases, six had connective tissue diseases (four rheumatoid arthritis, two lupus), three had hematologic malignancies (acute myelomonocytic leukemia, multiple myeloma, lymphocytic lymphoma), three had a chronic inflammatory disease (chronic active hepatitis, ulcerative colitis, and subacute bacterial endocarditis), and one had no associated disease. These skin lesions were usually papules or nodules over pressure points, and were located on the elbow in 80% of patients and on the digits in 40%. Approximately a third of the biopsies also demonstrated some histologic variant of vasculitis.

Chu et al. (355) have proposed the term "palisaded neutrophilic and granulomatous dermatitis of immune complex disease" to describe what they believe is the phenomenon noted by Finan and Winkelmann. They described the histopathologic findings in nine patients with collagen vascular disease and a symmetric papular eruption. Their findings suggest that granulomatous lesions in such patients may begin as leukocytoclastic vasculitis, develop palisaded granulomatous dermatitis with neutrophils, and resolve with fibrosis. While symmetrically distributed extremity papules are the usual clinical appearance of lesions with these histologic findings, linear bands and ulcerated plaques have also been reported to show these changes (355).

It is clear, then, that palisaded granuloma is not specific to Churg–Strauss syndrome. It has been suggested, but not proven, that immune complexes are essential to the genesis of such lesions. Even if this proves true, it is certainly far from proven that the pathogenesis of the main clinical and histologic features of Churg–Strauss syndrome is secondary to immune complex mechanisms.

LABORATORY MANIFESTATIONS

The characteristic laboratory finding in virtually all patients with allergic angiitis and granulomatosis is a striking eosinophilia (339,352,353). Eosinophilia reaches levels greater than 1,000 cells/μL in more than 80% of patients. While measured infrequently, IgE levels are usually elevated (352,353). This is a distinctive, intriguing, but nonspecific finding. ANCA testing is positive in 80% of patients, and is usually p-ANCA (70%, MPO specificity), but occasionally c-ANCA (10%, PR-3 specificity) (see Table 8.3).

Anemia and elevated leukocyte count, erythrocyte sedimentation rates, and rheumatoid factor are frequent nonspecific laboratory abnormalities (339,352). Other laboratory findings are similar to those of systemic PAN and reflect the organ systems involved.

DIFFERENTIAL DIAGNOSIS

Nonspecific manifestations of fever, malaise, anorexia, and weight loss are common to many systemic illnesses, including many vasculitides. The vasculitic syndromes most likely to be confused with allergic granulomatosis of Churg–Strauss are classic PAN, microscopic polyangiitis, and WG. Eosinophilia and eosinophilic tissue infiltration are striking in most patients with Churg–Strauss syndrome, and much less common in WG or PAN. Prominent pulmonary findings rule out classic PAN. The presence of severe renal disease would tend to favor WG or PAN over Churg–Strauss syndrome. Cutaneous lesions are frequent findings in Churg–Strauss syndrome and microscopic polyangiitis, less common in WG, and rare in classic PAN. The cutaneous lesions of Churg–Strauss syndrome frequently show prominent tissue infiltration, and are as likely to be nonpurpuric as purpuric, in contrast to microscopic polyangiitis or WG.

Features of Churg–Strauss syndrome and hypereosinophilic syndrome frequently overlap. Persistent peripheral blood eosinophilia is expected in both. Both can present with a Löffler prodrome of pulmonary infiltrates and peripheral eosinophilia (352). Both have a high frequency of cutaneous lesions, of elevated serum IgE levels, and of symptomatic pulmonary, cardiac, and gastrointestinal involvement (352,353,356). However, vasculitis is an expected finding in Churg–Strauss syndrome, whereas nonvasculitic perivascular inflammation or thrombosis is a more typical vascular finding in hypereosinophilic syndrome.

MANAGEMENT OF SKIN LESIONS AND PROGNOSIS

Survival was rare in the presteroid era, but Churg–Strauss syndrome responds well to corticosteroids. Five-year survival in the series of Chumbley et al. (351) was 62%, with a median survival of 9 years. The dose of corticosteroid is usually 40 to 60 mg prednisolone for several weeks, and tapering should be tailored to improvement in clinical findings. The response of the neuropathy is more gradual, and tapering is predicated on halting progression of nerve injury. Azathioprine, chlorambucil, or cyclophosphamide may be required (352). It may be prudent to use cyclophosphamide early in the severely ill patient who fails to respond to high-dose steroids, and to use azathioprine for maintenance therapy in refractory disease (338,352). Chlorambucil and plasma exchange are other therapies that may occasionally be effective in combination with steroid or immunosuppressants (338).

Abu-Shakra et al. (357) have reported a small series comparing PAN with Churg–Strauss syndrome. Cyclophosphamide therapy was required in seven of 13 patients with PAN, but only two of 12 patients with Churg–Strauss syndrome. They found that patients with PAN had a significantly worse prognosis with respect to organ damage, disability, and pain. At the time of this report, four (31%) patients with PAN had died, compared to only one (8%) patient with Churg–Strauss syndrome. However, this had not yet reached statistical significance.

Laboratory parameters that best indicate the response to treatment are the eosinophil count, total white blood cell count, and the erythrocyte sedimentation rate. Unlike classic PAN, the cause of death in Churg–Strauss syndrome is more likely to be related to pulmonary and cardiac disease as opposed to renal or gastrointestinal involvement.

Large-vessel Vasculitis: Temporal Arteritis (Giant Cell Arteritis)

Temporal arteritis, also referred to as cranial or giant cell arteritis, is an inflammation of medium- and large-sized arteries (358,359). It characteristically involves one or more branches of the carotid artery, particularly the temporal artery, hence the name cranial or temporal arteritis. However, it is a systemic disease that can involve arteries in multiple locations. Temporal arteritis often occurs in association with polymyalgia rheumatica, and both occur with an incidence ranging from one to 20 per 100,000 population per year, with the higher figures typical of populations 50 years of age or older (358,359). Both are rare before age 50, with peak prevalence in the seventh and eighth decades (358,359). Temporal arteritis occurs in all racial groups, but is rare in blacks. Women are affected approximately twice as often as men are, and familial aggregation has been reported.

The etiology of temporal arteritis is unknown, although cell-mediated immunity is implicated and immune complex vasculitis is not considered to play a role.

CUTANEOUS MANIFESTATIONS

Skin manifestations of temporal arteritis are uncommon. The two most frequent findings of temporal arteritis evident on skin examination are visible or palpable temporal arteries or aneurysms, and scalp tenderness, sometimes with scalp nodules or ulcers (360,361). The temporal arteries are tender, thickened, or nodular; they may pulsate early in the disease but may become occluded later. Rarely noted additional findings in the skin include urticaria, erythematous or violaceous edema, supravascular pallor, ecchymosis, vesicles or bullae overlying ischemic or necrotic areas (occasionally hemorrhagic), crusting, necrosis, ulceration, gangrene, alopecia, and hyperpigmentation (360). Most but not all cutaneous disease occurs on the scalp; lesions on arms and legs are extremely rare. Gangrene most often arises in the scalp regions supplied by the superficial temporal arteries, beginning as a band then rapidly enlarging and developing markedly irregular outlines (358). This complication is often bilateral, and may spare skin in the sagittal region. Oral manifestations include claudication or blanching of the tongue, gangrene of the tongue, glossitis, and temporomandibular pain (360).

Relationship Between Cutaneous and Systemic Features of Disease. Severe unilateral or bilateral headaches and scalp tenderness are the most common clinical findings, usually associated with fever, anemia, and a high sedimentation rate (358,359). Other manifestations include malaise, fatigue, anorexia, weight loss, sweats, and arthralgias. Temporal arteritis is closely associated with the polymyalgia rheumatica syndrome, also typically seen after 50 years of age and peaking between the ages of 70 and 80. Polymyalgia rheumatica is characterized by stiffness, aching, and pain in the muscles of the neck, shoulder, lower back, hips, and thighs and an erythrocyte sedimentation rate of more than 40 mm per hour. Diffuse swelling and pitting edema of the hands and feet have also been reported. Symptoms of polymyalgia rheumatica have been observed in 40% to 60% of patients with giant cell arteritis (359).

Temporal arteritis typically runs a three-stage course: a prodromal stage (primarily symptoms of polymyalgia rheumatica accompanied by worsening headaches), an acute stage, and a chronic stage (358,359). The acute stage is characterized by severe, bilateral headaches, accompanied by tender, edematous, and inflamed areas of affected scalp. Involvement of other cranial arteries often becomes evident at this stage, especially through activity-dependent pain of the masseter, pharynx, and tongue, or a variety of ophthalmologic symptoms or signs. Skin manifestations usually occur during this stage. If untreated, the chronic stage may develop. The headaches and systemic findings fade, the temporal arteries become narrow pulseless strands, and yet, areas of scalp ulceration, if present, tend to heal.

The well-recognized and dreaded complication of temporal arteritis, particularly in untreated patients, is due primarily to ischemic optic neuritis, which may lead to serious visual symptoms, even sudden blindness in some patients (359). Attention to symptoms relating to the head or eyes with institution of appropriate therapy will usually avoid this complication. Claudication of the extremities, strokes, myocardial infarctions, aortic aneurysms and dissections, and infarctions of visceral organs have been reported (358).

PATHOLOGY AND IMMUNOPATHOLOGY

The temporal artery is most frequently, but not necessarily, the only, medium- and large-sized artery involved in this disease (358,359). Because the characteristic arterial lesions are focal, the diagnosis may be missed on routine biopsy (358). Serial sectioning of biopsy specimens is recommended. Histologic findings include inflammatory mononuclear cell infiltrates within the vessel wall, frequent giant cells, proliferation of the intima, and fragmentation of the internal elastic lamina.

LABORATORY MANIFESTATIONS

The cardinal laboratory findings in temporal arteritis are an erythrocyte sedimentation rate above 50 mm per hour and an elevated C-reactive protein (358,359). Normochromic or slightly hypochromic anemia and liver function abnormalities are also common. Leukocytosis, thrombocytosis, low serum calcium, and elevated immunoglobulins or immune complexes are occasionally seen.

DIFFERENTIAL DIAGNOSIS

The diagnosis of temporal arteritis is usually made clinically, triggered by the findings of persistent headache in an elderly patient with or without symptoms of polymyalgia rheumatica. Fever, a high erythrocyte sedimentation rate, or anemia is frequently present at diagnosis. The diagnosis is confirmed by biopsy of the temporal artery. In some cases, a dramatic response to a therapeutic trial with corticosteroids provides strong support for this diagnosis. Polymyalgia rheumatica is the major consideration in the differential diagnosis. Biopsies of asymptomatic temporal arteries may reveal histologic findings of giant cell arteritis in up to 50% of patients with polymyalgia rheumatica, but an actual transition to temporal arteritis occurs in only 15% (315,359).

MANAGEMENT OF SKIN LESIONS AND PROGNOSIS

Temporal arteritis is usually exquisitely sensitive to corticosteroid therapy. Treatment should begin with prednisone, 40 to 100 mg per day, and usually in divided doses, followed by a gradual tapering (10% reduction every 1 to 2 weeks) to a maintenance dose of 7.5 to 10 mg per day (358,359). The headaches subside within days to weeks; the erythrocyte sedimentation rate normalizes within weeks (358). When ocular signs and symptoms occur, it is important that therapy be initiated or adjusted to control them. Initial pulsed intravenous doses of methylprednisolone (1 gm daily for 3 days) may be given to patients with recent visual loss or visual symptoms (359). Because of the possibility of relapse, therapy should be continued for at least 1 to 2 years (358,359). Calcium and vitamin D therapy are important in reducing bone loss. The prognosis is generally good, and most patients achieve complete remission, which is often maintained after withdrawal of therapy.

Large-Vessel Vasculitis: Takayasu Arteritis

Takayasu arteritis (pulseless disease) is a chronic inflammatory arteriopathy affecting predominantly the aorta and its main branches (362). It usually presents in younger women, especially of Asian descent, and seldom begins after age 40.

CUTANEOUS MANIFESTATIONS

Cutaneous involvement may be somewhat common in this syndrome, occurring in between 2.8% to 28% of patients, but this has been rarely reported in the dermatologic literature (363). Vasculitic lesions in the skin include erythema nodosum–like lesions, pyoderma gangrenosum–like lesions, purpura, and necrotic or ulcerated nodules (363). Other cutaneous manifestations include Raynaud phenomenon and livedo reticularis.

Relationship Between Cutaneous and Systemic Features of Disease. The disease typically presents with malaise, fever, myalgias, and weight loss. This is followed by a second stage of loss of pulses associated with inflammation of the media and adventitial layers of large vessels (363). Renal ischemia may present as high renin hypertension (362). Arm claudication is common, and bruits in the aortic arch vessels are frequent. Diagnosis is usually made by arteriographic demonstration of stenotic and obstructive lesions. Cutaneous lesions can be the presenting sign of this syndrome, and in the context of systemic symptoms, palpation of peripheral pulses or auscultation for bruits could rapidly suggest the correct diagnosis.

PATHOLOGY AND IMMUNOPATHOLOGY

Histopathologic studies have rarely been performed on cutaneous lesions in this syndrome. Necrotizing vasculitis, granulomatous vasculitis, and septal, lobular, and granulomatous panniculitis have been reported (363).

Larger vessel arteritis usually involves the outer part of the media and the adventitia in elastic-muscular type arteries. In the first stage, granulomatous changes with neovascularization between elastic fibers and lymphohistiocytic inflammation around the vasa vasorum are seen. This may be followed by diffuse inflammation with lymphocytes, plasma cells, and rare giant cells (363). Later stage disease shows arteriosclerotic changes with scarring in the media–adventitia junction.

LABORATORY MANIFESTATIONS

During the inflammatory phase, normochromic anemia, an elevated erythrocyte sedimentation rate, and thrombocytosis are frequently present, and hyperglobulinemia is occasionally seen (364). Subsequently, electrocardiographic findings of ischemia, radiographic findings of aortic widening, and aortographic findings of occlusion or aneurysm are expected.

DIFFERENTIAL DIAGNOSIS

The differential diagnosis of larger vessel disease includes carotid artery dissection, early arteriosclerosis, Ehlers–Danlos syndrome, giant cell arteritis, and sarcoidosis (362,364). The differential diagnosis of cutaneous lesions is suggested by their descriptions as noted previously.

MANAGEMENT OF SKIN LESIONS AND PROGNOSIS

Initial therapy is usually high-dose corticosteroid therapy, although this disease may be less responsive than giant cell arteritis (362). Methotrexate therapy has been advocated as a steroid-sparing agent. If scarring of larger vessels has occurred, vascular reconstructive surgery may be needed.

REFERENCES

1. Braverman I. The angiitides. *Skin signs of systemic disease,* 3rd ed. Philadelphia: WB Saunders, 1998:278–334.
2. Cupps TR, Fauci AS. The vasculitides. In: Smith LH JR, ed. *Major problems in internal medicine.* Vol. XXI. Philadelphia: WB Saunders; 1981:1–5.
3. Ryan TJ. Cutaneous vasculitis. In: Champion RH, Burton J, Burns D, Breathnach S, eds. *Textbook of dermatology,* 6th ed. Vol. 3. Oxford: Blackwell Science, 1998:2155–2225.
4. Rosenwasser L. The vasculitic syndromes. In: Goldman L, Bennett J, eds. *Cecil textbook of medicine,* 21st ed. Philadelphia: WB Saunders, 2000:1525–1527.
5. Le Boit PE. Vasculitis: The true and the near-true. *Am J Dermatophol* 2002; 24(3):267–269.
6. Zeek PM. Periarteritis nodosa and other forms of necrotizing angiitis. *N Engl J Med* 1953;248:764–772.
7. Winkelmann RK, Ditto WB. Cutaneous and visceral syndromes of necrotizing or "allergic" angiitis: a study of 38 cases. *Medicine* 1964;43:59–89.
8. Gilliam JN, Smiley JD. Cutaneous necrotizing vasculitis and related disorders. *Ann Allergy* 1976;37:328–339.
9. Sanchez NP, Van Hale HM, Su WPD. Clinical and histopathologic spectrum of necrotizing vasculitis: report of findings in 101 cases. *Arch Dermatol* 1985; 121:220–224.
10. Hunder GG, Arend WP, Bloch DA, et al. The American College of Rheumatology 1990 criteria for the classification of vasculitis. *Arthritis & Rheumatism* 1990;33:1065–1067.
11. Callen JP. Cutaneous vasculitis: relationship to systemic disease and therapy. *Curr Probl Dermatol* 1993;5:45–80.
12. Jennette CJ, Falk RJ, Andrassy K, et al. Nomenclature of systemic vasculitides. Proposal of an International Consensus Conference. *Arthritis Rheum* 1994;37:187–192.
13. Jennette CJ, Milling DM, Falk RJ. Vasculitis affecting the skin: a review. *Arch Dermatol* 1994;130:899–906.
14. McCluskey RT, Fienberg R. Vasculitis in primary vasculitides, granulomatoses, and connective tissue diseases. *Hum Pathol* 1983;14:305–315.
15. Bruce I, Bell A. A comparison of two nomenclature systems for primary systemic vasculitis. *Br J Rheumatol* 1997;36:453–458.
16. Schneider HA, Yonker RA, Katz P, et al. Rheumatoid vasculitis: experience with 13 patients and review of the literature. *Semin Arthritis Rheum* 1985;14:280–286.
17. Luqmani R, Robinson H. Introduction to, and classification of, the systemic vasculitides. *Best Pract Res Clin Rheumatol* 2001;15:187–202.
18. Watts R, Lane S, Bentham G, et al. Epidemiology of systemic vasculitis (SV)—a ten year study. *Arthritis Rheum* 2000;43:422–427.
19. Piette WW. The differential diagnosis of purpura from a morphologic perspective. *Adv Dermatol* 1994;9:3–24.
20. Sams Jr WM, Thorne EG. Leukocytoclastic vasculitis. *Arch Dermatol* 1976;112: 219–226.
21. Fan PT, Davis JA, Somer T, et al. A clinical approach to systemic vasculitis. *Semin Arthritis Rheum* 1980;9:248–302.
22. Chan LS, Cooper KD, Rasmussen JE. Koebnerization as a cutaneous manifestation of immune complex-mediated vasculitis. *J Am Acad Dermatol* 1990; 22:775–781.
23. Gower RG, Sams WM Jr Thorne EG, et al. Leukocytoclastic vasculitis—sequential appearance of immunoreactants and cellular changes in serial biopsies. *J Invest Dermatol* 1977;69:477–484.
24. Smoller BR, McNutt S, Contreras F. The natural history of vasculitis: what the histology tells us about pathogenesis. *Arch Dermatol* 1990;126:84–89.
25. Zax RH, Hodge SJ, Callen JP. Cutaneous leukocytoclastic vasculitis: serial histopathologic evaluation demonstrates the dynamic nature of the infiltrate. *Arch Dermatol* 1990;126:69–72.
26. Piette WW, Stone MS. A cutaneous sign of IgA-associated small dermal vessel leukocytoclastic vasculitis in adults (Henoch-Schönlein purpura). *Arch Dermatol* 1989;125:53–56.
27. Tencati JR, Novey HS. Hypersensitivity angiitis caused by fumes from heat-activated photocopy paper. *Ann Intern Med* 1983;98:320–322.
28. Naides S. Known causes of vasculitis in man. *Cleveland Clin J Med* 2002; 69[Suppl 2]:15–19.
29. Cohen Tervaert J. Infections in primary vasculitides. *Cleveland Clin J Med* 2002;69[Suppl 2]:24–26.
30. Ferri C, Zignego A, Giuggioli D, et al. HCV and cryoglobulinemic vasculitis. *Cleveland Clin J Med* 2002;69[Suppl 2]:20–23.
31. Cochrane CG, Koffler D. Immune complex disease in experimental animals and man. *Adv Immunol* 1973;16:185–264.
32. Braverman IM, Yen A. Demonstration of immune complexes in spontaneous and histamine-induced lesions and in normal skin of patients with leukocytoclastic angiitis. *J Invest Dermatol* 1975;64:105–112.
33. Spencer-Green G. The microvasculature. In: LeRoy EC, ed. *Systemic vasculitis: the biologic basis.* New York: Marcel Dekker, Inc., 1992:171–222.
34. Gauthier VJ, Mannik M. Immune complexes in the pathogenesis of vasculitis. In: LeRoy EC, ed. *Systemic vasculitis: the biologic basis.* New York: Marcel Dekker, Inc., 1992:401–420.
35. Lawley TJ, Kubota Y. Vasculitis. *Dermatol Clin* 1990;8:681–687.
36. Cid M, Vilardell C. Tissue targeting and disease patterns in systemic vasculitis. *Best Pract Res Clin Rheumatol* 2001;15:259–279.
37. Jennette J. Implications for pathogenesis of patterns of injury in small- and medium-sized-vessel vasculitis. *Cleveland Clin J Med* 2002;69[Suppl 2]:33–38.
38. Cid M. Endothelial cell biology, perivascular inflammation, and vasculitis. *Cleveland Clin J Med* 2002;69[Suppl 2]:45–49.
39. Gessner J, Heiken H, Tamm A, et al. The IgG Fc receptor family. *Ann Hematol* 1998;76:231–248.
40. Sunderkotter C, Seeliger S, Schonlau F, et al. Different pathways leading to cutaneous leukocytoclastic vasculitis in mice. *Exp Dermatol* 2001;10:391–404.
41. Ginsberg MH. Cell adhesion receptors and vasculitis. In: LeRoy EC, ed. *Systemic vasculitis: the biologic basis.* New York: Marcel Dekker, Inc., 1992:505–524.
42. Bender JR. Lymphocyte-endothelial interactions. In: LeRoy EC, ed. *Systemic vasculitis: the biologic basis.* New York: Marcel Dekker, Inc., 1992:93–128.
43. Davies D, Moran ME, Niall JF, et al. Segmental glomerulonephritis with antineutrophil antibody: possible arbovirus etiology. *BMJ* 1982;285:606.
44. Goeken JA. Antineutrophil cytoplasmic and anti-endothelial cell antibodies: new mechanisms for vasculitis. *Current Opin Dermatol* 1995:75–82.
45. Hall JB, Wadham B, Wood CJ, et al. Vasculitis and glomerulonephritis: a subgroup with anti-neutrophil cytoplasmic antibody. *Aust N Z J Med* 1984;14: 277–278.
46. van der Woude TJ, Rasmussen N, Lobatto S, et al. Autoantibodies against neutrophils and monocytes: tool for diagnosis and marker of disease activity in Wegener granulomatosis. *Lancet* 1985;1:425–429.
47. Nölle B, Specks U, Lüdemann J, et al. Anticytoplasmic antibodies: their immunodiagnostic value in Wegener granulomatosis. *Ann Intern Med* 1989; 111:28–40.
48. Jennette JC, Falk RJ. Anti-neutrophil cytoplasmic autoantibodies with specificity for myeloperoxidase in patients with systemic vasculitis and idiopathic necrotizing and crescentic glomerulonephritis. *N Engl J Med* 1988;318: 1651–1657.
49. Kallenberg CGM, Mulder AHL, Cohen Tervaert JW. Antineutrophil cytoplasmic antibodies: a still-growing class of autoantibodies in inflammatory disorders. *Am J Med* 1992;93:675–682.
50. Savige J, Gillis D, Benson E, et al. International consensus statement on testing and reporting of antineutrophil cytoplasmic antibodies (ANCA). *Am J Clin Pathol* 1999;111:507–513.
51. Hagen EC, Ballieux BEPB, van Es LA, et al. Antineutrophil cytoplasmic autoantibodies: A review of the antigens involved, the assays, and the clinical and possible pathogenetic consequences. *Blood* 1993;81:1996–2002.
52. Geffriaud-Ricouard C, Noel LH, Chauveau D, et al. Clinical spectrum of diseases associated with ANCA of defined antigen specificities in 98 selected cases. *Clin Nephrol* 1993;39:125–136.
53. Gross WL, Schmitt WH, Csernok E. ANCA and associated diseases: immunodiagnostic and pathogenetic aspects. *Clin Exp Immunol* 1993;91:1–12.
54. Hagen E, Daha M, Hermans J, et al. The diagnostic value of standardized assays for ANCA in idiopathic systemic vasculitis: results of an international collaborative study. *Kidney Int* 1998;53:743–753.
55. Mohan N, Kerr G. Diagnosis of vasculitis. *Best Pract Res Clin Rheumatol* 2001; 15:203–223.
56. D'Agati V. Antineutrophil cytoplasmic antibody and vasculitis: much more than a disease marker. *J Clin Invest* 2002;110:919–921.
57. Xiao H, al e. Antineutrophil cytoplasmic autoantibodies specific for myeloperoxidase cause glomerulonephritis and vasculitis in mice. *J Clin Invest* 2002;110:955–963.
58. Brons R, Kallenberg C, Cohen Tervaert J. Are antineutrophil cytoplasmic antibody-associated vasculitides pauci-immune? *Rheum Dis Clin N Am* 2001;27:833–848.
59. Aydintug AO, Tokgöz G, D'Cruz DP, et al. Antibodies to endothelial cells in patients with Behçet's disease. *Clin Immunol Immunopathol* 1993;67:157–162.
60. Lunardi C, Bambara LM, Biasi D, et al. Elimination diet in the treatment of selected patients with hypersensitivity vasculitis. *Clin Exp Rheumatol* 1992; 10:131–135.
61. Woodbury GR Jr, Fried W, Ertle JO, et al. Dapsone-associated agranulocytosis and severe anemia in a patient with leukocytoclastic vasculitis. *J Am Acad Dermatol* 1993;28(5 Pt 1):781–783.
62. Miyagawa S, Shiomi Y, Fukumoto T, et al. Recombinant granulocyte colony-stimulating factor for dapsone-induced agranulocytosis in leukocytoclastic vasculitis. *J Am Acad Dermatol* 1993;28:659–661.
63. Hazen PG, Michel B. Management of necrotizing vasculitis with colchicine: improvement in patients with cutaneous lesions and Behçet's syndrome. *Arch Dermatol* 1979;115:1303–1306.
64. Callen JP. Colchicine is effective in controlling chronic cutaneous leukocytoclastic vasculitis. *J Am Acad Dermatol* 1985;13:193–200.
65. Pyne D, Mootoo R, Bhanji A. Cochicine for the treatment of recurrent Henoch-Schönlein purpura in an adult [letter]. *Rheumatol* 2001;40:1430–1431.
66. Cupps TR, Springer RM, Fauci AS. Chronic, recurrent small-vessel cutaneous vasculitis: clinical experience in 13 patients. *J Am Med Assoc* 1982;247: 1994–1998.
67. Callen JP, Spencer LV, Burruss JB, et al. Azathioprine: an effective, corticosteroid-sparing therapy for patients with recalcitrant cutaneous lupus erythe-

matosus or with recalcitrant cutaneous leukocytoclastic vasculitis. *Arch Dermatol* 1991;127:515–522.
68. Heurkens AHM, Westedt ML, Breedveld FC. Prednisone plus azathioprine treatment in patients with rheumatoid arthritis complicated by vasculitis. *Arch Intern Med* 1991;151:2249–2254.
69. Haynes BF. Wegener's granulomatosis and midline granuloma. In: Wyngaarden JB, Smith Jr LH, Bennett JC, eds. *Cecil textbook of medicine,* 19th ed. Philadelphia: WB Saunders, 1992:1541–1544.
70. Haynes BF. Treatment of the granulomatous vasculitides: the spectrum of vasculitis: clinical, pathologic, immunologic, and therapeutic considerations. *Ann Intern Med* 1978;89:671–672.
71. Fauci AS, Haynes BF, Katz P, et al. Wegener's granulomatosis: prospective clinical and therapeutic experience with 85 patients for 21 years. *Ann Intern Med* 1983;98:76–85.
72. Chow CC, Li EK, Lai FM. Allergic granulomatosis and angiitis (Churg–Strauss syndrome): response to "pulse" intravenous cyclophosphamide. *Ann Rheum Dis* 1989;48:605–608.
73. Langford C. Management of systemic vasculitis. *Best Pract Res Clin Rheumatol* 2001;15:281–297.
74. Jayne D. Conventional treatment and outcome of Wegener's granulomatosis and microscopic polyangiitis. *Cleveland Clin J Med* 2002;69[Suppl 2]:110–116.
75. Levine S, Stone J. New approaches to treatment in systemic vasculitis: biological therapies. *Best Pract Res Clin Rheumatol* 2001;15:315–333.
76. Bartolucci P, Ramanoelina J, Cohen P, et al. Efficacy of the anti-TNF-α antibody infliximab against refractory systemic vasculitides: an open pilot study on 10 patients. *Rheumatol* 2002;41:1126–1132.
77. Zaja F, De Vita S, Russo D, et al. Rituximab for the treatment of type II mixed cryoglobulinemia. *Arthritis Rheum* 2002;46:2252–2264.
78. Ong C, Benson E. Successful treatment of chronic leukocytoclastic vasculitis and persistent ulceration with intravenous immunoglobulin. *Br J Dermatol* 2000;143:447–449.
79. McCombs RP. Systemic "allergic" vasculitis. *JAMA* 1965;194:1059.
80. Knowles HCJ, Zeek PM, Blankenhorn MA. Studies on necrotizing angiitis IV. Periarteritis nodasa and hypersensitivity angiitis. *Arch Intern Med* 1953;92: 789–805.
81. Parums DV. The arteritides. *Histopathol* 1994;25:1–20.
82. Ekenstam EAF, Callen JP. Cutaneous leukocytoclastic vasculitis: clinical and laboratory features of 82 patients seen in private practice. *Arch Dermatol* 1984; 120:484–489.
83. Handel DW, Roenigk JH, Shainoff J, et al. Necrotizing vasculitis. *Arch Dermatol* 1975;111:847–852.
84. Yermakov VM, Hitti IF, Sutton AL. Necrotizing vasculitis associated with diphenylhydantoin: two fatal cases. *Hum Pathol* 1983;13:182–184.
85. Haber MM, Marboe CC, Fenoglio JJ Jr. Vasculitis in drug reactions and serum sickness. In: Churg A, Churg J, eds. *Systemic vasculitis.* New York: Igaku-Shoin Medical Publishers, 1991:305–313.
86. Calabrese LH, Michel BA, Bloch DA, et al. The American College of Rheumatology 1990 criteria for the classification of hypersensitivity vasculitis. *Arthritis Rheum* 1990;33:1108–1113.
87. Michel BA, Hunder GG, Bloch DA, et al. Hypersensitivity vasculitis and Henoch-Schönlein purpura: a comparison between the 2 disorders. *J Rheumatol* 1992;19:721–728.
88. Cream JJ. Immunofluorescent studies of the skin in cryoglobulinaemic vasculitis. *Br J Dermatol* 1971;84:48–53.
89. Molina R, Provost TT, Alexander EL. Two types of inflammatory vascular disease in Sjögren's syndrome. *Arthritis Rheum* 1985;28:1251–1258.
90. Molina R, Provost TT, Arnett FC, al e. Primary Sjögren's syndrome in men: clinical, serologic, and immunogenetic features. *Am J Med* 1986;80:23–31.
91. Boom BW, Mommaas AM, Vermeer B. Presence and interpretation of vascular immune depositis in human skin: the value of direct immunofluorescence. *J Dermatol Sci* 1992;3:26–34.
92. Baart de la Faille-Kuyper EH, van der Meer JB, Baart de la Faille H. An immunohistochemical study of the skin of healthy individuals. *Acta Derm Venereol* 1974;54:271–274.
93. Dahl MV. *Clinical immunodermatology* Chicago: Year Book Medical Publishers, 1981.
94. Nieboer C. Immunofluorescence patterns in sun-exposed and non-sun-exposed skin of healthy individuals. *Acta Derm Venereol* 1981;61:471–479.
95. Schroeter AL, Powell FC. Cutaneous vascular immunofluorescence: a sensitivity and specificity study. In: McDonald DM, ed. *Immunodermatology.* London: Butterworth-Heineman, 1984:219–223.
96. Welbourn E, Champion RH, Parish WE. Hypersensitivity to bacteria in eczema, I: bacterial culture, skin tests and immunofluorescent detection of immunoglobulins and bacterial antigens. *Br J Dermatol* 1976;94:619–632.
97. Miller RAW, Griffiths WAD. Experimentally induced complement and immunoglobulin deposition along the basement membrane zone (BMZ) and in dermal blood vessels. *Br J Dermatol* 1982;106:275–279.
98. Longley S, Caldwell JR, Panush RS. Paraneoplastic vasculitis. *Am J Med* 1986; 80:1027–1030.
99. Sánchez-Geurrero J, Gutiérrez-Ureña S, Vidaller A, et al. Vasculitis as a paraneoplastic syndrome: report of 11 cases and review of the literature. *J Rheumatol* 1990;17:1458–1462.
100. Castro M, Conn DL, Su WPD, et al. Rheumatic manifestations in myelodysplastic syndromes. *J Rheumatol* 1991;18:721–727.
101. Bourantas K, Malamou-Mitsi VD, Christou L, et al. Cutaneous vasculitis as the initial manifestation in acute myelomonocytic leukemia. *Ann Intern Med* 1994;121:942–944.
102. Kurzrock R, Cohen PR, Markowitz A. Clinical manifestations of vasculitis in patients with solid tumors: a case report and review of the literature. *Arch Intern Med* 1994;154:334–340.
103. Soter NA, Mihm MC, Colten HR. Cutaneous necrotizing venulitis in patients with cystic fibrosis. *J Pediatr* 1979;95:197–201.
104. Finnegan MJ, Hinchcliffe J, Russell-Jones D, et al. Vasculitis complicating cystic fibrosis. *Q J Med* 1989;72:609–621.
105. Hilton AM, Hasleton PS, Bradlow A, et al. Cutaneous vasculitis and immune complexes in severe bronchiectasis. *Thorax* 1984;39:185–191.
106. Tanaka E, Tada K, Amitani R, et al. Systemic hypersensitivity vasculitis associated with bronchiectasis. *Chest* 1992;102:647–649.
107. Mackel SE, Jordan RE. Leukocytoclastic vasculitis. *Arch Dermatol* 1982;118: 296–301.
108. Wilkinson DS. Some clinical manifestations and associations of "allergic" vasculitis. *Br J Dermatol* 1965;77:186–192.
109. Alanko K, Stubb S, Kauppinen K. Cutaneous drug reactions: clinical types and causative agents: a five-year survey of in-patients. *Acta Derm Venereol (Stock)* 1989;69:223–226.
110. Ives TJ, Bentz EJ, Gwyther RE. Dermatologic adverse reactions in a family medicine setting. *Arch Fam Med* 1992;1:241–245.
111. Roujeau JC, Stern RS. Severe adverse cutaneous reactions to drugs. *N Engl J Med* 1994;331:1272–1285.
112. Mullick FG, McAllister HA, Wagner BM, et al. Drug related vasculitis. *Hum Pathol* 1979;10:313–325.
113. Lever WF, Schaumburg-Lever G. Eruptions due to drugs. *Histopathology of the skin,* 7th ed. Philadelphia: JB Lippincott Co, 1990:284–297.
114. ten Holder S, Joy M, Falk R. Cutaneous and systemic manifestations of drug-induced vasculitis. *Ann Pharmocotherap* 2002;36:130–147.
115. Lawley TJ, Bielory L, Gascon P, et al. A prospective clinical and immunologic analysis of patients with serum sickness. *N Engl J Med* 1984;311:1407–1413.
116. Bielory L, Yancey KB, Young NS, et al. Cutaneous manifestations of serum sickness in patients receiving antithymocyte globulin. *J Am Acad Dermatol* 1985;13:411–417.
117. Warrington RJ, Martens CJ, Rubin M, et al. Immunologic studies in subjects with a serum sickness-like illness after immunization with human diploid cell rabies vaccine. *J Allergy Clin Immunol* 1987;79:605–610.
118. Patel A, Prussick R, Buchanan WW, et al. Serum sickness-like illness and leukocytoclastic vasculitis after intravenous streptokinase. *J Am Acad Dermatol* 1991;24:652–653.
119. McDuffie FC, Sams WM Jr, Maldonado JE, et al. Hypocomplementemia with cutaneous vasculitis and arthritis. *Mayo Clin Proc* 1973;48:340–348.
120. Schwartz HR, McDuffie FC, Black LF, et al. Hypocomplementemic urticarial vasculitis: association with chronic obstructive pulmonary disease. *Mayo Clin Proc* 1982;57:231–238.
121. Soter NA, Mihm MC Jr, Gigli I, et al. Two distinct cellular patterns in cutaneous necrotizing angiitis. *J Invest Dermatol* 1976;66:344–350.
122. Mehregan DR, Hall MJ, Gibson LE. Urticarial vasculitis: a histopathologic and clinical review of 72 cases. *J Am Acad Dermatol* 1992;26:441–448.
123. Wiesnieski JJ, Baer AN, Christensen J, et al. Hypocomplementemic urticarial vasculitis syndrome. *Medicine* 1995;74:24–41.
124. Soter NA. Cutaneous necrotizing venulitis. In: Fitzpatrick TB, Eisen AZ, Wolff K, et al., eds. *Dermatology in general medicine.* Vol. 1. New York: McGraw-Hill, 1993:1501–1510.
125. Yasue T. Livedoid vasculitis and central nervous system involvement in systemic lupus erythematosus. *Arch Dermatol* 1986;122:66–70.
126. Provost TT, Zone JJ, Synkowski D, et al. Unusual cutaneous manifestations of systemic lupus erythematosus, I: Urticarial-like lesions—correlation with clinical and serological abnormalities. *J Invest Dermatol* 1980;75:495–499.
127. Asherson RA, Sontheimer R. Urticarial vasculitis and syndromes in association with connective tissue disease. *Ann Rheum Dis* 1991;50:743–744.
128. Asherson RA, D'Cruz D, Stephens CJM, et al. Urticarial vasculitis in a connective tissue disease clinic: patterns, presentations and treatment. *Semin Arthritis Rheum* 1991;20:285–296.
129. Davis M, Daoud M, Kirby B, et al. Clinicopathologic correlation of hypocomplementemic and normocomplementemic urticarial vasculitis. *J Am Acad Dermatol* 1998;38(6 Pt 1):899–905.
130. Kobza Black A. Urticarial vasculitis. *Clin Dermatol* 1999;17:565–569.
131. Jorizzo JL. Classification of vasculitis. *J Invest Dermatol* 1993;100:106S–110S.
132. Jorizzo JL, Solomon AR, Zanolli MD, et al. Neutrophilic vascular reactions. *J Am Acad Dermatol* 1988;19:983–1005.
133. Cohen P, Kurzrock R. Sweet's syndrome: a neutrophilic dermatosis classically associated with acute onset and fever. *Clin Dermatol* 2000;18:265–282.
134. Vignon-Pennamen M. The extracutaneous involvement in the neutrophilic dermatoses. *Clin Dermatol* 2000;18:339–347.
135. Weenig R, Davis M, Dahl P, et al. Skin ulcers misdiagnosed as pyoderma gangrenosum. *N Engl J Med* 2002;347:1412–1418.
136. Cream JJ. Vasculitis. *Curr Prob Dermatol* 1989;1:69–95.
137. Cupps TR. Infections and vasculitis: mechanisms considered. In: LeRoy EC, ed. *Systemic vasculitis, the biological basis.* New York: Marcel Dekker, Inc., 1992: 483–504.
138. Dodd HJ, Goldsmith HJ, Verbov JL. Necrotizing cutaneous vasculitis occurring as an early feature of "shunt nephritis." *Clin Exp Dermatol* 1985;10: 284–287.
139. Kingston ME, Mackey D. Skin clues in the diagnosis of life-threatening infections. *Rev Infect Dis* 1986;8:1–11.
140. Radcliffe-Crocker H, Williams C. Erythema elevatum diutinum. *Br J Dermatol* 1894;6:1–9.

141. Katz SI, Gallin JI, Hertz KC, et al. Erythema elevatum diutinum: skin and systemic manifestations, immunologic studies, and successful treatment with dapsone. *Medicine* 1977;56:443–455.
142. Fort SL, Rodman OG. Erythema elevatum diutinum. *Arch Dermatol* 1977;113: 819–822.
143. Muratori S, Carrera C, Gorani A, et al. Erythema elevatum diutinum and HIV infection: a report of five cases. *Br J Dermatol* 1999;141:335–338.
144. Mills JA, Michel BA, Bloch DA, et al. The American College of Rheumatology 1990 criteria for the classification of Henoch-Schönlein purpura. *Arthritis Rheum* 1990;33:1114–1121.
145. Allen M, Diamond LK, Howel DA. Anaphylactoid purpura in children. *Am J Dis Child* 1960;99:833–854.
146. Sterky G, Thilén A. A study on the onset and prognosis of acute vascular purpura (the Schönlein-Henoch syndrome) in children. *Acta Paediat* 1960;49: 217–229.
147. Nielsen HE. Epidemiology of Schönlein-Henoch purpura. *Acta Paediatr Scand* 1988;77:125–131.
148. Farley TA, Gillespie S, Rasoulpour M, et al. Epidemiology of a cluster of Henoch-Schönlein purpura. *Am J Dis Child* 1989;143:798–803.
149. Al-Sheyyab M, Batieha A, El-Shanti H, et al. Henoch-Schönlein purpura and streptococcal infection: a prospective case control study. *Ann Trop Paediatr* 1999;19:253–255.
150. Calvino M, Llorca J, Garcia-Porrua C, et al. Henoch-Schönlein purpura in children from northwestern Spain. *Medicine* 2001;80:279–290.
151. Saulsbury F. Epidemiology of Henoch-Schönlein purpura. *Cleveland Clin J Med* 2002;69[Suppl 2]:87–89.
152. Duquesnoy B. Henoch-Schönlein purpura. *Baillieres Clin Rheumatol* 1991;5: 253–261.
153. Watts R, Jolliffe V, Grattan C, et al. Cutaneous vasculitis in a defined population—clinical and epidemiological associations. *J Rheumatol* 1998;25:920–924.
154. Gonzalez-Gay M, Garcia-Porrua C. Systemic vasculitis in adults in northwestern Spain, 1988–1997. *Medicine* 1999;78:292–308.
155. Cream JJ, Gumpel JM, Peachey RDG. Schönlein-Henoch purpura in the adult: a study of 77 adults with anaphylactoid or Schönlein purpura. *Q J Med* 1970;156:461–484.
156. Heng MCY. Henoch-Schönlein purpura. *Br J Dermatol* 1985;112:235–240.
157. Talbot D, Craig R, Falconer S, et al. Henoch-Schönlein purpura secondary to trauma. *Arch Dis Child* 1988;63:1113–1115.
158. Meadow SR, Scott DG. Berger disease: Henoch-Schönlein syndrome without the rash. *J Pediatr* 1985;106:27–32.
159. Miyagawa S, Dohi K, Hanatani M, et al. Anaphylactoid purpura and familial IgA nephropathy. *Am J Med* 1989;86:340–342.
160. Sussman M, Jones JH, Almeida JD, et al. Deficiency of the second component of complement associated with anaphylactoid purpura and presence of *Mycoplasma* in the serum. *Clin Exp Immunol* 1973;14:531–539.
161. Einstein LP, Alper CA, Block KJ, al e. Biosynthetic deficiency in monocytes from human beings with genetic deficiency of the second component of complement. *N Engl J Med* 1975;292:1169–1171.
162. Gelfand EW, Clarkson JE, Minta JO. Selective deficiency of the second component of complement in a patient with anaphylactoid purpura. *Clin Immunol Immunopathol* 1975;4:269–274.
163. Ault BH, Stapleton B, Rivas ML, et al. Association of Henoch-Schönlein purpura glomerulonephritis with C4B deficiency. *J Pediatr* 1990;117:753–755.
164. McLean RH, Wyatt RJ, Julian BA. Complement phenotypes in glomerulonephritis: increased frequency of homozygous null C4 phenotypes in IgA nephropathy and Henoch-Schönlein purpura. *Kidney Int* 1984;26:855–860.
165. Wyatt RJ, Julian BA, Galla JH. Properdin deficiency with IgA nephropathy [letter]. *N Engl J Med* 1981;305:1097.
166. Welch TR, Berry A, Beischel LS. C4 isotype deficiency in IgA nephropathy. *Pediatr Nephrol* 1987;1:136–139.
167. Wyatt RJ, Schneider PD, Alpers CA, et al. C4B deficiency in two siblings with IgA nephropathy. *Am J Kidney Dis* 1990;15:66–71.
168. Wyatt RJ, Rivas ML, Schena FP, et al. Regional variation in C4 phenotype in patients with IgA nephropathy. *J Pediatr* 1990;116:72–77.
169. Kauffmann RH, Herrmann WA, Meÿer CJLM, et al. Circulating IgA-immune complexes in Henoch-Schönlein purpura: a longitudinal study of their relationship to disease activity and vascular deposition of IgA. *Am J Med* 1980;69: 859–866.
170. van Hale HM, Gibson LE, Schroeter AL. Henoch-Schönlein vasculitis: direct immunofluorescence study of uninvolved skin. *J Am Acad Dermatol* 1986; 15:665–670.
171. Hené RJ, Velthuis P, van de Wiel A, et al. The relevance of IgA deposits in vessel walls of clinically normal skin: a prospective study. *Arch Intern Med* 1986; 146:745–749.
172. Giangiacomo J, Tsai C. Dermal and glomerular deposition of IgA in anaphylactoid purpura. *Am J Dis Child* 1977;131:981–983.
173. Levinsky RJ, Barratt TM. IgA immune complexes in Henoch-Schönlein purpura. *Lancet* 1979;ii:1100–1103.
174. Kuno-Sakai H, Sakai H, Nomoto Y, et al. Increase of IgA-bearing peripheral blood lymphocytes in children with Henoch-Schönlein purpura. *Pediatrics* 1979;64:918–922.
175. Nussinovitch M, Prais D, Finkelstein Y, et al. Cutaneous manifestations of Henoch-Schönlein purpura in young children. *Pediatr Dermatol* 1998;15: 426–428.
176. Rauterburg EW, Lieberknecht H-M, Wingen A-M, et al. Complement membrane attack (MAC) in idiopathic IgA-glomerulonephritis. *Kidney Int* 1987;31: 820–829.
177. Boom Bw, Out-Luiting CJ, Baldwin WM, et al. Membrane attack complex of complement in leukocytoclastic vasculitis of the skin. *Arch Dermatol* 1987;123: 1191–1195.
178. Baart de la Faille-Kuyper EH, Kater L, Kooiker CJ, et al. IgA-deposits in cutaneous blood-vessel walls and mesangium in Henoch-Schönlein syndrome [letter]. *Lancet* 1973;1:892–893.
179. Baart de la Faille-Kuyper EH, van der Meer JB, Kater L, et al. Alternate pathway complement activation by IgA in Schönlein-Henoch syndrome. *Neth J Med* 1974;17:5–11.
180. Tsai CC, Giangiacomo J, Zuckner J. Dermal IgA deposits in Henoch-Schönlein purpura and Berger's nephritis. *Lancet* 1975;1:342–343.
181. Hiemstra PS, Gorter A, Stuurman ME, et al. Activation of the alternative pathway of complement by human serum IgA. *Eur J Immunol* 1987;17:321–326.
182. Sinniah R, Feng PH, Chen BTM. Henoch-Schönlein syndrome: a clinical and morphological study of renal biopsies. *Clin Nephrol* 1978;9:219–228.
183. Baart de la Faille-Kuyper EH, Kater L, Kuijten RH, et al. Occurrence of vascular IgA deposits in clinically normal skin of patients with renal disease. *Kidney Int* 1976;9:424–429.
184. Woodroffe AJ, Gormly AA, McKenzie PE, et al. Immunologic studies of ? in IgA nephropathy. *Kidney Int* 1980;18:366–374.
185. Nakamoto Y, Asano Y, Dohi K, et al. Primary IgA glomerulonephritis and Schönlein-Henoch purpura nephritis. *Q J Med* 1978;47:495–516.
186. Waldherr R, Ram Bausek M, Rauterberg W, et al. Immunohistochemical features of mesangial IgA glomerulonephritis. *Contrib Nephrol* 1984;40:99–106.
187. Roth DA, Wilz DR, Theil GB. Schönlein-Henoch syndrome in adults. *Q J Med* 1985;55:145–152.
188. Casaneuva B, Rodriguez-Valverde V, Farinas MC, et al. Autologous mixed lymphocyte reaction and T cell suppressor activity in patients with Henoch-Schönlein purpura and IgA nephropathy. *Nephron* 1990;54:224–228.
189. D'Amico G. The commonest glomerulonephritis in the world. *Q J Med* 1987;64:709–727.
190. Williams DG. IgA nephropathy. *BMJ* 1994;308:74–75.
191. Sinico R, Fornasieri A, Oreni N, et al. Polymeric IgA rheumatoid factor in idiopathic mesangial nephropathy (Berger's disease). *J Immunol* 1986;137: 536–541.
192. Saulsbury FT. IgA rheumatoid factor in Henoch-Schönlein purpura. *J Pediatr* 1986;108:71–76.
193. Tomino Y, Sakai H, Endoh M, et al. Cross-reactivity of eluted antibodies from renal tissues of patients with Henoch-Schönlein purpura nephritis and IgA nephropathy. *Am J Nephrol* 1983;3:315–318.
194. Nyulassy S, Buc M, Sasinska M, et al. The HLA system in glonerulonephritis. *Clin Immunol Immunopathol* 1977;7:319–323.
195. Berthoux FC, Gagne A, Sabatier JC, et al. HLA-BW35 and mesangial IgA glomerulonephritis [letter]. *N Engl J Med* 1978;298:1034–1035.
196. Amoli M, Thomson W, Hajeer A, et al. HLA-B35 association with nephritis in Henoch-Schönlein purpura. *J Rheumatol* 2002;29:948–949.
197. Tolkoff-Rubin NE, Cosimi AB, Fuller T, et al. IgA nephropathy in HLA identical siblings. *Transplantation* 1978;26:430–433.
198. Montoliu J, Darnell A, Torras A, et al. Familial IgA nephropathy: report of two cases and brief review of the literature. *Arch Int Med* 1980;140:1374–1375.
199. Julian BA, Quiggins PA, Thompson JS, et al. Familial IgA nephropathy: evidence of an inherited mechanism of disease. *N Engl J Med* 1985;312:202–208.
200. Egido J, Julian BA, Wyatt RJ. Genetic factors in primary IgA nephropathy. *Nephro Dial Transplant* 1987;2:134–142.
201. Montoliu J, Lens XM, Torras A, et al. Henoch-Schönlein purpura and IgA nephropathy in father and son. *Nephron* 1990;54:77–79.
202. D'Amico G. Influence of clinical and histological features on actuarial renal survival in adult patients with idiopathic IgA nephropathy, membranous nephropathy, and membranoproliferative glomerulonephritis: survey of the recent literature. *Am J Kidney Dis* 1992;20:315–323.
203. Van den Wall Bakke AWL, Daha MR, Radl J, et al. The bone marrow as production site of the IgA deposited in the kidneys of patients with IgA nephropathy. *Clin Exp Immunol* 1988;72:321–325.
204. Egido J, Biasco R, Lozano J, et al. Immunological abnormalities in the tonsils of patients with IgA nephropathy: inversion in the ratio of IgA: IgG bearing lymphocytes and increased polymeric IgA synthesis. *Clin Exp Immunol* 1984; 57:101–106.
205. André C, Berthoux FC, André F, et al. Prevalence of IgA2 deposits in IgA nephropathies. *N Engl J Med* 1980;23:1343–1346.
206. Williams DG. Pathogenesis of idiopathic IgA nephropathy. *Pediatr Nephrol* 1993;7:303–311.
207. Hirschel-Scholz S, Hunziker N. Acute hemorrhagic edema of the infant (Finkelstein's disease) [letter]. *Pediatr Dermatol* 1990;7:323.
208. Snow IM. Purpura, urticaria and angioneurotic edema of the hands and feet in a nursing baby. *J Am Med Assoc* 1913;61:18–19.
209. Dubin BA, Bronson DM, Eng AM. Acute hemorrhagic edema of childhood: An unusual variant of leukocytoclastic vasculitis. *J Am Acad Dermatol* 1990; 23:347–350.
210. Legrain V, Lejean S, Taïeb A, et al. Infantile acute hemorrhagic edema skin: study of ten cases. *J Am Acad Dermatol* 1991;24:17–22.
211. Cox NH. Seidlmayer's syndrome: Postinfectious cockade purpura of early childhood. *J Am Acad Dermatol* 1992;26:275.
212. Saraçlar Y, Tinaztepe K, Adalioglu G, et al. Acute hemorrhagic edema of infancy (AHEI)—a variant of Henoch-Schönlein purpura or a distinct clinical entity? *J All Clin Immunol* 1990;86:473–483.
213. Saraçlar Y, Tinaztepe K. Infantile acute hemorrhagic edema of the skin [letter]. *J Am Acad Dermatol* 1992;26:275–276.

214. Gonggryp L, Todd G. Acute haemorrhagic edema of childhood. *Pediatr Dermatol* 1998;15:91–96.
215. Dillon M. Henoch-Schönlein purpura (treatment and outcome). *Cleveland Clin J Med* 2002;69[Suppl 2]:121–123.
216. Goraya J, Kaur S. Acute infantile hemorrhagic edema and Henoch-Schönlein purpura: is IgA the missing link? [letter]. *J Am Acad Dermatol* 2002; 47:801.
217. Peeters AJ, van den Wall Bake AWL, Daha MR, et al. Inflammatory bowel disease and ankylosing spondylitis associated with cutaneous vasculitis, glomerulonephritis, and circulating IgA immune complexes. *Ann Rheum Dis* 1990;49:638–640.
218. Bruneau C, Villiaumey J, Avouac B, et al. Seronegative spondyloarthropathies and IgA glomerulonephritis: a report of four cases and a review of the literature. *Sem Arthritis Rheum* 1986;15:179–184.
219. Choong C, Beasley S. Intra-abdominal manifestations of Henoch-Schönlein purpura. *J Pediatr Child Health* 1998;34:405–409.
220. Levy M, Broyer M, Arsan A, et al. Anaphylactoid purpura nephritis in childhood: natural history and immunopathology. In: Hamburger J, Crosnier J, Maxwell MH, eds. *Advances in nephrology.* New York: Year Book Medical Publishers, 1976:183–228.
221. Cybulsky AV, Jothy S, Seely JF. Late development of purpura in a patient with glomerulonephritis. *Can Med Assoc J* 1984;130:149–152.
222. Sano H, Izumida M, Shimizu H, et al. Risk factors of renal involvement and significant proteinuria in Henoch-Schönlein purpura. *Eur J Pediatr* 2002;161: 196–201.
223. Counehan R, Cameron JS. Henoch-Schönlein nephritis. *Contrib Nephrol* 1977; 7:143–165.
224. Tancrede-Bohin E, Ochonisky S, Vignon-Pennamen M, et al. Schönlein - Henoch purpura in adult patients. *Arch Dermatol* 1997;133:438–442.
225. Piette W. Schönlein-Henoch purpura—why should we care? *Arch Dermatol* 1997;133.
226. Blanco R, Martinez-Taboada V, Rodriguez-Valverde V, et al. Henoch-Schönlein purpura in adulthood and childhood: two different expressions of the same syndrome. *Arthritis Rheum* 1997;40:859–864.
227. Pillebout E, Thervet E, Hill G, et al. Henoch-Schönlein purpura in adults: outcome and prognostic factors. *J Am Soc Nephrol* 2002;13:1271–1278.
228. Flynn J, Smoyer W, Bunchman T, et al. Treatment of Henoch-Schönlein purpura glomerulonephritis in children with high-dose corticosteroids plus oral cyclophosphamide. *Am J Nephrol* 2001;21:128–133.
229. Singh S, Devidayal, Kumar L, Joshi K, Minz R, Datta U. Severe Henoch-Schönlein nephritis: resolution with azathioprine and steroids. *Rheumatol Int* 2002;22:133–137.
230. Ronkainen J, Nuutinen M, Koskimies O. The adult kidney 24 years after childhood Henoch-Schönlein purpura: a retrospective cohort study. *Lancet* 2002;360:666–670.
231. Goldstein AR, White RHR, Akuse R, et al. Long-term follow-up of childhood Henoch-Schönlein nephritis. *Lancet* 1992;339:280–282.
232. Knight JF, Cameron JS. Henoch-Schönlein nephritis in adults: a report from the UK glomerulonephritis registry. *Nephro Dial Transplant* 1987;2:415.
233. Byrn JR, Fitzgerald JF, Northway JD, et al. Unusual manifestations of Henoch-Schönlein syndrome. *Am J Dis Child* 1976;130:1335–1337.
234. Hasegawa A, Kawamura T, Ito H, et al. Fate of renal grafts with recurrent Henoch-Schönlein purpura nephritis in children. *Transplant Proc* 1989;21: 2130–2133.
235. van de Wiel A, Valentijn RM, Schuurman HJ, et al. Circulating IgA immune complexes and skin IgA deposits in liver disease: relation to liver histopathology. *Dig Dis Sci* 1988;33:678–684.
236. Aggarwal M, Manske CL, Lynch PJ, et al. Henoch-Schönlein vasculitis as a manifestation of IgA-associated disease in cirrhosis. *Am J Kidney Dis* 1992; 20:400–402.
237. Harvey JG, Colditz PB. Henoch-Schönlein purpura: A surgical review. *Aust Paediatr J* 1984;20:13–16.
238. Saulsbury FT. Henoch-Schönlein purpura. *Pediatr Dermatol* 1984;1:195–201.
239. Hall RP, Stachura I, Cason J, et al. IgA-containing circulating immune complexes in patients with nephropathy. *Am J Med* 1983;74:56–63.
240. Arrese Estrada J, Goffin F, Cornil F, et al. Dendrocytoclasis in Henoch-Schönlein purpura. *Acta Derm Venereol* 1991;71:358–359.
241. Saulsbury FT. Heavy and light chain composition of serum IgA and IgA rheumatoid factor in Henoch-Schönlein purpura. *Arthritis Rheum* 1992;35: 1377–1380.
242. Brown J, Melinkovich P. Schönlein-Henoch purpura misdiagnosed as suspected child abuse: a case report and literature review. *J Am Med Assoc* 1986;256:617–618.
243. McNairy SL, Millns JL, Phyliky RL, et al. Vitamin K-responsive coagulopathy in Henoch-Schönlein purpura. *Mayo Clin Proc* 1977;52:746–747.
244. Ledermann JA, Hoffbrand BI. Dapsone in allergic vasculitis: its use in Henoch-Schönlein disease following vaccination. *J Royal Soc Med* 1983;76: 613–614.
245. Utani A, Ohta M, Shinya A, et al. Successful treatment of adult Henoch-Schönlein purpura with factor XIII concentrate. *J Am Acad Dermatol* 1991; 24:438–442.
246. Karges HE, Clemens R. Factor XIII: enzymatic and clinical aspects. *Behring Inst Mitt* 1988;82:43–58.
247. Kamitsuji H, Tani K, Yasui M, et al. Activity of blood coagulation factor XIII as a prognostic indicator in patients with Henoch-Schönlein purpura: efficacy of factor XIII substitution. *Eur J Pedatr* 1987;146:519–523.
248. van Ypersele de Strihou C. Fish oil for IgA nephropathy [editorial]? *N Engl J Med* 1994;331:1227–1229.
249. Donadio JV, Bergstralh EJ, Offord KP, et al. Clinical and histopathologic associations with impaired renal function in IgA nephropathy. *Clin Nephrol* 1994; 41:65–71.
250. Donadio JJV, Bergstralh MS, Offord KP, et al. A controlled trial of fish oil in IgA nephropathy. *N Engl J Med* 1994;331:1194–1199.
251. Brouet JC, Clauvel JP, Danon F, et al. Biologic and clinical significance of cryoglobulins: a report of 86 cases. *Am J Med* 1974;57:775–788.
252. Gorevic PD, Kassab HJ, Levo Y, et al. Mixed cryoglobulinemia: clinical aspects and long-term follow-up of 40 patients. *Am J Med* 1980;69:287–308.
253. Cohen SJ, Pittelkow MR, Su WPD. Cutaneous manifestations of cryoglobulinemia: clinical and histopathologic study of seventy-two patients. *J Am Acad Dermatol* 1991;25:21–27.
254. Cattaneo R, Fenini MG, Facchetti F. The cryoglobulinemic vasculitis. *Ric Clin Lab* 1986;16:327–333.
255. Hundt M, Zielinska-Skowronek M, Schmidt RE. Fcg receptor activation of neutrophils in cryoglobulin-induced leukocytoclastic vasculitis. *Arthritis Rheum* 1993;36:974–982.
256. Stone MS, Piette WW, Davey WP. Cutaneous necrosis at sites of transfusion: cold agglutinin disease [letter]. *J Am Acad Dermatol* 1988;19:356–357.
257. Lawley TJ, Gorevic PD, Hamburger MI, et al. Multiple types of immune complexes in patients with mixed cryoglobulinemia. *J Invest Dermatol* 1980;75: 297–301.
258. Gorevic PD. Cryopathies: cryoglobulins and cryofibrinogenemia. In: Samter M, ed. *Immunological diseases,* 4th ed. Vol. 2: Little, Brown and Company, 1988: 1687–1713.
259. Kaufman LD. The skin and vasculitis. In: LeRoy EC, ed. *Systemic vasculitis: the biologic basis.* New York: Marcel Dekker, Inc., 1992:249–272.
260. Schimmer BM, Bloch KJ. Mixed IgM-IgG cryoglobulinaemia terminating in polyarteritis nodosa. *J Rheumatol* 1975;2:241–250.
261. Garcia-Bracado F, Fernandez JM, Navarro C, et al. Peripheral neuropathy in essential mixed cryoglobulinemia. *Arch Neurol* 1988;45:1210–1214.
262. Meltzer M, Franklin EC. Cryoglobulinemia: a study of 29 patients, I: IgG and IgM cryoglobuins and factors affecting cryoprecipitability. *Am J Med* 1966; 40:828–836.
263. Fauci AS, Haynes BF, Katz P. The spectrum of vasculitis: clinical, pathologic, immunologic, and therapeutic considerations. *Ann Intern Med* 1978;89: 660–676.
264. Winfield JB. Cryoglobulinemia. *Human Pathol* 1983;14:350–354.
265. Ellis FA. The cutaneous manifestation of cryoglobulinemia. *Arch Dermatol* 1964;89:690–697.
266. Inman RD, Hodge M, Johnston MEA, et al. Arthritis, vasculitis, and cryoglobulinemia associated with relapsing hepatitis A virus infection. *Ann Intern Med* 1986;105:700–703.
267. Dan M, Yaniv R. Cholestatic hepatitis, cutaneous vasculitis, and vascular deposits of immunoglobulin M and complement associated with hepatitis A virus infection. *Am J Med* 1990;89:103–104.
268. Ilan Y, Hillman M, Oren R, et al. Vasculitis and cryoglobulinemia associated with persisting cholestatic hepatitis A virus infection. *Am J Gastroenterol* 1990;85:586–587.
269. Levo Y, Gorevic PD, Kassab HJ, et al. The association between hepatitis B virus and essential mixed cryoglobulinemia. *N Engl J Med* 1977;296: 1501–1504.
270. Gocke DJ, McIntosh RM. Cryoprecipitates containing hepatitis B antigen (HBsAg) in patients with liver disease. *Gastroenterology* 1973;65:542.
271. Misiani R, Bellavita P, Fenili D. Hepatitis C virus infection in patients with essential mixed cryoglobulinemia. *Ann Intern Med* 1992;117:573–577.
272. Ferri C, Greco F, Longombardo G, et al. Association between hepatitis C virus and mixed cryoglobulinemia. *Clin Exp Rheumatol* 1991;9:621–624.
273. Agnello V, Chung RT, Kaplan LM. A role for hepatitis C virus infection in type II cryoglobulinemia. *N Engl J Med* 1992;327:1490–1495.
274. Pawlotsky JM, Roudot-Thoraval F, Simmonds P, et al. Extrahepatic immunologic manifestations in chronic hepatitis C and hepatitis C virus serotypes. *Ann Intern Med* 1995;122:169–173.
275. Cacoub P, Lunel Fabiani F, Musset L, et al. Mixed cryoglobulinemia and hepatitis C virus. *Am J Med* 1994;96:124–132.
276. Pawlotsky J-M, Yahia M, Andre C, et al. Immunological disorders in C virus chronic active hepatitis: a prospective case-control study. *Hepatology* 1994; 19:841–848.
277. Alexander EL, Arnett FC, Provost TT, et al. Sjögren's syndrome: association of anti-Ro (SS-A) antibodies with vasculitis, hematologic abnormalities, and serologic hyperreactivity. *Ann Intern Med* 1983;98:155–159.
278. Lamprecht P, Gause A, Gross W. Cryoglobulinemic vasculitis. *Arthritis Rheum* 1999;42:2507–2516.
279. Tarantino A, De Vecchi A, Montagnino G, et al. Renal disease in essential mixed cryoglobulinaemia. *Q J Med* 1981;50:1–30.
280. Pusey CD, Schifferli JA, Lockwood CM, et al. Use of plasma exchange in the management of mixed essential cryoglobulinaemia. *Artif Organs* 1981;5 [Suppl]:183–187.
281. Boom BW, Brand A, Bavinck JNB, et al. Severe leukocytoclastic vasculitis of the skin in a patient with essential mixed cryoglobulinemia treated with high-dose g-globulin intravenously. *Arch Dermatol* 1988;124:1550–1553.
282. Levey JM, Bjornsson B, Banner B, et al. Mixed cryoglobulinemia in chronic hepatitis C infection: a clinicopathologic analysis of 10 cases and review of recent literature. *Medicine* 1994;73:53–67.

283. Bloch KJ. Cryoglobulinemia and hepatitis C virus. *N Engl J Med* 1992;327: 1521–1522.
284. Casato M, Laganà B, Antonelli G, et al. Long-term results of therapy with interferon-A for type II essential mixed cryoglobulinaemia. *Blood* 1991;78: 3142–3147.
285. Mazzaro C, Pozzato G, Moretti M, et al. Long-term effects of alpha-interferon therapy for type II mixed cryoglobulinemia. *Haematologica* 1994;79:342–349.
286. Misiani R, Bellavita P, Fenili D, et al. Interferon alfa-2a therapy in cryoglobulinemia associated with hepatitis C virus. *N Engl J Med* 1994;330:751–756.
287. Zimmermann R, König V, Bauditz J, et al. Interferon alpha in leukocytoclastic vasculitis, mixed cryoglobulinaemia, and chronic hepatitis C [letter]. *Lancet* 1993;341:561–562.
288. Lauer G, Walker B. Medical progress: hepatitis C virus infection. *N Engl J Med* 2001;345:41–52.
289. Cacoub P, Lidove O, Maisonobe T, et al. Interferon-alpha and ribavirin treatment in patients with hepatitis C virus-related systemic vasculitis. *Arthritis Rheum* 2002;46:3317–3326.
290. Homas PB, David-Bajar KM, Fitzpatrick JE, et al. Microscopic polyarteritis: report of a case with cutaneous involvement and antimyeloperoxidase antibodies. *Arch Dermatol* 1992;128:1223–1228.
291. Savage CO, Winearls CG, Evans DJ, et al. Microscopic polyarteritis: presentation, pathology, and prognosis. *Q J Med* 1985;56:467–483.
292. Rodgers H, Gutherie JA, Brownjohn AM, et al. Microscopic polyarteritis: clinical features and treatment. *Postgrad Med J* 1989;65:515–518.
293. Andrassy K, Koderish J, Rufer M, et al. Detection and clinical implication of anti-neutrophil cytoplasm antibodies in Wegener's granulomatosis and rapidly progressive glomerulonephritis. *Clin Nephrol* 1989;32:159–167.
294. Minkowitz G, Smoller BR, McNutt S. Benign cutaneous polyarteritis nodosa: relationship to systemic polyarteritis nodosa and to hepatitis B infection. *Arch Dermatol* 1991;127:1520–1523.
295. Thomas RHM, Black MM. The wide clinical spectrum of polyarteritis nodosa with cutaneous involvement. *Clin Exp Dermatol* 1983;8:47–59.
296. Borrie P. Cutaneous polyarteritis nodosa. *Br J Dermatol* 1972;87:87–95.
297. Siberry GK, Cohen BA, Johnson B. Cutaneous polyarteritis nodosa: Reports of two cases in children and review of the literature. *Arch Dermatol* 1994;130: 884–889.
298. Stone MS, Oslon RR, Weismann DN, et al. Cutaneous vasculitis in the newborn of a mother with cutaneous polyarteritis nodosa. *J Am Acad Dermatol* 1993;28:101–105.
299. Sheth AP, Olson JC, Esterly NB. Cutaneous polyarteritis nodosa of childhood. *J Am Acad Dermatol* 1995;31:561–566.
300. Cohen RD, Conn DL, Ilstrup DM. Clinical features, prognosis and response to treatment in polyarteritis. *Mayo Clin Proc* 1980;55:146–155.
301. Guillevin L, Le THD, Godeau P, et al. Clinical findings and prognosis of polyarteritis nodosa and Churg–Strauss angiitis: a study in 165 patients. *Br J Rheumatol* 1988;27:258–264.
302. Leib ES, Restivo C, Paulus HE. Immunosuppressive and corticosteroid therapy of polyarteritis nodosa. *Am J Med* 1979;67:941–947.
303. Citron BP, Halpern M, McCarron M, et al. Necrotizing angiitis associated with drug abuse. *N Engl J Med* 1970;283:1003–1011.
304. Sergent JS, Christian CL. Necrotizing vasculitis after acute serous otitis media. *Ann Intern Med* 1974;81:195–199.
305. Calabrese LH. Vasculitis and infection with the human immunodeficiency virus. *Rheum Dis Clin North Am* 1991;17:131–147.
306. Ozen S, Besbas N, Saatci U, et al. Diagnostic criteria for periarteritis in childhood. *J Pediatr* 1992;120:206–209.
307. Finkel TH, Toeroek TJ, Ferguson PJ, et al. Chronic parvovirus B19 infection and systemic necrotising vasculitis: opportunistic infection or aetiological agent? *Lancet* 1994;343:1255–1258.
308. Weinstein A. Systemic hairy cell leukemia. *J Rheumatol* 1982;9:349–350.
309. Spann CR, Callen JP, Yam LT, et al. Cutaneous leukocytoclastic vasculitis complicating hairy cell leukemia. *Arch Dermatol* 1986;122:1057–1059.
310. Komadina KH, Houk RW. Polyarteritis nodosa presenting as recurrent pneumonia following splenectomy for hairy-cell leukemia. *Semin Arthritis Rheum* 1989;18:252–257.
311. Trepo CG, Zuckerman AJ, Bird RC, et al. The role of circulating hepatitis B antigen/antibody immune complexes in the pathogenesis of vascular and hepatic manifestations in polyarteritis nodosa. *J Clin Pathol* 1974;27:863–868.
312. Guillevin L, Lhote F, Jarrousse B, et al. Polyarteritis nodosa related to hepatitis B virus: a retrospective study of 66 patients. *Ann Med Interne* 1992;143 [Suppl 1]:63–74.
313. Chen KR. Cutaneous polyarteritis nodosa: a clinical and histopathological study of 20 cases. *J Dermatol* 1989;16:429–442.
314. Moreland LW, Ball GV. Cutaneous polyarteritis nodosa. *Am J Med* 1990; 88:426–430.
315. van de Pette JEW, Jarvis JM, Wilton JMA, et al. Cutaneous periarteritis nodosa. *Arch Dermatol* 1984;120:109–111.
316. Gudbjörnsson B, Hällgren R. Cutaneous polyarteritis. *J Rheumatol* 1990;17: 386–390.
317. Chiu G, Rajapakse CNA. Cutaneous polyarteritis nodosa and ulcerative colitis. *J Rheumatol* 1991;18:769–770.
318. Dyer NH, Dawson AM, Verbov JL, et al. Cutaneous polyarteritis nodosa associated with Crohn's disease. *Lancet* 1970;1:647–650.
319. Lever WF, Schaumburg-Lever G. Vascular diseases. In: Lever W, Schaumberg-Lever G, eds. *Histopathology of the skin,* 7th ed. Philadelphia: JB Lippincott Co., 1990:185–209.
320. Diaz-Perez JL, Winkelmann RK. Cutaneous periarteritis nodosa. *Arch Dermatol* 1974;110:407–414.
321. Hauschild S, Csernok E, Schmitt WH, et al. Antineutrophil cytoplasmic antibodies in systemic polyarteritis nodosa with and without hepatitis virus infection and Churg–Strauss syndrome-62 patients [letter and reply]. *J Rheumatol* 1994;21:1173–1174.
322. Fortin PR, Larson MG, Watters AK, et al. Prognostic factors in systemic necrotizing vasculitis of the polyarteritis nodosa group: a review of 45 cases. *J Rheumatol* 1995;22:78–84.
323. Nachman P, Hogan S, Jennette J, et al. Treatment response and relapse in antineutrophil cytoplasmic autoantibody-associated microscopic polyangiitis and glomerulonephritis. *J Am Soc Nephrol* 1996;7:33–39.
324. Guillevin L, Lhote F, Sauvaget F, et al. Treatment of polyarteritis nodosa related to hepatitis B virus with interferon-alpha and plasma exchanges. *Ann Rheum Dis* 1994;53:334–337.
325. Carpenter MT, West SG. Polyarteritis nodosa in hairy cell leukemia: treatment with interferon-Alpha. *J Rheumatol* 1994;21:1150–1152.
326. Hoffman G. Classification of the systemic vasculitides: antineutrophil cytoplasmic antibodies, consensus and controversy. *Clin Exp Dermatol* 1998;16: 111–115.
327. Anderson G, Coles ET, Crane M, et al. Wegener's granuloma: a series of 265 British cases seen between 1975 and 1985—a report by a sub-committee of the British Thoracic Society Research Committee. *Q J Med* 1992;83:427–438.
328. Daoud MS, Gibson LE, DeRemee RA, et al. Cutaneous Wegener's granulomatosis: clinical, histopathologic, and immunopathologic features of thirty patients. *J Am Acad Dermatol* 1994;31:605–612.
329. Reinhold-Keller E, Beuge N, Latza U, et al. An interdisciplinary approach to the care of patients with Wegener's granulomatosis. *Arthritis Rheum* 2000;43: 1021–1032.
330. Patten SF, Tomecki KJ. Wegener's granulomatosis: cutaneous and oral mucosal disease. *J Am Acad Dermatol* 1993;28:710–718.
331. Francès C, Du LHT, Piette JC, et al. Wegener's granulomatosis: dermatological manifestations in 75 cases with clinicopathologic correlation. *Arch Dermatol* 1994;130:861–867.
332. Mangold MC, Callen JP. Cutaneous leukocytoclastic vasculitis associated with active Wegener's granulomatosis. *J Am Acad Dermatol* 1992;26:579–584.
333. Hoffman GS, Kerr GS, Leavitt RY, et al. Wegener's granulomatosis: an analysis of 158 patients. *Ann Intern Med* 1992;116:488–498.
334. Hu CH, O'Loughlin S, Winkelmann RK. Cutaneous manifestations of Wegener's granulomatosis. *Arch Dermatol* 1977;113:175–182.
335. Spigel GT, Krall RA, Hilal A. Limited Wegener's granulomatosos: unusual cutaneous, radiographic, and pathologic manifestations. *Cutis* 1983;32:41–51.
336. Reed WB, Jensen AK, Konwaler BFE, et al. The cutaneous manifestations in Wegener's granulomatosis. *Acta Derm Venereol* 1963;43:250–264.
337. Handfield-Jones SE, Parker SC, Fenton DA, et al. Wegener's granulomatosis presenting as pyoderma gangrenosum. *Clin Exp Dermatol* 1992;17:197–200.
338. Schwartz RA, Churg J. Churg–Strauss syndrome. *Br J Dermatol* 1992;127: 199–204.
339. Crotty CP, DeRemee RA, Winkelmann RK. Cutaneous clinicopathologic correlation of allergic granulomatosis. *J Am Acad Dermatol* 1981;5:571–581.
340. Finan MC, Winkelmann RK. The cutaneous extravascular necrotizing granuloma (Churg–Strauss granuloma) and systemic disease: a review of 27 cases. *Medicine* 1983;62:142–158.
341. Finan MC. Rheumatoid papule: cutaneous, extravascular necrotizing granuloma, and Churg–Strauss granuloma—are they the same entity? *J Am Acad Dermatol* 1990;22:142–143.
342. Sheahan P, Donnelly M, O'Reilly S, et al. T/NK cell non-Hodgkin's lymphoma of the sinonasal tract. *J Laryngol Otology* 2001;115:1032–1035.
343. Trimarchi M, Gregorini G, Facchetti F, et al. Cocaine-induced midline destructive lesions: clinical, radiographic, histopathologic, and serologic features and their differentiation from Wegener's granulomatosis. *Medicine* 2001;80:391–404.
344. Leavitt RY, Fauci AS, Bloch DA, et al. The American College of Rheumatology 1990 criteria for the classification of Wegener's granulomatosis. *Arthritis Rheum* 1990;33:1101–1107.
345. Nishino H, DeRemee RA, Rubino FA, et al. Wegener's granulomatosis associated with vasculitis of the temporal artery: report of five cases. *Mayo Clinic Proc* 1993;68:115–121.
346. Matteson EL, Palella TD. Alpha-methyldopa-induced systemic vasculitis confused with Wegener's granulomatosis [letter]. *Arthritis Rheum* 1989;32: 356–367.
347. DeRemee RA, McDonald TJ, Weiland LH. Wegener's granulomatosis: observations on treatment with antimicrobial agents. *Mayo Clin Proc* 1985;60:27–32.
348. DeRemee RA. The treatment of Wegener's granulomatosis with trimethoprim/sulfamethoxazole: Illusion or vision? *Arthritis Rheum* 1988;31:1068–1072.
349. Israel HL. Sulfamethoxazole-trimethoprim therapy for Wegener's granulomatosis. *Arch Intern Med* 1988;148:2293–2295.
350. Churg J, Strauss L. Allergic granulomatosis, allergic angiitis, and periarteritis nodosa. *Am J Pathol* 1951;27:277–301.
351. Chumbley LC, Harrison EG Jr, DeRemee RA. Allergic granulomatosis and angiitis (Churg–Strauss syndrome): report and analysis of 30 cases. *Mayo Clin Proc* 1977;52:477–484.
352. Lanham JG, Elkon KB, Pusey CD, et al. Systemic vasculitis with asthma and eosinophilia: a clinical approach to the Churg–Strauss syndrome. *Medicine (Baltimore)* 1984;63:65–81.
353. Masi AT, Hunder GG, Lie JT, et al. The American College of Rheumatology

1990 criteria for the classification of Churg–Strauss syndrome (allergic granulomatosis and angiitis). *Arthritis Rheum* 1990;33:1094–1100.
354. Jamaleddine G, Diab K, Tabbara Z, et al. Leukotriene antagonists and the Churg–Strauss syndrome. *Semin Arthritis Rheum* 2002;31:218–227.
355. Chu P, Connolly MK, LeBoit PE. The histopathologic spectrum of palisaded neutrohilic and granulomatous dermatitis in patients with collagen vascular disease. *Arch Dermatol* 1994;130:1278–1283.
356. Weller PF. The idiopathic hypereosinophilic syndrome. *Blood* 1994;83: 2759–2779.
357. Abu-Shakra M, Smythe H, Lewtas J, et al. Outcome of polyarteritis nodosa and Churg–Strauss syndrome. *Arthritis Rheum* 1994;37:1798–1803.
358. Fritsch PO. Giant cell arteritis. In: Fitzpatrick TB, Eisen AZ, Wolff K, et al., eds. *Dermatology in general medicine* Vol. 1. New York: McGraw-Hill, 1993: 2178–2181.
359. Salvarani C, Cantini F, Boiardi L, et al. Polymyalgia rheumatica and giant cell arteritis. *N Engl J Med* 2002;347:261–271.
360. Hitch JM. Dermatologic manifestations of giant-cell (temporal, cranial) arteritis. *Arch Dermatol* 1970;101:409–415.
361. Distler O, Muller-Ladner U, Gluck T. Clinical images: skin necrosis in giant cell arteritis. *Arthritis Rheum* 1999;42:1296.
362. Mandell B, Hoffman G. Systemic necrotizing arteritis. In: Freedberg I, Eisen A, Wolff K, et al., eds. *Dermatology in general medicine,* 5th ed. Vol. 2. New York: McGraw-Hill; 1999:2034–2044.
363. Skaria A, Ruffieux P, Piletta P, et al. Takayasu arteritis and cutaneous necrotizing vasculitis. *Dermatology* 2000;200:139–143.
364. Hunder G. Vasculitis: clinical and laboratory features. In: Klippel J, ed. *Primer on the rheumatic diseases,* 11th ed. Atlanta: Arthritis Foundation; 1997:294–300.

CHAPTER 9

Psoriatic Arthritis and Reiter Syndrome

Andrew G. Franks, Jr.

PSORIATIC ARTHRITIS

Although the association of psoriasis with arthritis was made in 1818, it was not until 1959 that the term "psoriatic arthritis" was conceived and distinguished from rheumatoid arthritis and osteoarthritis (1). The demonstration of rheumatoid factor in 1948, the finding that most people with psoriasis and arthritis were "seronegative," and the different clinical patterns and unique radiographic features ultimately suggested that the arthritis of psoriasis be separately classified (2). More recently, the inclusion of psoriatic arthritis as one of the *seronegative spondyloarthropathies*, has been accepted (3). The spondyloarthropathies are a group of related disorders, which include ankylosing spondylitis, Reiter syndrome/reactive arthritis, psoriatic arthritis, inflammatory bowel–related arthritis, and undifferentiated spondyloarthropathy, that share common genetics and pathophysiology (see later).

Epidemiology

Psoriasis affects over 2% of the U.S. population, but because criteria for evaluating arthritis in psoriasis are not applied uniformly, there is no general agreement on the frequency of psoriatic arthritis. Reports suggest that from 10% to 20% of those individuals with skin psoriasis may develop features of psoriatic arthritis (3).

The male-to-female ratio appears to be about equal, in contrast to the predilection of rheumatoid arthritis for woman. However, there are gender differences in the pattern of joint involvement. Distal joint involvement, oligoarthritis, and symptomatic spondyloarthritis appear more common in men, whereas symmetric polyarthritis resembling rheumatoid arthritis appears more common in women (4). Psoriatic arthritis may occur at any age, but peaks between the fourth and fifth decades (5).

Genetics

Family studies have suggested a multifactorial mode of inheritance, as in skin psoriasis, with environmental triggers in some individuals (6). Psoriasis and psoriatic arthritis are associated with both class I (B13, B17, B38, B 39, B27, Cw6) and class II (DR4, DR7, DQw3) HLA antigens, whereas rheumatoid arthritis is associated only with class II antigens (DR4, DQw3) (7,8). HLA-B38 is most highly associated with peripheral disease and appears to be relatively specific, because it is not found in either seropositive rheumatoid arthritis or Reiter disease (9). HLA-B27 occurs less frequently in psoriatic spondyloarthropathy (50%) than in idiopathic ankylosing spondylitis (90%) or Reiter syndrome (80%), revealing more polygenetic influence (10). HLA typing may provide important information that may be useful in combination with clinical variables when choosing treatment algorithms (see later) (11,12).

Pathogenesis

An understanding of the role of pathogenic T cells in generating cytokines that induce keratinocyte and endothelial cell growth factors in the skin and joints of individuals with psoriasis supports the concept that psoriasis and psoriatic arthritis are immune-/inflammatory-mediated disorders, although the exact mechanisms remain unknown (13,14).

In addition to these genetic and immunologic factors, environmental triggers, particularly infections, are thought to be prominent in the development and perpetuation of the disease (15). The de novo development or exacerbation of psoriasis with streptococcal infection, as well as psoriatic arthritis with human immunodeficiency virus (HIV) infection has been documented (16).

Diagnosis

Many different definitions of psoriatic arthritis have been suggested, and provisional criteria have been proposed, but none is universally accepted. However, because patients with psoriatic arthritis may differ from those with rheumatoid arthritis, on the basis of the clinical pattern of arthritic involvement, the absence of rheumatoid factor, the presence of different radiographic features, the association with HLA-B27, and the presence of an enthesopathy (see later), psoriatic arthritis is classified as a seronegative spondyloarthropathy (17).

Clinical Manifestations

JOINT DISEASE

Psoriatic arthritis may be present with or without skin lesions or there may be only nail malformation or scalp lesions. In most instances, the psoriasis precedes the arthritis, occasionally by as much as 20 years. However, in some patients, the arthritis may appear before the psoriasis (18). If the latter is the case, a family history of psoriasis may reveal a hereditary pattern prompting a change in diagnosis from seronegative rheumatoid arthritis to psoriatic arthritis.

Initial symptoms may be acute, and when localized to the toes or foot may be mistaken for gout, tendonitis, or sports injury. Alternatively, patients may only experience stiffness and pain with few objective findings. Recently, the possibility that there is less joint tenderness with psoriatic arthritis than with rheumatoid

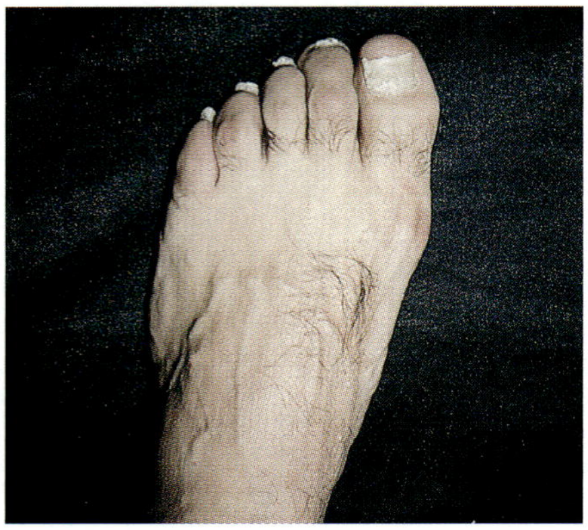

Figure 9.1. Psoriatic arthritis of the foot with dactylitis causing "sausaging." Onychodystrophy is present. (Courtesy of the Andrew G. Franks Jr. collection.)

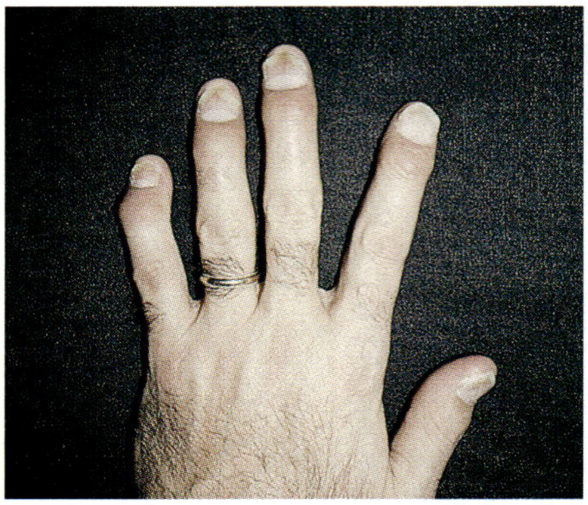

Figure 9.3. Psoriatic arthritis with distal interphalangeal joint involvement, and associated nail and paronychial changes. (Courtesy of the Andrew G. Franks Jr. collection.)

arthritis has been emphasized (19). Enthesopathy or enthesitis, which is an insertional tendonitis, is considered a major component of the clinical symptoms and signs. Fibromyalgia-like soft-tissue symptoms may overlap the insertional tendonitis features.

The clinical manifestations of psoriatic arthritis fall into several subtypes that may overlap one another and change with time in the individual patient:

1. *Asymmetric oligoarthritis.* This common pattern may occur in up to half of male patients. Usually, the digits of the hands and feet are affected first, with inflammation of the flexor tendon and synovium occurring simultaneously, leading to the typical "sausage" appearance (Fig. 9.1). Usually, fewer than five joints are affected at any one time (20).
2. *Symmetric polyarthritis.* This rheumatoid-like pattern is the most common type in women. The hands, ankles, and feet may be involved, as in seropositive rheumatoid arthritis, and also the wrists, but the latter are not usually targeted as early or as symptomatically. It is differentiated from rheumatoid arthritis by the presence of distal interphalangeal (DIP) joint involvement, less involvement of the ulnar styloid and wrist, the absence of subcutaneous "rheumatoid" nodules, and a negative test for rheumatoid factor (Fig. 9.2) (21).
3. *DIP joint.* DIP joint involvement is the "classic" type of psoriatic arthritis. It occurs in its symmetric form in less than 5% of patients, primarily men, and may mimic the Heberden nodes of primary osteoarthritis. However, DIP involvement is often identified more commonly in an asymmetric pattern overlapping the oligoarthritic or rheumatoid-like types. Involvement of the nail with significant inflammation of the paronychia and swelling of the digital tuft may be prominent (Fig. 9.3) (22).
4. *Arthritis mutilans.* Resorption of bone (osteolysis) with dissolution of the joint, seen as the "pencil-in-cup" radiographic finding (Fig 9.4) (23), leads to redundant overlying skin with a "telescoping" motion of the digit. This "opera-glass hand" is more common in men, and is more frequent in early-onset disease (Fig. 9.5).
5. *Spondylitis.* The neck, thoracic, and lumbosacral spine may be involved in an "axial" pattern. Asymmetric sacroiliitis predominates, in contrast to the symmetric sacroiliitis of de novo ankylosing spondylitis (24). Mild or asymptomatic spondylitis often is identified along with all other patterns of peripheral joint involvement. However, when axial involvement predominates, this psoriatic arthritis spondylitis may mimic true ankylosing spondylitis with significant deformity and extracutaneous manifestations (25). HLA-B27 is present in most of these patients (26).

A recent review has suggested an alternative clinical classification based on the impression that symmetric polyarthritis occurs in most patients with psoriatic arthritis and at

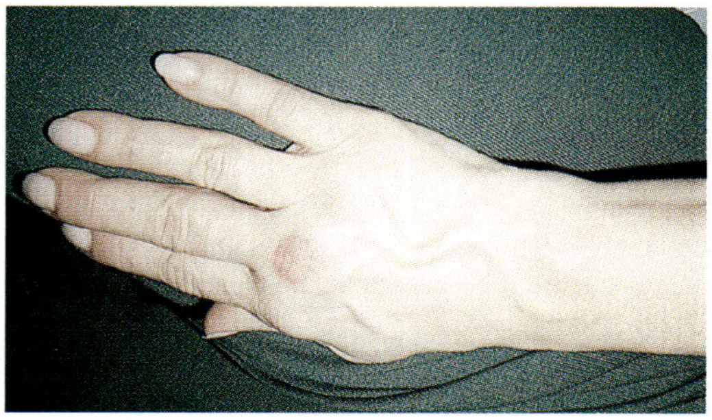

Figure 9.2. Psoriatic arthritis resembling rheumatoid arthritis with symmetric involvement and early "swan-neck" deformity. Note the distal interphalangeal involvement. (Courtesy of the Andrew G. Franks Jr. collection.)

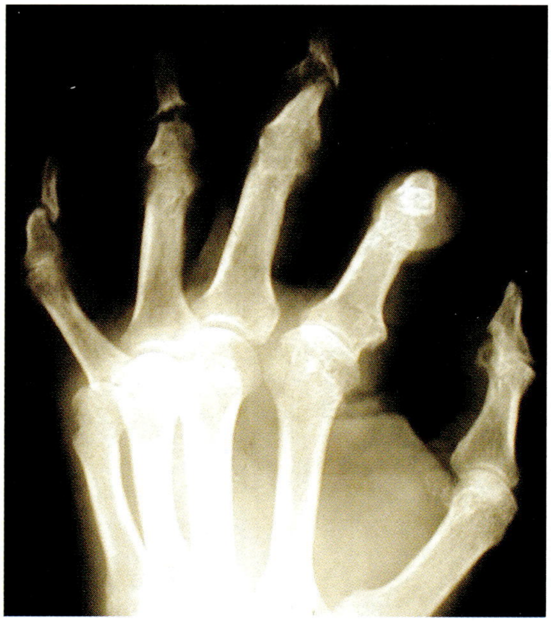

Figure 9.4. Radiograph demonstrating "pencil-in-cup" deformity of the distal interphalangeal joint in psoriatic "arthritis mutilans." (Courtesy of the Andrew G. Franks Jr. collection.)

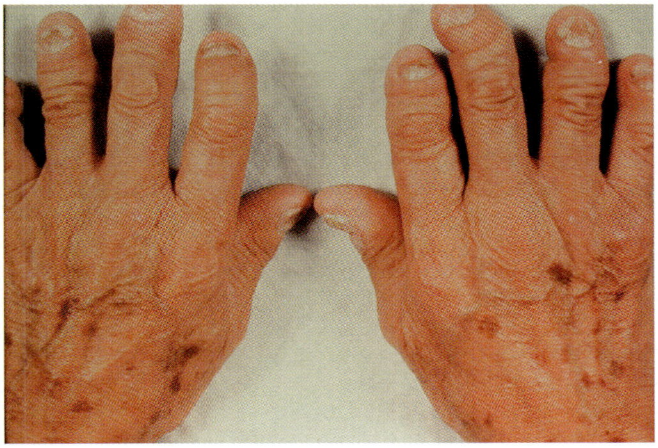

Figure 9.5. Psoriatic arthritis causing osteolysis and resorption of bone (arthritis mutilans), with "telescoping" of the digits. (Courtesy of the Andrew G. Franks Jr. collection.)

times, it may be indistinguishable from rheumatoid arthritis (27):

1. Peripheral arthritis, which includes DIP joint involvement, dactylitis, arthritis mutilans, enthesopathy, and rheumatoid-like disease
2. Spondylitis with asymmetric sacroiliitis, syndesmophytes, and paravertebral ossification
3. Extraarticular bone manifestations, including SAPHO syndrome (synovitis, acne, pustulosis, hyperostosis, and osteitis) and psoriatic onychopachydermoperiostitis (see later)

SKIN DISEASE

Classic psoriasis appears as papules and plaques with layers of scales; the individual lesion is erythematous, covered with layers of silver–white scale, and rather sharply demarcated from adjacent uninvolved skin. Removing the scale results in punctate bleeding that reflects rupture of the superficial blood vessels in the tips of the dermal papillae (Auspitz sign). Individual lesions may heal with transient hyperpigmentation or hypopigmentation. Psoriasis may occur over any portion of the skin, especially the elbows, knees, lumbosacral area, scalp, gluteal cleft, and genitalia. The glans penis is frequently affected, the oral mucosa is infrequently involved, and the tongue is rarely affected. At times, there are considerable numbers of droplike plaques designated as "guttate psoriasis," which may occur after infections. The skin lesions often appear at sites of trauma (Köebner reaction or isomorphic phenomenon). Generalized erythroderma or exfoliative dermatitis may develop spontaneously or occur after systemic illness, the administration of medication, or acute sunburn. Pustular types of psoriasis are less common and occur in two forms: One is generalized, and the other is localized to the palms and soles. Patients with generalized pustular psoriasis manifest an extensive sterile pustular eruption that may also involve the mucous membranes. The skin lesions consist of superficial pustules that may evolve into large purulent areas; preexisting psoriatic plaques may also develop sterile pustules. Localized pustular psoriasis of the palms and soles is usually bilateral. There are increased numbers of *Staphylococcus aureus* on lesional skin of patients with psoriasis. Surgical intervention through psoriatic plaques, such as in prosthetic joint replacement, has been associated with increased risk of local infection (30).

Although no distinctive pattern of skin involvement suggests a particular form of psoriatic arthritis, certain features can be helpful in classifying the condition. Thus, up to one third of patients with generalized pustular psoriasis has arthritis, which is usually severe and predominantly affects the spine (28). Localized pustular psoriasis starting at the fingertips (acrodermatitis continua) may be associated with severe peripheral arthritis and extracutaneous manifestations that overlap with Reiter disease (29). An increased incidence of patients with SAPHO syndrome with arthritis and sclerosis of the sternum (chest wall syndrome) is described in association with pustular psoriasis of the palms and soles (pustulosis palmoplantaris) (31). Despite these associations, patients with severe arthritis may only have mild psoriasis lying in one of the "hidden" areas such as the scalp, axillae, umbilicus, perineum, or gluteal fold, so called "inverse psoriasis."

NAIL CHANGES

The presence of nail psoriasis is much more common than skin psoriasis alone in patients with psoriatic arthritis, occurring in more than 80% of cases (32). DIP joint involvement and nail changes often occur simultaneously. Other patterns of psoriatic arthritis are also more common in patients with nail deformity.

The most characteristic nail change in psoriasis is pitting of the nail plate. Other commonly recognized signs are onycholysis with either pitting or transverse ridges (Beau lines), the "oil droplet" appearance beginning at the junction of the nail bed, and distal onycholysis. Stippling, loss of transparency, yellowing, and subungual keratosis also occur. Paronychial reaction may be prominent, with swelling, redness, and scale. The combination of pitting with one or more additional nail changes is highly suggestive of psoriasis (Fig. 9.6). (33).

Psoriatic nail dystrophy, soft-tissue periungual swelling, and exuberant periosteal reaction in the terminal phalanx sparing the DIP joint ("ivory phalanx") is termed "psoriatic onychopachydermoperiostitis" (34). This rare disorder may result in marked deformity and pain in the terminal digits of the hands or feet and may be difficult to differentiate from infection or tumor.

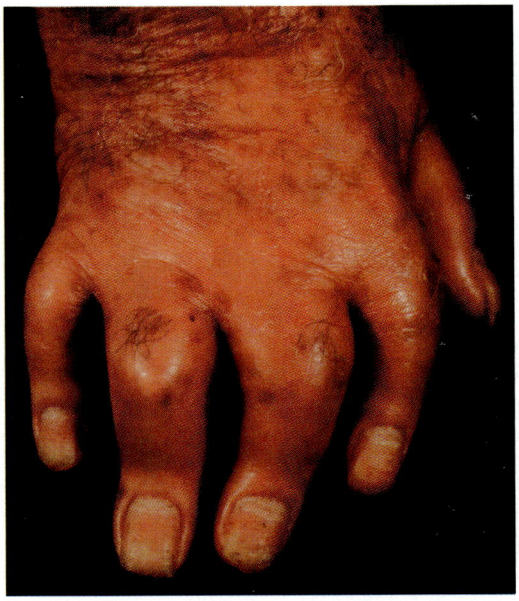

Figure 9.6. Psoriatic arthritis with dactylitis and characteristic nail pitting and onycholysis. (Courtesy of the Andrew G. Franks Jr. collection.)

MISCELLANEOUS FEATURES

There is an overlap of extracutaneous features in the "seronegative" group of diseases including Reiter disease, Behçet disease, and idiopathic ankylosing spondylitis. Eye involvement may be found in almost one third of patients with psoriatic arthritis, less commonly than in Reiter disease. These eye conditions include conjunctivitis, iritis, keratoconjunctivitis sicca, and episcleritis. HLA-B27 is increased in patients with iritis and spondylitis (35).

Laboratory Findings

Although no blood study specifically identifies psoriatic arthritis, the absence of rheumatoid factor is most important in the diagnosis. A positive test for rheumatoid factor in a patient with psoriasis and arthritis may either be the concurrence of two common diseases, psoriasis and rheumatoid arthritis, or if the pattern of joint involvement is most consistent with psoriatic arthritis, the known occurrence of seropositivity in up to 5% of the general population. Antinuclear antibodies may be found in up to 10% of patients (36).

An elevated sedimentation rate and other acute-phase reactants, especially C-reactive protein, may be found during flares of the disease (37). Anemia and leukocytosis may occur with erythrodermic and pustular flares. Hyperuricemia may be a result of increased purine metabolism due to rapid skin turnover in psoriasis per se and may be further elevated by low-dose salicylate therapy that interferes with urate metabolism by the kidneys, both leading to confusion with gout.

Analysis of synovial fluid often reveals a group II inflammatory fluid with neutrophils predominating. Uric acid crystals are not found unless gout coexists (38).

Prognosis

Until recently, psoriatic arthritis had been generally considered a milder disease than rheumatoid arthritis. However, several factors influence the severity of the disease, including the clinical subset (arthritis mutilans, symmetric polyarthritis), early age of onset, severity of skin involvement, female sex, family history of arthritis, and the presence of HLA-DR4 and HLA-DR7. Thus, new evidence suggests that psoriatic arthritis may be as disabling and destructive as rheumatoid arthritis when the appropriate comparisons are made, and treatment may need to be more aggressive in those individuals. HLA-DR4 may predispose the patient to a more progressive rheumatoid-like course (39).

Treatment

Rapid expansion in our knowledge about the immunologic basis for psoriasis will dramatically change therapeutics for psoriatic arthritis. The following is a brief overview of current options.

It is important that the disease be recognized early so that appropriate treatment may be initiated with the intent of reduction in day-to-day symptoms and interdiction of progressive joint deformity and destruction with the use of remittive or disease-modifying agents, similar to the therapeutic algorithms invoked for rheumatoid arthritis. This is especially important because evidence suggests that there is less tenderness and pain in severely affected psoriatic joints than in rheumatoid joints, allowing disease progression to occur unrecognized by both patient and physician. The initial treatment of psoriatic arthritis is usually symptomatic with nonsteroidal antiinflammatory drugs (NSAIDs). The choice of agent depends on a number of factors, as is the case for any rheumatic disorder. However, there are some issues with skin psoriasis and psoriatic arthritis that should be noted. The approach to therapy of psoriatic arthritis should include treatment for both the skin and the joints. Although no specific data are available, some patients' rheumatic symptoms abate when the skin component is in remission. Furthermore, if the skin disease is fulminant, such as with generalized pustular psoriasis, systemic agents that treat the skin and the joints concomitantly usually take precedence in a treatment algorithm. The photosensitivity potential of individual medications needs to be recognized in view of the potential unpredictable effects when concomitant light therapy is being administered. Some drugs may exacerbate skin psoriasis whereas others may have a beneficial effect on the skin. The interaction of individual NSAIDs with other systemic agents is also important to consider when second- and third-line multiple-therapy regimens are instituted. Therefore, physicians who care for patients with psoriatic arthritis should be aware of the treatments of the skin disease as well as the interaction of these agents to more specifically define therapy.

Second-line therapy should be instituted when progressive, erosive deforming disease is probable or imminent. As noted, if the skin disease is aggressive, the systemic agents of choice for the skin per se are often also second-line agents for the joints. The most commonly used second-line agents include sulfasalazine, retinoic acid derivatives, methotrexate, and cyclosporine. Additional agents include antimalarials [which may induce cutaneous flare of psoriasis including erythroderma (40,41)], gold, azathioprine, mycophenolate mofetil, hydroxyurea, and psoralen-UV-A (PUVA). Of note, it is important to avoid systemic corticosteroids in patients with psoriatic arthritis to diminish potential skin transformation to generalized pustular psoriasis or erythroderma. In the past, massive loss of fluids via the skin has been documented in some patients with psoriasis treated with systemic corticosteroids (42,43).

Very recently, anti–tumor necrosis factor-α (TNF-α) therapies, including the biologic response modifiers infliximab and etanercept, have been used in the treatment of psoriasis and psoriatic arthritis. Infliximab, a monoclonal antibody against TNF-α, is a chimera of a human antibody bound to a murine binding site for TNF-α. Because of the murine portion, infliximab is immunogenic, leading to the formation of human antichimeric antibodies. Therefore, low-dose methotrexate is used concomitantly to suppress antibody formation. Etanercept is a fusion protein that acts as a false TNF receptor, binding soluble and cell-bound TNF-α. Both these agents are U.S. Food and Drug Administration–approved for use in rheumatoid arthritis, and etanercept is approved for psoriatic arthritis as well (44,45).

REITER SYNDROME

Reiter syndrome is the eponym used to describe a syndrome classically defined as the clinical triad of arthritis, conjunctivitis, and nongonococcal urethritis first described by Han Reiter in 1916 (46). It is strongly associated with HLA-B27, which is present in more than 80% of cases (47). It has an incomplete form in which only two typical findings are required for the diagnosis (48). Alternately, peripheral arthritis lasting longer than 1 month, associated with urethritis *or* cervicitis *or* diarrhea has been described. Moreover, the original triad has been expanded into a sextet including mucosal ulcerations, circinate balanitis, and keratoderma blennorrhagicum. It is considered part of the family of seronegative spondyloarthropathies (ankylosing spondylitis, psoriatic arthritis, Reiter syndrome/reactive arthritis, inflammatory bowel–related arthritis, and undifferentiated spondyloarthropathy) precipitated by an extraarticular bacterial infection in a genetically susceptible host (49).

Epidemiology

Because of the variable clinical manifestations and the multiplicity of precipitating infectious agents, it has been difficult to obtain accurate epidemiologic data but its estimated frequency is three to four per 100,000 (50). However, two environmental settings are regularly found: the epidemic or postdysenteric form following infection of the gastrointestinal tract, and the endemic sexually transmitted venereal form following infection of the genitourinary tract. Some authors have suggested that Reiter syndrome may also occur in association with HIV and be part of the *HIV-associated rheumatic disease syndrome* (51).

The incidence of the disease in the general U.S. population is difficult to ascertain but is probably lower than rheumatoid arthritis. Its worldwide occurrence appears to relate to the prevalence of HLA-B27 in each population. The age range of most common occurrence is 20 to 30 years. Most reported cases of Reiter disease are in men, except in the postdysenteric reactive form, which is equally distributed among men and women (52).

Genetics

There is a strong association with HLA-B27, but not all individuals have this marker and there is recent evidence to suggest other genetic factors may be prevalent in certain populations. Theories about the relationship between HLA-B27 and arthritis-causing bacteria have been proposed, including mimicry between HLA-B27 and bacterial macromolecules. HLA-B27–negative patients may have less frequent sacroiliitis and uveitis and a milder clinical course (53).

Pathogenesis

A wide variety of bacterial species has been implicated in the pathogenesis of the disease. Nongonococcal urethritis caused by *Chlamydia* species is the most common sporadic form of Reiter syndrome, and postdysenteric outbreaks have been reported with *Shigella*, *Salmonella*, *Campylobacter*, and *Yersinia* species (54). Although these organisms cannot be cultured from the joint fluid or synovium, which emphasizes the "reactive" nature of the disease, recent evidence suggests that some bacteria can survive in the synovium in metabolically quiescent states, supporting the need for modification of current diagnostic criteria (55).

Diagnosis

The diagnosis may be unequivocal in a young man with recent sexual exposure and nongonococcal urethritis who suddenly develops the classic triad. However, the broad array of clinical manifestations, the disparate temporal sequence in developing the extraarticular manifestations, and the wide overlap with other forms of "reactive arthritis," as well as the seronegative spondyloarthritis, may make the diagnosis in the individual patient difficult to confirm (56). Because gonococcal arthritis is the most important differential diagnosis and may even be present simultaneously, an early attempt at finding the possible precipitating infectious agent should be made.

Psoriatic arthritis and Reiter syndrome overlap in several manifestations. Pustular psoriasis, particularly of the palms and soles, *palmoplantar pustulosis*, may be indistinguishable from keratoderma blennorrhagicum but usually does not involve the mucous membranes (57).

Clinical Manifestations

In most instances, arthritis and conjunctivitis begin within 1 to 3 weeks of the initial urethritis or diarrhea. However, the interval between the first clinical manifestation and subsequent ones may vary from days to months. It may be difficult to decide whether the reactive arthritis is postvenereal or postdysenteric, because it is not uncommon for a patient with postdysenteric arthritis to develop a sterile urethritis within 1 to 2 weeks of the initial bout of diarrhea (58). Constitutional symptoms include low-grade fever, malaise, and weight loss.

JOINT DISEASE

Acute, asymmetric arthritis of the knees, ankles, and feet is the most common initial joint manifestation, usually subsequent to urethritis and conjunctivitis. After a few weeks, the disease usually settles into a few joints, lasting from 2 to 12 months. Most patients experience recurrent episodes of arthritis for several years. The intensity of the inflammation varies from mild to severe, and joint effusions tend to be larger than in other rheumatic diseases, especially of the knees. Periarticular features may be prominent, reflecting the pattern of insertional tendonitis or enthesopathy, which is characteristic of the disease. This soft-tissue swelling is similar to that seen in psoriatic arthritis and causes diffuse inflammation or "sausaging" of the digit involved (dactylitis) (Fig. 9.7). Painful heels secondary to Achilles tendonitis, plantar fasciitis, and calcaneal periostitis ("lover's heel") are common (59).

Axial involvement may begin in the initial phase with lower back pain, which radiates to the buttock and thigh, reflecting inflammation of the sacroiliac joint. It is often unilateral, worse in the morning, and exacerbated by rest. The disease may ascend to the cervical spine with interval skip areas sometimes prominent. Paravertebral calcification and syndesmophytes may be seen (60).

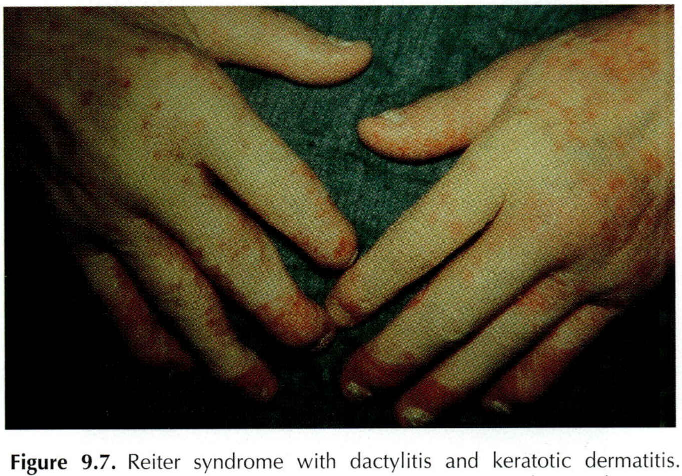

Figure 9.7. Reiter syndrome with dactylitis and keratotic dermatitis. Although nail dystrophy is prominent, there is no evidence of pitting. (Courtesy of the Andrew G. Franks Jr. collection.)

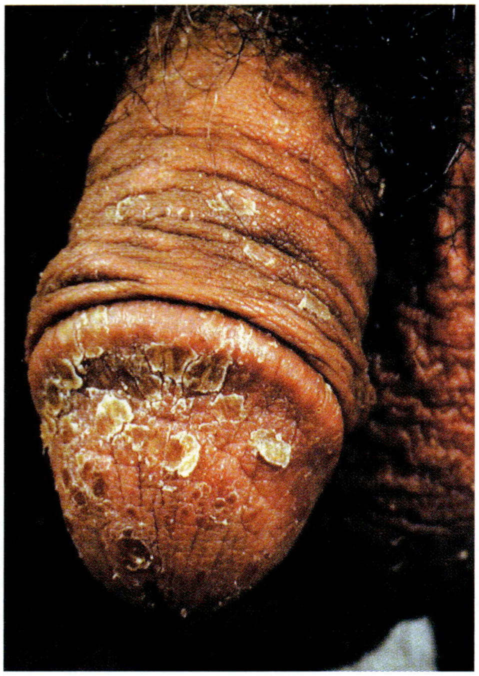

Figure 9.8. Reiter syndrome of the glans penis with psoriasiform scale–crust. (Courtesy of the Andrew G. Franks Jr. collection.)

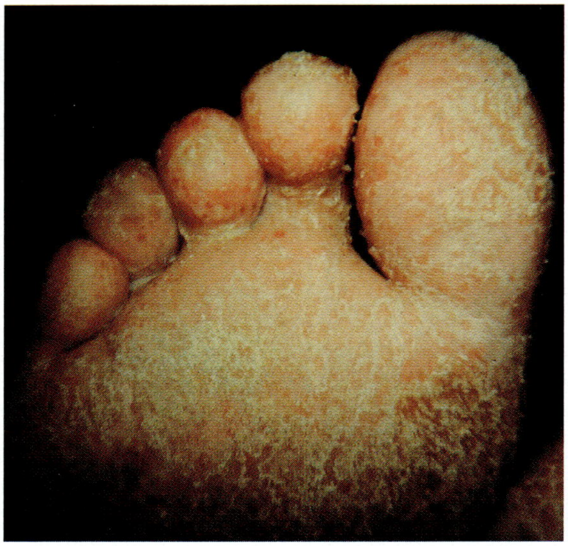

Figure 9.10. Reiter syndrome characterized by the hyperkeratotic lesions on the sole of the foot (keratoderma blennorrhagica). (Courtesy of the Andrew G. Franks Jr. collection.)

SKIN DISEASE

Erythema progressing to pinpoint erosive papules and pustules with subsequent superficial ulceration may be found around the external meatus and corona. Circinate balanitis, a coalescence of these lesions on the glans penis, often with a ragged or scalloped border, may be identified in about 25% of patients with either the venereal or dysenteric form. Scale crust, which is reminiscent of psoriasis, may be prominent in the circumcised patient (Fig. 9.8). Moist vesicles and erosions in the uncircumcised patient may mimic *Candida* species or herpes simplex. Involvement of the skin is most common on the palms (Fig. 9.9) and soles. The initial lesion is an erythematous macule evolving into a small papule that rapidly develops a vesicopustular, keratotic appearance (see Fig. 9. 9). Individual lesions may coalesce producing large areas of thick keratotic scale crust. These thick yellow–to–reddish-brown lesions, characteristically found on the soles, are termed "keratoderma blennorrhagica" and usually develop several weeks after onset of other manifestations of the disease (Fig. 9.10).

Scaling plaques may develop on the scalp as well as over the knees and elbows, again mimicking psoriasis. The skin disease in these two disorders is often difficult or impossible to distinguish clinically or histologically. Subungual hyperkeratosis is a form of keratoderma blennorrhagicum that may also closely resemble psoriasis. The nails may be thickened with ridges. Pitting is usually absent. Scaling of the skin may

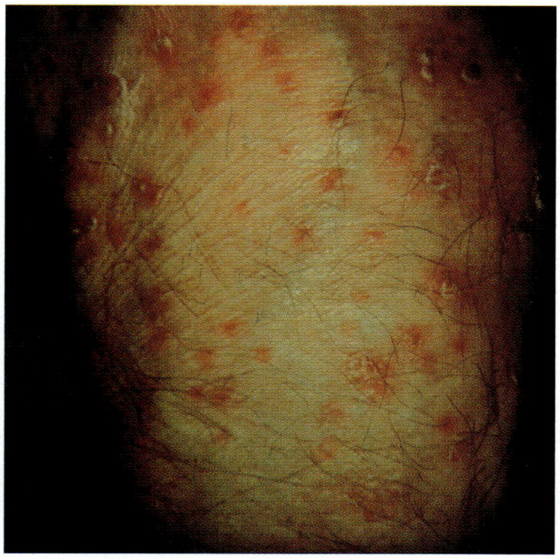

Figure 9.9. Reiter syndrome with rapidly developing vesicopustules with characteristic keratotic borders. (Courtesy of the Andrew G. Franks Jr. collection.)

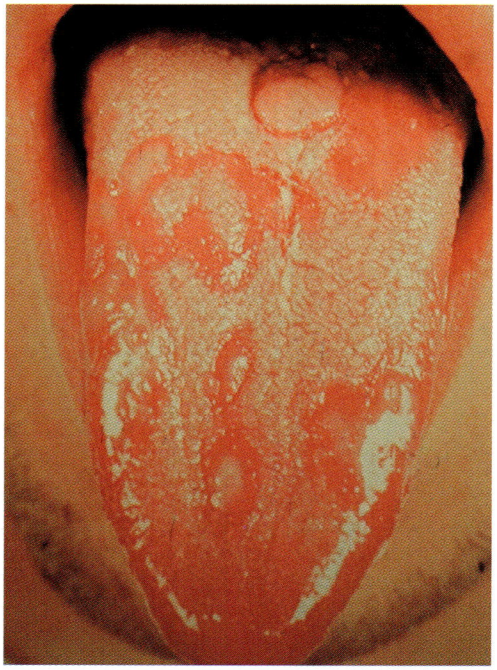

Figure 9.11. Reiter syndrome with superficial, painless erosions on the tongue. (Courtesy of the Andrew G. Franks Jr. collection.)

be the only residual manifestation of these lesions, which are self-limiting, nonscarring, and resolve spontaneously within several weeks.

Superficial, painless ulcerations with an erythematous base are frequently seen on the buccal mucosa, tongue, and palate. They may be quite evanescent and vary from a few millimeters to a centimeter in diameter (Fig. 9.11) (61).

GENITOURINARY DISEASE

A transient watery-to-mucopurulent discharge is characteristic, with dysuria varying from nearly asymptomatic to severe frequency and burning. Prostatitis may often accompany the urethritis, and less commonly, hemorrhagic cystitis may cause suprapubic pain. In women, vulvovaginitis, cervicitis, and, salpingitis have been reported.

OCULAR DISEASE

Conjunctivitis is the most common eye disease and is usually bilateral, mild, and evanescent. There may be slight burning, and a mucoid discharge with chemosis and photophobia may also occur. Anterior uveitis (iritis) is less common, usually unilateral, and often associated with more severe disease, especially when the sacroiliac joints are involved (62).

GASTROINTESTINAL DISEASE

Diarrhea is most often mild and brief, but occasionally is severe, bloody, and protracted. Epidemic dysentery may be associated with erythema nodosum when precipitated by *Yersinia* species.

Erythema nodosum is most common in Scandinavian women, especially those who are HLA-B27–negative, and is associated with either mild or no arthritic component (63).

MISCELLANEOUS FEATURES

Aortic insufficiency has been reported as a late sequela, though it is uncommon. However, conduction abnormalities, particularly a prolonged PR interval, may occur early, along with pericarditis and myocarditis (64). Unusual cranial and peripheral neuropathies have been rarely reported (65).

Laboratory Findings

An attempt to document a specific bacterial infection should be made, with cultures of the urethra, cervix, synovial fluid, blood, and stool. Gonococcal arthritis must be ruled out and stool cultures may confirm the presence of bacillary dysentery. Because *Chlamydia* species cannot be grown on artificial media, nonculture tests are also necessary including direct fluorescent antibody, enzyme-linked immunosorbent assay, and polymerase chain reaction.

The white blood count is usually elevated along with the erythrocyte sedimentation rate or C-reactive protein level. Rheumatoid factor and antinuclear antibody are usually negative. Anemia may occur in patients with protracted illnesses. Those at risk should be tested for the presence of HIV.

Synovial analysis most often reveals a group III fluid with large numbers of neutrophils, and may reveal prominent macrophages that have ingested neutrophilic debris (Reiter cells) (66).

Prognosis

The course of the disease is highly variable and may depend on the precipitating infection and the presence of the HLA-B27 antigen. Acute signs and symptoms usually resolve within 6 months, but up to 50% of patients may have recurrent episodes of arthritis. In addition, soft-tissue complaints, including tendonitis and fasciitis, may persist or progress to more chronic disease in up to 30%, particularly in those individuals with chlamydial infection. The postdysentery form appears to have a better prognosis. The long-term use of antibiotics may improve the outcome in some of these patients (see later) (67).

Treatment

Because genital infections with *Chlamydia trachomatis* are frequently asymptomatic, especially in women, empiric treatment of cervicitis or urethritis with antibiotics such as doxycycline and ciprofloxacin hydrochloride should be considered after appropriate cultures have been taken. Antibiotics are generally not recommended for the postdysentery forms of the disease.

Symptomatic treatment of the rheumatic symptoms is similar to that for psoriatic arthritis, (see before) including the NSAIDs, with a historic bias toward the indoleacetic acid group. If NSAIDS alone are ineffective, sulfasalazine is a useful choice. Occasionally, a short course of corticosteroids may be used, especially after appropriate antibiotics have been completed.

Second-line agents include methotrexate, azathioprine, leflunomide, hydroxychloroquine, cyclosporine, and others. Recently, several of the anti–TNF-α *biologic response modifiers*, including etanercept and infliximab, have shown effectiveness in treating Reiter syndrome similar to that shown in psoriatic arthritis (see before) (68).

REFERENCES

1. Wright V. Psoriasis and arthritis. *Ann Rheum Dis* 1956;15:348.
2. Wright V. Psoriatic arthritis: a comparative radiographic study of rheumatoid arthritis and arthritis associated with psoriasis. *Ann Rheum Dis* 1961;20:123.
3. Kahn MA, van der Linden SM. A wider spectrum of spondyloarthropathies. *Semin Arthritis Rheum* 1990;20:107.
4. Hellgren L. Association between rheumatoid arthritis and psoriasis in total populations. *Acta Rheum Scand* 1969;15:316.
5. Stern RS. The epidemiology of joint complaints in patients with psoriasis. *J Rheumatol* 1985;12:315.
6. Vasey FB. Psoriatic arthritis. In: Schumacher HR Jr, Klippel JH, Koopman WJ, et al., eds. *Primer on the rheumatic diseases,* 10th ed. Atlanta: Arthritis Foundation 1993;10:161.
7. Gladman DD, Shuckett R, Russell ML, et al. Psoriatic arthritis: an analysis of 220 patients. *Q J Med* 1987;62:127–141.
8. Gladman DD. Toward unraveling the mystery of psoriatic arthritis. *Arthritis Rheum* 1993;36:88.
9. Espinoza LR, Vasey FB, Oh JH, et al. Association between HLA-BW38 and peripheral psoriatic arthritis. *Arthritis Rheum* 1978;21:72.
10. Kantor SM, Hsu SH, Bias WB, et al. Clinical and immunogenic subsets of psoriatic arthritis. *Clin Exp Rheumatol* 1984;2:105.
11. Gladman DD, Farewell VT. The role of HLA antigens as indicators of progression in psoriatic arthritis (PSA): multivariate relative risk model. *Arthritis Rheum* 1995;38:845.
12. McHugh NJ, Laurent MR, Treadwell BL, et al. Psoriatic arthritis: clinical subgroups and histocompatibility antigens. *Ann Rheum Dis* 1987;46:184.
13. Wrone-Smith T, Nickoloff BJ. Dermal injection of immunocytes induces psoriasis. *J Clin Invest* 1996;98:1878–1887.
14. Robert C, Kupper TS. Inflammatory skin diseases, T cells, and immune surveillance. *N Engl J Med* 1999;341:1817–1828.
15. Gladman DD. Psoriatic arthritis: recent advances in pathogenesis and treatment. *Rheum Dis Clin North Am* 1992;18:247.
16. Reveille JD, Conant MA, Davic M. Human immunodeficiency virus-associated psoriasis, psoriatic arthritis and Reiter's syndrome: a disease continuum?*Arthritis Rheum* 1990;33:1574.
17. Torre Alonso JC, Rodriguez Perez A, Arribas Castrillo JM, et al. Psoriatic arthritis: a clinical, immunological and radiological study of 180 patients. *Br J Rheumatol* 1991;30:245.
18. Moll JM, Wright V. Psoriatic arthritis. *Semin Arthritis Rheum* 1973;3:55.
19. Buskila D, Langevitz P, Gladman DD, et al. Patients with rheumatoid arthritis are more tender than those with psoriatic arthritis. *J Rheumatol* 1992;19:1115.
20. Aguilar JL, Espinoza LR. Psoriatic arthritis: a current perspective. *J Musculoskel Med* 1989;11–28.
21. Gladman DD, Shuckett R, Russell ML, et al. Psoriatic arthritis (PSA): an analysis of 220 patients. *Q J Med* 1987;62:127.
22. Scarpa R, Biondi C, Oriente P. The classification of psoriatic arthritis: what will happen in the future? *J Am Acad Dermatol* 1997;36:78–83.

23. Avila R, Pugh DG, Slocumb CH, et al. Psoriatic arthritis: a roentgenologic study. *Radiology* 1960;75:691.
24. Wilke WS, Sayers ME. Psoriatic arthritis. In: Camisa C, ed. *Psoriasis,* 1st ed. Cambridge, MA: Blackwell Scientific, 1994:109–163.
25. Roberts ME, Wright V, Hill AG, et al. Psoriatic arthritis: follow-up study. *Ann Rheum Dis* 1976;35:206.
26. Hanly JG, Russell ML, Gladman DD. Psoriatic spondyloarthropathy: a long term prospective study. *Ann Rheum Dis* 1988;47:386.
27. Helliwell P, Marchesoni A, Peters M, et al. A re-evaluation of the osteoarthritic manifestations of psoriasis. *Br J Rheumatol* 1991;30:339–345.
28. Zelickson BD, Muller SA. Generalized pustular psoriasis: a review of 63 cases. *Arch Dermatol* 1991;127:1339.
29. Szanto E, Linse U. Arthropathy associated with palmoplantar pustulosis. *Clin Rheumatol* 1991;10:130.
30. Soter NA, Franks AG Jr. Cutaneous manifestations of rheumatic diseases. In: Kelley WN, Harris ED Jr, Ruddy S, et al., eds. *Textbook of rheumatology,* 5th ed. Philadelphia: WB Saunders, 1997:497–510.
31. Kahn MF, Kahn MA. SAPHO syndrome. *Baillieres Clin Rheumatol* 1994;8:333–362.
32. Laurent MR. Psoriatic arthritis. *Clin Rheum Dis* 1985;11:61–85.
33. Eastmond CJ, Wright V. The nail dystrophy of psoriatic arthritis. *Ann Rheum Dis* 1979;38:226.
34. Goupille P, Laulan J, Vedere V, et al. Psoriatic onycho-periostitis: report of three cases. *Scand J Rheumatol* 1995;24:53–54.
35. Kammer GM, Soter NA, Gibson DJ, et al. Psoriatic arthritis: a clinical, immunologic, and HLA study of 100 patients. *Semin Arthritis Rheum* 1979;9: 75–97.
36. Calzavara PG, Cattaneo R, Franceschini F, et al. Antinuclear antibodies in psoriatic arthritis and its subgroups. *Acta Derm Venereol* 1989;146[suppl]:31.
37. Helliwell PS, Marchesoni A, Peters M, et al. Cytidine deaminase activity, C-reactive protein, histidine, and erythrocyte sedimentation rate as measures of disease activity in psoriatic arthritis. *Ann Rheum Dis* 1991;50:362.
38. Franks Jr. AG. Synovial fluid analysis. In: Scott WN, ed. *Arthroscopy of the knee: diagnosis and therapy.* New York: WB Saunders, 1990:43–48.
39. Gladman DD, Farewell VT, Kopciuk K, et al. HLA antigens and progression in psoriatic arthritis. *J Rheumatol* 1998; 25:730.
40. Slagel GA, James WD. Plaquenil-induced erythroderma. *J Am Acad Dermatol* 1985;12:857–862.
41. Luzar MJ. Hydroxychloroquine in psoriatic arthropathy: exacerbations of psoriatic skin lesions. *J Rheumatol* 1982;9:462–464.
42. Baker H, Ryan TJ. Generalized pustular psoriasis: a clinical and epidemiological study of 104 cases. *Br J Dermatol* 1968;80:771–793.
43. Braverman IM, Cohen I, O'Keefe E. Metabolic and ultrastructural studies in a patient with pustular psoriasis (von Zumbusch). *Arch Dermatol* 1972;105:189–196.
44. Lebwohl M, Ali S. Treatment of psoriasis, II: systemic therapies. *J Am Acad Dermatol* 2001;45:649–661.
45. Krueger JG. The immunologic basis for the treatment of psoriasis with new biologic agents. *J Am Acad Dermatol* 2002;46:1–23.
46. Bauer W, Engelman EP. A syndrome of unknown etiology characterized by urethritis, conjunctivitis, and arthritis (so-called Reiter's disease). *Trans Assoc Am Phys* 1942;57:307.
47. Brewerton DA, Caffrey M, Nicholls A, et al. Reiter's disease and HLA 27. *Lancet* 1973;2:996.
48. Arnett FC, McClusky E, Schacter BZ, et al. Incomplete Reiter's syndrome: discriminating features and HLA-W27 in diagnosis. *Ann Intern Med* 1976;84:8–12.
49. Hughes RA, Keat AC. Reiter's syndrome and reactive arthritis: a current view. *Semin Arthritis Rheum* 1994;24:190.
50. Fan PT, Yu DTY. Reiter's syndrome. In: Kelley WN, Harris ED Jr, Ruddy S, et al., eds. *Textbook of rheumatology,* 4th ed. Philadelphia: WB Saunders, 1993:961.
51. Winchester R, Bernstein DH, Fischer HD, et al. The co-occurrence of Reiter's syndrome and acquired immunodeficiency. *Ann Intern Med* 1987;106:19.
52. Michet CJ, Machado EBV, Ballard DJ, et al. Epidemiology of Reiter's syndrome in Rochester, Minnesota: 1950-1980. *Arthritis Rheum* 1988;31:428.
53. Arnett FC, Hochberg MC, Bias WB. Cross-reactive HLA antigens in B27-negative Reiter's syndrome and sacroiliitis. *Johns Hopkins Med J* 1977;141:193.
54. Amor B. Reiter's syndrome: diagnosis and clinical features. *Rheum Dis Clin North Am* 1998;24:677–695.
55. Inman RD, Whittum-Hudson JP, Schumacher HR, et al. *Chlamydia* and associated arthritis. *Curr Opin Rheumatol.* 2000;12:254–262.
56. Keat AC. Reiter's syndrome and reactive arthritis in perspective. *N Engl J Med* 1983;309:1606.
57. Weinberger HS, Ropes MW, Kulka JP, et al. Reiter's syndrome, clinical and pathologic observations. *Medicine* 1962;41:35.
58. Lahesmanaa-Rantala R, Toivanen A. Clinical spectrum of reactive arthritis. In: Toivanen A, Toivanen P, eds. *Reactive arthritis.* Boca Raton, FL: CRC Press, 1988:1–13.
59. Fox R, Calin A, Gerber RC, et al. The chronicity of symptoms and disability in Reiter's syndrome: an analysis of 131 consecutive patients. *Ann Intern Med* 1979;91:190.
60. Resnik D. Reiter's syndrome. In: Resnik D, Niwayama G, eds. *Diagnosis of bone and joint disorders,* 4th ed. Philadelphia: WB Saunders, 1988:1110–1126p.
61. Winchester R. Cutaneous manifestations of multisystem diseases: Reiter's syndrome. In: Fitzpatrick TB, Eisen AZ, Wolff K, et al., eds. *Dermatology in general medicine,* 6th ed. New York: McGraw-Hill, 1993:1769–1776.
62. Belz J, Breneman DL, Nordlund W, et al. Characterization of uveitis associated with spondyloarthritis. *J Am Acad Dermatol* 1989;20:898.
63. Granfors K, Jalkanen S, von Essen R, et al. *Yersinia* antigens in synovial fluid cells from patients with reactive arthritis. *N Engl J Med* 1989;320:216.
64. Bergfeldt L, Insulander P, Lindblom D, et al. HLA-B27: an important genetic risk factor for lone aortic regurgitation and severe conduction system abnormalities. *Am J Med* 1988;85:12.
65. Oates JK, Hancock JAH. Neurological symptoms and lesions occurring in the course of Reiter's disease. *Am J Med Sci* 1959;238:79.
66. Franks Jr. AG: Inflammatory arthritis of the knee. In: Insall J, ed. *Surgery of the knee.* Philadelphia: Churchill Livingstone, 2001:1089–1102.
67. West SG, Lawless OJ. The chronic disability of Reiter's syndrome in the US Army. *Arthritis Rheum* 1981;24:S78.
68. Boeger CA, Wittwer H, Schattenkirchner M, et al. Treatment of ankylosing spondylitis with infliximab. *Ann Rheum Dis* 2001;60:1159–1160.

CHAPTER 10

Miscellaneous Rheumatic Diseases That Can Involve the Skin

Samuel L. Moschella

MIXED (OR UNDIFFERENTIATED) CONNECTIVE TISSUE DISEASE

Some rheumatic diseases do not fit the traditional classification criteria, and a diagnosis cannot be made. These conditions have been described as undifferentiated connective tissue diseases. Some of the patients with these conditions have disease that fits the entity reported as mixed connective tissue disease, other patients have disease that is in an indistinguishable phase in the evolution of a more recognizable rheumatic disorder, and still other patients continue to have clinical signs that permit a more definitive progressive diagnosis such as systemic sclerosis or part of the spectrum of systemic lupus erythematosus (SLE) (1,2).

In 1972, Sharp et al. (3) described 25 patients who had a combination of clinical characteristics of SLE, progressive systemic sclerosis, and dermatomyositis, as well as the presence of a significant amount of antibodies to saline extractable nuclear protein. They called this entity mixed connective tissue disease (MCTD). These anti–U_1 ribonucleic protein (RNP) antibodies are present without anti-Sm antibodies. Other autoantibodies reported are anti-U_2RNP, anti-Ku, and anti-70K. The unifying features reported are not only the presence of significant titers of U_1RNP antibodies but also a more benign course and a dramatic response of the disease to corticosteroids.

Clinical Manifestations

The prevalence of MCTD is not known (4,5). It appears to be less frequent than SLE but more frequent than progressive systemic sclerosis and dermatomyositis. It favors females, especially in the second and third decades of life. No racial or ethnic predilection exists, and no distinctive HLA association has been appreciated. Sunlight and drugs have not been described as precipitants. Fever is a prominent feature. Arthralgia and morning stiffness are universal complaints. Arthritis is present in about 60% of patients. Deformities of the hand are mostly caused by extensor flexor tenosynovitis.

The mucocutaneous lesions seen in MCTD are puffy hands (Fig. 10.1), Raynaud phenomenon, sclerodactyly, skin ulceration, malar rash, discoid lupus erythematosus, telangiectasia, heliotrope eyelids, calcinosis cutis, Gottron papules, buccal mucosa ulceration, and nasal septal perforation. Raynaud phenomenon and edematous (puffy) fingers are found not only in MCTD; they are also found in early progressive systemic sclerosis, rheumatoid arthritis, SLE, and dermatomyositis.

Pleurisy is a common clinical manifestation. Pulmonary hypertension is the most common cause of death. Myocarditis can also occur. Esophageal dysmotility and gastroesophageal reflux occur in about 80% of patients. Although it has been suggested that high titers of anti-RNP antibodies protect against severe renal disease, this complication has been reported in about 25% of patients. Central nervous system involvement is unusual.

Diagnosis

Guidelines for diagnosing MCTD are listed in Table 10.1.

Pathology

The pathogenesis is believed to be a vasculopathy of small- and medium-sized vessels characterized by proliferative intimal hyperplasia. Upregulation by anti-U_1RNP autoantibodies of proliferative cytokine associated with vascular endothelial cells may play a role in the immunopathologic process leading to the characteristic proliferative vasculopathy of MCTD (6).

Immunogenetics and Immunologic Parameters

Immunogenetic studies have demonstrated most frequently the presence of HLA types DR4 and/or DR2 (7). The immunologic parameters reported are high levels of immunoglobulins and C-reactive protein and increased serum levels of interleukin-10 (IL-10), interferon-γ, and tumor necrosis factor-α (8).

Treatment

Because severe renal disease and life-threatening central nervous system disease occur infrequently, the major cause of death is cardiac complications resulting from pulmonary hypertension.

No therapeutic cure exists. Treatment of the patient requires a continuous assessment of the ever-changing status of the disease and a constant awareness of the iatrogenic effect of therapy. The selection and intensity of therapy with antiinflammatory drugs, such as aspirin, antimalarials, prednisone, and other

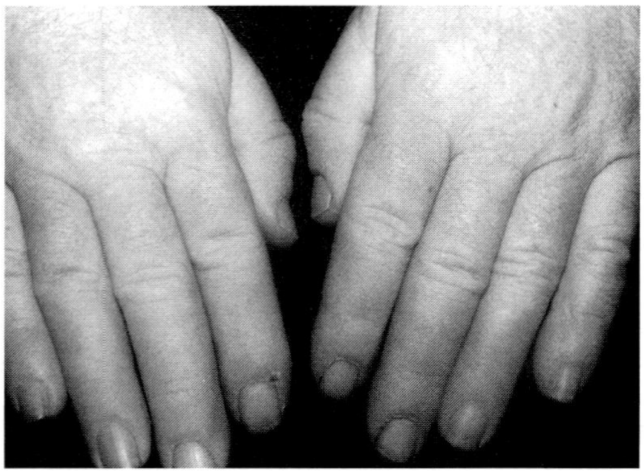

Figure 10.1. "Sausage" fingers seen in patients with mixed connective tissue disease as well as the edematous stage of the sclerodactyly of the localized type of systemic sclerosis.

immunosuppressants, depend on the extent and severity of systemic involvement.

Prognosis

The course of MCTD is unpredictable. Patients with a high titer of anti-RNP antibodies have a low prevalence of serious renal disease and life-threatening neurologic problems. The major cause of mortality is progressive pulmonary hypertension and its associated cardiac sequelae.

At the present time, the best evidence suggests that the MCTD is generally a dynamic transient state. For example, a 10-year follow-up of the original patients of Sharp et al. (3) and Nimelstein et al. (5) indicated that most patients had evolved into a scleroderma-like presentation. Other studies suggest that the HLA phenotype of the patient with MCTD influences the final clinical presentation. For example, most patients with MCTD and an HLA-DR3 phenotype evolve toward a clinical designation of SLE with features of Sjögren syndrome and interstitial lung disease; HLA-DR5–positive patients evolve toward a scleroderma-like picture and in general, those patients with MCTD who are HLA-DR2 and HLA-DR4 remain classified as having an undifferentiated connective tissue disease (7a).

TABLE 10.1. Guidelines for Diagnosing Mixed Connective Tissue Disease

General
Clinical features of a diffuse connective tissue disorder
Serologic
Positive antinuclear antibody, speckled pattern, titer > 1:1000
Antibodies of U_1RNP, U_1-70 kDa polypeptide of RNP
Absence of antibodies to double-stranded DNA, histones, Sm, Scl_{70}, PMScl, Ro, La, and other specificities
Commonly: hypergammaglobulinemia and positive rheumatoid factor
Clinical
Sequential evolution of overlap features over course of several years, including Raynaud phenomenon, serositis, gastrointestinal dysmotility, myositis, arthritis, sclerodactyly, skin rashes, and an abnormal diffusing capacity of the lung for carbon monoxide on pulmonary function tests
Absence of truncal scleroderma, severe renal disease, and severe central nervous system involvement
A nailfold capillary pattern identical to that seen in progressive systemic sclerosis (dropout and dilated vessels)

From Bennett RM. Mixed connective tissue disease and other overlap syndromes. In: Kelly WN, Harris ED Jr, et al. eds. *Textbook of rheumatology,* 3rd ed. Philadelphia: WB Saunders, 1989:1150, with permission.

ADULT-ONSET STILL DISEASE

In 1971, Bywaters (9) described 14 adult patients with an acute febrile polyarthritis that resembled systemic juvenile rheumatoid arthritis or juvenile-onset Still disease. Systemic juvenile rheumatoid arthritis is characterized by age at onset (< 16 years old), arthritis, intermittent fever, a characteristic evanescent rash, visceral disease (hepatosplenomegaly, lymphadenopathy), and the exclusion of other diseases. Unfortunately, the pathogenesis of systemic juvenile rheumatoid arthritis and adult-onset Still disease (ASD) are unknown.

Clinical Manifestations

The disease is slightly more common in women (10–12). High spiking fevers are almost always present. Most patients have a single daily spike, and the fever can continue from 8 weeks to 8 months. The characteristic so-called "rheumatoid rash" is a salmon-pink color, evanescent, urticarial, or measles-like eruption found mainly on the trunk, extremities, and areas of pressure, and rarely on the face, palms, and soles. It is occasionally pruritic. The rash and fever usually peak in the afternoon. Subcutaneous nodules are not present. A sore throat is described in about 40% of patients and consists of mild congestion with diffuse redness. Bacterial cultures of the throat reveal no growth of organisms. The pharyngitis does not respond to antibiotics but does respond to antiinflammatory drugs. Arthritis and arthralgia have been reported in 85% of patients. They can be mild and fleeting, affecting a few joints, or more extensive, although rarely progressively erosive. The knees, wrists, and metacarpophalangeal and proximal interphalangeal joints are usually affected. Lymphadenopathy, involving especially the cervical and submandibular chains, occurs in about 45% of patients, and splenomegaly is present in about 40% of patients. Hepatomegaly with serum abnormalities occurs in about 35% of patients. Pleural infiltrates in about 10% and pericarditis in 20% of patients have been reported. Involvement of the central nervous system and peripheral nerves has been seen infrequently. When a patient is seen with fever and polyarthralgia without joint swelling, the diagnosis is suspected in the presence of the characteristic rash. Generalized myalgias have been seen early in the course of the disease. The coexistence of polymyositis with or without rhabdomyolysis has been reported and successfully treated with methotrexate and corticosteroids (13). Renal amyloidosis should be suspected in patients with unexplained proteinuria (14).

Laboratory Studies

Histologically, the rheumatoid rash reveals a superficial perivascular neutrophilic infiltration without evidence of vasculitis. Hematologically, 90% of patients have a normocytic, normochromic anemia and leukocytosis with neutrophilia. It is associated with high erythrocyte sedimentation rate, increased level of serum ferritin, and negative rheumatoid factor and antinuclear antibody tests. The systemic overproduction of IL-18 may be closely related to the pathogenesis of ASD and the activity of disease appears to be related to the levels of IL-18 and its specific inhibitors (15).

Diagnosis

Because ASD presents as a multisystem disease and is underappreciated, many diagnostic and expensive evaluations are performed. Reginato et al. (10) proposed criteria for guidance in the diagnosis of ASD (Table 10.2).

TABLE 10.2. Criteria Proposed for Guidelines in the Diagnosis of Adult-Onset Still Disease

Major manifestations
- Persistent or intermittent fever
- Evanescent erythematous maculopapular rash
- Polyarthritis or oligoarthritis
- Neutrophilic leukocytosis

Minor manifestations
- Serositis
- Sore throat
- Hepatic dysfunction
- Lymph node enlargement
- Splenomegaly
- Other organ involvement

Negative studies of synovial fluid for microorganisms and crystals, as well as negative blood cultures and nondiagnostic serologic and bacteriologic studies for known bacterial, parasitic, fungal, and viral infections

Exclusion of other connective tissue diseases, hematologic or rheumatic diseases included in the exclusion list of the American Rheumatism Association criteria for rheumatoid arthritis. Rheumatoid factor in a significant titer should be absent

Absence of monoclonal gammopathy and absence of specific findings for other diseases on histopathologic studies of skin, synovium, lymph nodes, and any other involved organ

Chronic and/or recurrent clinical course

Radiographic articular changes in the carpal joints similar to those observed in childhood Still disease may further support the diagnosis and quality as classic adult-onset Still disease

All four major criteria are suggested to establish a diagnosis of definite adult-onset Still disease

Fever, arthritis, one other major, and one or more minor criteria would indicate probable adult-onset Still disease

From Reginato AJ, Schumacher HR Jr, Baker DG, et al. Adult onset Still disease: experience in 23 patients and literature review with emphasis on organ failure. *Semin Arthritis Rheum* 1987;17:39–54, with permission.

Treatment

About 25% of patients experience adequate control of fever and other systemic complaints in 2 to 3 weeks with adequate acetylsalicylic acid therapy. Other patients who fail to respond or who are intolerant to aspirin respond to nonsteroidal anti-inflammatory drugs. Other drugs used in nonresponsive disease are prednisone, parenteral gold, antimalarials, and penicillamine. In some patients whose disease is severely steroid-resistant, immunosuppressants, such as methotrexate, cyclophosphamide, azathioprine, mechlorethamine, and intravenous immunoglobulin, have been used with adequate immediate response, but long-term follow-up results are not available.

RHEUMATIC FEVER

In children, several poststreptococcal syndromes with arthritis have been described such as acute rheumatic fever (ARF), poststreptococcal reactive arthritis, and polyarteritis nodosa.

Poststreptococcal reactive arthritis occurs also in adults and favors females. It has a nonmigratory type of arthritis and may be associated with erythema nodosum and erythema multiforme. The patient may have cholestatic hepatitis. There is an absence of carditis and it is rarely complicated by vasculitis, pneumonitis, or acute glomerulonephritis (16).

Rheumatic fever is an inflammatory disease that occurs after a pharyngeal group A streptococcal infection and involves principally the joints, heart, central nervous system, skin, and subcutaneous tissues. It does not complicate cutaneous streptococcal infections.

In the 18th century, rheumatic fever was included in the broad diagnostic category of rheumatism (17). In 1812, Wells linked heart disease with rheumatism. In 1889, Cheadle described, in a schema, the various manifestations of the rheumatic state (i.e., tonsillitis, arthritis, pleurisy, chorea, erythematous rashes, and subcutaneous nodules) (17). In 1944, Jones created a mathematic approach to the clinical diagnosis by using the so-called Jones criteria as reported by Denny (18).

Etiologic Factors and Pathogenesis

The precise roles of bacteria, the human host, and the environment need more investigation. Evidence that group A streptococci are the etiologic agents is indirect because the organism is not recovered from the lesions, and no experimental model is available. The three main observations that support the etiologic role of group A streptococci are the following: (a) rheumatic fever is often preceded by a sore throat, but about one half of patients deny it; (b) initial (primary) or recurrent (secondary) rheumatic fever is always associated with a streptococcal antibody response (antistreptolysin O, anti-DNAse B, or antihyaluronidase titers); and (c) initial attacks and recurrences can be prevented by prompt and effective penicillin therapy. Other factors suspected of contributing generally to the attack rate are the site of infection (the lymphatic connections between the pharynx and the heart), the severity of the sore throat, and the magnitude of the streptococcal antibody response. The existence of "rheumatogenic" strains of group A streptococci is supported by some investigators. Patients with rheumatic fever have exhibited statistically significant increased humoral and cellular immune responses to all streptococcal antigens (19).

Pathology

The presence of Aschoff nodules is pathognomonic. They can be found in the collagen of the connective tissues of the heart and the subcutaneous tissue of the skin (the subcutaneous nodules). They consist of a central zone of fibrinoid necrosis of collagen surrounded by histiocytes and fibroblasts and lymphocytes and polymorphonuclear cells about the small blood vessels. The lesions heal rapidly and leave no scars.

Clinical Manifestations

The acute febrile disease usually occurs in children between the ages of 5 and 15 years in the northeastern United States during the spring and in the southwestern United States during the fall (20). No single sign, symptom, or laboratory test is diagnostic, but several combinations are diagnostic. The Jones criteria established for its diagnosis are based on a combination of major and minor manifestations and are used to prevent overdiagnosis and to deliver more appropriate therapy. The probability of the presence of rheumatic fever is high when the patient has an antecedent streptococcal infection, an increased titer of streptococcal antibodies, and evidence of two major, or one major and two minor, manifestations (Table 10.3). The latent period between the onset of pharyngitis and acute rheumatic fever is about 3 weeks.

Erythema marginatum (erythema annulare and erythema papulatum) is relatively specific for rheumatic fever and is characterized by rapidly spreading ringed lesions that can be flat (erythema marginatum) or raised (papular variant, erythema annulare) and are asymptomatic. They are usually pre-

TABLE 10.3. Jones Criteria for the Diagnosis of Rheumatic Fever

Major Manifestations	Minor Manifestations
Carditis	Fever
Polyarthritis	Arthralgia
Chorea	Previous rheumatic fever or rheumatic heart disease
Erythema marginatum	Elevated erythrocyte sedimentation rate or positive C-reactive protein
Subcutaneous nodules	Prolonged PR interval

Two major criteria or one major and two minor criteria indicate a high probability of the presence of rheumatic fever with supporting evidence of preceding streptococcal infection: history of recent scarlet fever, positive throat culture for group A streptococcus, increased antistreptolysin O titer or other streptococcal antibodies. From Stollerman GH. Rheumatic fever. In: Wilson JD, Braunwald E, Isselbacher KJ, et al., eds. *Harrison's principles of internal medicine,* 12th ed. New York: McGraw-Hill, 1991:935, with permission.

sent when the disease is active but can occur during periods of inactivity, are usually associated with carditis, and are unaffected by antiinflammatory therapy. The lesions start as erythematous macules or papules that expand peripherally with central clearing and result in complete or incomplete rings that meet, forming polycyclic patterns. The rapid spread from 2 to 7 mm in 12 hours is an essential feature. They appear in crops on the trunk and proximal parts of the extremities, and rarely on the face and about the hands. The eruption may appear only in the axillary vault. The duration of the lesions may be 2 hours to several days. The center of the spreading lesions may be pale or hypopigmented. On histopathologic examination, the presence of a perivascular infiltrate of neutrophils in the papillary dermis supports the clinical diagnosis (21).

Erythema papulatum rarely occurs. It consists of asymptomatic macules or papules that are 3 to 4 mm in diameter, appear in crops on the extremities (especially the flexor surface of the elbows or knees) and the buttocks, may last 6 to 8 days, do not form rings, and, histopathologically, exhibit nonspecific superficial dermatitis.

Subcutaneous nodules, which are one of the major cutaneous manifestations, appear late in the disease, are associated more often with carditis, and appear rarely with erythema marginatum. The subcutaneous nodules are firm, freely movable, and painless. They measure 0.5 to 2 cm. They appear in crops over bony prominences and particularly the tendons of the hands and feet. The scalp (especially the occiput), elbows, knees, wrists, ankles, and the vertebral spines are the other sites. The nodules tend to be smaller, less persistent, and histologically more "exudative" than rheumatoid nodules. They usually last a week or two but can disappear in a few days.

Differential Diagnosis

Among the diseases to be considered in the differential diagnosis are rheumatoid arthritis, SLE, serum sickness, urticarial vasculitis, renal diseases with or without myocarditis, and Henoch–Schönlein purpura.

Therapy

About 70% to 80% of the acute attacks subside in 6 weeks; 90% of patients recover in 12 weeks, and 5% of attacks last 6 months or more. The manifestations and severity of the disease determine the nature and intensity of treatment, which consists of bed rest, primary and secondary antibiotic prophylaxis, and antirheumatic therapy.

GOUT

Gout is used to describe a metabolic heterogenous group of diseases that are usually acquired but can be transmitted genetically. When gout is fully developed, patients have hyperuricemia, acute and recurrent inflammatory arthritis caused by monosodium urate crystals, tophi (aggregated deposits of these crystals) around joints and in soft tissue, renal disease, and uric acid nephrolithiasis.

History

The disease was recognized by Hippocrates in the fifth century BC (22–27). In the 13th century, de Vielehardouin originated the term "gout"; in 1848, Wollaston described the presence of urate in tophi; and in 1899, Freudweiler reported that urate crystals caused gouty arthritis (22,23).

Epidemiology and Pathogenesis

A serum urate level about 7.0 mg/dL represents supersaturation and carries an increased risk for gout and kidney stones (24,25). Familial hyperuricemia appears to be polygenic and multifactorial. Serum urate values correlate positively with weight and body surface, body bulk, protein intake, social position, educational achievement, and alcohol ingestion. The urate crystals precipitate from saturated body fluids and stimulate production of IL-1 by monocytes and macrophages, which mediate inflammation by activation of neutrophils with their subsequent phagocytosis, chemotaxis, and complement activation. The neutrophils release lysosomes creating further inflammation and tissue damage (26).

Gout is found in all races, but especially in Filipinos, the Maoris of New Zealand, and natives of Mariana Islands. During World Wars I and II, acute gouty arthritis was uncommon, presumably because of the lack of dietary protein. The prevalence of gout in Europe and the United States is about 0.13% to 0.37%. Primary gout is chiefly a disease of adult men. It is seen infrequently in women and, if so, is present mainly in postmenopausal women.

The concentration of plasma urate depends on the balance between absorption and production, destruction, and excretion of purines. Hyperuricemia and gout can be classified as primary or secondary. Primary gout can be idiopathic or associated with specific enzyme or metabolic defects, such as two sex-linked heritable deficiencies of ribose-phosphate pyrophosphokinase, protein synthetase, and hypoxanthine guanine phosphoribosyltransferase, which represent less than 1% of gout. The secondary type of gout is associated with increased de novo purine biosynthesis, as in the increased nucleic acid turnover in chronic hemolysis, polycythemia, myeloid metaplasia, chemotherapy, Lesch–Nyhan syndrome, and glycogen storage disease type 2 (von Gierke disease), and in the decreased clearance of uric acid or renal failure, (i.e., associated with medications such as thiazide diuretics). Lesch–Nyhan syndrome is an X-linked recessive disorder characterized by hyperuricemia, choreoathetosis, spasticity, mental retardation, and self-mutilation (27).

Clinical Manifestations

The four clinical expressions of gout are acute arthritis, tophaceous gout, urate nephropathy, and urate urolithiasis (31). The acute arthritis is initially monoarthritic with few constitutional symptoms and may be associated with lymphangitis; later in the disease process, it may be polyarticular and symptomatic. Frequently, the first metatarsophalangeal joint (podagra) is involved (28). The overlying skin is initially erythematous, warm, and tender; it resembles a cellulitis or an association with an underlying septic joint. Later, the skin becomes violaceous and scaly (Fig. 10.2). The acute attack gradually subsides over a few days to weeks with complete recovery. The acute attack can be precipitated by trauma, surgery, infection, alcohol, dietary excess, and starvation.

Hyperuricemia may occur in psoriasis because of the increased metabolism of purines in the skin. Patients with psoriasis have had recurrent gouty attacks. Because psoriatic arthritis may mimic gout, the synovial fluid should be examined for crystals to establish the diagnosis, to help estimate the association of gout and psoriasis, and to assess the latter as a kind of triggering mechanism (29).

The onset of tophaceous gout depends on the degree of hyperuricemia, severity of renal impairment, and duration of the disease (on average, about 12 years). It results from progressive failure to dispose of urate as rapidly as it is produced. Hyperuricemia and tophus formation can occur without gouty arthritis (30). Urate crystals tend to deposit in avascular tissue, such as the helix and antihelix of the ear; the olecranon (Fig. 10.3); the prepatellar bursae; and the tendons of the fingers (Fig. 10.4), wrists, toes, ankles, and heels. Subcutaneous deposits may produce yellow–white infiltrates, which are seen in the fingertips, toes, palms, and soles. These tophi may produce painless nodular or saccular swellings around joints, tendons, and bursae (31). The overlying skin frequently becomes thin, vascular, and orange-colored and can ulcerate and discharge white chalky or creamy material. Unusual locations of tophi are the heart valves, eyes, finger pads, larynx, nose, and breast. Destruction of cartilage and bone resulting from crystalline urate deposits produces the punched-out lesions and corticoid erosions with the characteristic "overhanging margins" seen on radiographic studies (32). It affects about 3% to 10% of patients with gout. Tophi appearing at the initial attack are usually secondary to a myeloproliferative disorder. Patients with tophaceous gout tend to have milder and less frequent attacks of acute gouty arthritis. Since the onset of effective antiuricemic therapy, attacks are less frequent, and tophi develop in fewer patients.

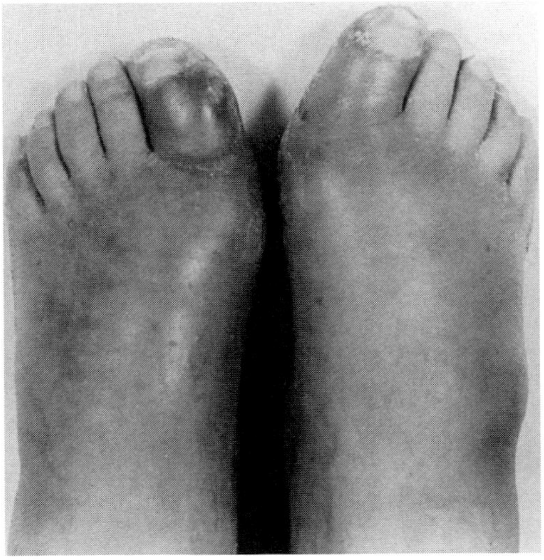

Figure 10.2. Bilateral pseudocellulitis of acute podagra.

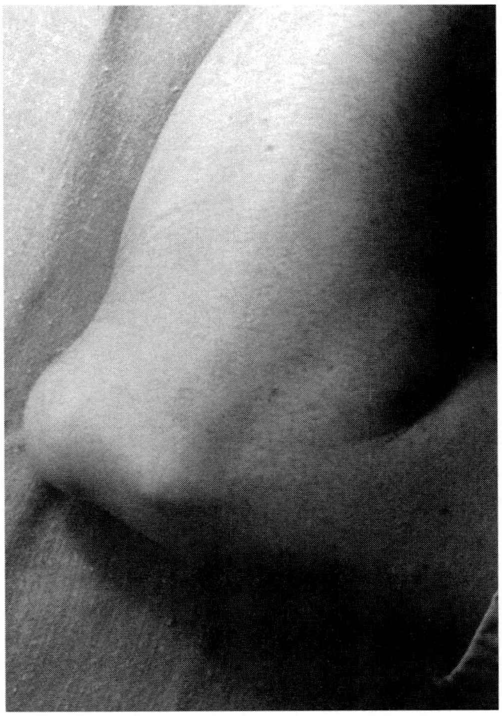

Figure 10.3. Acute gouty olecranon bursitis.

Among the soft-tissue lesions to be considered in the differential diagnosis are tendon xanthomas, rheumatoid nodules, multicentric reticulohistiocytosis, calcinosis cutis, giant cell tumor of tendon sheaths, pretibial myxedema (Fig. 10.5), and ganglions.

Urate nephropathy may result from an interstitial nephropathy caused by the presence of sodium urate crystals in the medulla or pyramids or from an obstructive uropathy from the precipitation of uric acid crystals in collecting tubules, pelvis, or ureters. Nephrolithiasis results from the hyperuricemia and contributing factors, such as undue acidity, increased concentration of urine, and possibly from abnormalities of urinary constituents stones that can affect the solubility of uric acid. Because urate stones are radiolucent, contrast medium is necessary to reveal them on radiographs.

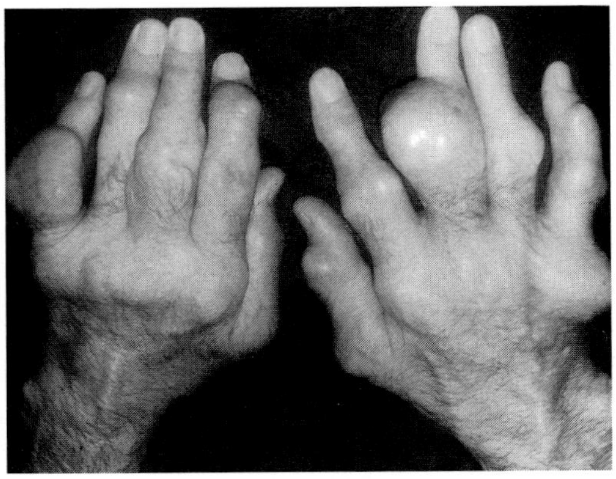

Figure 10.4. Severe tophaceous gout of hands.

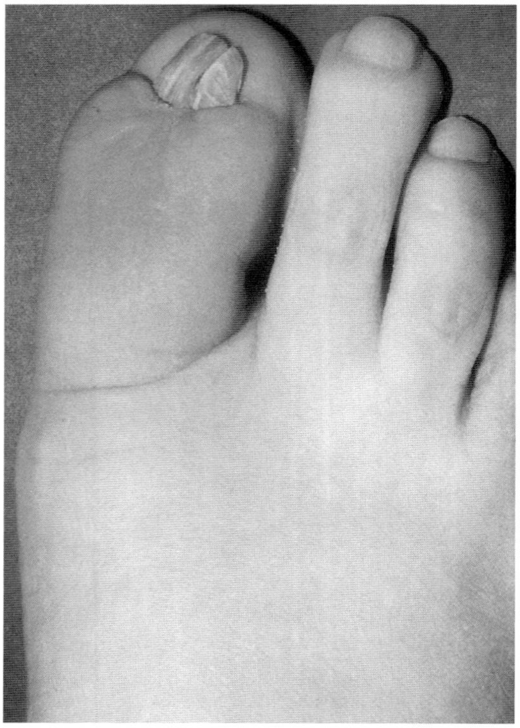

Figure 10.5. Pseudocellulitic changes of pretibial myxedema resembling acute podagra.

Pathology

To appreciate the presence of needle-shaped urate crystals, fixation of tissue in alcohol is necessary. The crystals appear brownish and are doubly refractive on polariscopic examination. The aggregates of crystals are surrounded characteristically by foreign-body giant cells. The sodium urate crystals can become secondarily calcified. Even with formalin fixation, the diagnosis can be suggested by the presence of amorphous brownish material surrounded by foreign giant cells and macrophages. An ethanol-based fixative is necessary to preserve crystals. The De Galantha stain stains the crystals brown/black.

Diagnosis

The diagnosis is not difficult to establish when the classic clinical presentation of podagra is appreciated. Negatively birefringent needle-shaped crystals of sodium urate in the leukocytes from the aspirated synovial fluid is diagnostic. If the presence of urates is suspected around the joint, bursa, or other sites, the chalky material should be expressed and examined for urates optically, chemically (murexide test), by ultraviolet spectrophotometry, or by degradation by uricase. The demonstration of tophi in visible body surface (Fig. 10.6) or punched-out destructive bone lesions establishes the presence of chronic tophaceous gout (Fig. 10.7). A rapid therapeutic response of arthritis to colchicine supports the diagnosis of gout.

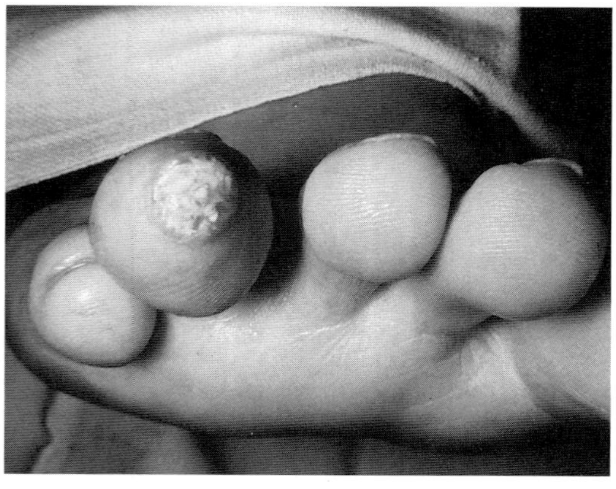

Figure 10.6. Draining dermal tophus.

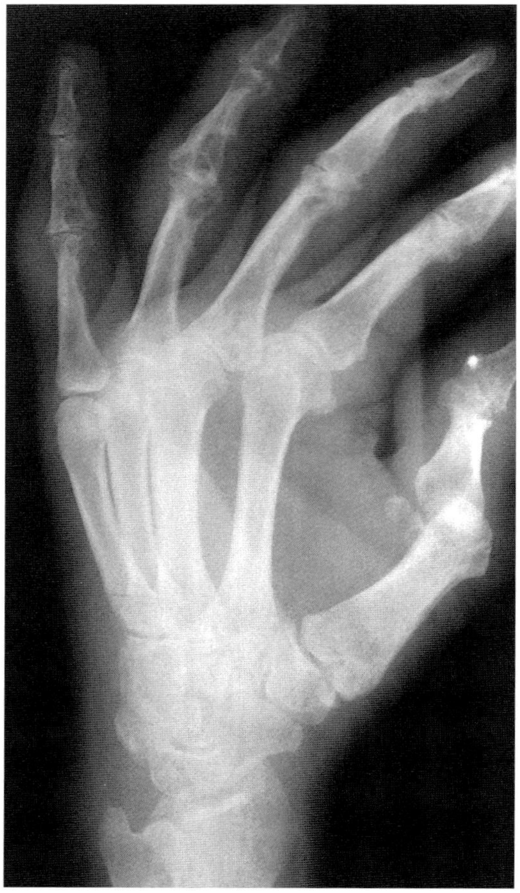

Figure 10.7. Punched-out digital osseous lesions of gout.

Treatment

The therapeutic approaches are to terminate acute gouty arthritis with colchicine, nonsteroidal antiinflammatory drugs, or a systemic corticosteroid and to prevent recurrences or reverse deposits of urates and kidney stone formation with a low-purine diet, high fluid intake, and allopurinol (33,34).

HYPERTROPHIC OSTEOARTHROPATHY

Hypertrophic osteoarthropathy (HOA) is a syndrome characterized by the presence of chronic proliferative periostitis of the long bones; clubbing of fingers, toes, or both; and oligosynovitis or polysynovitis. HOA can be classified as primary, which may be heritable or idiopathic, or secondary, which may be associated with pulmonary, cardiovascular, and gastrointestinal diseases and neoplasms, and a miscellaneous group, including connective tissue disease and thyroid acropathy (35).

Clubbing was described in the writings of Hippocrates in about 400 BC (35). An association of clubbing and arthritis with chronic lung and heart disease was made by Bamberger in 1891 (36) and Marie in 1890 (37).

In this syndrome, vascular proliferation associated with platelet/endothelial cell activation are recognized and one or more growth factors such as vascular endothelial growth factor may fit in with the pathogenesis of HOA (38).

Clinical Manifestations

Among the clinical syndromes are pachydermoperiostosis, idiopathic HOA, and familial and idiopathic clubbing (39–43). In a review of the literature, 125 patients were classified as having pachydermoperiostosis, primary HOA, and familial HOA. Table 10.4 lists the outstanding clinical features. A bimodal distribution has been described, with one peak occurring during first year of life and another at age 15 years. Familial clustering occurs. Effusion occurs in the knee, ankle, and wrist joints. Periostitis most frequently affects the tibia and fibula. Because of thickening of the bones, the hands can become spadelike (Fig. 10.8), and the limbs, cylindric. The fingers and toes may undergo acroosteolysis. Among the conditions to be considered in the differential diagnosis are acromegaly and thyroid acropathy.

The two cutaneous manifestations are hypertrophy of the soft tissues, such as coarse facial features with blepharostasis, elephant feet, and cutis verticis gyrata (Fig. 10.9), and glandular abnormalities, such as acne, hyperhidrosis, and seborrhea. It has been suggested that HOA is not a synovial disease, that the synovitis is a sympathetic reaction, and that a genetically controlled growth-promoting factor different from the growth hormone plays a role in the pathogenesis of this syndrome. The skin and bone changes may progress for more than 5 to 10 years and then stabilize; rarely, they may continue, especially the skin changes. Some patients may have sparse facial and pubic hair and gynecomastia without evidence of an underlying endocrinopathy. These patients may also be mentally retarded.

Clubbing of the fingers and toes may be familial, idiopathic, or part of HOA. The disease usually occurs insidiously over a period of months to years and is asymptomatic. The more rapid onset in adults is usually associated with chronic infections or neoplasms. Clubbing of the toes alone has been described in patients with patent ductus arteriosus. Unilateral clubbing has been described with aneurysms of the large arteries of the chest, apical pulmonary or axillary neoplasms, aortic insufficiency, venous incompetence in the arm, and hemiplegia. Clubbing has the following clinical characteristics: fluctuance and softening of the nail bed with periungual erythema, enlargement of the distal volar pad, a loss of the normal 15-degree angle between the nail and the cuticle (Lovibond angle); an accentuation of nail convexity; a clubbed appearance of the fingertips, which are warm and sweaty; and a shiny, glossy change of the nail with longitudinal striations (Fig. 10.10).

Secondary HOA characterized by periostitis, clubbing, and polyarthritis is associated with pulmonary conditions such as bronchogenic carcinoma, mesotheliomas, chronic bronchitis, bronchiectasis, cystic fibrosis, pulmonary fibrosis, and pneumoconiosis. Associated cardiovascular conditions include bacterial endocarditis, cyanotic congenital heart disease, patent ductus arteriosus, aortic aneurysm, and aortic prosthesis. Gastrointestinal tract conditions include carcinoma of the esophagus, liver, or colon; amebic dysentery; biliary cirrhosis; cirrhosis; and inflammatory bowel disease. Neoplasms often include intrathoracic metastases. The most commonly related condition is bronchogenic carcinoma.

Secondary HOA occurs predominantly in men between the ages of 30 and 70 years. The underlying disease is usually already present, but the osteoarthropathy may precede the symptoms of the associated condition by months.

The bone changes of secondary HOA develop more quickly than the primary type and tend to be more painful. The skin changes may be relatively mild or absent. The distal parts of the extremities often have tender, firm, pitting edema. Effective

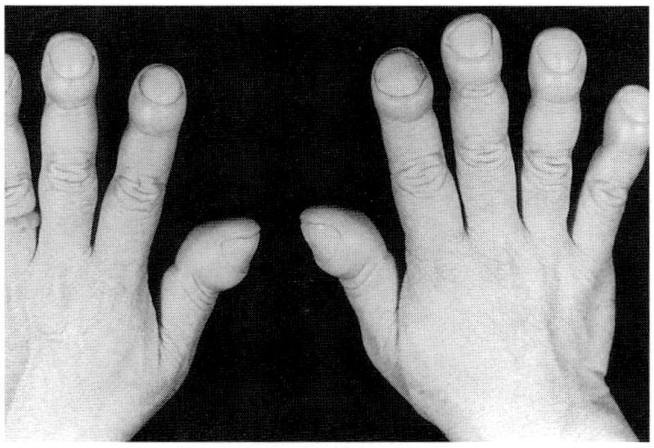

Figure 10.8. Spadelike changes of patient with pachydermoperiostosis.

TABLE 10.4. Outstanding Clinical Features of 125 Patients with Primary Hypertrophic Osteoarthropathy Described in the Literature

Finding	%
Men	89
Positive family history	38
Digital clubbing	89
Radiographic periostitis	97
Synovial effusion	41
Skin involvement	
Hypertrophic skin changes	73
Coarse facial features	61
Cutis verticis gyrata	24
"Elephant feet"	24
Hyperhydrosis	36
Seborrhea	33
Acne	13

From Martinez-Lavin M, Pineda C, Valdez T, et al. Primary hypertrophic osteoarthropathy. *Semin Arthritis Rheum* 1988;17:156–162, with permission.

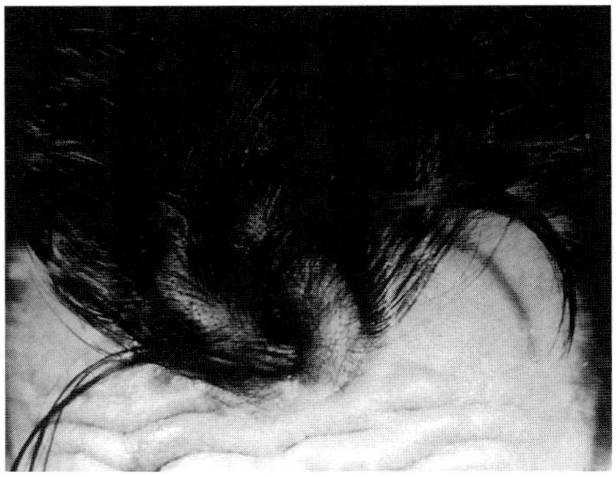

Figure 10.9. Cutis vertis gyrata in patient with pachydermoperiostosis.

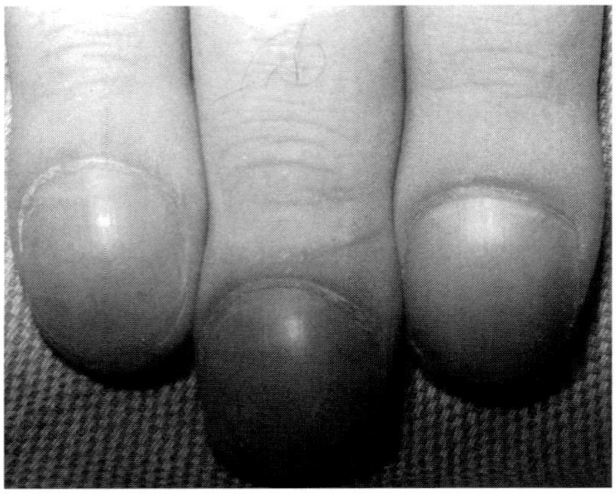

Figure 10.10. Clubbing of fingers in patient with chronic bronchiectasis.

TABLE 10.5. Criteria for the Diagnosis of Relapsing Polychondritis

Initial criteria[a]
Recurrent chondritis of both auricles with tragal and conchal bowl involvement but sparing of the helix and the antihelix
Nonerosive inflammatory arthritis
Chondritis of the nasal cartilage
Ocular inflammation
Chondritis of the larynx, trachea, or both
Damage to the cochlea, vestibule, or both, with hearing loss and tinnitus or vertigo, or both
Modified criteria
Three or more of the initial criteria, with no histologic confirmation necessary
One or more of the initial criteria, with histologic confirmation
Chondritis in two or more anatomic locations, with a response to corticosteroids, dapsone, or both

[a]At least three of the criteria must be met to establish the diagnosis.

treatment of the underlying condition can result in regression of the bone and skin changes.

Laboratory Findings

The abnormal laboratory findings of primary and secondary HOA may include an elevated sedimentation rate, an elevated alkaline phosphatase level, and noninflammatory synovial fluid. The histopathology reveals an increase in the amount and size of collagen bundles and fibroblasts and ground substance extending into subcutaneous tissue and glandular (eccrine and sebaceous) hypertrophy.

Diagnosis

Primary pachydermoperiostosis can be differentiated from the secondary type by the family history, age of onset, sex, rate of progression, nature of the periostitis, absence of a pulmonary lesion, and greater frequency of cutaneous changes. The periostitis of primary HOA is less symptomatic and on radiographic study, appears thicker, denser, and smoother. Other conditions to be considered in the differential diagnosis are acromegaly and thyroid acropathy.

Management

Primary HOA is rarely symptomatic, and if so, aspirin and nonsteroidal antiinflammatory drugs may be helpful. The most effective therapy for symptomatic changes of secondary HOA is the removal or cure of the underlying condition. Antiinflammatory drugs have been effective in reducing pain and discomfort.

RELAPSING POLYCHONDRITIS (ATROPHIC POLYCHONDRITIS, SYSTEMIC CHONDROMALACIA)

In 1923, relapsing polychondritis was described by Jaksch-Wartenhorst (44) as "polychondropathica," and subsequently as "chondromalacia" by Altherr (45) and von Mayenburg in 1936 (46). Pearson et al. (46) suggested the name "relapsing polychondritis." In 1976, McAdam et al. (47) proposed the diagnostic criteria.

Etiologic Factors and Pathogenesis

The etiology and pathogenesis are not established. Current evidence suggests that a hypersensitivity reaction results in the release of proteolytic enzymes with a dissolution of the cartilage mucopolysaccharides. The evidence advanced to support an immunopathogenic concept is (a) the demonstration of antibodies to cartilage and type II cartilage by indirect immunofluorescence, (b) the presence of immune complexes supported by the demonstration of deposits of immunoglobulin and C3 at the chondrofibrous junction by direct immunofluorescence, (c) the detection of abnormalities of cell-mediated immunity, and (d), in 25% to 30% of the patients, an association with a preceding or coexistent rheumatic or autoimmune disease, such as rheumatoid arthritis, SLE, vasculitis, Behçet disease [mouth and genital ulcers with inflamed cartilage (MAGIC syndrome)], or Hashimoto disease.

McAdam et al. (47) suggested that the diagnosis could be made in the presence of the combination of three of the clinical criteria and a histologic report of chondritis. The diagnostic clinical criteria include bilateral auricular chondritis, nonerosive seronegative inflammatory polyarthritis, nasal chondritis, ocular inflammation, respiratory chondritis, and vestibular damage. These clinical diagnostic criteria were modified by Damiani and Levine (48) in 1979 to include histologic features and therapeutic response.

Recent studies suggest that in unusual cases, relapsing polychondritis may be a paraneoplastic disease associated with a myelodysplastic disorder (47a,47b). The criteria for the diagnosis of relapsing polychondritis are shown in Table 10.5 (48).

Clinical Manifestations

Relapsing polychondritis affects both sexes equally, and usually patients are in the third to fifth decades of life (49–51). No familial predisposition is known. Fever usually occurs in about 40% of the patients. The frequencies of clinical expressions of the disease are as follows: auricular involvement (100%), oligoarthritis or polyarthritis (80%), nasal chondritis (70%), ocular inflammation (55%), respiratory tract involvement (14%), vestibular damage (6%), cardiac valvular involvement (3%), and other skin lesions (28%).

The most frequent clinical presentation is an acute patchy or diffuse redness, swelling, and pain of both external ears; earlobes are spared. The involved ears ultimately become "floppy" or "cauliflower" in appearance (Fig. 10.11).

The nasal involvement can result in the characteristic saddle nose deformity (Fig. 10.12). The nasal changes may be asymptomatic or associated with stuffiness, rhinorrhea, and hemor-

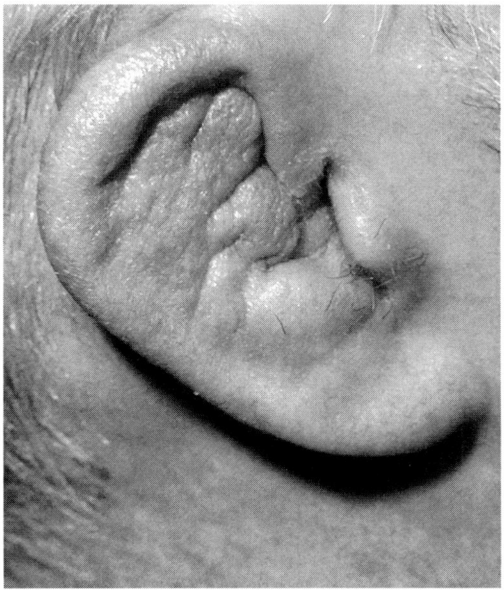

Figure 10.11. Advanced auricular involvement of patient with chronic relapsing polychondritis resembling "cauliflower" ears.

rhagic crusting. The ocular findings include episcleritis or scleritis, often with a nongranulomatous uveitis. The arthropathy is usually episodic, asymmetric, and nonerosive and monoarticular or polyarticular. The condition can be active for several days or weeks. Tenosynovitis may be present. The main cardiovascular change is valvular damage, especially in the aorta, which may occur from 6 months to 20 years after the onset of the disease and may cause death. Focal or disseminated vasculitis of medium and large vessels may occur, which may be indolent or fulminant and fatal. The other rheumatic diseases that may antedate, follow, or appear in conjunction with relapsing polychondritis are rheumatoid arthritis and its variants, Reiter syndrome, subacute cutaneous lupus erythematosus, psoriatic arthritis, Sjögren syndrome, and ankylosing spondylitis.

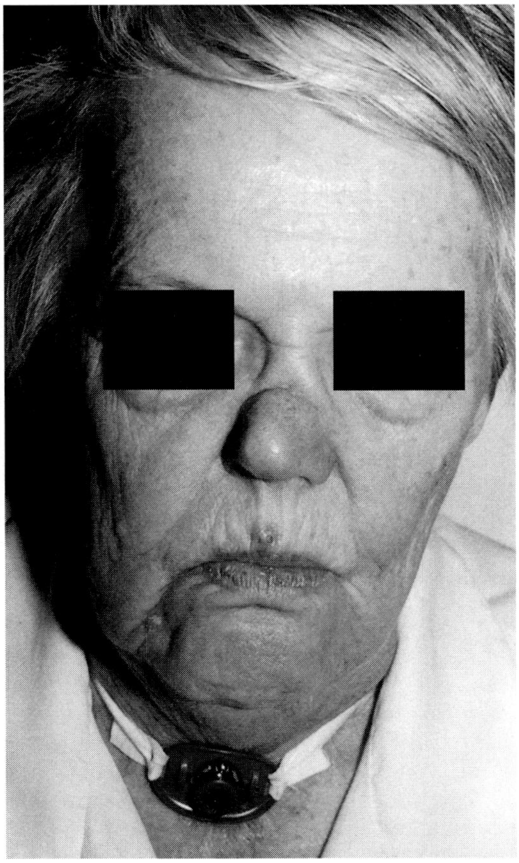

Figure 10.12. Saddle nose deformity of patient with relapsing polychondritis. Note the tracheostomy for severe laryngeal involvement.

Among the other dermatologic manifestations in patients with relapsing polychondritis without associated disease are purpura due to leukocytoclastic or lymphocytic vasculitis, livedo reticularis from leukocytoclastic vasculitis, urticarial papules from leukocytoclastic or lymphocytic vasculitis, bluish-red papules from aseptic neutrophilic infiltrate, erythema elevatum diutinum, nodules on limbs from septal panniculitis, deep neutrophilic infiltrate, vascular thrombosis and leukocytoclastic vasculitis, superficial phlebitis, sterile pustules, ulcerations on limbs from thrombosis vessels, leukocytoclastic vasculitis, pyoderma gangrenosum–like changes, and distal necrosis (52).

An overlap syndrome has been described as MAGIC syndrome (features of both relapsing polychondritis and Behçet disease) (53).

Laboratory Features

The histopathologic changes described include a loss of basophilia of the cartilage, peripherally damaged chondrocytes, and a perichondrial encroachment by inflammatory cells. With recurrent or chronic attacks, granulation tissue and fibrosis are seen.

The laboratory findings are an elevated sedimentation rate; a slight leukocytosis; a mild chronic normocytic, normochromic anemia; and eosinophilia. Serologic studies reveal the presence of rheumatoid factor and antinuclear antibodies, usually of the diffuse staining pattern.

Magnetic resonance imaging is a useful adjunct in the diagnosis and treatment of problems with the respiratory tract, especially the larynx in relapsing polychondritis (54).

Treatment

The clinical course is variable and may be punctuated by periodic flares, or it may be smoldering, or fulminant with a rapid downhill course (55). The most frequent causes of death are infection, cardiac failure, and systemic vasculitis. The clinical parameters that favor a more guarded prognosis are 50 years of age or older, nasal chondritis, laryngotracheal involvement, valvular heart disease, large-vessel aneurysm, and vasculitis, especially with microscopic hematuria.

Mild disease may be controlled by such antiinflammatory drugs as aspirin, nonsteroidal antiinflammatory drugs, and dapsone (56). In severe acute attacks, glucocorticosteroids are usually effective in suppressing the acute aspects and in controlling and reducing the frequency of recurrence. In severe attacks that do not respond to steroids, a trial of adjunctive immunosuppressive drugs, azathioprine or cyclophosphamide, methotrexate, anti-CD4 monoclonal antibodies, and cyclosporine may be instituted.

WHIPPLE DISEASE

In Chapter 11, infectious diseases that affect the skin and joints are described. Whipple disease is a rare infectious multisystem disease with pathologic changes occurring in the gastrointestinal tract causing a severe malabsorption syndrome and affecting other organ systems such as joints, lymph nodes, skin, heart, and central nervous system.

History

In 1907, Whipple (57) made a comprehensive description of the disease. In 1958, Black-Schaffer (58) reported that the foamy pink macrophages in the lamina propria of the small intestine and mesenteric lymph nodes stained a brilliant magenta with periodic acid–Schiff reagent, which indicated the presence of mucopolysaccharide and permitted the appreciation of the systemic nature of the disorder. Since that time the infectious nature was established. In 1959, antibiotic therapy was reported to result in remission (59). In the 1960s, a characteristic rod-shaped bacillus was found, but could not be reproducibly cultured. Electron microscopic and immunofluorescent data demonstrated the presence of a single bacterium (60); this was further confirmed by refined genetic techniques. It is a gram-positive actinomycetic-like bacteria, with the proposed name of *Tropheryma whippelii.* It is closely related to aerobic soil organisms. Initiation or promotion of the disease may be in part a result of host susceptibility due to immune deficiency, the nature of which has not been established.

Diagnosis

Patients who present clinically with seronegative arthritis and diarrhea with malabsorption and weight loss could have Whipple disease. The diagnosis is established by the demonstration in the intestinal or extraintestinal lesional biopsy, which reveals the presence of gram-positive, acid fast–negative bacilli. Polymerase chain reaction–based diagnostic assay may be useful for diagnosis and monitoring therapy. The differential diagnosis is celiac disease, intraabdominal lymphoma, and infection with *Mycobacterium avium.*

Cutaneous Manifestations

Cutaneous involvements are hyperpigmentation of the skin, erythema nodosum, and subcutaneous nodules, which contain macrophages containing degenerative bacilli (61–64). The hyperpigmentation is the most common skin change and is best appreciated in the sun-exposed areas and scars, occurs in the absence of adrenal insufficiency, and has been attributed to the malabsorption. When the subcutaneous nodules are present, they are either the erythematous tender lesions on the limbs consistent clinically and histologically with erythema nodosum or the red–brown painful subcutaneous nodules of the neck and limbs, which on biopsy reveal a subcutaneous septal panniculitis containing the classic inflammatory changes of Whipple disease (65).

Treatment

Before corticosteroids and antibiotics, Whipple disease was uniformly fatal. The treatments of choice are trimethoprim–sulfamethoxazole for 1 year or procaine penicillin G and streptomycin (parenterally) for 2 weeks, plus trimethoprim–sulfamethoxazole for 1 year (66). Alternative therapies are penicillin, ampicillin, or chloramphenicol for 1 year.

SCHNITZLER SYNDROME

Schnitzler syndrome is a rare and underdiagnosed constellation of clinical and investigative studies (67,68). The diagnostic criteria are an urticarial rash, monoclonal IgM component, and at least two of the following clinical and laboratory criteria: fever, arthralgia, arthritis, bone pain, palpable nodes, liver or spleen enlargement, elevated sedimentation rate, leukocytosis, and abnormal findings on bone marrow studies.

The eruption is characterized by a chronic, pale rose maculopapular eruption, is monomorphic, can coalesce, and can be pruritic. The lesions favor the trunk and limbs and last 12 to 24 hours. The eruption is refractory to treatment. Angioedema is rarely seen. Histopathology of the skin lesions reveals neutrophilic urticarial changes without evidence of vasculitis.

The differential diagnosis is ASD, hypocomplemententemic vasculitis, SLE, lymphoma, and Waldenström disease. The most frequent complications are severe anemia of chronic disease and the evolution to a lymphoplasmacytic malignancy that can complicate the syndrome 20 years later.

The constitutional symptoms of fever, arthralgia, and bone marrow pain may respond to nonsteroidal antiinflammatory drugs; however, patients with more severe refractory symptoms and anemia may require systemic steroids and immunotherapy.

METABOLIC DISEASES ASSOCIATED WITH ARTHRITIS AND SKIN ERUPTIONS ARE AS FOLLOWS:

1. Hemochromatosis
2. Scurvy
3. Diabetes mellitus
4. Lipoprotein disorders
5. Ochronosis
6. Andersen–Fabry disease
7. Farber disease

HEMOCHROMATOSIS

Hemochromatosis is a chronic disease characterized by excessive iron deposition and fibrosis in many organs and tissues with ultimate functional impairment in untreated patients. There is a genetic type (previously called primary or idiopathic), which is an autosomal recessive disease characterized by an inappropriate high intestinal absorption of iron with pathologic deposition of iron in the parenchymal cells (69). There is an increased frequency of HLA-A3 or HLA-B14 phenotypes. Recently, the hemochromatosis gene (*HFE*) has been localized to the short arm of chromosome 6. Two point mutations, a cystine to tyrosine at amino acid 282 and a histidine for aspartic acid at amino acid 63, have been identified (69a).

Secondary iron overload conditions associated with increased iron from parenteral or oral routes include ineffective erythropoiesis (hereditary hemolytic anemias), inherited defects of iron transport and metabolism, porphyria cutanea tarda, and liver disease (i.e., alcoholic liver disease) (70).

Clinical Features

Genetic hemochromatosis usually occurs in 40- to 60-year-old men. There is no predictable pattern of organ involvement. The classic triad of cirrhosis, diabetes, and pigmentation (bronze diabetes) rarely occurs and is a late manifestation. In iron storage disease, the common target organs are the liver, pancreas, skin, joints, heart, and pituitary gland.

Table 10.6 presents a list of the frequency of clinical features at the time of diagnosis in patients with genetic hemochromatosis (71).

TABLE 10.6. Diagnostic Signs and Symptoms of Genetic Hemochromatosis and their Frequency at Initial Examination

Sign/Symptom	%
Weakness, lethargy	80
Hepatomegaly	80
Pigmentation	70
Abdominal pain	55
Arthralgia	45
Loss of libido or sexual potency	35
Electrocardiographic changes	35
Loss of body hair	15
Secondary amenorrhea	15
Dyspnea exertion	10
Esophageal varices	10
Splenomegaly	10
Peripheral edema	10
Jaundice	10
Gynecomastia	5
Ascites	5
Neurologic symptoms	5

From Niedereau C, Fischer R, Purschel A, et al. Long-term survival in patients with hereditary hemochromatosis. *Gastroenterology* 1996;110:1107, with permission.

The hyperpigmentation is due to increased deposition of melanin and dermal iron (Fig 10.13A). The skin coloration can be slate gray to brown and is most prominent in light-exposed areas, external genitalia, nipple areola, and flexures. The diabetes results from insulin depletion. The cardiomyopathy is associated with dysrhythmia and heart failure.

The deposition of iron in the gonadotropic cells of the pituitary results in testicular atrophy and low testosterone resulting in impotence and loss of libido. Secondary amenorrhea has been described in women.

The arthropathy occurs in 50% or more of the cases of genetic hemochromatosis but is uncommon in other forms of iron storage disease. The diagnostic features of the arthropathy of hemochromatosis are degenerative with prominent involvement of the metacarpophalangeal and proximal and distal interphalangeal joints, hips, and knees; chondrocalcinosis; and iron deposition in the synovial lining cells.

The diagnostic features of hemochromatosis are as follows (72,73):

1. Cirrhosis with iron deposition predominantly in parenchymal cells (see Fig. 10.13B)
2. Iron deposition in other organs causing cardiomyopathy, diabetes, or other endocrine deficiencies
3. Increased skin pigmentation, largely by melanin
4. Elevated serum iron concentration and saturated iron-binding capacity

The combination of an increased serum ferritin level and transferrin saturation of greater than 50% is approximately 95% sensitive and 85% specific for the diagnosis of genetic hemochromatosis. Direct measurement of iron in a liver biopsy specimen makes a definitive diagnosis.

Treatment

The treatment of genetic hemochromatosis is to remove excessive iron by phlebotomy. In secondary iron overload, phlebotomy is effective; however, in diseases associated with anemia, deferoxamine, an iron-chelating agent, may be administered by subcutaneous injection or intravenous infusion to remove the excess iron.

SCURVY

Scurvy is a rare disorder caused by vitamin C deficiency and is seen in populations with predisposing risk factors such as alcoholism, poor nutrition, malabsorption disorders, cancer, dialysis, and poverty. The diagnosis is made on the basis of the presence of the characteristic skin and mucosal changes, diet history, and inability to detect serum vitamin C levels (74).

Vitamin C is involved physiologically as a cofactor in the formation of collagen and consequently defective collagen molecules result in capillary fragility characterized clinically by petechiae, purpura, ecchymosis, gum swelling and bleeding, dystrophic hair lesions presenting clinically as enlarged hyperkeratotic follicles with hemorrhagic and fractured and coiled hair, delayed wound healing, and bone fragility (Fig. 10.14A–C). Scurvy also alters the metabolism of iron and the depletion of active tetrahydrofolate, which results in an anemia that may be microcytic, or megaloblastic.

Other nonspecific classic findings are fever, arthralgia, myalgia, and easy fatigability. Among the late-stage complications are hemarthrosis, intramuscular hemorrhage, central nervous system hemorrhage, and gastrointestinal bleeding (75,76).

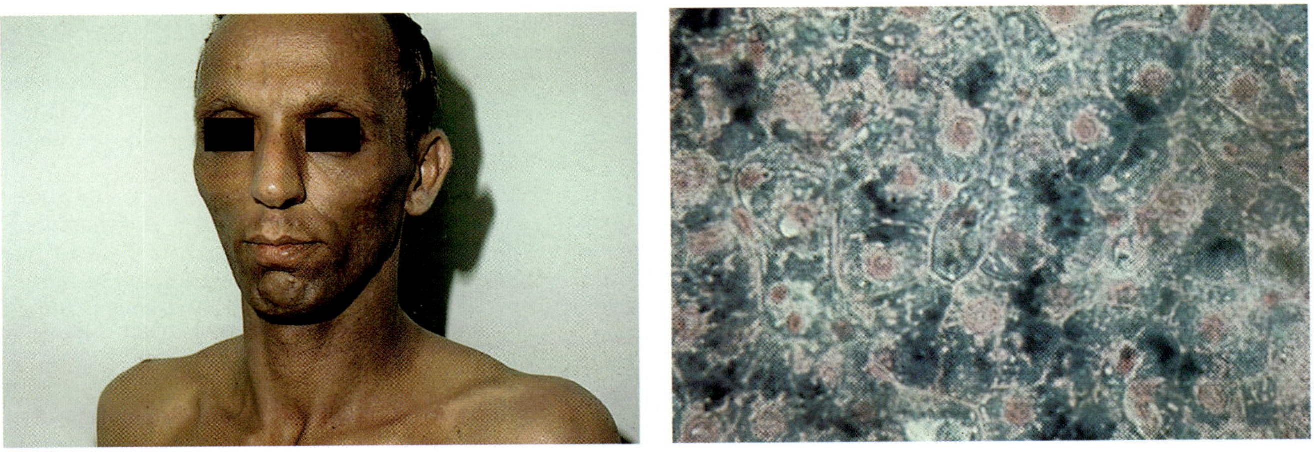

A B

Figure 10.13. A: Hyperpigmentation especially in the light-exposed areas in patient with hemochromatosis. **B:** Positive Pearl stain in liver biopsy revealing saturation of liver with iron.

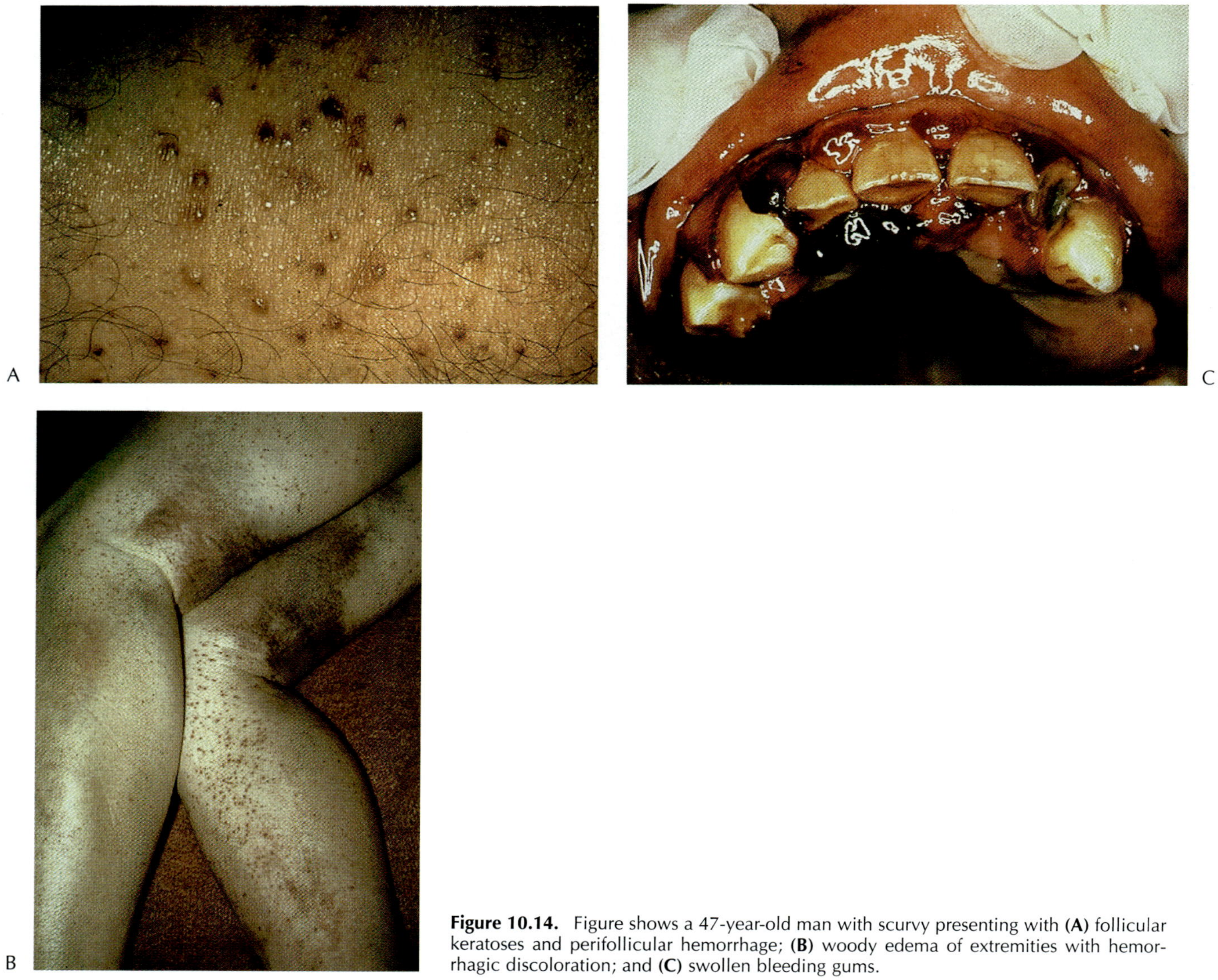

Figure 10.14. Figure shows a 47-year-old man with scurvy presenting with **(A)** follicular keratoses and perifollicular hemorrhage; **(B)** woody edema of extremities with hemorrhagic discoloration; and **(C)** swollen bleeding gums.

The goal of therapy is to replenish the vitamin C deficiency and to preserve the vitamin C stores. The initial dose of vitamin C is 1 g ascorbic acid per day until resolution of signs and symptoms and then 10 mg daily.

DIABETES MELLITUS

The more familiar dermatologic conditions associated with diabetes mellitus are pruritus, necrobiosis lipoidica diabeticorum, and granuloma annulare. The musculoskeletal and neurologic complications of diabetes may not be appreciated by those who are unfamiliar with musculoskeletal and neurologic diseases. The genesis of these disorders may be neuropathic changes, ischemic vascular disease, proliferation of fibrous tissue, or a combination (77,78).

Among those changes that are primarily the result of neuropathic changes are destructive arthropathies of ankle and forefoot (Charcot joints) (79), reflex sympathetic dystrophy of the hand or arm, carpal or tarsal tunnel syndrome, interosseous wasting, and proximal muscle weakness and atrophy. Other clinical signs of neuropathy are peripheral sensory neuropathy with a stocking-and-glove anesthesia, decreased vibratory and position sense, and reduced or absent deep tendon reflexes. Insensitivity of the hands and foot invites frequent wounding of these parts with the development of ulcerations (i.e., malum perforans of the foot). A mononeuropathy affecting most commonly the third and sixth cranial nerves occurs and, less frequently, the fourth and seventh nerves. Autonomic nervous system involvement can result in localized or widespread hypohidrosis or anhidrosis, orthostatic hypotension, impotence, and diarrhea.

There are a group of conditions characterized by proliferation of fibrous tissue probably caused by excessive glycosylation of collagen and decreased collagen degeneration and removal. However, diabetic microvasculopathy is closely associated with these fibrotic changes. The thick shiny skin of the hands, sclerodactyly, may resemble scleroderma, but the nailfold capillaroscopy is normal. The diabetic stiff hand syndrome results from progressive thickening of tendons, joint capsules, and subcutaneous tissue, which are responsible for the stiffness and flexion contractures and the "prayer sign" of the hands (80). These changes, which occur in long-standing diabetics (30%), are predictive of other diabetic complications such as those of the kidney and retina. Dupuytren contracture can occur in about 30% of patients with diabetes alone or with diabetic stiff hand syndrome (81).

LIPOPROTEIN DISORDERS

Lipoprotein disorders result from a defect in the synthesis or catabolism of lipoproteins and have been called the hyperlipoproteinemias.

Clinical Manifestations

Familial hypercholesterolemia, type IIA hyperlipoproteinemia is an autosomal dominant disorder resulting from mutation in the gene encoding the low-density lipoprotein recessive protein.

In the homozygotes, there is a high concentration of low-density lipoprotein in the connective tissue and arterial walls resulting in xanthoma and arthrosclerosis (82). There is a prevalence of one in a million. Before 10 years of age, orange–yellow xanthomas appear within the webbing of the fingers. They also typically present with skin-colored or yellowish nodules of the extensor tendons of the hands, Achilles tendon, and subperiosteal olecranon and tibial areas, as well as cutaneous tuberous subcutaneous nodules elsewhere (Fig. 10.15). Within the second decade, coronary artery disease usually occurs. The patients may experience oligoarthritis or polyarthritis favoring the knees and ankles and several joints of the hands or feet (83). The arthritis, as well as the tenosynovitis, may be presenting symptoms of the lipoprotein disorder. The joints are tender, swollen, and red. The attacks, like those in gout, are self-limited and last few to 10 days without permanent damage.

The heterozygote of familial hypercholesterolemia occurs in about one of 500 people. By the second decade, they may experience tendon xanthomas and after the third decade, manifestations of coronary artery disease appear. About 40% of the patients experience at least one episode of tenosynovitis, oligoarticular or polyarticular arthritis, or rheumatic fever–like arthritis.

Patients with so-called type IV hyperlipoproteinemia, characterized by elevated levels of very low-density lipoprotein and triglycerides, have been reported to have an associated polyarthritis (84–86). The arthritis is a persistent oligoarthritis, which is bilateral and asymptomatic with minimal deformity. They have eruptive xanthomas of the buttock, back, and shoulders. Tendon and tuberous xanthomas may be present.

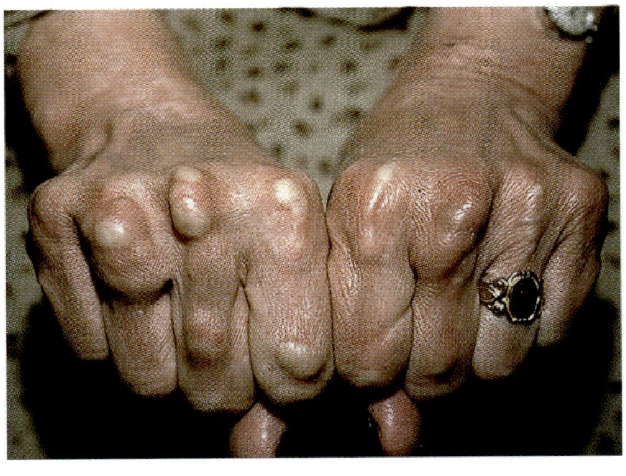

Figure 10.15. Patient with homozygous familial hypercholesterolemia with extensor tendon xanthomas of the hands.

ALKAPTONURIA AND OCHRONOSIS

Alkaptonuria is a symptomless, rare, autosomal recessive disorder of homogenetic acid (HGA) catabolism resulting from the lack of renal and hepatic HGA oxidase activity (1). Patients who have alkaptonuria and live to the fourth decade almost invariably develop ochronosis, which describes a bluish pigmentation due to a melanin-like product binding irreversibly to collagen and cartilage. The human gene responsible for alkaptonuria has been mapped to chromosome 3q2 (87).

Clinical Manifestations

Patients with alkaptonuria will notice that his or her urine turns black when alkalinized or on standing and when the urine is tested for sugar by Benedict–Hopkins–Cole reagent, it produces a yellow–orange precipitate (88,89). Eventually, ochronosis and ochronotic arthropathy develop. With a decrease in renal function, there is a significant increase in HGA levels, which results in pigmentation of cartilage, skin, and sclera; ochronotic spondylosis; peripheral arthropathy; prostate calculi; and cardiovascular involvement.

The concha and antihelix of ears have a slate-blue discoloration; the cartilage is irregularly thickened and inflexible and the opaque pigmented area becomes more prominent when transilluminated (Fig 10.16A). Not only the cerumen, but also the tympanic membrane and ossicles can become grayish-black; there may be tinnitus and hearing loss. The sclera frequently exhibits a small, pigmented patch halfway between either canthi or the cornea, which has been called Osler sign. The most common sites of hyperpigmentation are the ears, axillae, and groin. These are sites where the skin is thin and overlie cartilage and tendons.

The major skeletal changes are osteoporosis, abnormal calcification and ossification, and arthropathy. The abnormal calcification and ossification are most evident in the intervertebral discs of the lumbar spine (see Fig 10.16B); they also occur in helix of the ear, peripheral tendons, and ligaments. The degenerative arthropathy affects the peripheral skeleton, knees, hips, and shoulders. The cardiac valves can be involved with resultant deformity. Prostate calculi may be palpated rectally.

Diagnosis

Clinical and pathologic correlations are used to make a diagnosis. There are presumptive, but nonspecific tests that are based on color reaction resulting from the reducing properties of homogenetic acid. Molybdate reduction produces a deep blue color (Brigg test). A black spot appears on photographic paper when a drop of urine is placed on it due to reduction of silver. Darkening of urine occurs with the addition of sodium hydroxide due to oxidation of homogenetic acid (see Fig. 10.16C). A specific enzymatic test has been developed to quantitate the homogenetic acid in urine and blood.

Treatment

There is neither gene therapy nor any effective dietary or drug therapy available. Joint replacements and cardiac valve surgery have been successful.

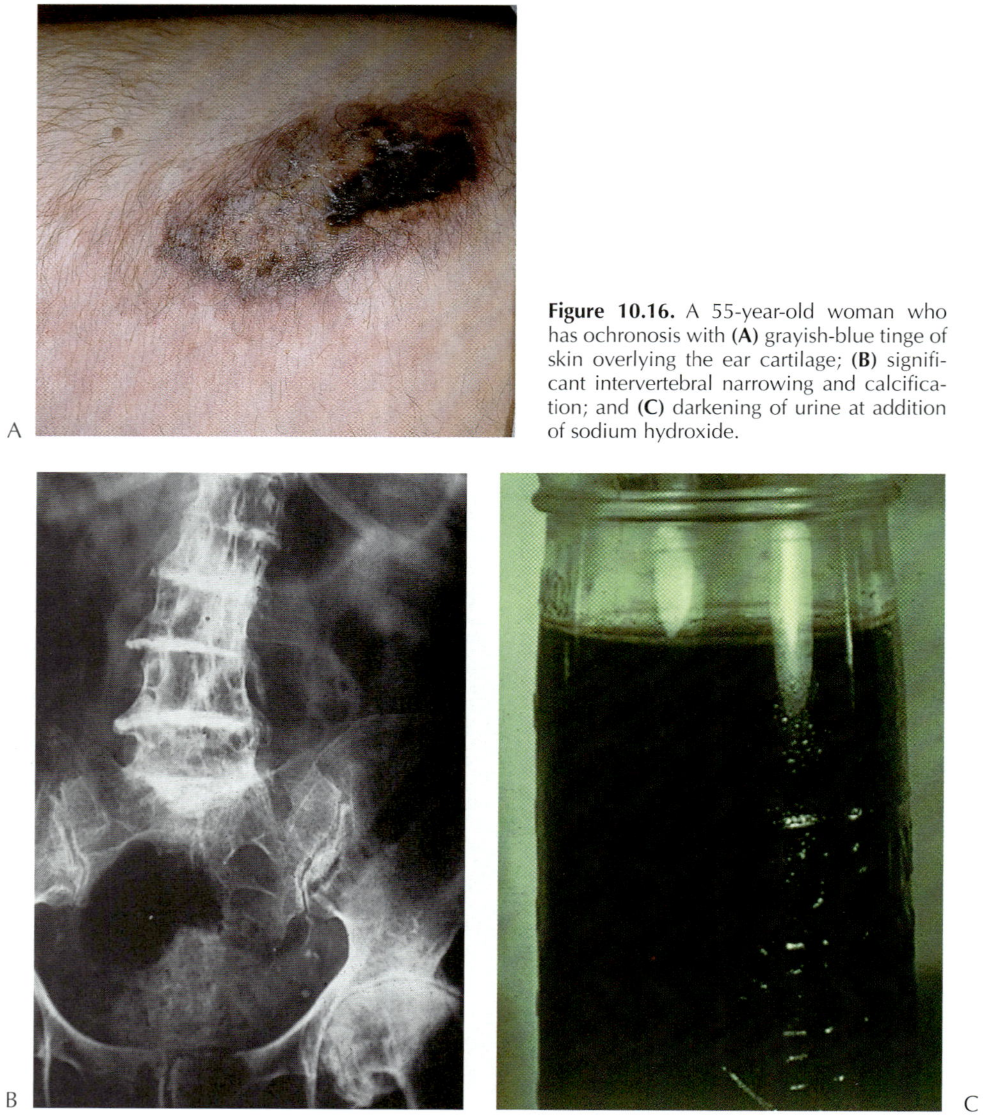

Figure 10.16. A 55-year-old woman who has ochronosis with (A) grayish-blue tinge of skin overlying the ear cartilage; (B) significant intervertebral narrowing and calcification; and (C) darkening of urine at addition of sodium hydroxide.

ANDERSEN–FABRY DISEASE

Andersen–Fabry disease is a rare X-linked inborn error of glycosphingolipid metabolism resulting from deficient α-galactosidase A activity and the pathologic accumulation of globotriaosylceramide and related glycosphingolipids primarily in vascular endothelial lysosomes and in a variety of other tissues such as the heart, kidney, nerves, cornea, and synovium (90–92). The responsible gene is localized on the long arm of the X chromosome at Xq22. The heterozygous female presents with milder clinical manifestation; the disease can be diagnosed by slit-lamp examination demonstrating corneal opacities (whorl-like epithelial dystrophy).

The skin lesions are telangiectasias and/or angiokeratomas and favor the area between the umbilicus and knees, are bilaterally symmetric, and increase with age. The mucosa and conjunctivae may be involved. Anhidrosis or more common hypohidrosis are usually early findings.

Among the other clinical manifestations of the classic Fabry disease are fever, acroparesthesia, eye lesions (corneal opacities, retina ischemia, lenticular opacities, conjunctival vascular lesions), cardiac disease (ischemia, infarction, decompensation, arrhythmia), central nervous system lesions (cerebrovascular accident; dysfunction of the trigeminal, eighth, and/or hypoglossal nerves), kidney disorders (hypertension, proteinemia, renal failure), gastrointestinal symptoms (diarrhea, malabsorption, nausea, vomiting, pain), and respiratory disorders (cough, dyspnea, wheeze). Among skeletal manifestations are polyarteritis, flexion contractures of the interphalangeal joints, bone pain with or without aseptic necrosis, and acromegalic-like facies.

Heterozygote patients may have angiokeratomas (30%), corneal dystrophy (70%), acroparesthesias (< 10%), and less than 1% may exhibit hypohidrosis and central nervous system, renal, or cardiac involvement.

In men, the diagnosis can be made by demonstrating low activity of α-galactosidase A in plasma, leukocytes, or cultured fibroblasts. In the heterozygote female, the diagnosis can only be established by genetic examination.

Because there is no specific treatment, patients are treated symptomatically. Among the new therapeutic developments and approaches are enzyme replacement (93), enzyme stabilization, gene therapy, and bone marrow transplantation.

FARBER DISEASE

Farber disease (lipogranulomatosis) is a rare autosomal recessive disorder resulting from the accumulation of ceramide in tissues and caused by lysosomal acid ceramidase deficiency (94–96). It manifests itself within a few months after birth and is characterized by a clinical triad of erythematous papules and subcutaneous nodules (lipogranulomata), which are periauricular and over pressure sites; progressive painful deformed joints; and laryngeal lesions. Similar skin lesions occur on the ears, neck, and trunk. Lesions of the larynx and epiglottis may be seen and can result in disturbances of respiration and swallowing. Involvement of the heart, lungs, lymph nodes, and nervous system with gross mental and motor impairment can occur. Patients may experience intermittent fever. The arthropathy may simulate systemic polyarticular juvenile rheumatoid arthritis (97). The diagnosis is made by demonstrating a reduction of the functional activity of the enzyme in cultured skin fibroblasts or leukocytes. There is no specific or effective therapy.

REFERENCES

1. LeRoy EC, Maricq HR, Kahaleh MB. Undifferentiated connective tissue syndrome. *Arthritis Rheum* 1980;23:341–343.
2. Lazaro MA, Maldonado Cocco JA, et al. Clinical and serologic characteristics of patients with overlap syndrome: is mixed connective tissue disease a distinct clinical entity? *Medicine* 1989;68:58–65.
3. Sharp GC, Irvin WS, Tan EM, et al. Mixed connective tissue disease: an apparently distinct rheumatic disease syndrome associated with a specific antibody to an extractable nuclear antigen (ENA). *Am J Med* 1972;52:148–159.
4. Bennett RM, O'Connell DJ. Mixed connective tissue disease: a clinicopathologic study of 20 cases. *Semin Arthritis Rheum* 1980;10:25–51.
5. Nimelstein SH, Brody S, McShane D, et al. Mixed connective tissue disease: a subsequent evaluation of the original 25 patients. *Medicine* 1980;59:239–248.
6. Okawa-Takatsuj M, Aotsuka S, Kinoshita M, et al. Increase of cytokine production by pulmonary artery endothelial cells induced by supernatants from monocytes stimulated with autoantibodies against U1-ribounucleoprotien. *Clin Exp Rheumatol* 1999;17:705–712.
7. Kaneoka H, Hsu K-C, Takeda Y, et al. Molecular genetic analysis of HLA-DR and HLA-DQ genes among anti-U1-70kd autoantibodies positive connective tissue disease patients. *Arthritis Rheum* 1992;35:83–94.

7a. Gendi H, Welsh KI, Van Venrooij WJ, et al. HLA type as a predictor of mixed connective tissue disease differentiation: ten-year clinical and immunogenetic followup of 46 patients. *Arthritis Rheum* 1995;38:259–266.

8. Bakritlassan A, Ronnelid J, Gunnarsson I, et al. Increase serum levels of immunoglobulins, C-reactive protein and type 1 and type 2 cytokines in patients with mixed connective tissue disease. *J Autoimmune* 1998;11:503–508.
9. Bywaters EG. Still's disease in the adult. *Ann Rheum Dis* 1971;30:121–133.
10. Reginato AJ, Schumacher HR Jr, Baker DG, et al. Adult onset Still's disease: experience in 23 patients and literature review with emphasis on organ failure. *Semin Arthritis Rheum* 1987;17:39–54.
11. Wouters JM, van de Putte LB. Adult-onset Still's disease: clinical and laboratory features, treatment and prognosis of 45 cases. *Q J Med* 1986;61:1055–1065.
12. Ohta A, Yamaguchi M, Kaneoka H, et al. Adult Still's disease: review of 228 cases from the literature. *J Rheumatol* 1987;14:1139–1146.
13. Samuels AJ, Berney SN, Tourtellotte CD, et al. Coexistence of adult onset Still's disease and polymyositis with rhabdomyolysis successfully treated with methotrexate and corticosteroids. *J Rheumatol* 1989;16:685–687.
14. Oh YB, Bae SC, Jung JH, et al. Secondary amyloidosis in adult onset Still's disease: case report and review of literature. *Korean J Intern Med* 2000;15:131–134.
15. Kawashima M, Yamamura M, Taniai M, et al. Levels of interleukin-18 and its binding inhibitors in the blood circulation of patients with adult-onset Still's disease. *Arthritis Rheum* 2001;44:550–560.
16. Bout L, Brus F, Dijkman-Neerinex RHM, et al. The clinical spectrum of post-streptococcal syndromes with arthritis in children. *Clin Exp Rheumatol* 1998;16:750–752.
17. English PC. Emergence of rheumatic fever in the nineteenth century. *Milbank Q* 1989;67[Suppl 1]:33–49.
18. Denny FW. T. Duckett Jones and rheumatic fever in 1986: T. Duckett Jones Memorial Lecture. *Circulation* 1987;76:963–970.
19. Cairns LM. The immunology of rheumatic fever. *N Z Med J* 1988;101(847 Pt 2):388–391.
20. Stollerman GH. Rheumatic fever. In: Wilson JD, Braunwald E, Isselbacher KJ, et al., eds. *Harrison's principles of internal medicine,* 12th ed. Vol. 1. New York: McGraw-Hill, 1991:933–938.
21. Troyer C, Grossman ME, Silvers DN. Erythema marginatum in rheumatic fever: early diagnosis by skin biopsy. *J Am Acad Dermatol* 1983;8:724–728.
22. Copeman WSC. *A short history of the gout.* Berkeley: University of California Press, 1964.
23. Kelley WN, Fox IH, Palella TD. Gout and related disorders of purine metabolism. In: Kelley WN, Harris ED Jr, Ruddy S, et al., eds. *Textbook of rheumatology,* 3rd ed. Philadelphia: WB Saunders, 1989:1395–1448.
24. Wyngaarden JD, Kelley WN. *Gout and hyperuricemia.* New York: Grune & Stratton, 1976.
25. Arnold WJ, Grobner W. Clinical manifestations of hyperuricemia. *Clin Rheum Dis* 1977;3:51.
26. Touart DM, San P. Cutaneous deposition diseases, II. *J Am Acad Dermatol* 1998;39:527–544.
27. Wood MH, Fox RM, Vincent L, et al. The Lesch-Nyhan syndrome: report of three cases. *Aust N Z J Med* 1972;2:57–64.
28. McCarty DJ. The gouty toe: a multifactorial condition [editorial]. *Ann Intern Med* 86:234–236.
29. Fordham JN, Storey GO. Psoriasis and gout. *Postgrad Med J* 1982;58:477–480.
30. Hollingworth P, Scott JT, Burry HC. Nonarticular gout: hyperuricemia and tophus formation without gouty arthritis. *Arthritis Rheum* 1983;26:98–101.
31. Canoso JJ, Yood RA. Acute gouty bursitis: report of 15 cases. *Ann Rheum Dis* 1979;38:326–328.
32. Nakayama DA, Barthelemy C, Carrera G, et al. Tophaceous gout: a clinical and radiographic assessment. *Arthritis Rheum* 1984;27:468–471.
33. Wallace SL. Colchicine and new antiinflammatory drugs for the treatment of acute gout. *Arthritis Rheum* 1975;185:847–851.
34. Kelley WN, Schumacher MR Jr. Gout. In: Kelley WN, Harris ED Jr, Ruddy S, et al., eds. *Textbook of rheumatology,* 4th ed. Philadelphia: WB Saunders, 1993:1319–1336.
35. Martinez-Lavin M, Pineda C, Valdez T, et al. Primary hypertrophic osteoarthropathy. *Semin Arthritis Rheum* 1988;17:156–162.
36. Bamberger E. Ueber knochenveranderungen bei chronischen lungenund herzkrankheiten. *Z Klin Med* 1891;18:193–217.
37. Marie P. De l'osteoarthropathie hypertrophiante pneumique. *Rev Med (Paris)* 1890;10:1–36.
38. Silveira LH, Martinez-Lavin M, Pineda C, et al. Vascular endothelial growth factor and hypertrophic osteoarthropathy. *Clin Exp Rheumatol* 2000;18:57–62.
39. Brugsch H. Acropachydermia with pachyperiostitis: report of a case. *Arch Intern Med* 1941;68:687–700.
40. Findlay GH, Oosthuizen WJ. Pachydermoperiostosis: syndrome of Touraine, Solente and Golé. *S Afr Med J* 1951;25:747–752.
41. Herman MA, Massaro D, Katz S, et al. Pachydermoperiostosis: clinical spectrum. *Arch Intern Med* 1965;116:918–923.
42. Kerber RE, Vogl A. Pachydermoperiostosis: peripheral circulatory studies. *Arch Intern Med* 1973;132:245–248.
43. Rimoin DL. Pachydermoperiostosis (idiopathic clubbing and periostosis): genetic and physiologic considerations. *N Engl J Med* 1965;272:923–931.
44. Jaksch-Wartenhorst R. Polychondropathia. *Arch f. Inn Med (Vienna)* 1923;6:93–100.
45. Altherr F. Uber einen Fall von systematisierter Chondromalacie. *Virchows Arch f path Anat* 1936;297:445–479.
46. Pearson CM, Kline HM, Newcomer VD. Relapsing polychondritis. *N Engl J Med* 1960;263:51–58.
47. McAdam LP, O'Hanlan MA, Bluestone R, et al. Relapsing polychondritis: prospective review of 23 patients and review of the literature. *Medicine* 1976;55:193–215.

47a. Diebold J, Rauh G, Jager K, et al. Bone marrow pathology in relapsing polychondritis: high frequency of myelodysplastic syndromes. *Br J Haematol* 1995;89:820–830.

47b. Hebbar M, Brouillard M, Wattel E, et al. Association of myelodysplastic syndrome and relapsing polychondritis. *Leukemia* 1995:9:731—733.

48. Damiani J, Levine H. Weekly clinicopathological exercise: case records of the Massachusetts General Hospital—case 32-1999. *N Engl J Med* 1999;341:192–199.
49. Damiani JM, Levine HL. Relapsing polychondritis: report of 10 cases. *Laryngoscope* 1979;89:929–946.
50. Kaye RL, Sones DA. Relapsing polychondritis: clinical and pathologic features in fourteen cases. *Ann Intern Med* 1964;60:653–664.
51. Hughes RA, Berry CL, Seifert M, et al. Relapsing polychondritis: three cases with clinico-pathological study and literature review. *Q J Med* 1972;41:363–380.
52. Frances C, el Rossi R, Laporte JL, et al. Dermatologic manifestations of relapsing polychondritis: a study of 200 cases at a single center. *Medicine* 2001;80:173–179.
53. Firestein GS, Gruber HE, Weisman MH, et al. Mouth and genital ulcers with inflamed cartilage: MAGIC syndrome-five patients with features of relapsing polychondritis and Behçet's disease. *Am J Med* 1985;79:65–72.
54. Heman-Ackah YD, Remley KB, Goding GS Jr. A new role for magnetic resonance imaging in the diagnosis of laryngeal relapsing polychondritis. *Head Neck* 1999;21:484–489.
55. White JW Jr. Relapsing polychondritis. *South Med J* 1985;78:448–451.
56. Barranco VP, Minor DB, Soloman H. Treatment of relapsing polychondritis with dapsone. *Arch Dermatol* 1976;112:1286–1288.
57. Whipple GH: A hitherto undescribed disease characterized anatomically by deposit of fat and fatty acids in the intestinal and mesenteric lymphatic tissues. *Bull Johns Hopkins Hosp* 1907;18:382–391.
58. Black-Schaffer B. Tinctorial demonstration of glycoprotein in Whipple's disease: observations in systemic involvement. *Arch Pathol* 1958;66:464–467.

59. Sieracki JC, Fine G. Whipple's disease—observations in systemic involvement, II: gross and histologic observations. *Arch Pathol* 1959;67:81–93.
60. Yardley JH, Hendrix TR. Combined electron and light microscopy in Whipple's disease. *Bull John Hopkins Hosp* 1961;109-80–98.
61. Silva MT, Macedo PM, Nunes JF. Ultrastructure of bacilli and bacillary origin of the macrophage inclusions in Whipple's disease. *J Gen Microbiol* 1985;131: 101–103.
62. Good A, Beals T, Simmons JL. A subcutaneous nodule with Whipple's disease key to early diagnosis. *Arthritis Rheum* 1980;23:856–859.
63. Kwee D, Fields JP, King LE. Subcutaneous Whipple's disease. *J Am Acad Dermatol* 1987;16:188–190.
64. Balestrieri GP, Villanacci V, Battocchio S, et al. Cutaneous involvement in Whipple's disease. *Br J Dermatol* 1996;135:652–668.
65. Tarroch X, Vives P, Slas A, et al. Subcutaneous nodules in Whipple's disease. *J Cutan Pathol* 2001;28:368–370.
66. Keinath RD, Merrel DE, Vlietstra R, et al. Antibiotic treatment and relapse in Whipple's disease: long-term follow-up of 85 patients. *Gastroenterology* 1985; 88:1867–1873.
67. Berdy SS, Block KJ. Schnitzler's syndrome: a broader clinical spectrum. *J Allergy Clin Immunol* 1991;87:849–854.
68. Lipsker D, Vernan Y, Grunenberger F, et al. The Schnitzler syndrome: four new cases and review of the literature. *Medicine* 2001;80:37–44.
69. Schumacher HR Jr. Ochronosis, hemochromatosis, and Wilson's disease. In: Ruddy S, Harris ED JR, Sledge CB, eds. *Kelley's textbook of rheumatology,* 6th ed. Philadelphia: WB Saunders, 2000:2437–2444.
69a. Hanson EH, Imperatore G, Burke W. HFE gene and heriditary hemachromatosus: a HuGE review—human genome epidemiology. *Am J Epidemiol* 2001;154:193–206.
70. Bottomly SS. Secondary iron overload disorders. *Semin Hematol* 1998;35:77–86.
71. Niederau C, Fischer R, Purschel A, et al. Long-term survival in patients with hereditary hemochromatosis. *Gastroenterology* 1996;110:1107–1119.
72. Lambert RE. Iron storage disease. In: Ruddy S, Harris ED Jr, Sledge CB, eds. *Kelley's textbook of rheumatology,* 6th ed. Philadelphia: WB Saunders, 2000:1550–1566.
73. Smith LH Jr. Overview of hemochromatosis. *West J Med* 1990;153:296–308.
74. Reuler JB, Broudy VC, Cooney TG. Adult scurvy. *JAMA* 1985;253:805–807.
75. Leone J, Delhinger V, Maes D, et al. Rheumatic manifestations of scurvy: a report of two cases. *Rev Rheum Engl Ed* 1997;64:428–431.
76. Pangan AL, Robinson D. Hemarthrosis as initial presentation of scurvy. *J Rheumatol* 23001;28:1923–1925.
77. Sergent JS. Arthritis accompanying endocrine and metabolic disorders. In: Ruddy S, Harris ED Jr, Sledge CB, eds. *Kelley's textbook of rheumatology,* 6th ed. Philadelphia: WB Saunders, 2000:1581–1582.
78. Thomas PK. Classification, differential diagnosis, and staging of diabetic peripheral neuropathy. *Diabetes,* 1997;46[Suppl 2]:554.
79. Armstrong DG, Lavery LA. Acute Charcot's foot. *Rays* 1997;22:524.
80. Wasaki T, Kohama T, Howjou S, et al. Diabetic scleroderma and scleroderma-like changes in a patient with maturity onset type diabetes of young people. *Dermatology* 1994;188:228.
81. Chammas M, Bousquet P, Renard E, et al. Dupuytren's disease, carpal tunnel syndrome, trigger finger, and diabetic mellitus. *J Hand Surg Am* 1995;20:1109.
82. Goldstein JL, Hobbs HH, Brun MS. Familial hypercholesterolemia. In: Screwer CR, Beaudet AC, Sly WS, et al., eds. *The metabolic and molecular bases of inherited disease,* 7th ed. New York: McGraw-Hill, 1995;1981–2030.
83. Rimon D, Cohen L. Hypercholesterolemia (type II hyperlipoproteinemia) arthritis. *J Rheumatol* 1989;16:703–705.
84. Goldman JA, Glueck CJ Abrams RR, et al. Musculoskeletal disorders associated with type IV hyperlipoproteinemia. *Lancet* 1972;2:449–453.
85. Kemp P, Holland AM, Magoos FL, et al. Musculoskeletal manifestations in hyperlipidemia: a controlled study. *Am Rheum Dis* 1983;42:519–523.
86. Buckingham RB, Bale GG, Bassett DR, et al. Polyarthritis associated with type IV hyperlipoproteinemia. *Arch Intern Med* 1975;135:289–290.
87. Schumacher HR Jr. Ochronosis, hemochromatosis, and Wilson's disease. In: Ruddy S, Harris ED Jr, Sledge CB, eds. *Kelley's textbook of rheumatology,* 6th ed. Philadelphia: WB Saunders, 2000:2437–2444.
88. Tonart DM, San P. Cutaneous deposition diseases, II. *J Am Acad Dermatol* 1998; 39:527–544.
89. Albers SE, Brozena SJ, Glass LF, et al. Alkaptonuria and ochronosis: case report and review. *J Am Acad Dermatol* 1992;27:609–614.
90. Peters FPJ, Vermeulen A, Ichot L. Anderson-Fabry's disease: alpha galactosidase deficiency. *Lancet* 2001;357:138–140.
91. Peters FPJ, Sommer A, Vermealen A, et al. Fabry's disease: a multidisciplinary disorder. *Postgrad Med J* 1997;73:710–712.
92. Desnick RJ, Ioannou YA, Eng CM. Alpha galactoside A deficiency Fabry disease. In: Scriver CR, Beaudet AL, Sly WS, et al., eds. *The metabolic and molecular basis of inherited disease,* 6th ed. New York: McGraw-Hill, 1996:2741–2784.
93. Schiffmann R, Koop JB, Ansten HM, et al. Enzyme replacement therapy in Fabry disease. *JAMA* 2001;285:2743–2749.
94. Farber S. Lipid metabolic disorder-disseminated lipogranulomatosis a syndrome with similarity to, and important difference from, Neiman-Pick and Hand-Schuller-Christian Disease. *Am J Dis Child* 1952;84:449–500.
95. Heck LW Jr. Arthritis associated with hematologic disorders, storage diseases of lipid metabolism and dysproteinemias. In: Koopinean WJ, ed. *Arthritis and allied conditions,* 14th ed. Philadelphia: Lippincott Williams & Wilkins, 2001:1918.
96. Dulaney JT, Milunsky A, Sidbury JB, et al. Diagnosis of lipogranulomatosis (Farber's disease) by use of cultured fibroblasts. *J Pediatr* 1976;89:59–61.
97. Jameson RA, Holt PJL, Keen JH. Farber's disease (lysosomal and ceramide deficiency). *Ann Rheum Dis* 1987;46:559–561.

CHAPTER 11

Miscellaneous Disorders That Commonly Affect Both Skin and Joints

Jeffrey P. Callen

NEUTROPHILIC DERMATOSES

The neutrophilic dermatoses are a group of noninfectious disorders characterized by the presence of an angiocentric, vessel-based, primary neutrophilic inflammatory cell infiltrate (1) (Table 11.1). These disorders can be further divided into those that lead to vessel wall destruction (vasculitis) and those that do not destroy the vessels. The disorders to be discussed in this chapter will be those in which the vessel wall is not destroyed. These disorders are linked by similar associated processes, cutaneous neutrophilic infiltrate, overlapping clinical features, and similar approaches to therapy.

SWEET SYNDROME (ACUTE FEBRILE NEUTROPHILIC DERMATOSIS)

In 1964, R.D. Sweet described a group of patients with one or more attacks of painful, erythematous plaques, accompanied by fever, arthralgias, and leukocytosis (2). The histopathologic correlate was a massive neutrophilic infiltration of the dermis in the absence of vessel wall destruction or demonstrable infection. Sweet termed the process "acute febrile neutrophilic dermatosis" (AFND), but it has most often been called "Sweet syndrome."

This syndrome is more frequent in women (4:1) between the ages of 30 and 60 years. The disease may be preceded by symptoms suggestive of an upper respiratory tract infection. The skin lesions are believed to be distinctive, but may simulate several other processes. The characteristic lesion is a well-defined, erythematous plaque with a mamillated surface, which may give the clinical impression of microvesiculation (Fig. 11.1). There is rarely any accompanying epidermal change or ulceration, and the lesions heal without scar formation. Pustules may stud the surface or may be a major feature of the process. The lesions occur in crops, and may be initiated by a variety of traumatic injuries (pathergy) such as a needle stick, wound débridement, or burn (Fig. 11.2). The lesions are accompanied by fever and malaise in most patients, and myalgias and/or arthralgias in about one half of the patients. Headache, nausea, vomiting, diarrhea, and/or conjunctivitis may also occur in some patients. Untreated lesions self-resolve over a period of 6 to 8 weeks; however, many patients continue to produce lesions on a chronic or a recurrent basis.

Several clinical variants of Sweet syndrome have been described. Sweet syndrome has been reported in a number of patients who have a septal panniculitis. Some authors have suggested that this represents two separate but related processes, acute febrile neutrophilic dermatosis, and erythema nodosum (EN) (3), whereas others would call this deeper process "Sweet panniculitis" (4). A patient of mine with acute myelogenous leukemia had typical Sweet syndrome; following resolution of his typical lesions, he developed subcutaneous tender nodules on the legs and abdomen (5). Biopsy revealed an intense neutrophilic septal panniculitis, which I would interpret as Sweet panniculitis. Cohen et al. (3) reported a patient with this combination of typical Sweet syndrome and subcutaneous nodules and reviewed the eight previously reported patients. They highlighted the similar nature of associated conditions that have been reported with both Sweet syndrome and EN.

Another possible variant of Sweet syndrome is one that simulates facial erysipelas (6). Sweet syndrome often mimics a cellulitis, but in these patients, the lesions are located on the face, are edematous, and are sharply marginated. Some lesions have been described as vesiculated/pseudovesiculated (7,8) or purpuric. Most of these patients have had an associated myelogenous leukemia (9). This variant closely resembles an atypical bullous pyoderma gangrenosum.

Sweet syndrome has been reported in a number of children. Most of the features seen in adults also occur in children. However, several children with secondary localized cutis laxa have been reported (10), and several patients with presumed pulmonary involvement have also been reported (11).

Involvement of the female genital tract (12), as well as perianal involvement (13), has been reported. However, the lesions in these areas are almost always reported to be erosive or ulcerative and thus it may be better to classify these patients as having vulvar pyoderma gangrenosum.

Sweet, in his initial report, focused on the cutaneous aspects of the disease. However, this neutrophilic vascular reaction is a systemic process. At least a third of the patients have polyarthralgias, with many having a nondestructive polyarthritis. The inflammatory involvement of the joints almost always correlates with the cutaneous disease. Oral lesions have also been reported. Conjunctivitis has been reported in some patients as has peripheral ulcerative keratitis (14). Pulmonary involvement may occur in rare individuals (15,16). In several instances, lung biopsy has

TABLE 11.1. Noninfectious Neutrophilic Dermatoses

Nonangiocentric
Psoriasis
Reiter syndrome
Subcorneal pustular dermatosis
Acne fulminans
Blastomycosis-like pyoderma (pyoderma vegetans)
Angiocentric
Vessel wall destruction
Leukocytoclastic vasculitis
Polyarteritis nodosa
No vessel wall destruction
Acute febrile neutrophilic dermatosis (Sweet syndrome)
Typical
Atypical (cancer-associated) variant
Pyoderma gangrenosum
Typical
Atypical (cancer-associated) variant
"Pustular vasculitis"
Behçet disease
Bowel-associated dermatosis–arthritis syndrome
Rheumatoid neutrophilic dermatosis
Pyostomatitis vegetans
Pustular eruption of ulcerative colitis
Familial Mediterranean fever

From Jorrizo JL. Neutrophilic dermatoses: Sweet's syndrome and pyoderma gangrenosum. In: Gallin JI, Goldstein IM, Synderman NR, eds. *Inflammation: basic principles and clinical correlates.* New York: Raven Press, 1988:785–802, with permission.

been performed and has revealed a prominent neutrophilic infiltrate (17,18). Cardiac involvement is possible and may be due to infiltration of the heart muscle by neutrophils (19). Neutrophilic infiltration of the bones may also occur; this process is known as multifocal sterile osteomyelitis (20).

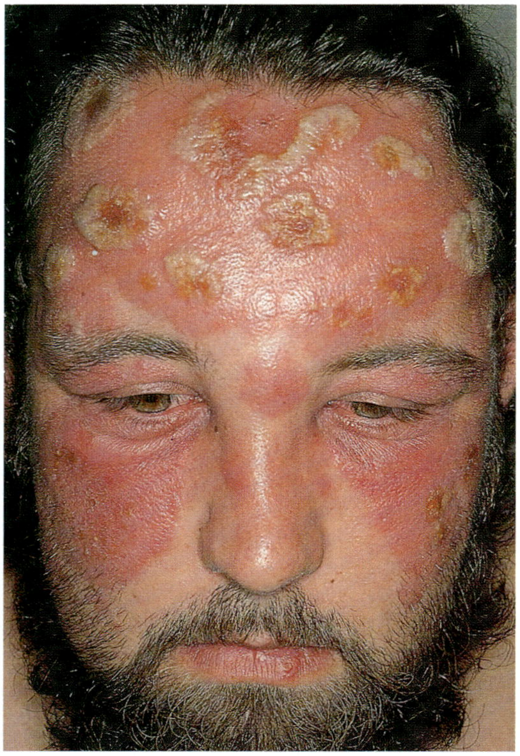

Figure 11.1. Sweet syndrome. This patient acutely developed erythematous plaques with a central mamillated "microvesicular" surface.

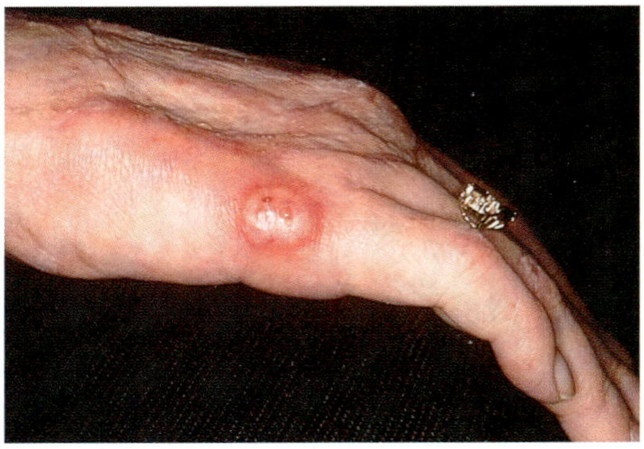

Figure 11.2. This patient's pustular lesion on an erythematous base was initiated after a kitchen accident in which boiling water splattered on her hand.

The laboratory findings include a leukocytosis, which is composed of mature neutrophils. White blood cell counts generally range from 10,000 to 20,000 cells/mm^3. The remainder of the blood count is within normal limits, except in patients who have Sweet syndrome associated with leukemia. Histopathologically there is a dense dermal infiltrate composed of mature polymorphonuclear leukocytes. The infiltrate may be more pronounced in perivascular areas, and leukocytoclasia is frequent, but the vessel walls generally are spared (Fig. 11.3). In a recent study, Malone et al. (21) demonstrated that vascular inflammation is frequent and correlates with the age of the lesion. Edema in the papillary dermis may be intense, coinciding with the microvesicular lesions observed clinically. Findings at immunofluorescence microscopy have been negative in the limited number of cases in which it has been reported.

Sweet syndrome has been reported with a variety of diseases (Table 11.2), but the most frequent association is with myelogenous leukemia or preleukemia (22,23). Sweet syndrome is not clinically or histopathologically different in the presence of leukemia, but patients more frequently tend to be anemic or thrombocytopenic (Fig. 11.4). Sweet syndrome has also been reported in conjunction with lupus erythematosus (LE) (24), rheumatoid arthritis (25–27), Sjögren syndrome (28), inflammatory bowel disease (29), pregnancy (30), Behçet disease (31), benign monoclonal gammopathy, multiple myeloma (32), lymphoma, myelodysplastic disorders, and several solid tumors (33,34). It is not known how frequently myeloproliferative disease is associated with Sweet syndrome, but most authorities quote a figure ranging from 10% to 15%. However, this figure

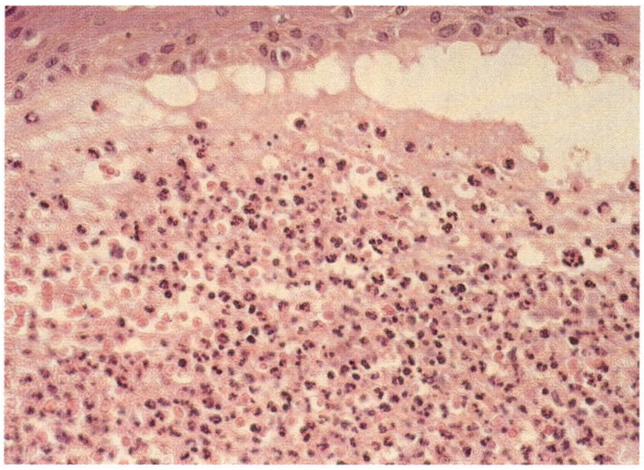

Figure 11.3. Massive infiltrate of mature neutrophils. This biopsy was taken from the patient pictured in Fig. 11.2.

TABLE 11.2. Acute Febrile Neutrophilic Dermatosis (Sweet Syndrome): Associated Diseases and Phenomena

Myeloproliferative disorders
Myelodysplasia (agnogenic myeloid metaplasia)
Acute myelocytic leukemia
Hematologic disorders
Acute myelogenous leukemia
Chronic myelogenous leukemia
Myelodysplasia
Multiple myeloma
Other malignancies (variety of individual reports)
Sarcoidosis
Inflammatory bowel disease
Crohn disease
Ulcerative colitis
Rheumatoid arthritis
Lupus erythematosus
Sjögren syndrome
Immunizations
Pregnancy
Postinfectious: bacterial, fungal, parasitic
Behçet disease
Drug-induced
Administration of leukocyte colony-stimulating factors
Hashimoto thyroiditis

may not be realistic because a reporting bias may exist, with disease associated with malignancy more frequently reported. In a "large" series of 29 patients, Kemmett and Hunter (35) reported two (6.7%) patients with leukemia-associated Sweet syndrome; in one patient, the leukemia was a late complication and may not have been present at the time of the active Sweet syndrome.

Neutrophilic dermatoses have been reported with the administration of various hematopoietic colony-stimulating factors such as granulocyte colony-stimulating factor (G-CSF) (36) and granulocyte-macrophage-CSF (GM-CSF) (37). It has been postulated that the up-regulation of neutrophil function and secondary release of cytokines may be responsible for these complications. Furthermore, most of the patients reported have had an associated malignancy, which was being treated with chemotherapy. The G-CSF or GM-CSF was usually being administered for the associated neutropenia. Also, therapy with all-*trans* retinoic acid, an agent that induces differentiation and maturation of myeloid precursors, has been associated with the development of Sweet syndrome in several leukemic patients (37–39).

The pathogenesis of Sweet syndrome is not known. Studies for circulating immune complexes, tissue-bound immunoglobulins, or complement have generally been negative. Kemmett and Hunter (35) reported antineutrophil cytoplasmic antibodies in six patients with Sweet syndrome, but this may be an epiphenomenon. Studies of neutrophil function have not shown a consistent abnormality.

Sweet syndrome (in the absence of leukemia or bowel disease) is usually an acute, steroid-responsive, self-limited disease. In general, a 2-week tapering course of oral prednisone (40 to 60 mg per day) is effective. One or more exacerbations requiring brief reinstitution of corticosteroids are common. Within Sweet's initial report, and in multiple subsequent reports, were patients in whom the process followed a chronic or recurrent course. In these patients, consideration of a steroid-sparing agent should occur (12). In individual reports, dapsone, potassium iodide, indomethacin, clofazimine, doxycycline, colchicine, isotretinoin, methotrexate, chlorambucil, pulse methylprednisolone, and cyclosporine have been used successfully (40–46).

PYODERMA GANGRENOSUM

Pyoderma gangrenosum (PG) is an uncommon ulcerative cutaneous condition with distinctive clinical characteristics (47). Frequently there is an associated systemic disease. The diagnosis is made by exclusion of other processes, which may cause cutaneous ulcers. Like patients with Sweet syndrome, patients with PG are often pathergic, with lesions sometimes developing after minor trauma.

Two variants account for most of the cases of PG—the typical (classic) form and the atypical, more superficial form (48). These two differ in their clinical manifestations, their associations with systemic diseases, and their responsiveness to corticosteroids.

The ulcerations of classic PG frequently are clinically characteristic. The border is well defined with a deep erythematous to violaceous coloration. The lesion extends peripherally and often the border overhangs the ulceration (undermined) as the inflammatory process spreads within the dermis, only secondarily causing necrosis of the epidermis (Fig. 11.5). The lesions may be single or may occur in crops, often beginning as a discrete pustule with a surrounding inflammatory erythema. The lesions may occur on any surface but are most common on the legs. Pain is a prominent feature and is sometimes so severe that narcotics are required for symptomatic relief. As the lesion heals, scar formation occurs and the resulting scar is often described as cribriform (Fig. 11.6).

Several variants of PG have been described. The pustular eruption of *ulcerative colitis* was first reported by O'Loughlin and

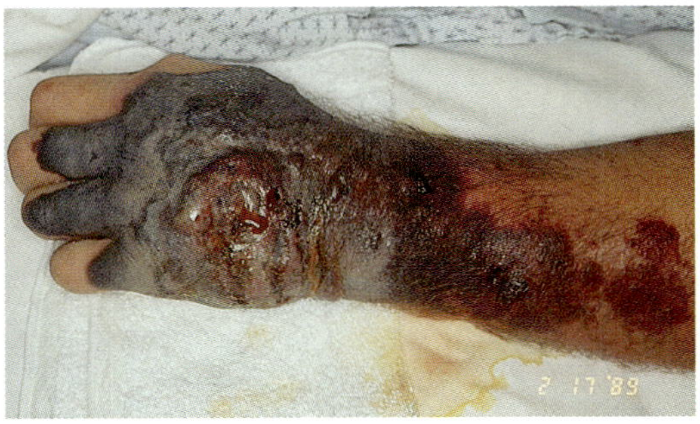

Figure 11.4. Sweet syndrome in a patient with acute myelogenous leukemia. The purpura is due to bleeding into the lesions associated with thrombocytopenia.

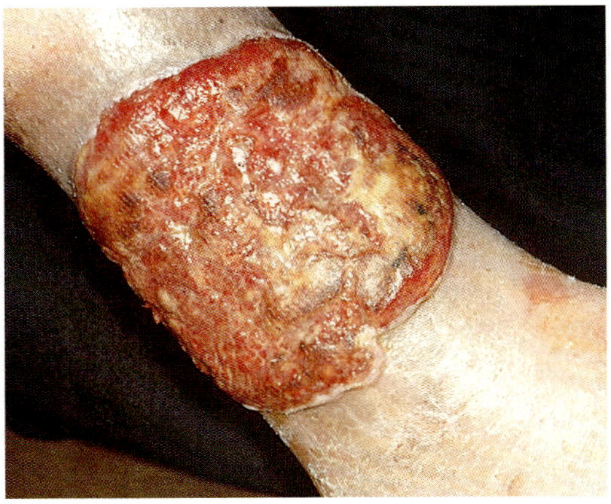

Figure 11.5. Pyoderma gangrenosum. Typical large ulceration with an undermined violaceous border.

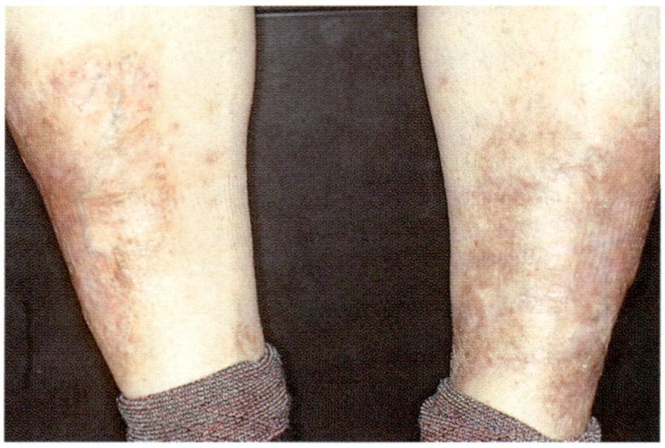

Figure 11.6. Healed lesion of pyoderma gangrenosum.

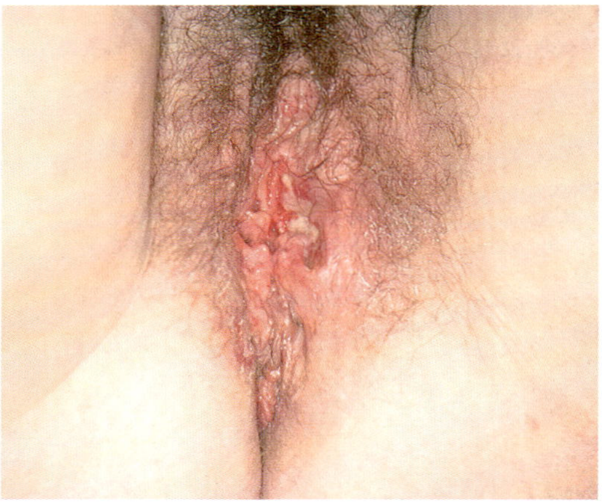

Figure 11.8. Vulvar pyoderma gangrenosum.

Perry (49). In this process, the patient is acutely ill with fever and develops multiple sterile pustules (50,51). The lesions may regress without scarring, or some may progress into a typical lesion of PG. Biopsy of the early lesion reveals sheets of mature polymorphonuclear leukocytes. Thus, this condition seems to represent an overlap between Sweet syndrome and PG.

Peristomal pyoderma gangrenosum has been described in a number of patients (Fig. 11.7). This variant occurs primarily in patients with inflammatory bowel disease, either ulcerative colitis or Crohn disease, but may also occur in patients who have had abdominal surgery for cancer with the creation of an ileostomy, colostomy or urostomy (52–54). The ulceration may occur as an early or late phenomenon. Perhaps irritation from the ileostomy or colostomy appliance is involved in the induction of this process (pathergy). These ulcerations must be differentiated from infection, dermatitis, or extension of the underlying bowel disease (Crohn disease only). Patients with this variant may have active inflammation of the bowel; thus, even those with a history of ulcerative colitis whose entire colon has been resected or those patients that develop the process after cancer surgery should be studied for the possibility that Crohn disease is present. These patients may respond to excision of actively inflamed bowel (54), to antibiotics such as dapsone or metronidazole, to topical agents such as superpotent corticosteroids or tacrolimus (53), or to infliximab as used for Crohn disease. However, they may require therapies that are more aggressive.

Vulvar pyoderma gangrenosum (Fig. 11.8) has been described in several reports (55,56). Often these ulcerations are débrided, which leads to spread of the disease. Other causes of mucosal ulceration must be excluded. Therapy with systemic corticosteroids has been successful in the previously reported cases. I have recently seen a patient with vulvar PG who failed to improve with minocycline, dapsone, prednisone, and methotrexate therapy. Chlorambucil therapy 4 mg per day led to control of her disease.

PG may occur in children. The associated diseases are similar to those seen in adults. Infants tend not to have any underlying systemic illness, whereas older children usually have an associated process. Graham et al. (57) have reviewed 46 cases of PG in children. They noted that infants tended to have perineal or perianal ulcerations. Treatment is generally similar to that for adults.

Another variant is *pyostomatitis vegetans* This process is one in which chronic, pustular, eventually vegetative erosions develop on the mucous membranes (Fig. 11.9), most notably in the oral cavity (58). Most of these patients have had inflammatory bowel disease, and some have had ulcerative or vegetating skin lesions similar to PG.

A condition known as *malignant pyoderma* is distinguished from PG by three features: (a) lesions predominantly on the head and neck (atypical for PG), (b) lack of associated systemic diseases, and (c) the absence of undermined borders and surrounding erythema (59). The distinctiveness of this variant has been questioned (60).

Lastly, there is a variant known as *atypical* or *bullous* PG. In this variation, the ulceration is more superficial, there is often a bullous, blue–gray margin, and the upper extremities (Fig. 11.10) and face are more commonly affected (61,62). An entity termed "pustular vasculitis of the dorsal hands" (later termed "neutrophilic dermatosis of the dorsal hands") is in my view a vari-

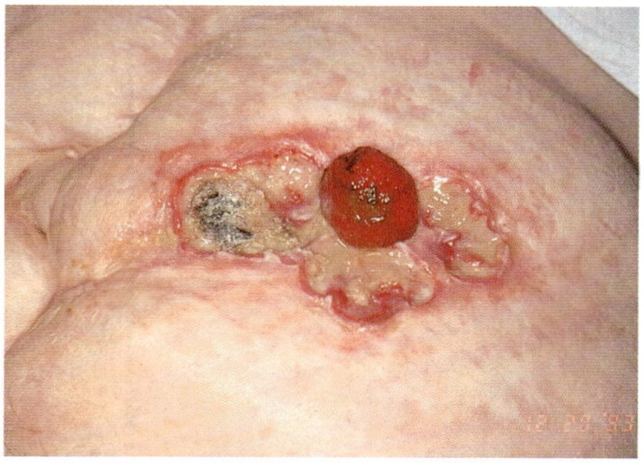

Figure 11.7. Peristomal pyoderma gangrenosum.

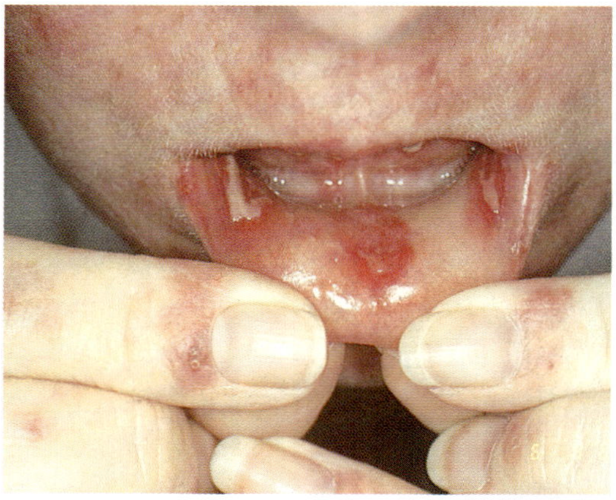

Figure 11.9. Pyostomatitis vegetans. This vegetative ulceration occurred in a patient with ulcerative colitis.

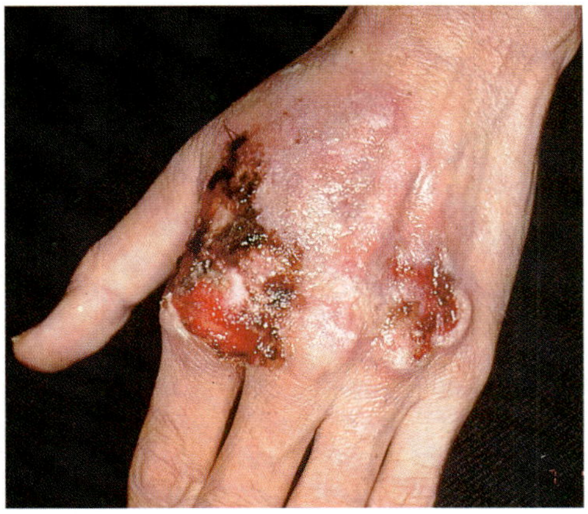

Figure 11.10. Atypical pyoderma gangrenosum in a patient with preleukemic state. The lesion is a shallow ulcer with a bullous blue–gray border.

ant of atypical PG (63). This variant has been reported with hematologic disease, specifically preleukemic conditions such as myeloid metaplasia (48,64) or acute myelogenous leukemia. At times, the separation of atypical PG from leukemia-associated Sweet syndrome is difficult.

The histopathology of PG is not specific but is useful in ruling out other causes of cutaneous ulceration. Controversy exists over the initial histopathologic change, with some classifying the process as a neutrophilic dermatosis (1), and others believing that the initial changes involve lymphocytic infiltrate, endothelial cell swelling, and fibrinoid necrosis of the vessel wall (a lymphocytic vasculitis) (65). Regardless, the histopathology does not involve a leukocytoclastic vasculitis, nor is granuloma formation compatible with a diagnosis of PG.

The etiology and pathogenesis of PG are not understood, but a variety of abnormalities of the immune system has been described. Although associated conditions are common (Table 11.3), perhaps one fourth to one half of the patients have "idiopathic" disease. The most common associated conditions are inflammatory bowel disease, arthritis, paraproteinemia, and hematologic malignancy.

Initial reports of PG focused on its association with ulcerative colitis (66). Over time, it has been recognized that regional enteritis and Crohn disease (granulomatous colitis) account for about 50% of patients with inflammatory bowel disease and PG (67,68). In the most recent literature, inflammatory bowel disease has represented about 15% to 20% of the associated phenomena. In addition, early reports stressed the relationship of PG to the activity of the bowel disease, and even suggested that some patients' PG lesions may benefit from surgical resection of the inflamed bowel (ulcerative colitis only). Callen et al. (69) have reported PG in association with inactive terminal ileitis, and Talansky et al. (70) also have reported lack of effect of bowel resection in some patients with PG and ulcerative colitis.

Arthritis is a frequent finding with PG. In some of the recent reports, arthritis has been the most common associated condition (48,67,68). Five of the nine patients with arthritis reported by Prystowsky et al. (68) had arthritis associated with inflammatory bowel disease. In general, the arthritis associated with PG is a symmetric polyarthritis, which may be rheumatoid factor–negative or –positive. Spondylitis, which may occur with inflammatory bowel disease, has not been reported to be independently associated with PG.

Various malignancies have been reported with PG, most commonly myelogenous leukemia or preleukemia. This association may be more common with the atypical variants of PG. Although several kinds of solid tumors have been reported, their presence is probably coincidental.

Paraproteinemia, in general a benign variant, has been reported with PG. With newer techniques of protein separation, it appears that 15% of patients with PG may have a benign monoclonal gammopathy, most often of IgA variety (68,71). The development of myeloma in PG appears to be a very rare occurrence.

As with Sweet syndrome, there have been several reports of pulmonary involvement in PG (56). Additionally, one patient has been reported with a neutrophilic carditis, bullous pyoderma gangrenosum, and myelodysplasia (72).

The diagnostic evaluation (Table 11.4) of the patient presumed to have PG has two objectives: (a) to rule out other causes of cutaneous ulceration and (b) to determine whether there is a treatable systemic associated disorder. There is not a specific laboratory or histopathologic test that is diagnostic of PG. Moreover, some of the associated disease processes may be clinically silent.

TABLE 11.3. Diseases Associated with Pyoderma Gangrenosum

Common associations
Inflammatory bowel disease
Chronic ulcerative colitis
Regional enteritis, granulomatous colitis (Crohn disease)
Arthritis
Seronegative with inflammatory bowel disease
Seronegative without inflammatory bowel disease
Rheumatoid arthritis
Spondylitis
Osteoarthritis
Hematologic diseases
Myelocytic leukemias
Hairy cell leukemia
Myelofibrosis, agnogenic myeloid metaplasia
Monoclonal gammopathy (IgA)
Rarely reported associations
Chronic active hepatitis
Myeloma
Polycythemia rubra vera
Paroxysmal nocturnal hemoglobinuria
Takayasu arteritis
Primary biliary cirrhosis
Systemic lupus erythematosus
Wegener granulomatosis
Hidradenitis suppurativa
Acne conglobata
Malignancy: various sites and cell types
Thyroid disease
Pulmonary disease
Sarcoidosis
Diabetes mellitus
Human immunodeficiency virus infection
Other pustular dermatosis, particularly Behçet disease

TABLE 11.4. Diagnostic Evaluation of the Patient with Pyoderma Gangrenosum

Careful history and thorough physical examination
Skin biopsy with tissue taken for cultures (bacterial, viral, fungal, and so on)
Studies of the gastrointestinal tract
Studies for possible abnormal serum proteins
Complete blood count, examination of the peripheral smear, and possibly a bone marrow examination

The differential diagnoses of ulcerative cutaneous lesions include (a) infectious diseases such as tuberculosis, deep fungal infections (73,74), bacterial infections, viral infections, and, in light of acquired immunodeficiency syndrome, rare opportunistic microorganisms; (b) halogenodermas; (c) vasculitis; (d) insect bites, in particular the bite of the brown recluse spider; (e) venous or arterial insufficiency; and (f) factitial ulcerations. Culture from both exudate and tissue sources should be performed.

To evaluate for the presence of an associated disorder, another series of examinations is indicated. A thorough historical evaluation for gastrointestinal disease should be performed. Examination of the gastrointestinal tract should be undertaken in conjunction with a gastroenterologist only in selected cases. Radiographic procedures may include an upper gastrointestinal series and a barium enema. Flexible sigmoidoscopy or colonoscopy, or both, may also be performed, with appropriate biopsies taken. A complete blood count, careful evaluation of the peripheral smear, and possibly a bone marrow aspirate or biopsy will help to rule out the presence of an associated malignant hematologic process. Serum protein electrophoresis, serum immunodiffusion studies, and, possibly, serum and urine immunoelectrophoresis will help to eliminate a diagnosis of an associated monoclonal gammopathy or myeloma.

There is not a specific, uniformly effective treatment for PG. Although systemic treatment may affect the underlying disease process in some patients with ulcerative colitis (75), it sometimes becomes necessary to address the advisability of colectomy. Some patients' skin lesions will respond to bowel resection, but there are patients in whom total colectomy, including removal of the rectosigmoid colon, does not lead to a remission (70). In one report, a patient developed PG 10 years after total colectomy (76). Additionally, there are patients without large bowels who develop peristomal PG.

In mild cases, local measures such as dressings, elevation, rest, topical agents, or intralesional injections may be sufficient to control the disease process. Compresses, wet-to-dry dressings, or the newer biooclusive semipermeable dressings may be useful. Cleansing or therapy with antibacterial agents such as hydrogen peroxide or benzoyl peroxide has been reported to be beneficial in a few patients. Hyperbaric oxygen has also been reported to be effective in a limited number of cases. Superpotent topical corticosteroids or topical tacrolimus might be beneficial, particularly in those patients with peristomal PG (53). Intralesional injections of corticosteroids may be beneficial in some patients, but care must be taken to avoid introducing an infection, to limit the potential systemic effects of corticosteroids that arise from injecting large doses, and to avoid spread of the lesion due to pathergy (77). In general, the periphery of the lesion is injected, but the ulcer base may also be injected. Two of my patients have responded to intralesional therapy. Other topical approaches are the use of sodium cromoglycate, topical 5-aminosalicylic acid, and topical nitrogen mustard (78,79).

In patients who do not respond to topical or local therapies, or whose severe rapid course warrants the use of a systemic agent, sulfonamides, sulfones, or corticosteroids have been the most commonly used agents. Perry (66) has reported that oral sulfasalazine is effective in patients with inflammatory bowel disease and in those without accompanying bowel disease.

Dapsone in doses of up to 400 mg per day has often been used as a monotherapy or as an adjunctive steroid-sparing agent. Usually the drug is administered in lower doses (100 to 150 mg per day), and the usual precautions and pretherapy evaluation are necessary. The mechanism of action of the sulfas and sulfones in this process is not understood, but effects on the polymorphonuclear leukocytes may be a factor. Another antileprosy agent, clofazimine, has also been reported to be successful in some patients with PG. Finally, several other antibiotics have been used successfully in individual cases, including minocycline and rifampin. Other nonsteroidal nonimmunosuppressive therapies reported to be effective include potassium iodide and splenectomy (80,81).

Systemic corticosteroids have been used extensively in patients with PG and its variants and are generally believed to be very effective. Usually, large doses (40 to 120 mg per day) are necessary to induce a remission of the disease. These doses, used over the long term, will frequently result in steroid-related side effects. In the studies by Holt et al. (82), six of 12 patients treated with corticosteroids developed serious steroid complications, and four of these six patients died as a result of the therapy. To avoid the complications of long-term steroid use, Johnson and Lazarus (83), and subsequently others, have used pulse therapy with 1 g of methylprednisolone administered intravenously each day for a period of 5 days. Maintenance of the remission was accomplished with oral corticosteroids every other day. Prystowsky et al. (68) have reported the same experience as Johnson and Lazarus, with an additional eight patients. They found that remissions occurred in five of the patients, and that they were usually able to discontinue oral corticosteroid therapy and often lower the dose of other therapies. Pulse therapy is not without side effects, which can include sudden death. In the hands of Prystowsky et al., and my experience with three patients, this therapy has primarily resulted in transient hyperglycemia; however, this therapy should only be used with great caution and proper monitoring.

Cytotoxic/immunosuppressive agents have been suggested for use in patients who fail to respond to other therapies, particularly systemic corticosteroids, or who develop steroid-related side effects. Individual reports using azathioprine, oral and intravenous cyclophosphamide (84), chlorambucil (45), or A1 cyclosporine, tacrolimus, or high-dose immunoglobulin have suggested that at least in some patients, these agents may be used successfully (45,84–88). Multiple reports have documented the usefulness of cyclosporine for PG. Regardless of the clinical features or associated phenomena, most patients have responded to cyclosporine 5 mg/kg daily. The usual response time varies between 5 and 24 months. The mode of action of the immunosuppressive agents is not understood, but they may alter the immunologic aberrations that may be present in the patient with PG. Recently thalidomide has been reported to be useful for pyoderma gangrenosum (89,90).

With the introduction of biologic agents for inflammatory bowel disease and arthritis, there are now reports of the effectiveness of the anti–tumor necrosis factor-α (TNF-α) monoclonal antibody (infliximab) for patients with PG (91). Lastly, although generally surgery is contraindicated, some patients have been successfully grafted with bioengineered skin when pretreated with an immunosuppressive agent (92).

RHEUMATOID NEUTROPHILIC DERMATITIS

Ackerman (93) described a neutrophilic dermatosis in patients with rheumatoid arthritis. Scherbenske et al. (94) reported a patient with severe seropositive rheumatoid arthritis and fixed urticarial plaques on the trunk, shoulders, and posterior neck. Histopathologic examination revealed a dense neutrophilic infiltrate without vasculitis or leukocytoclasia. Sanchez and Cruz (95) reported three cases of what they considered to be rheumatoid neutrophilic dermatitis (RND); however, although there was no vasculitis, leukocytoclasis was present on biopsy specimen. Lowe et al. (96) have reported an additional three patients. The lesions of RND tend to be symmetric erythematous papules and plaques usually on the elbows, dorsal surface of the hands, or extensor surface of the forearms (Fig. 11.11).

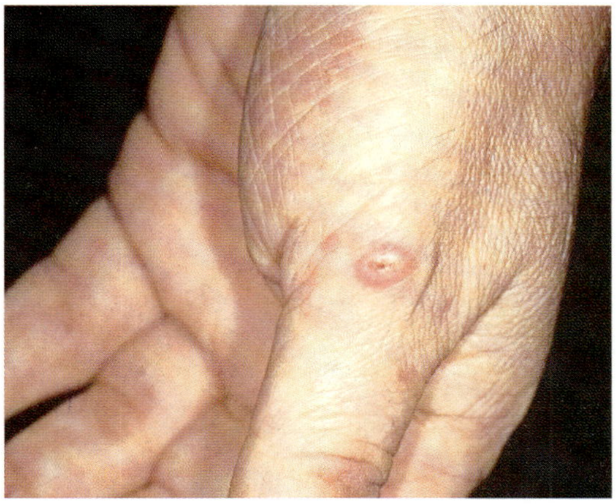

Figure 11.11. Rheumatoid neutrophilic dermatosis.

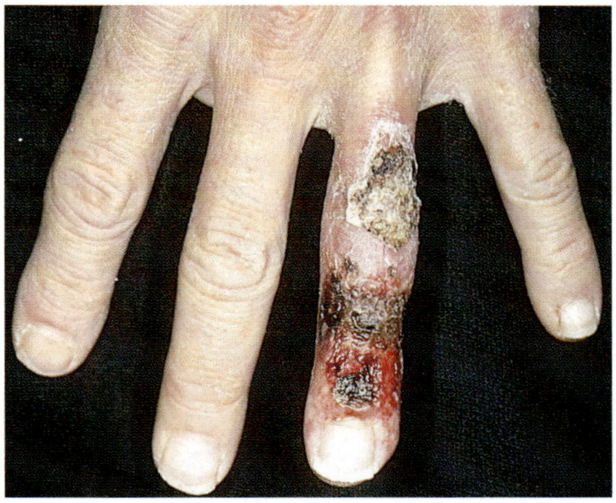

Figure 11.12. Bowel bypass syndrome secondary to Roux-en-Y anastomosis.

Most patients have seropositive rheumatoid arthritis, but recent reports by Gay-Crosier et al. (97) and Brown et al. (98) suggest that the process may occur in seronegative patients. It is not clear whether this condition is clinically or histopathologically distinct, specifically, whether it can be differentiated from Sweet syndrome. Therapies that may be effective include corticosteroids, dapsone, or colchicine; additionally, spontaneous resolution can occur.

BOWEL-ASSOCIATED DERMATOSIS–ARTHRITIS SYNDROME

Patients who had undergone bowel bypass surgery for morbid obesity were noted on occasion to develop scattered pustular lesions with arthritis. This became known as the bowel bypass syndrome, and was believed to represent an immune complex disease caused by bacterial overgrowth in the blind loop. Treatment with antibiotics was often effective in clearing the cutaneous lesions and improving the joint symptoms. Later, Jorizzo et al. (99) coined the term "bowel bypass syndrome without bowel bypass or bowel-associated dermatosis–arthritis syndrome." They reported four patients with this syndrome of whom two had blind loops due to Billroth II procedures, one had ulcerative colitis, and one had Crohn disease. Dicken (100) reported two similar patients who had had Roux-en-Y procedures with resultant blind loops. Clinically, these patients presented with a widespread eruption characterized by pustules on an erythematous or necrotic base (Fig. 11.12). The lesions may be few, or they may be extensive. Ulceration seems to occur rarely. The appearance of the lesions is often accompanied by fever, arthralgias or a true inflammatory arthropathy, and myalgias. The arthritis that accompanies this process is generally symmetric, nondeforming, and most frequently involves the small joints such as the wrists, metacarpophalangeal joints, proximal interphalangeal joints, ankles, and metatarsophalangeal joints. Histopathologically the disease resembles Sweet syndrome. In fact, only after the report by Jorizzo et al. (99) did we recognize that a patient reported by our group (101) probably would have been more correctly diagnosed as having the bowel-associated dermatosis-arthritis syndrome rather than Sweet syndrome, because of his prior Billroth II procedure. This disease is presumed to be due to immune complexes (102), and although antiinflammatory therapy is at times helpful, antibiotics, in particular oral metronidazole, frequently control the process or bowel surgery to remove "blind" loops will reverse the process.

NEUTROPHILIC ECCRINE HIDRADENITIS

Neutrophilic eccrine hidradenitis is a recently described entity that is characterized by erythematosus papules, plaques, or nodules, most often on acral skin (103). Several additional presentations are possible including periorbital inflammation, pustular lesions, and disseminated disease. The histopathology of this entity is characterized by neutrophilic infiltration surrounding the eccrine glands. The process is primarily linked to acute myelogenous leukemia and usually occurs during chemotherapy. Some cases have been reported in which this condition heralded the onset of the leukemia. Recently a patient with Behçet disease has been reported to have neutrophilic eccrine hidradenitis (104). The process is self-limiting and usually does not require specific therapy.

PANNICULITIS

Panniculitis refers to inflammation within the subcutaneous fat. Panniculitis is most likely a dynamic process that progresses through inflammation with neutrophils to lymphocytes to histiocytes and ends with fibrosis (105,106). It can become granulomatous in the histiocytic phase. The exact nature of the infiltrate perhaps depends on the timing of the biopsy in relation to the age of the lesion. Panniculitis has been broken down into four categories on the basis of histopathologic criteria: (a) septal panniculitis, (b) lobular panniculitis, (c) mixed with septal and lobular components, or (d) vasculitic panniculitis. Unfortunately, in practice, there is often not such a clear-cut histopathologic picture and the clinical–pathologic correlation becomes important to best classify and treat these patients (107–110). Table 11.5 presents one of the currently accepted classification schemas for the types of panniculitis. Frequently, panniculitis is associated with systemic disease. Often the separation of one syndrome from another is made only over a period of observation.

Panniculitis can affect all ages, including children. The peak age for EN is varied, but Weber–Christian disease and lupus erythematosus panniculitis tend to occur in young adults. Most types of panniculitis are more prevalent in women, but the reasons for this sex distribution are unclear. These entities are rare

TABLE 11.5. Classification of the Panniculitides

I. Septal panniculitis
  A. Erythema nodosum
  B. Vilanova disease (subacute nodular migratory panniculitis)
II. Lobular panniculitis
  A. Weber–Christian disease (relapsing febrile nodular nonsuppurative panniculitis)
  B. Rothman–Makai syndrome (lipogranulomatosis subcutanea)
  C. Subcutaneous fat necrosis of the newborn
  D. Poststeroid panniculitis
  E. Enzymatic panniculitis
    1. Pancreatic
    2. α_1-Antitrypsin deficiency
  F. Physical or factitial panniculitis
  G. Histiocytic cytophagic panniculitis (subcutaneous T-cell lymphoma)
  H. Lipodystrophy syndromes
  I. Connective tissue panniculitis (scleroderma or myositis)
  J. Lipodermatosclerosis or sclerosing panniculitis (probably a manifestation of venous stasis)
  K. Calcifying panniculitis associated with renal failure (often hemodialysis), also known as calciphylaxis
III. Mixed panniculitis
  A. Lupus profundus (lupus erythematosus panniculitis)
IV. Panniculitis with vasculitis
  A. Small-vessel vasculitis (postcapillary venule), leukocytoclastic vasculitis
  B. Medium-sized vessel vasculitis (arterioles or small arteries)
    1. Polyarteritis nodosa
    2. Erythema induratum

and thus no racial or genetic associations have been clearly identified (Table 11.6).

The prototypic *septal panniculitis* is EN. A relatively common process, EN is usually acute and self-limited (111). The typical clinical presentation is the sudden onset of one or more tender, erythematous nodules on the anterior tibial surface (Fig. 11.13). The lesions are deep nodules, which are more easily palpated than visualized. As the lesions age they may soften and develop an ecchymotic appearance. Over a 4- to 6-week period, the lesions heal without scar formation. Ulceration of the primary process is extremely rare. Whereas other symptoms may be present, they are usually those of an associated condition.

Although EN is usually an acute process, patients with chronic processes have been described. Terms such as "chronic erythema," " erythema nodosum migrans," "subacute nodular migratory panniculitis" (Villanova disease), or "septal granulomatous panniculitis" have been used to characterize these patients. The patient with EN migrans tends to be a middle-aged woman (mean age, 45 to 50 years). The disease is often present for several years and is most common on the legs. As with EN, accompanying symptoms may be present, but are usually those of an associated condition.

Etiologic or associated conditions are present in about 50% of patients with either acute or chronic variants of EN (112). The associated conditions can be broken into three broad categories: infections, drugs, or systemic diseases (usually inflammatory disorders). A partial list of the known associations is found in Table 11.7. The infectious agents associated with EN tend to primarily affect the respiratory or gastrointestinal tract and are most often bacterial or fungal in origin. The most common drugs are antibiotics or birth control pills. Pregnancy, particularly in its second trimester, is a known association, and the EN will recur with subsequent pregnancies or with the administration of oral contraceptives. A specific variant of sarcoidosis associated with EN is known as Löfgren syndrome (113). This is an acute, most often self-resolving, variant of sarcoidosis, in which EN occurs with asymptomatic bilateral hilar lymphadenopathy, arthritis, and/or anterior uveitis. Granulomatous colitis (Crohn disease), regional enteritis, and ulcerative colitis have been associated with EN. In patients with inflammatory bowel disease, it appears that the EN parallels the activity of the bowel disease. Panniculitis can occur with the collagen-vascular disease, but it may not be best to classify the process as EN (see later). At least half of the cases of EN do not have an associated or underlying process.

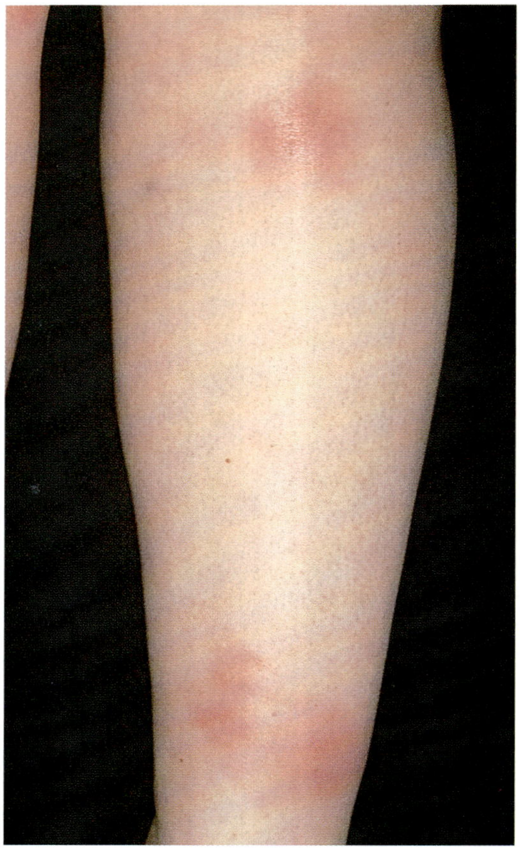

Figure 11.13. Erythema nodosum. Tender, red nodules on the anterior tibial surface.

TABLE 11.6. Epidemiology of the Major Panniculitides

	EN	WCD	LEP
Peak age, y	None	37	27
Sex distribution (M:F)	1:9	3:7	1:9
Prevalence (per 100,000)	<1	<1	<1
Annual incidence (per 100,000)	<1	<1	<1
Racial predilection	None	None	Unknown
Genetic associations	Unknown	Unknown	Unknown

EN, erythema nodosum; F, female; LEP, lupus erythematosus panniculitis; M, male; WCD, Weber–Christian disease.

TABLE 11.7. Some Etiologic Factors or Associations with Erythema Nodosum

Infections
- Streptococcal pharyngitis
- Tuberculosis
- Valley fever (coccidioidomycosis)
- Blastomycosis
- Histoplasmosis
- Psittacosis
- *Yersinia* colitis
- *Salmonella* gastroenteritis
- Cat scratch fever
- Leprosy
- Lyme disease

Drugs
- Antibiotics: penicillins, sulfonamides
- Birth control pills

Systemic diseases
- Pregnancy
- Sarcoidosis
- Inflammatory bowel disease
- Collagen-vascular disorders: dermatomyositis, lupus erythematosus, scleroderma
- Malignancy (rare)
- Sweet syndrome

Idiopathic

Types of Panniculitis

WEBER–CHRISTIAN DISEASE

Weber–Christian disease (WCD) is characterized by multiple recurrent subcutaneous nodules with accompanying fever (Fig. 11.14) (114). On biopsy, the change is characterized by a lobular panniculitis with an early neutrophilic infiltrate with fat degeneration, foamy histiocytes, and giant cell formation. Eventually fibrosis occurs, and this plus the destruction of fat results in the clinical finding of an atrophic scar. Some of the patients with WCD have had multiple surgical procedures due to the presence of an acute inflammatory lesion with fever. Other clinical features that commonly occur are arthralgias and myalgias. Some patients also have recurrent abdominal pain. In addition to the skin lesions, any area of the body containing fat can be affected by WCD. Several cases of mesenteric panniculitis have been reported, but involvement of the heart (115), lungs, liver, and/or kidneys has also been noted. The disease is chronic but can result in death in 10% to 15% of cases.

The laboratory abnormalities associated with WCD include an elevated sedimentation rate, anemia, leukopenia or leukocytosis, depression of complement components, and evidence of circulating immune complexes. In addition, there have been several reports of α_1-antitrypsin deficiency in patients with WCD; however, the meaning of this finding is not clear. Patients have been misclassified as having WCD who actually have LE or pancreatic disease. In these patients, accompanying laboratory abnormalities would be those associated with the underlying process.

PANNICULITIS WITH α_1-ANTITRYPSIN DEFICIENCY

Several groups of patients with a lobular or septal panniculitis have been found to have a deficiency of α_1-antitrypsin. In a study of 96 patients with panniculitis, Smith et al. (116) found 15 patients with α_1-antitrypsin deficiency. There were differences in the clinical and histopathologic manifestations, but very little difference was noted regarding the associated conditions present in either group. Specifically, the group with α_1-antitrypsin deficiency was more likely to have ulceration and drainage, and correspondingly had greater amounts of fat necrosis and elastic tissue destruction. Furthermore, Smith et al. believed that induction of lesions by trauma was more likely in the antitrypsin-deficient group. Recognition of these patients may be important on several grounds. First, débridement of the lesion should be avoided. Second, in patients believed to have factitial panniculitis, α_1-antitrypsin deficiency should be considered. Third, these patients should be evaluated for pulmonary disease and should be counseled to avoid smoking. Fourth, therapy with α_1-proteinase inhibitor concentrate may be helpful and, recently, liver transplantation, which replaces the missing enzyme, have been reported to give a long-term remission (117). Several reports have documented the effectiveness of doxycycline and postulated that its effects were mediated through its anticollagenase properties (118,119).

PANCREATIC PANNICULITIS

Some patients with pancreatic diseases develop subcutaneous fat necrosis (lobular panniculitis) (Fig. 11.15) with accompanying polyarthritis and osseous intramedullary fat necrosis. Many pancreatic pathologic changes have been implicated in the development of this process, including pancreatitis, pancreatic carcinoma (acinar cell), pancreatitis secondary to cholelithiasis, posttraumatic lesions, pancreatic ischemia, pancreatic pseudocyst, and pancreatic diffusum (a congenital pancreatic abnormality) (120). In at least one recently reported patient, the onset of polyarthritis and panniculitis led to the discovery of chronic pancreatitis (121). It is not clear whether the elevated lipase in the circulation is primarily involved in the pathogenesis of the fat necrosis, or whether its presence follows the fat necrosis. Histopathologically,

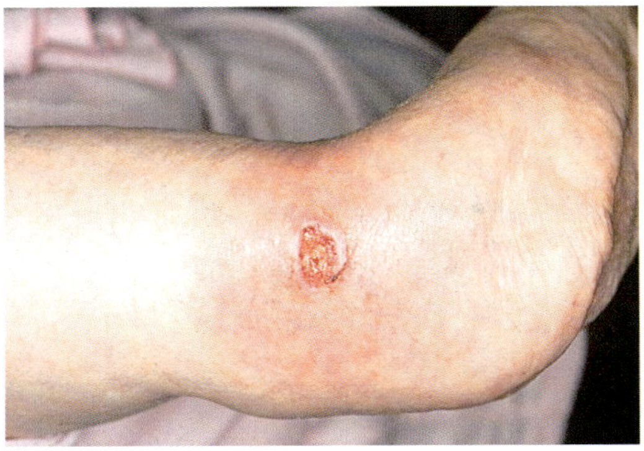

Figure 11.14. Weber–Christian disease. Tender, deep erythematous nodule.

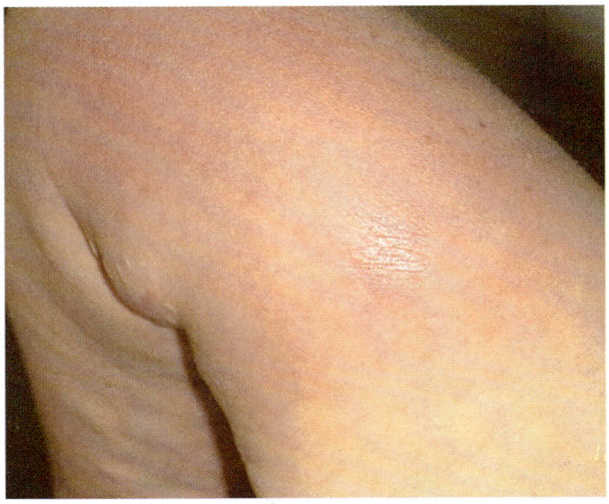

Figure 11.15. Pancreatic panniculitis.

there is extensive fat necrosis with a basophilic alteration of lipocytes. Ghost cells with absent nuclei are also common.

POSTSTEROID PANNICULITIS

Panniculitis following withdrawal of corticosteroid therapy is a rare entity that seems to be limited to children (122). Patients have been treated with corticosteroids for a wide array of conditions including leukemia, nephrotic syndrome, rheumatic carditis, and encephalopathy. Interestingly, the panniculitis may clear with readministration of the corticosteroids. The pathogenesis of this rare complication is not understood.

LIPOATROPHIC PANNICULITIS

Several conditions that often result in lipoatrophy following the inflammatory reaction have been described in children. There exists a spectrum, which may include Rothman–Makai syndrome (lipogranulomatosis subcutanea), lipoatrophic panniculitis, lipophagic panniculitis of childhood, and localized lipoatrophy (atrophic connective tissue disease panniculitis) (123). These children tend to have multiple erythematous lesions, most commonly on the extremities, which resolve with subcutaneous atrophy (Fig. 11.16). The patients often manifest fever. They may have associated "autoimmune" phenomena such as juvenile rheumatoid arthritis, Hashimoto thyroiditis, or diabetes mellitus. There is no known effective therapy, but some patients have responded to oral administration of corticosteroids, antimalarial drugs, or dapsone.

CYTOPHAGIC HISTIOCYTIC PANNICULITIS

Cytophagic histiocytic panniculitis was described by Crotty and Winkelmann (124) as a chronic histiocytic disease of the subcutaneous fat, with accompanying inflammatory panniculitis, fever, serositis, and "reticuloendotheliomegaly." This is an extremely rare entity, reported in only a limited number of patients. Patients frequently have fever, hepatosplenomegaly, pancytopenia, and serositis. Two distinct entities have been suggested to be present under this term: a primary panniculitis for which the cause is unknown, or an infiltrative T-cell lymphoma known as subcutaneous T-cell lymphoma (125). Hemorrhagic complications, perhaps due to thrombocytopenia, have occurred in 50% of patients. I have recently treated a patient who was initially diagnosed as lupus panniculitis that evolved into subcutaneous T-cell lymphoma (126). This entity is often difficult to diagnose at its onset. Alegre and Winkelmann (127), and subsequently Pettersson et al. (128), have suggested using aggressive therapy with cytotoxic agents early in this process.

FACTITIAL PANNICULITIS

Factitial panniculitis from external trauma of the injection of foreign substances is not uncommon, and should be considered in any patient with panniculitis and unusual clinical (Fig. 11.17) or histopathologic features. In traumatic lesions, there is often an

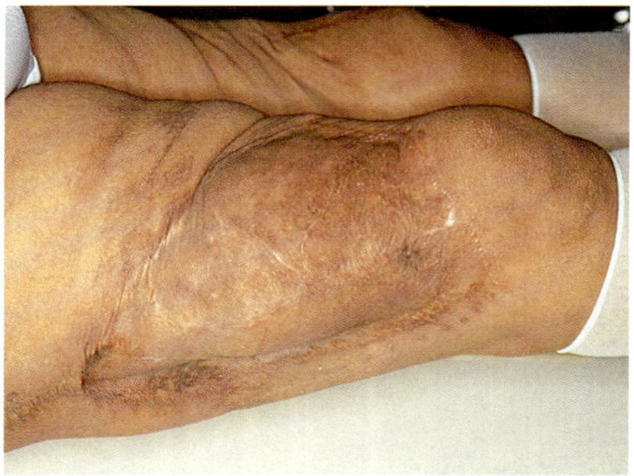

Figure 11.17. Factitial panniculitis. Multiple scars are present in this patient who was injecting a foreign substance into her subcutaneous tissue.

organizing hematoma demonstrated histologically; whereas with injections, one encounters refractile bodies or a "Swiss cheese" effect. Occasionally, spectroscopic and/or chromatographic techniques are necessary to identify the causative injected material.

LUPUS ERYTHEMATOSUS PANNICULITIS (LUPUS PROFUNDUS)

Lupus erythematosus panniculitis (LEP) is a rare manifestation of LE, occurring in less than 3% of cases of systemic lupus erythematosus (SLE) and in less than 1% of cases with cutaneous LE (129,130). The lesions are tender, red–blue subcutaneous nodules, which may eventually ulcerate (Fig. 11.18). They tend to occur on the face, upper arms, and/or buttocks. The lesions may underlie a typical lesion of discoid LE. Histopathologic changes include a panniculitis, which is both lobular and septal. Only when the overlying epidermis and dermis demonstrate changes of LE can the diagnosis of LEP be histologically confirmed. Twice as many patients with LEP do not have systemic

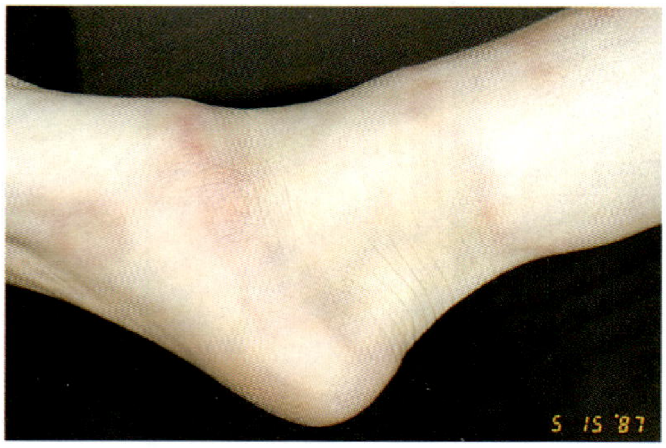

Figure 11.16. Lipoatrophic panniculitis in childhood.

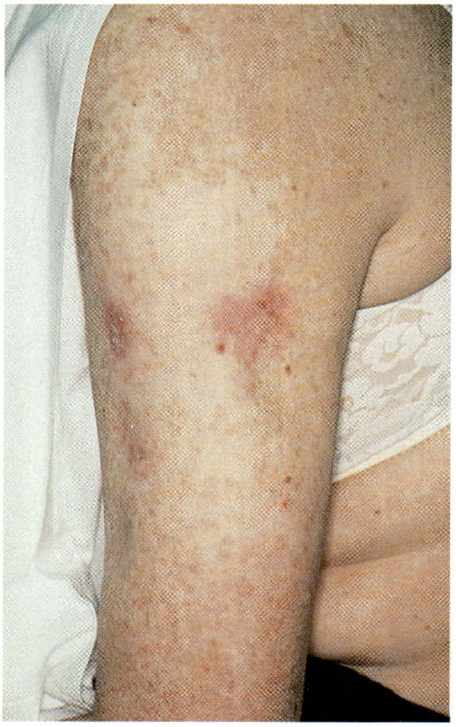

Figure 11.18. Lupus erythematosus panniculitis.

disease as have systemic disease. It has been postulated that renal disease in the patient with LEP is rarely present, and when present, it is among the more benign forms. Patients with LEP generally respond well to antimalarial therapy (131).

COLD PANNICULITIS

Cold panniculitis appears to be a condition of early childhood (132), mostly occurring in infants under the age of 9 months. This condition is rare and is induced by exposure to cold air or after contact with cold objects including ice cubes, ice bags, or popsicles. There is no underlying disorder such as cryoglobulinemia, cold agglutinins, or other laboratory abnormality. The process occurs in otherwise healthy infants who remain healthy following resolution of the process. The disease almost always occurs on the cheek(s) (Fig. 11.19). Histopathologic examination reveals necrosis, fibrosis, and inflammation of the adipose tissue. Resolution is usually rapid and occurs without sequelae.

SCLEROSING PANNICULITIS (LIPODERMATOSCLEROSIS OR HYPODERMITIS SCLERODERMAFORMIS)

Sclerosing panniculitis, a recently described entity, is a condition found on the lower legs that is characterized by erythema, telangiectasia, edema, hyperpigmentation, and woody induration (133). Ulceration may also occur in some patients. The process is usually seen in women over age 40. It is chronic and poorly responsive to therapy. While there is evidence of inflammation in the panniculus and dermal sclerosis, there has been a suggestion that venous stasis and previous thrombophlebitis play a role in pathogenesis. I believe that this process is common and represents an unusual stage of venous insufficiency. Response to therapy is poor with the exception of gradient support stockings (30 to 40 mm Hg gradient) (134).

CALCIFYING PANNICULITIS

Calcifying panniculitis is a rare condition that generally occurs in patients with end-stage renal disease who develop calciphylaxis (135). Calciphylaxis is the acute calcification of soft tissue. The patient usually has abnormally high calcium–phosphorus product and secondary hyperparathyroidism. After a "precipitating" event occurs, such as trauma or injection of various medications, patients develop tender, indurated plaques or nodules (Fig. 11.20). Progression to necrosis or ulceration is relatively common. Histopathologic examination reveals a lobular panniculitis, fat necrosis, and calcification of the vessel walls. Treatment of the metabolic disorder combined with local care seems most appropriate (136). A role for antiinflammatory drug therapy has not been established.

Recent studies suggest that vascular mural calcification is an early and essential process in the development of a calciphylaxis plaque. Furthermore, protein C and/or protein S deficiency may play an etiologic role (reviewed in Au and Crawford [136a]).

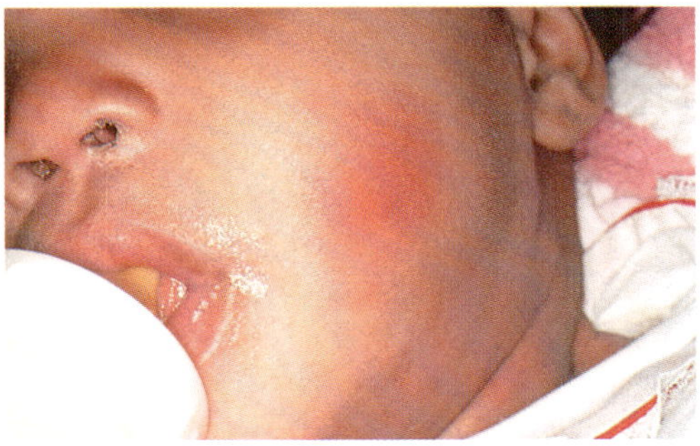

Figure 11.19. Cold panniculitis.

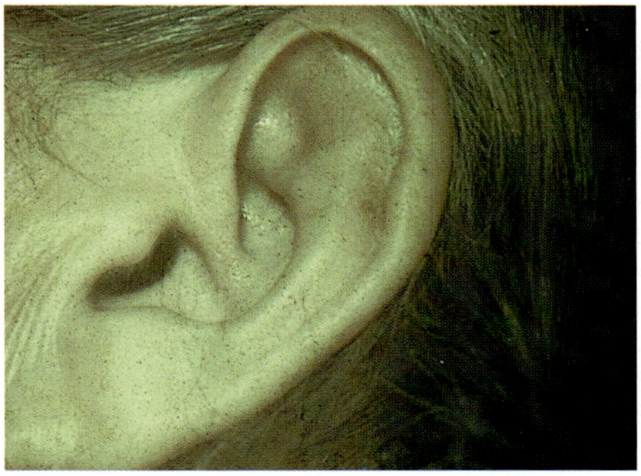

Figure 11.20. Calciphylaxis (calcifying panniculitis).

PANNICULITIS WITH VASCULITIS

Nodular vasculitis, polyarteritis nodosa (both cutaneous and systemic varieties), and small-vessel vasculitis may involve subcutaneous vessels and result in inflammatory or ischemic changes in the subcutaneous fat. Erythema induratum is a form of nodular vasculitis caused by tuberculosis.

Evaluation of the Patient with Panniculitis

The evaluation of the patient with panniculitis should include a careful history and physical examination. The possibility of infection of the upper respiratory tract should be considered, and a throat swab for a rapid strep screen, a purified protein derivative test, and a radiograph of the chest should be performed. In general, neither inflammatory bowel disease nor infectious enteritis is asymptomatic and thus it is not necessary to perform endoscopic or radiographic procedures in these patients. Tests for enzymatic abnormalities such as amylase, lipase, or α_1-antitrypsin deficiency should be ordered. The possibility of a coexistent collagen-vascular disease should be considered.

The differential diagnosis of EN involves distinguishing it from (a) other forms of panniculitis (all of which may present with tender subcutaneous nodules), (b) insect bites, (c) thrombophlebitis, or (d) cellulitis. Insect bites may be tender, red, infiltrated lesions. The distribution is dependent on the type of bite, and in general, if the patient lacks associated symptomatology. Often there is a puncture site within the lesion. Cellulitis rarely manifests as subcutaneous nodules. The lesion of cellulitis may be tender and erythematous, but often there is an accompanying fever and a lymphangitic streak ascending from the primary area of involvement. When the diagnosis is in question, a wedge biopsy or deep punch biopsy that includes subcutaneous fat will be helpful.

The differential diagnosis of WCD includes other types of lobular panniculitis, EN, and LEP (lupus profundus). EN can be separated on clinical and histopathologic grounds. Lupus profundus occurs in conjunction with typical LE skin lesions or in patients with SLE. This latter group may be difficult to distinguish from those with WCD, particularly in view of the reports of WCD in some patients with SLE. Perhaps the diagnosis of WCD should be made only in the absence of associated disorders such as LE, scleroderma, dermatomyositis, malignancy, pancreatic disease, sarcoidosis, or factitial panniculitis.

Treatment of the Patient with Panniculitis

The treatment of EN and other types of panniculitis first involves assessment of a causative disease and its treatment. In the absence of a treatable disorder, therapy is symptomatic. Acute EN is often self-limited; thus, nontoxic therapies are advised. Bed rest and leg elevation are very useful in controlling symptoms. In patients who need to continue to be ambulatory, support stockings or tights may be helpful. Aspirin or other nonsteroidal anti-inflammatory drugs (NSAIDs) may provide relief. My experience with aspirin has not produced results before toxicity and therefore my choice is to use oral indomethacin in a dose of 25 to 75 mg per day.

In patients with chronic EN or frequent recurrences, oral potassium iodide (saturated solution of potassium iodide or tablets) 300 to 900 mg per day has been useful in open clinical trials. In my experience, treatment with oral potassium iodide for 10 of my patients with EN yielded control of the disease in eight patients (J.P.C., unpublished observation). In some of the patients who responded, the disease relapsed when the drug was stopped or the dosage was lowered, but the patients responded again with reinstitution of therapy. Other therapy that may be considered includes oral corticosteroids, colchicine, or an immunosuppressive agent. Systemic corticosteroids, which are usually effective, are often complicated by iatrogenic Cushing syndrome, a common adverse reaction. Colchicine has not been effective in any of the patients that I have treated. Azathioprine and cyclosporine have been used successfully in some patients. One adjunctive therapy that can be helpful is intralesionally injected triamcinolone acetonide (3 to 5 mg/mL).

There is no specific therapy for WCD. Reports have centered on the use of antiinflammatory agents including aspirin, NSAIDs, oral corticosteroids, antimalarials, and immunosuppressives including cyclophosphamide and cyclosporine. In addition, colchicine, dapsone, and potassium iodide may be effective in some cases.

Patients with LEP may respond to antimalarials. Corticosteroids and/or immunosuppressives are rarely necessary for LEP.

Panniculitis forms a wide array of syndromes, which perhaps can be separated on the basis of clinical features, associated disorders, and/or histopathologic features. Unfortunately, several of the syndromes seem to have overlapping features, the pathogenesis is not understood for most, and the therapeutic options are similar for all the syndromes. The differential diagnosis often depends on an adequate specimen for histopathologic investigation. Thus, a fusiform incisional biopsy or a wedge biopsy should be performed. Furthermore, the youngest lesion should be biopsied. Sections should be serially cut to identify the pattern of the panniculitis: lobular, septal, vasculitic, or mixed. Evaluation for underlying process should be performed and includes ingestants, infections, malignancy, and autoimmune disorders. Treatment, in the absence of an underlying disease, is aimed at control of the inflammatory reaction with agents such as NSAIDs, corticosteroids, dapsone, potassium iodide, antimalarials, colchicine, or cytotoxic/immunosuppressive agents.

BEHÇET DISEASE

Behçet disease is a multisystem disorder described by the Turkish dermatologist, Hulusi Behçet in the 1930s. There are no pathognomonic clinical or laboratory findings, and thus the diagnosis is based upon fulfillment of a set of clinical criteria (Table 11.8) (137). Other causes of disease such as inflammatory bowel disease, which can be associated with aphthae, EN, and pathergy, must be ruled out.

The pathogenesis of Behçet disease is unknown. The disease may be more common in patients with HLA-B5 and HLA-Bw51 or HLA-DRw52 genes (138). This genetic predisposition may predispose the patient to an abnormal immunologic response to infections (viral or other). However, no consistent abnormalities of humoral or cellular immunity have been observed.

TABLE 11.8. Diagnostic Criteria for Behçet DIisease

Criteria	Comment
Recurrent oral aphthous ulcers	At least three episodes per year
Plus two of the following:	
1. Recurrent genital ulceration	
2. Ocular lesions	Uveitis, retinal vasculitis
3. Skin lesions	Erythema nodosum–like lesions, papulopustular lesions, "acneiform" lesions
4. Pathergy	Test or observation

The diagnosis of Behçet disease requires oral aphthae plus at least two other criteria. Other causes of disease must be ruled out.
From Ter Poorten MC, Thiers BH. Panniculitis [review]. *Dermatol Clin* 2002;20: 421–433, with permission.

The earliest mucocutaneous lesions in Behçet disease represent a neutrophilic vascular reaction or fully developed leukocytoclastic vasculitis (LCV) (139). There is some support for a role for immune complex–mediated vessel damage in lesional pathogenesis. Studies of neutrophil function show that a heat-stable serum factor in patients with Behçet disease enhances the *in vitro* migration of neutrophils. In addition, there may be defective fibrinolysis. These two factors may explain the frequent vascular involvement observed in Behçet disease (140).

Behçet disease affects both sexes and is primarily a disease of young adults. Men may have more severe involvement than women. The disease occurs worldwide but is more prevalent in Asia and the Mediterranean countries.

The hallmark of Behçet disease is recurrent oral aphthous ulcerations. The oral aphthae are identical to those observed in patients with simple oral aphthosis, except that they occur in crops and more are frequently multiple. These lesions are the presenting manifestation in 25% to 75% of patients. The lesions occur most commonly on the lips, tongue, and buccal mucosa and occasionally on the gums, palate, and posterior pharynx. They are characterized by a yellow, necrotic base with a sharply demarcated, erythematous border (Fig. 11.21). Untreated, the lesions persist for 10 to 14 days, and resolution occurs without residua or scar formation. These lesions must be distinguished from simple aphthosis (major or minor variants), herpes simplex infection, primary syphilis, erythema multiforme, pemphigus vulgaris, and Reiter syndrome.

The genital ulcerations are similar to the oral lesions (Figs. 10.22 and 10.23). They are more often single lesions. Genital

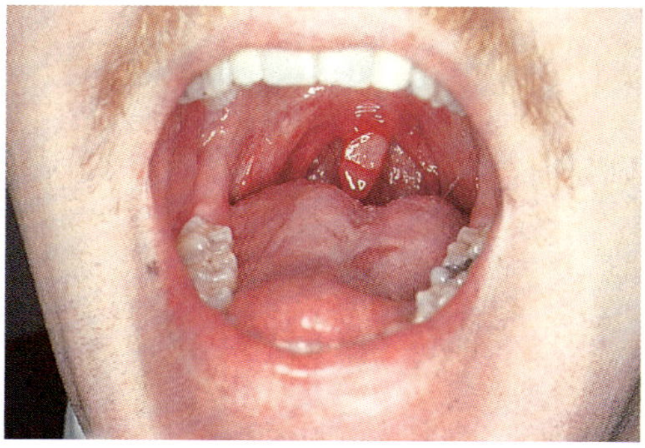

Figure 11.21. Aphthous ulceration on the uvula.

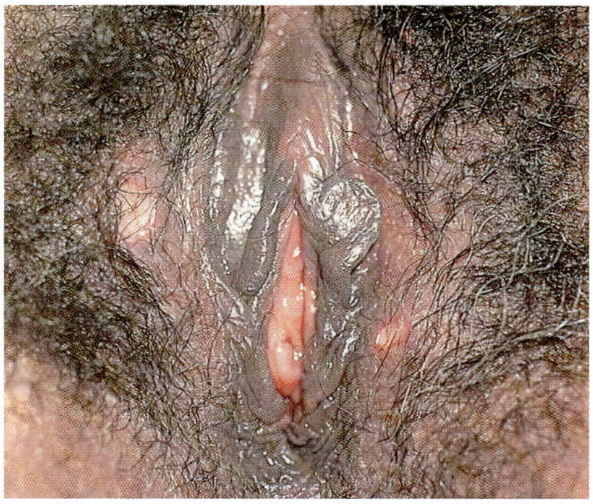

Figure 11.22. Vulvar ulceration in Behçet disease. (Courtesy of Kenneth Greer, M.D., University of Virginia, with permission.)

ulcers occur in 60% to 80% of patients with Behçet disease at some time in their course. The lesions may occur in the vulva, vagina, penis, scrotum, or perianal skin. These lesions must be differentiated from infections such as herpes simplex, syphilis, and chancroid. In addition, inflammatory bowel disease should be excluded.

Pathergy, the development of cutaneous papulopustular lesions 2 to 4 hours after cutaneous trauma (e.g., by a needle prick or intradermal injection), is a characteristic feature seen in many patients with Behçet disease (40% to 80%). Histopathologic examination of this lesion reveals the infiltration of polymorphonuclear leukocytes into the skin. Jorizzo et al. (141) have termed this phenomenon a "pustular vasculitis." Pathergy can also occur in patients with Sweet syndrome, pyoderma gangrenosum, and bowel-associated dermatosis–arthritis syndrome.

A variety of skin lesions occurs in Behçet disease, including papulopustular lesions (Fig. 11.24), acneiform "eruptions," and EN-like lesions (Fig. 11.25). The lesions observed are not those of folliculitis or acne vulgaris, but are rather a pustular vasculitis. The EN-like lesion is clinically indistinguishable from EN. Chun et al. (142) have studied the histopathology of these EN-like lesions and found a spectrum of change including both septal and lobular panniculitis.

Ocular disease occurs in 25% to 90% of patients with Behçet disease (143). The disease usually affects both eyes and can

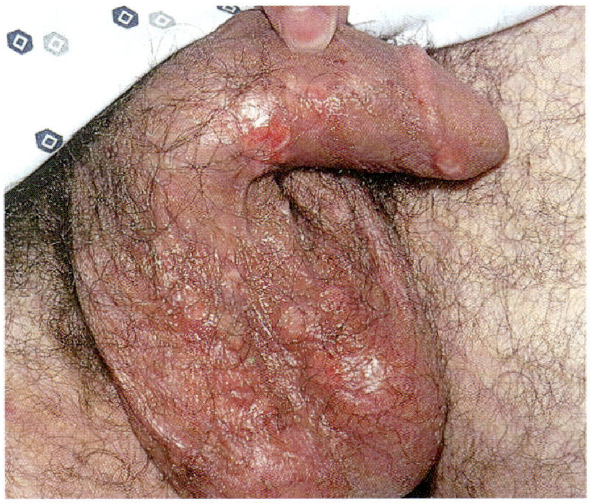

Figure 11.23. Multiple scrotal ulcers in Behçet disease. (Courtesy of Robert Soderstrom, M.D., Flint, Michigan, with permission.)

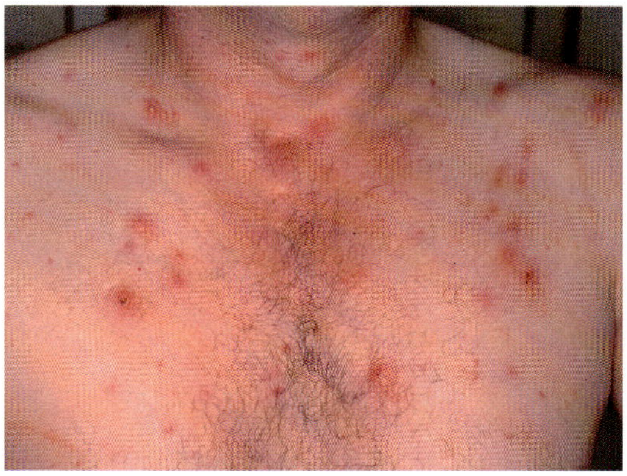

Figure 11.24. Multiple papulopustular lesions in Behçet disease.

result in visual loss (144). Both the anterior and posterior segments may be affected. Involvement includes anterior and/or posterior uveitis, iridocyclitis, retinal vasculitis, and hypopyon. The presence of ocular disease correlates closely with neurologic involvement.

Behçet disease is a multisystem disease. About 40% of patients will have a recurrent arthritis. In general, articular manifestations are nondeforming, seronegative and symmetrically involve a limited number of the larger joints such as the elbows, knees, ankles, and wrists. Neurologic involvement occurs in 10% to 30% of patients and is characterized by a variety of manifestations including meningoencephalitis, vasculitis with ischemic changes, psychiatric disorder, dementia, and peripheral or autonomic neuropathy. Behçet disease is characterized by vascular inflammation or occlusion. All sizes of vessels can be affected.

The course of Behçet disease is extremely variable. Many patients suffer frequent painful bouts of oral and genital aphthae and arthritis over a period of years. The progression of ocular disease (specifically posterior uveitis) to blindness is a major cause of morbidity. Death can occur from cerebrovascular involvement, bowel perforation, or large-vessel occlusion.

Before selecting a treatment, it is necessary to assess the extent of the disease. This often involves several subspecialists, including dermatologists, rheumatologists, ophthalmologists, neurologists, gastroenterologists, infectious disease specialists, and others. Selection of the appropriate therapy must be based on the organ systems involved and the severity of the involvement. Therapeutic agents routinely used in patients with Behçet disease along with their indications, dosage, and potential toxicity are presented in Table 11.9. A discussion of approaches to treatment by organ system follows.

It is possible to simplify the therapeutic approach to the patient with Behçet disease. For patients with non–life-threat-

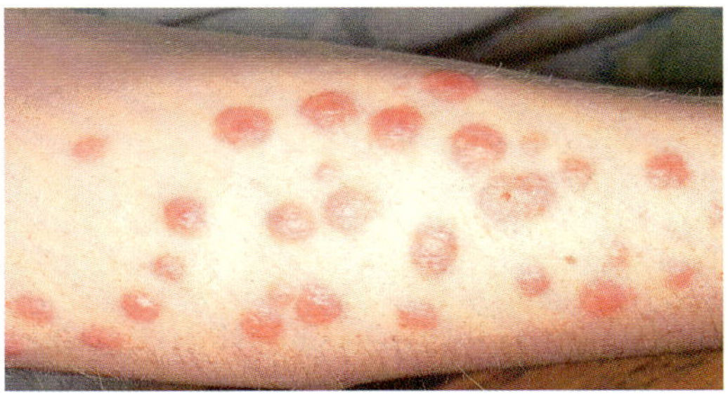

Figure 11.25. Multiple erythematous, tender nodules in a patient with Behçet disease.

Table 11.9 Therapeutic Options for Behçet's Disease

Drug	Indications	Dosage	Increased Risk Factors	Toxicity
Colchicine	Aphthae Cutaneous pustular vasculitis	0.6 mg b.i.d.–t.i.d.		Diarrhea, nausea, bone marrow suppression Teratogenicity
Dapsone	Aphthae Cutaneous pustular vasculitis	50–200 mg/day	G6PD deficiency	Hemolytic anemia Peripheral neuropathy Mononucleosis-like syndrome
Thalidomide	Mucocutaneous disease Arthritis Possibly uveitis	50–300 mg/day (given at bedtime)		Teratogenicity Peripheral neuropathy Somnolence
Sulfonamides	Aphthae Cutaneous pustular vasculitis	Varies by agent		Drug eruption
Prednisone	Severe mucocutaneous disease Severe arthritis Ocular involvement Central nervous system disease	0.5–1 mg/kg/day		Osteoporosis Cataract formation Hypertension Diabetes mellitus Iatrogenic Cushing's syndrome
Methotrexate	Severe mucocutaneous disease Severe arthritis	5–15 mg/week	Reduced renal function Alcoholism Concomitant use of trimethoprim	Hepatotoxicity Diarrhea, nausea Bone marrow suppression Pneumonitis Immunosuppression
Azathioprine	Posterior uveitis CNS involvement	1–2.5 mg/kg/day	Thiopurine methyltransferase deficiency	Bone marrow suppression Drug-induced fever Pancreatitis
Mycophenolate mofetil	Mucocutaneous disease	1–1.5 gm b.i.d.		Bone marrow suppression Diarrhea, nausea
Chlorambucil	Posterior uveitis CNS involvement Severe vascular involvement	Initial–2 mg/day, maximum varies depending on the need to control the disease		Bone marrow suppression Nausea, diarrhea Risk of malignancy—squamous cell carcinoma of the skin and lymphoma/leukemia Sterility (at times irreversible)
Cyclophosphamide	Posterior uveitis CNS involvement Severe vascular involvement	1–2 mg/kg/day (given early in the day with adequate hydration) Monthly IV pulses may be considered		Bone marrow suppression Nausea, diarrhea Risk of subsequent malignancy—lymphoma/leukemia Sterility (at times irreversible) Hemorrhagic cystitis
Cyclosporine	Posterior uveitis	5 mg/kg/day	Hypertension Reduced renal function Drugs that affect cytochrome P450	Nephrotoxicity Immunosuppression Possible subsequent neoplasia
Interferon–α2a	Mucocutaneous disease	3–12 million units, 3 times/week (subcutaneous administration)		Fever Flu-like symptoms
Infliximab	Mucocutaneous disease	5 mg/kg/intravenous infusion, given at 2–4 week intervals		Autoantibody induction Collagen vascular disease Demyelinating neurologic disease

ening disease, the therapy involves topical agents, NSAIDs, antihistamines, dapsone, colchicine, possibly TNF-α antagonists, and occasionally low-dose weekly methotrexate or low doses of oral prednisone. In patients with ocular disease that can lead to blindness, central nervous system disease, or involvement of large vessels, high doses of prednisone with or without an immunosuppressive agent can control the disease. Newer agents such as recombinant interferon-α-2A (IFN-α-2A), interleukin-2 receptor antagonist, or interleukin-10 may be effective and less toxic than agents such as chlorambucil, cyclosporin, tacrolimus, or cyclophosphamide. Unfortunately, data on cytokine therapy have not yet demonstrated its effectiveness or safety.

Mucocutaneous Disease

The therapy of oral and genital aphthae as well as cutaneous pustular lesions is similar. These lesions rarely respond to topical therapy with corticosteroids. Intralesional triamcinolone acetonide is at times temporarily beneficial, but its administration can be traumatic and can result in a spread of the lesion via the phenomenon of pathergy. When adequate relief is not obtained with topical or intralesional corticosteroid therapy, oral colchicine 0.6 mg twice daily may be tried (145). This drug results in an improvement within days to weeks. If it is not effective within 2 weeks, the dosage may be increased or the drug abandoned. Oral dapsone is a second-line systemic agent

(146). After an appropriate pretherapy evaluation, dapsone is begun at a dose of 25 mg per day. The dose can gradually be raised to 200 mg per day if laboratory and/or other clinical evidence of toxicity do not occur. A randomized, double blind, placebo-controlled trial of thalidomide has demonstrated that significant reduction in oral and genital aphthae occurs, and that the effect was not dose-related (147). However, four of the 32 patients who received thalidomide developed a polyneuropathy. An open trial has demonstrated benefits from oral pentoxyfylline for oral aphthae. Lastly, several recent case reports have documented a possible role for infliximab in the treatment of mucocutaneous lesions (148).

Although oral corticosteroids are effective for the mucocutaneous manifestations of Behçet disease, their long-term administration is associated with multiple side effects. If dapsone and/or colchicine are ineffective as steroid-sparing agents, the use of low-dose weekly methotrexate should be considered. Methotrexate may be given in doses of 5 to 25 mg per week. After a complete assessment, methotrexate can be begun at a low dose that is raised weekly or biweekly following determinations of complete blood counts and liver function tests (149). Long-term usage may be required, but whether or not a liver biopsy should be used to monitor patients with Behçet disease has not been determined. The guidelines of the American College of Rheumatology for methotrexate usage in patients with rheumatoid arthritis should be followed.

Another agent that can be considered for mucocutaneous disease is IFN-α-2A (450). Alpsoy et al. studied IFN-α-2A in an open-label trial (150). They initially administered 3 million units of subcutaneous IFN-α-2A three times per week, but gradually increased the dose to 12 million units three times per week. The study period was 2 months, but treatment with 9 million units three times per week was continued in seven of the 14 patients for 6 months. All patients became symptom-free by the end of the 2-month treatment period, and in some, this symptom-free period was maintained even after the cessation of therapy. The most dramatic response was noted for the oral and genital ulcerations and the pustular vasculitis, but positive effects on arthritic complaints and eye disease were also noted. There were too few patients with serious vascular or central nervous system involvement to study the use of IFN in this subset. The usual toxic reaction of a flulike syndrome was noted in the early phases of the treatment, but was controlled with the administration of oral acetaminophen.

Synovitis

Arthritis occurs in approximately half the patients with Behçet disease. Joint involvement is typically oligoarthritic and nonerosive and the disease may affect large or small joints. Initial therapy should include NSAIDs and possibly sulfasalazine. IFN-α is also effective. Low-dose corticosteroids with or without agents such as azathioprine or methotrexate may be effective in patients who do not respond well to less toxic agents.

Uveitis

Uveitis occurs in half the patients with Behçet disease, and the potential for blindness is the most important morbidity that occurs from the disease. Uveitis may affect the anterior or posterior segment. Anterior uveitis may be treated with topical applications of corticosteroids and, if necessary, agents to reduce ocular pressure. Posterior uveitis is believed to be the results of a retinal vasculitis and tends to be closely linked to disease in the central nervous system. Posterior uveal involvement is the primary cause of blindness. The ability to reduce the risk of blindness is justification for the use of therapeutic agents associated with potential toxicity.

Systemic corticosteroids, such as high-dose prednisone (1 to 2 mg/kg per day), have traditionally been the initial treatment of choice for patients with Behçet disease. However, corticosteroids often are not sufficient to adequately suppress retinal disease, and immunosuppressive/cytotoxic agents are usually recommended early in the course of the disease. Recently, Demiroglu et al. (151) reported that the use of IFN-α-2B with colchicine and benzathine penicillin was significantly more effective in controlling ocular disease and in preventing new attacks than treatment with colchicine and benzathine penicillin. They also noted that there were fewer episodes of arthritis, mucocutaneous lesions, and vascular events in those patients who received IFN. Toxicity was minimal in that study. Azathioprine, chlorambucil, cyclophosphamide, mycophenolate mofetil, cyclosporine, and tacrolimus are available and have been suggested as disease-altering, steroid-sparing agents for serious ocular and/or central nervous system involvement (152–157). Unfortunately, there are few adequately controlled trials that compare these agents. Thus, recommendations are largely empiric and are often based on familiarity with the drug and dependent on the institution within which the treating physician trained.

Azathioprine is given in a single morning dose of 2 to 3 mg/kg per day. In a recent double-blind, placebo-controlled trial, azathioprine was demonstrated to prevent the development of ocular disease in patients without ocular involvement and to prevent the development of involvement of the second eye in patients with unilateral involvement. However, the drug was not effective in improving the visual acuity in treated patients. Furthermore, there are little if any data that can indicate that azathioprine can effect a long-term remission. Therefore, although azathioprine is less toxic than the other available agents, it is apparently less efficacious.

Chlorambucil is administered in a dosage of 2 mg per day initially and raised by 2 mg per day weekly until the disease becomes quiescent, or there is evidence of toxicity. This therapy is usually effective within 3 to 9 months and has been associated with improvement of visual acuity and long-term remissions. After ocular disease is controlled, chlorambucil dose can be reduced and often stopped. Relapses generally will respond to readministration of the drug. Chlorambucil may be used with corticosteroids, in which case the corticosteroids are usually tapered and stopped before tapering the chlorambucil, or it can be used as the sole therapy in selected patients. Long-term low-dose therapy is at times necessary. The unfortunate risks of neoplasia (leukemia or lymphoma) and permanent sterility (azospermia or anovulation) must be considered and discussed with the patient at the onset of therapy.

Cyclophosphamide, another alkylating agent, has also been demonstrated to be effective in some patients with Behçet disease. It has been less well studied than chlorambucil, but would be predicted to carry roughly the same benefits based on its pharmacology. However, in addition to the risks of subsequent malignancy and sterility, hemorrhagic cystitis is also associated with its administration. Recently, cyclophosphamide has been administered via an intermittent high-dose pulse therapy, and it has demonstrated benefits for severe uveitis and central nervous system disease.

Cyclosporine has also been used for treatment of patients with uveitis due to Behçet disease. It has been demonstrated to reduce the number of ocular attacks and improve visual acuity, but its use has not resulted in long-term remissions. In addition, cyclosporine has seemingly not been effective for therapy of central nervous system involvement, intestinal involvement, or vascular lesions.

Tacrolimus (FK-506) and mycophenolate mofetil are the newest immunosuppressive agents used for the prevention of transplant rejection. However, there are no reports documenting the efficacious use in patients with Behçet disease.

Central Nervous Disease and Systemic Vascular Involvement

Treatment of central nervous disease and systemic vascular involvement is identical to that for posterior uveal tract involvement. Therapy involves the use of an immunosuppressive/cytotoxic agent with or without high-dose corticosteroids.

THE MAGIC SYNDROME

Several patients have been reported with features of Behçet syndrome and relapsing polychondritis. Firestein et al. (158) reported five patients with oral and genital ulceration, arthritis, chondritis, and ocular disease. They coined the term "mouth and genital ulcers with inflamed cartilage" (MAGIC) syndrome to encompass the overlapping features of these patients. At least one patient has been reported in whom an antiphospholipid antibody was found (159). A subsequent report detailed the possibility of vascular involvement and the usefulness of immunosuppressive therapy (160). Lastly, a patient has been successfully treated with methotrexate (5 mg per week) and pentoxyfylline (300 mg per day) for control of her oral ulcers, EN-like lesions, and arthritis (161).

ERYTHEMA ELEVATUM DIUTINUM

Erythema elevatum diutinum is an unusual form of cutaneous vasculitis characterized by persistent, erythematous, violaceous and/or yellow papules, plaques, and/or nodules (Fig. 11.26) (162). The lesions often occur over bony prominences, are most often on acral or extensor skin surfaces, and are distributed symmetrically. Occasionally the patients may have arthralgias, but other systemic manifestations associated with necrotizing vasculitis are not observed. The cause is unknown, but some of the patients with erythema elevatum diutinum have a paraprotein, usually IgA, but occasionally IgM (163). Other associated processes recently observed in several patients with erythema elevatum diutinum have been HIV infection and Crohn disease (164,165). Erythema elevatum diutinum appears to be resistant to usual therapies for vasculitis but reportedly responds well to oral dapsone (100 to 200 mg per day).

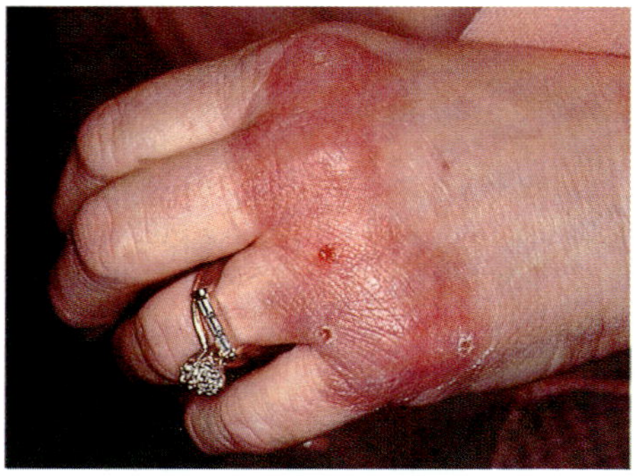

Figure 11.26. Erythema elevatum diutinum. Erythematous plaques in the metacarpophalangeal joints.

MUSCULOSKELETAL SYNDROMES ASSOCIATED WITH ACNE AND HIDRADENITIS

Burns and Colville (166) first called attention to the possibility of arthritis as a complication of severe acne in 1959. Since then, there have been multiple reports of individual patients as well as several studies involving an additional 100 to 150 patients (167,168). Almost all patients with arthritis have had severe forms of acne, either acne conglobata or acne fulminans (169). Acne conglobata may be part of the "follicular triad," which additionally consists of hidradenitis suppurativa and dissecting cellulitis of the scalp. Interestingly, only a few cases of arthropathy associated with hidradenitis have been reported (170).

The term *acne fulminans* is believed to have been coined by Plewig and Kligman (171) to describe patients with acute ulcerative and necrotic acne accompanied by fever and other systemic symptoms such as weight loss, arthralgia/arthritis, and myalgia. Most patients are in their teenage years and are white males; most cases begin with mild papulopustular or cystic acne. Acne fulminans usually involves the face (Fig. 11.27) and is usually widespread, involving the chest and/or back. Patients are often on therapy with antibiotics at the time acne fulminans develops. Also, some patients have developed acne fulminans while on isotretinoin. The pathogenesis of acne fulminans is unknown, but it has been postulated that either drug-induced or immunologic aberrations may be involved in initiating the reaction.

Musculoskeletal symptoms are a hallmark of acne fulminans and are temporally related to the skin lesions. Painful bone lesions are a distinctive feature of acne fulminans and are found in about 40% of those patients. In about one half of those with painful bone lesions, osseous defects are observed on radiographic studies or bone scans. Biopsies of osteolytic lesions have failed to reveal infection, but do reveal a nonspecific inflammatory response. Arthritis occurs in about one third of

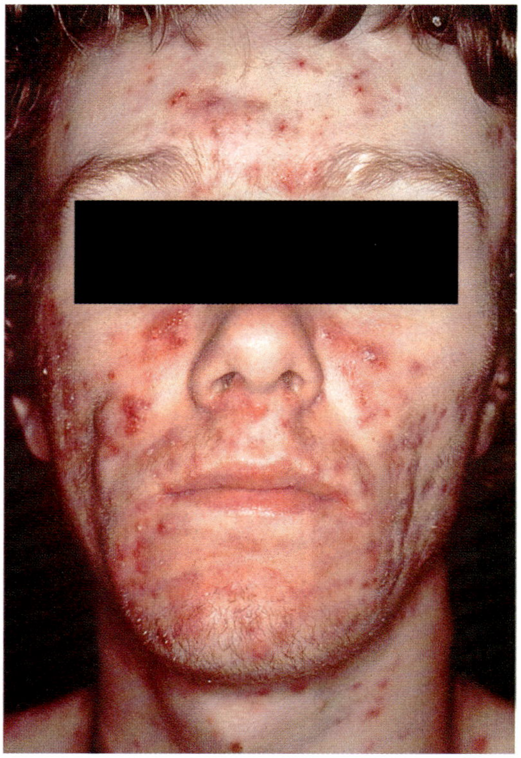

Figure 11.27. Acne fulminans. (Courtesy of Steve Estes, M.D., with permission Cincinnati, Ohio.)

patients with acne fulminans and has a predilection for the larger joints, particularly the knees. The arthritis is nondeforming. Arthralgias and/or myalgias occur in 80% to 90% of patients.

Treatment of acne fulminans almost always involves the use of systemic corticosteroids with oral isotretinoin added after about 4 weeks of therapy. Individual cases have responded to antibiotics, dapsone, NSAIDs, clofazimine, azathioprine, and isotretinoin. In general, prednisone 0.5 to 1 mg/kg per day given in a single morning dose is effective in calming the severe skin lesions, controlling the fever, and improving the musculoskeletal symptoms. Isotretinoin 0.5 mg/kg per day is added after 4 weeks of prednisone (172). Corticosteroids should be withdrawn slowly over a period of 2 to 3 months to minimize recurrence. Eventually the disease regresses, but relapses often occur prior to regression.

Acne conglobata consists of polyporous comedonal cysts, deep inflammatory cysts, draining sinus tracts, and bridging scars (Fig. 11.28). This process may occur alone or in the presence of hidradenitis suppurativa and dissecting cellulitis of the scalp. The occurrence of all three conditions is known as the follicular occlusion triad.

The prevalence of musculoskeletal disease in acne conglobata or follicular occlusion triad has not been well studied. Eighty-one percent of patients with acne conglobata–associated musculoskeletal syndrome are black and 75% are women. The musculoskeletal findings are different from acne fulminans in patients with acne conglobata. The patients with acne conglobata or follicular occlusion triad tend to have arthralgias and/or arthritis. Peripheral joints are more commonly involved, and symmetric involvement occurs 60% of the time. Spondyloarthropathy may also occur. Constitutional findings such as fever or weight loss do not complicate acne conglobata. The joint involvement may well follow the course of the disease and may be responsive to usual acne therapies combined with NSAIDs.

Isotretinoin is a commonly used drug for treatment of severe acne vulgaris and acne conglobata as well as a variety of other conditions. Among its side effects are musculoskeletal symptoms. Arthralgias and/or myalgias may occur in up to a third of treated patients. Arthritis may occur but is a rare phenomenon (173). Skeletal hyperostosis, often of the cervical spine, may occur but is dose-related. This process appears to be identical to diffuse idiopathic skeletal hyperostosis (DISH) and is usually asymptomatic. Musculoskeletal symptoms other than DISH resolve with discontinuation of the drug. During therapy, symptomatic treatment with NSAIDs may be helpful.

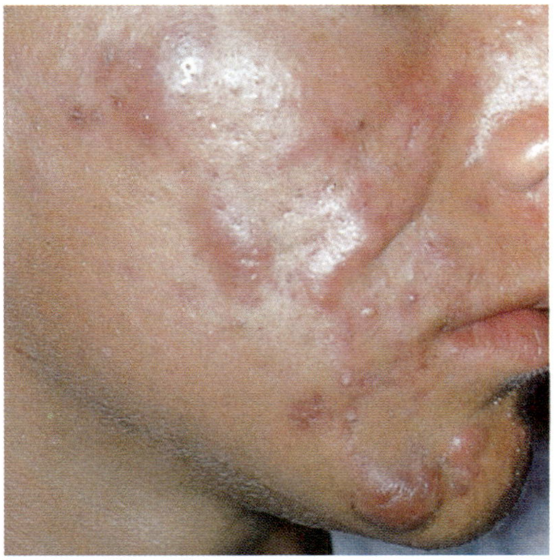

Figure 11.28. Acne conglobata.

Palmoplantar pustulosis may be associated on rare occasion with an unusual bone and joint condition, which may involve the peripheral joints or the sternoclavicular joints. This condition has been termed "pustulotic arthroosteitis" (PAO) or *synovitis, acne, pustulosis, hyperostosis, osteitis* (SAPHO syndrome) (174–176). This disorder has been more frequently reported in Japanese or Scandinavian patients, but several reports from Europe and the United States have been published. The SAPHO syndrome may occur in patients with psoriasis, acne, or palmoplantar pustular dermatitis. Some patients have also had multifocal sterile osteomyelitis, Sweet syndrome, and pyoderma gangrenosum (176). The arthritis is not infectious and is believed to be distinct from psoriatic arthritis since typical psoriatic skin or nail lesions are not seen and no HLA association has been demonstrated. The joint symptoms do seem to correlate with the activity of the skin disease. Reportedly, symptomatic therapy with NSAIDs or low-dose oral corticosteroids is effective.

FAMILIAL MEDITERRANEAN FEVER

Familial Mediterranean fever (FMF) is characterized by recurrent self-limited abdominal pain, chest pain, erysipelas-like erythema, and/or arthritis accompanied by fever in people of "Mediterranean" ancestry. The disease has a predilection for Ashkenazi and Sephardic Jews, Armenians, Arabs, and Anatolian Turks. The inheritance pattern is autosomal recessive (OMIM*249100), but a rare autosomal dominant form (OMIM*134610) has been observed in several families. The recessive form has been mapped to 16p13. Pras et al. (177) have suggested diagnostic criteria (Table 11.10). Abdominal pain due to peritonitis occurs in 90% of patients and is the presenting manifestation in 68%. Pleuritis and pericarditis are the causes of chest pain. Synovitis of large joints occurs in 75% of patients, but is a rare presenting manifestation. Cutaneous disease has been reported in 43% of children with FMF (178). An erysipelas-like erythema is the characteristic cutaneous change in FMF, but palpable purpura consistent with Henoch–Schönlein purpura has been regularly reported. The pathogenesis of FMF is not known. Diagnosis may be confirmed by intravenous infusion of 10 mg of metaraminol bitartrate, which simulates a mild attack. There are multiple genetic variants that have been identified. This disorder may be simulated by an inherited syndrome known as the tumor necrosis factor receptor–associated periodic syndrome (OMIM*191190) (179). Therapy with oral colchicine is effective in reducing the frequency and severity of attacks. In addition, chronic long-term administration of colchicine has effectively prevented the development of nephropathic amyloidosis and the complication of renal failure.

TABLE 11.10. Diagnostic Criteria for Familial Mediterranean Fever

1. Self-limited attacks of fever (39°C–40°C) at irregular intervals
2. Painful inflammation of the abdomen, chest, joints, and/or skin associated with the fever[a]
3. Nephropathic amyloidosis
4. Autosomal recessive inheritance
5. Ethnic restriction

[a]Exclusion of other causes of disease.

SARCOIDOSIS

Sarcoidosis is a multisystem disorder of unknown etiology. It most commonly involves the lungs, lymph nodes, liver, spleen, skin, eyes, glandular tissues, and bones. Involvement of the skin is relatively common in chronic sarcoidosis. Bone involvement has also been reported to be a frequent accompaniment of chronic cutaneous sarcoidosis. This involvement is that of bone cysts or destructive lesions. Arthritis occurs in acute sarcoidosis in association with EN (see before) and is generally self-limited. In addition, muscle involvement may occur. Sarcoidal granulomas may be found in muscle, but usually there are no symptoms. A full discussion of this multisystem disorder is beyond the scope of this text.

MULTICENTRIC RETICULOHISTIOCYTOSIS

The term "multicentric reticulohistiocytosis" was coined by Goltz and Laymon (180) in 1954 to describe patients who had a destructive arthritis with multiple cutaneous nodules in which the histopathologic change consists of histiocytic multinucleated giant cells with eosinophilic ground-glass cytoplasm. This condition is rare, with fewer than 100 cases reported in the world literature (181). The disease occurs in mid life (mean age at onset, 43 years) and affects women more often than men (2:1). It is seen mostly in whites, but it has been reported in all races.

Multicentric reticulohistiocytosis is characterized by a destructive polyarthritis. The arthritis is frequently among the presenting manifestations and occurs as the sole manifestation in 45% and with cutaneous lesions (30%). The disease manifests findings that are similar to those of rheumatoid arthritis, but has a predilection to affect the distal interphalangeal joints. Synovial fluid analysis demonstrates an inflammatory picture, and synovial biopsy reveals lipid-laden giant cells and histiocytes similar to those observed on skin biopsy.

The classic skin lesions are multiple nodules that have a predilection for the hands but may occur on any body surface (Fig. 11.29). The nodules may be skin colored or may have a yellow or red–brown color. They vary from 1 to 10 mm in size and can coalesce to form a cobblestone appearance or plaques. In addition, about one third of the patients have had xanthelasma. The nodules grow slowly, but do not seem to ulcerate. Regression may occur spontaneously or in relation to therapy.

Although multicentric reticulohistiocytosis is primarily a disease of the skin and joints, a variety of other systemic features can occur. Orkin et al. (182) reported pulmonary involvement in 20% of patients with multicentric reticulohistiocytosis. Cardiac involvement is a rare complication (183). Additionally, widespread infiltration of the serosal surfaces, lymphoreticular tissues, and glandular tissues can occur (183,184).

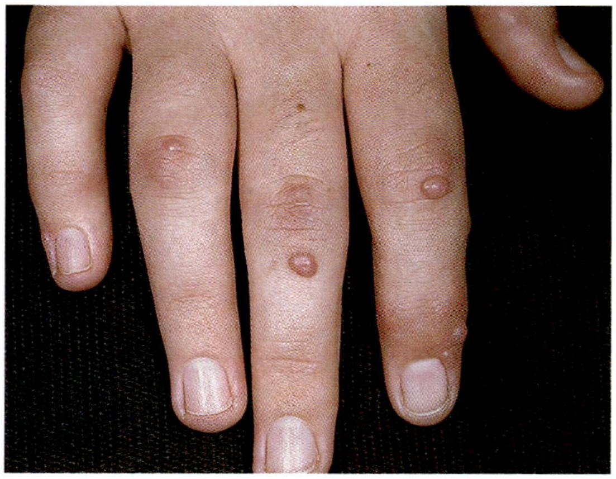

Figure 11.29. Multicentric reticulohistiocytosis.

Multicentric reticulohistiocytosis has been associated with a variety of conditions. About half the patients will have hypercholesterolemia. Between 10% and 25% of patients have a malignancy, which is frequently recognized at diagnosis. In some cases, removal of the malignancy has resulted in resolution of the arthritis and skin lesions (185). Various malignancies have been reported including breast, colon, bronchus, cervix, stomach, and ovary (usually adenocarcinoma), as well as cases of melanoma, sarcoma, leukemia, and lymphoma (186). The features of multicentric reticulohistiocytosis associated with malignancy do not differ from those seen in patients without associated malignancy. Other associations noted in individual cases include diabetes mellitus, hypothyroidism, Sjögren syndrome, primary biliary cirrhosis, myopathy, and pregnancy.

Multicentric reticulohistiocytosis must be differentiated from a variety of other cutaneous and rheumatologic disorders. The diagnosis is confirmed by skin biopsy and/or synovial biopsy when other histiocytic disorders are ruled out. The differential diagnosis generally includes rheumatoid arthritis with rheumatoid nodulosis, sarcoidosis, xanthomata, dermatomyositis, Langerhans cell histiocytosis, nonhistiocytosis, lepromatous leprosy, and gout.

While the disease may spontaneously "burn out," the patient can be left with residual severe joint deformities. Various pharmacologic agents have been recommended, including corticosteroids, antimalarials, and cytotoxic agents. No therapy has been consistently effective; however, there are many reports that suggest that cytotoxic agents are the most predictable in their effects (181–184). Ginsburg et al. (187) suggested that the use of cyclophosphamide or chlorambucil was effective in a small group of patients. Others have found that methotrexate was effective in a patient (188,189). Recommendations for therapy are not exact, but early and aggressive treatment may prevent the devastating arthropathy and disfiguring cutaneous sequelae.

REFERENCES

1. Jorizzo JL. Neutrophilic dermatoses: Sweet's syndrome and pyoderma gangrenosum. In: Gallin JI, Goldstein IM, Synderma NR, eds. *Inflammation: basic principles and clinical correlates.* New York: Raven Press, 1988:785–802.
2. Sweet RD. An acute febrile neutrophilic dermatosis. *Br J Dermatol* 1964;76: 349–356.
3. Cohen PR, Holder WR, Rapini RP. Concurrent Sweet's syndrome and erythema nodosum: a report, world literature review and mechanism of pathogenesis. *J Rheumatol* 1992;19:814–820.
4. Cullity J, Maguire B, Gebauer K. Sweet's panniculitis. *Australas J Dermatol* 1991;32:61–64.
5. Morgan KW, Callen JP. Sweet's syndrome in acute myelogenous leukemia presenting as periorbital cellulitis with an infiltrate of leukemic cells. *J Am Acad Dermatol* 2001;45:590.
6. Dompmartin A, Trowsard X, Lorier E, et al. Sweet syndrome associated with acute myelogenous leukemia: atypical form simulating facial erysipelas. *Int J Dermatol* 1991;30:644–647.
7. Bulengo-Ransby SM, Brown MD, Dubin HV, et al. Sweet's syndrome presenting as an unusual periorbital eruption. *J Am Acad Dermatol* 1991;24: 140–141.
8. Torri O, Laeille B, Ruto F, et al. Cellulite faciale febrile: tableau grave et trompeur d'une dermatose aigne neutrophique au cours d'une leucemia myeloide chronique. *Ann Dermatol Venereol* 1993;120:803–805.
9. Tercedor J, Rodenas JM, Henraz MD, et al. Facial cellulitis-like Sweet's syndrome in acute myelogenous leukemia. *Int J Dermatol* 1992;31:598–599.
10. Kibbi AG, Zaynoun ST, Kurban AK, et al. Acute febrile neutrophilic dermatosis (Sweet's syndrome): case report and review of the literature. *Pediatr Dermatol* 1985;3:40–44.
11. Collins P, Rogers S, Keenan P, et al. Acute febrile neutrophilic dermatosis in childhood (Sweet's syndrome). *Br J Dermatol* 1985;3:40–44.

12. Delke I, Veridiano MP, Tancer MI, et al. Sweet syndrome with involvement of the female genital tract. *Obstet Gynecol* 1981;58:394–396.
13. Banet DE, McClave SA, Callen JP. Oral metronidazole is an effective treatment for Sweet's syndrome: a case report in a patient with associated inflammatory bowel disease. *J Rheumatol* 1994;21:1766–1768.
14. Wilson DM, John GR, Callen JP. Peripheral ulcerative keratitis—an extracutaneous neutrophilic disorder: report of a patient with rheumatoid arthritis, pustular vasculitis, pyoderma gangrenosum, and Sweet's syndrome with an excellent response to cyclosporine therapy. *J Am Acad Dermatol* 1999;40: 331–334.
15. Takimoto CH, Warnock M, Golden JA. Sweet's syndrome with lung involvement. *Am Rev Respir Dis* 1991;143:177–179.
16. Brown TS, Marshall GS, Callen JP. Cavitating pulmonary infiltrate in an adolescent with pyoderma gangrenosum: a rarely recognized extracutaneous manifestation of a neutrophilic dermatosis. *J Am Acad Dermatol* 2000;43: 108–112.
17. Bourke SJ, Quinn AG, Farr PM, et al. Neutrophilic alveolitis in Sweet's syndrome. *Thorax* 1992;47:572–573.
18. Kar PM, Aronoff G, Schuette P. Bronchopulmonary disease: an association with ulcerative colitis and pyoderma gangrenosum. *J Ky Med Assoc* 1993;91: 320–323.
19. Rodriquez de la Serna A, Domingo-Pedrol P, Blanch-Torra L, et al. Acute febrile neutrophilic dermatosis (Sweet's syndrome) associated with post-myocardial infarction syndrome (Dressler's syndrome). *Arch Intern Med* 1985;145:1522–1524.
20. Nurre LD, Rabalais GP, Callen JP. Neutrophilic dermatosis-associated sterile chronic multifocal osteomyelitis in pediatric patients: case report and review. *Pediatr Dermatol* 1999;16:214–216.
21. Malone JC, Slone SP, Willis-Frank LA, et al. Vascular inflammation (vasculitis) in Sweet's syndrome: a clinicopathologic study of 28 biopsies from 21 patients. *Arch Dermatol* 2002;138:345–349.
22. Cooper PH, Innes DJ Jr, Greer KE. Acute febrile neutrophilic dermatosis (Sweet's syndrome) and myeloproliferative disorders. *Cancer* 1983;51: 1518–1526.
23. Cohen PR, Talpaz T, Kurzock R. Malignancy associated Sweet's syndrome: review of the literature. *J Clin Oncol* 1988;6:1887–1897.
24. Goette DK. Sweet's syndrome in subacute cutaneous lupus erythematosus. *Arch Dermatol* 1985;121:789–791.
25. Harary AM. Sweet's syndrome associated with rheumatoid arthritis. *Arch Intern Med* 1983;143:1993–1995.
26. Delaporte E, Gaveau DJ, Piette FA, et al. Acute febrile neutrophilic dermatosis (Sweet's syndrome): association with rheumatoid vasculitis. *Arch Dermatol* 1989;125:1101–1106.
27. Trentham DE, Masi AT, Bale GF. Arthritis with an inflammatory dermatoses resembling Sweet's syndrome: report of a unique case and review of the literature on arthritis associated with the inflammatory dermatoses. *Am J Med* 1976;61:424–432.
28. Romano J, Safai B. Pyoderma gangrenosum and myeloproliferative disorders. *Arch Intern Med* 1979;139:932–934.
29. Benton EC, Rutherford D, Hunter JAA. Sweet's syndrome and pyoderma gangrenosum associated with ulcerative colitis. *Acta Derm Venereol* 1985;65: 77–80.
30. Satra K, Zalka A, Cohen PR, et al. Sweet's syndrome and pregnancy. *J Am Acad Dermatol* 1994;30:297–300.
31. Oguz O, Serdaraglus A, Tuzun Y, et al. Acute febrile neutrophilic dermatosis (Sweet's syndrome) associated with Behçet's disease. *Int J Dermatol* 1992;31: 645–646.
32. Torralbo A, Herrero JA, del Rio E, et al. Sweet's syndrome associated with multiple myeloma. *Int J Dermatol* 1992;31:297–298.
33. Uchida H, Ikari Y, Hashizume S, et al. A case of Sweet's syndrome with early gastric cancer. *Dermatologica* 1990;181:224–227.
34. Ehrsam EPJ, et al. Sweet's syndrome associated with ovarian carcinoma. *J Eur Acad Dermatol Venereol* 1993;2:235–238.
35. Kemmett D, Hunter JAA. Sweet's syndrome: a clinicopathologic review of twenty-nine cases. *J Am Acad Dermatol* 1990;23:503–507.
36. Park JW, Mehrota B, Barnett B, et al. The Sweet syndrome during therapy with granulocyte colony-stimulating factor. *Ann Intern Med* 1992;116:996–998.
37. Johnson ML, Grimwood RE. Leukocyte colony-stimulating factors. *Arch Dermatol* 1994;130:77–81.
38. Piette WW, Trapp JF, O'Donnell MJ, et al. Acute neutrophilic dermatosis with myeloblastic infiltrate in a leukemia patient receiving all-trans-retinoic acid therapy. *J Am Acad Dermatol* 1994;30:293–297.
39. Cox NH, O'Brien HAW. Sweet's syndrome associated with trans-retinoic acid treatment in acute promyelocytic leukaemia. *Clin Exp Dermatol* 1994;19: 51–52.
40. Aram H. Acute febrile neutrophilic dermatosis (Sweet's syndrome): response to dapsone. *Arch Dermatol* 1984;120:245–247.
41. Horio T, Immamura S, Danno K, et al. Treatment of acute febrile neutrophilic dermatosis (Sweet's syndrome) with potassium iodide. *Dermatologica* 1980; 160:341–347.
42. Hoffman GS. Treatment of Sweet's syndrome (acute febrile neutrophilic dermatosis) with indomethacin. *J Rheumatol* 1977;4:201–206.
43. Subhisa S, Tagam H, Inque F, et al. Colchicine in the treatment of acute febrile neutrophilic dermatosis (Sweet's syndrome). *Br J Dermatol* 1983;108:99–101.
44. Joshi RK, Atukorala DN, Abanmi A, et al. Successful treatment of Sweet's syndrome with doxycycline. *Br J Dermatol* 1993;128:584–586.
45. Case JD, Smith SZ, Callen JP. The use of pulse methylprednisolone and chlorambucil in the treatment of Sweet's syndrome. *Cutis* 1969;44:125–129.
46. Bourke JF, Berth-Jones J, Graham-Brown RAC. Sweet's syndrome responding to cyclosporin. *Br J Dermatol* 1992;127:36–38.
47. Callen JP. Pyoderma gangrenosum. *Lancet* 1998;351:581–585.
48. Bennett ML, Jackson JM, Jorizzo JL, et al. Pyoderma gangrenosum: a comparison of typical and atypical forms with an emphasis on time to remission—case review of 86 patients from 2 institutions. *Medicine (Baltimore)* 2000;79:37–46.
49. O'Loughlin S, Perry HO. A diffuse pustular eruption associated with ulcerative colitis. *Arch Dermatol* 1978;114:1061–1064.
50. Fenske NA, Gern JE, Pierce D, et al. Vesiculopustular eruption of ulcerative colitis. *Arch Dermatol* 1983;119:664–669.
51. Callen JP, Woo TY. Vesiculopustular eruption in a patient with ulcerative colitis. *Arch Dermatol* 1985;121:339–404.
52. Hughes AP, Jackson MJ, Callen JP. Clinical features and treatment of peristomal pyoderma gangrenosum. *JAMA* 2000;284:1546–1548.
53. Lyon CC, Smith AJ, Beck MH, et al. Parastomal pyoderma gangrenosum: clinical features and management. *J Am Acad Dermatol* 2000;42:992–1002.
54. Sheldon DG, Sawchuck LL, Kozarek RA, et al. Twenty cases of peristomal pyoderma gangrenosum. Diagnostic implications and management. *Arch Surg* 2000;135:564–569.
55. McCalmont CS, Leshin B, White WL, et al. Vulvar pyoderma gangrenosum. *Int J Gynecol Obstet* 1991;35:175–178.
56. Lebbe C, Moulonguet-Michau I, Perrin P, et al. Steroid-responsive pyoderma gangrenosum with vulvar and pulmonary involvement. *J Am Acad Dermatol* 1992;27:623–625.
57. Graham JA, Hansen KK, Rabinowitz LG, et al. Pyoderma gangrenosum in infants and children. *Pediatr Dermatol* 1994;11:10–17.
58. VanHale HM, Rogers RS, Zone JJ, et al. Pyostomatitis vegetans: a reactive mucosal marker for inflammatory disease of the gut. *Arch Dermatol* 1985;121: 94–98.
59. Perry HO, Winklemann RK, Muller SA, et al. Malignant pyoderma. *Arch Dermatol* 1968;98:561–567.
60. Wernikoff S, Merritt C, Briggaman RA, et al. Malignant pyoderma or pyoderma gangrenosum of the head and neck? *Arch Dermatol* 1987;123:371–375.
61. Perry HO, Winkelmann RK. Bullous pyoderma gangrenosum and leukemia. *Arch Dermatol* 1972;106:901–905.
62. Romano J, Safai B. Pyoderma gangrenosum and myeloproliferative disorders. *Arch Intern Med* 1979;932–934.
63. Galaria NA, Junkins-Hopkins JM, Kligman D, et al. Neutrophilic dermatosis of the dorsal hands: pustular vasculitis revisited. *J Am Acad Dermatol* 2000;43: 870–874.
64. Callen JP, Dubin HV, Gherke CF. Pyoderma gangrenosum and agnogenic myeloid metaplasia. *Arch Dermatol* 1976;113:1585–1586.
65. Su WPD, Schroeter AL, Perry HO, et al. Histopathologic and immunopathologic study of pyoderma gangrenosum. *J Cutan Pathol* 1986;13:323–330.
66. Perry HO. Pyoderma gangrenosum. *South Med J* 1959;62:899–908.
67. Powell FC, Schroeter AL, Su WPD, et al. Pyoderma gangrenosum: a review of 86 patients. *Q J Med* 1985;55:173–186.
68. Prystowsky SD, Fye KH, Goette KD, et al. AFND (Sweet's syndrome) associated with Sjogren's syndrome. *Arch Dermatol* 1978;114:1234–1235.
69. Callen JP, Case JD, Sager D. Chlorambucil: an effective corticosteroid-sparing therapy for pyoderma gangrenosum. *J Am Acad Dermatol* 1989;21:515–519.
70. Talansky AL, Myers S, Greenstein AJ, et al. Does intestinal resection heal the pyoderma gangrenosum of inflammatory bowel disease? *J Clin Gastroenterol* 1983;108:580–581.
71. Murray JC. Pyoderma gangrenosum and IgA gammopathy. *Cutis* 1983;32: 477–486.
72. Koester G, Tarnower A, Levisohn D, et al. Bullous pyoderma gangrenosum. *J Am Acad Dermatol* 1993;29:875–878.
73. Harmon CB, Su WPD, Peters MS. Cutaneous aspergillosis complicating pyoderma gangrenosum. *J Am Acad Dermatol* 1993;29:656–658.
74. Wan-Qing L, Yu-lin Z, Zhen SJ. Sporotrichosis presenting as pyoderma gangrenosum. *Mycopathologica* 1991;116:165–168.
75. Mir-Madjlessi SH, Taylor JS, Farmer RG. Clinical course and evolution of erythema nodosum and pyoderma gangrenosum in chronic ulcerative colitis: a study of 42 patients. *Am J Gastroenterol* 1985;80:615–620.
76. Cox NH, Peebles-Brown A, Mackie RM. Pyoderma gangrenosum occurring 10 years after protocolectomy for ulcerative colitis. *Br J Hosp Med* 1986;36:363.
77. Gardner LW, Acker DW. Triamcinolone and pyoderma gangrenosum. *Arch Dermatol* 1972;106:599–600.
78. Sanders CJG, Hulsman RFHJ. Successful treatment of pyoderma gangrenosum with topical 5-aminosalicylic acid. *Cutis* 1993;262:264.
79. Tsele E, Yu RCH, Chu AC. Pyoderma gangrenosum: response to topical nitrogen mustard. *Clin Exp Dermatol* 1992;17:437–440.
80. Richardson JB, Callen JP. Pyoderma gangrenosum treated successfully with potassium iodide. *J Am Acad Dermatol* 1993;28:1005–1007.
81. Campbell DA, Corman LC, Williams RC Jr. Splenectomy as treatment for non-healing soft tissue defect after total knee arthroplasty in a patient with Felty's syndrome. *J Rheumatol* 1992;19:1126–1129.
82. Holt PJA, Davies MG, Saunders KC, et al. Pyoderma gangrenosum. *Medicine* 1980;59:114–133.
83. Johnson RB, Lazarus GS. Pulse therapy. *Arch Dematol* 1983;118:76–84.
84. Newell LM, Malkinson FD. Pyoderma gangrenosum: response to cyclophosphamide therapy. *Arch Dermatol* 1983;119:495–497.

85. Curley RK, MacFarlane AW, Vickers CFH. Pyoderma gangrenosum treated with cyclosporin A. *Br J Dermatol* 1985;113:601–604.
86. Matis WL, Ellis CN, Griffiths CEM, et al. Treatment of pyoderma gangrenosum with cyclosporine. *Arch Dermatol* 1992;128:1060–1064.
87. Abu-Elmagd K, Jegasothy BV, Ackerman CD, et al. Efficacy of FK 506 in the treatment of recalcitrant pyoderma gangrenosum. *Transplant Proc* 1991;23: 3328–3329.
88. Gupta AK, Shear NH, Sauder DN. Efficacy of human intravenous immune globulin in pyoderma gangrenosum. *J Am Acad Dermatol* 1995;32:140–142.
89. Hecker MS, Lebwohl MG. Recalcitrant pyoderma gangrenosum: treatment with thalidomide. *J Am Acad Dermatol* 1998;38:490–1.
90. Federman CL, Federman DG. Recalcitrant pyoderma gangrenosum treated with thalidomide. *Mayo Clin Proc* 2000;75:842–844.
91. Tan MH, Gordon M, Lebwohl O, et al. Improvement of Pyoderma gangrenosum and psoriasis associated with Crohn disease with anti-tumor necrosis factor α monoclonal antibody. *Arch Dermatol* 2001;137:930–933.
92. de Imus G, Golomb C, Wilkel C, et al. Accelerated healing of pyoderma gangrenosum treated with bioengineered skin and concomitant immunosuppression. *J Am Acad Dermatol* 2001;44:61–66.
93. Ackerman A. *Histologic diagnosis of inflammatory skin diseases: a method by pattern analysis.* Philadelphia: Lea & Febiger, 1988:449–450.
94. Scherbenske JM, Benson PM, Lupton GP. Rheumatoid neutrophilic dermatitis. *Arch Dermatol* 1989;125:1105–1108.
95. Sanchez JL, Cruz A. Rheumatoid neutrophilic dermatosis. *J Am Acad Dermatol* 1990;22:922–925.
96. Lowe L, Kornfeld B, Clayman J, et al. Rheumatoid neutrophilic dermatitis. *J Cutan Pathol* 1992;19:48–53.
97. Gay-Crosier F, Dayer JM, Chavaz P, et al. Rheumatoid neutrophilic dermatitis/sweet's syndrome in a patient with seronegative rheumatoid arthritis. *Dermatology* 2000;201:185–187.
98. Brown TS, Fearneyhough PK, Burruss JB, et al. Rheumatoid neutrophilic dermatitis in a woman with seronegative rheumatoid arthritis. *J Am Acad Dermatol* 2001;45:596–600.
99. Jorizzo JL, Schmalstieg FC, Dinehart SM, et al. Bowel-associated dermatosis-arthritis syndrome: immune complex-mediated vessel damage and increased neutrophil migration. *Arch Intern Med* 1984;144:738–740.
100. Dicken CH. Bowel-associated dermatosis-arthritis syndrome: bowel bypass syndrome without bowel bypass. *Mayo Clin Proc* 1984;49:43–46.
101. Bechtel MA, Callen JP. Acute febrile neutrophilic dermatosis (Sweet's syndrome). *Arch Dermatol* 1982;117:664–666.
102. Jorizzo JL, Apisarnthanarax P, Sulent P, et al. Bowel bypass syndrome without bowel bypass: bowel-associated dermatosis-arthritis syndrome. *Arch Intern Med* 1983;143:457–461.
103. Bachmeyer C, Arbactingi S. Neutrophilic eccrine hidradentitis. *Clin Dermatol* 2000;18:319–330.
104. Bilic M, Mutasim DF. Neutrophilic eccrine hidradenitis in a patient with Behçet's disease. *Cutis* 2001;68:107–111.
105. Black MM. Panniculitis: problems with diagnosis. *Australas J Dermatol* 1988; 29:79–84.
106. Patterson JW. Panniculitis: a guide to differential diagnosis. *J Assoc Milit Dermatol* 1983;9:36–39.
107. Requena L, Yus ES. Panniculitis, I: mostly septal panniculitis. *J Am Acad Dermatol* 2001;45:163–183.
108. Requena L, Sanchez Yus E. Panniculitis, II: mostly lobular panniculitis.*J Am Acad Dermatol* 2001;45:325–361.
109. Phelps RG, Shoji T. Update on Panniculitis. *Mt Sinai Med J* 2001;68:262–267.
110. Ter Poorten MC, Thiers BH. Panniculitis [review]. *Dermatol Clin* 2002;20: 421–433.
111. Weinstein L. Erythema nodosum. *Dis Mon* 1969;June:1–30.
112. Garcia-Porrua C, Gonzalez-Gay MA, Vazquez-Caruncho M, et al. Erythema nodosum: etiologic and predictive factors in a defined population (errata appears in *Arthritis Rheum* 2000;43:1061). *Arthritis Rheum* 2000;43:584–592.
113. Mana J, Gomez-Vaquero C, Montero A, et al. Lofgren's syndrome revisited: a study of 186 patients. *Am J Med* 1999;107:240–245
114. Panush RS, Vonker RA, Diesk A, et al. Weber-Christian disease. *Medicine* 1985;64:181–190.
115. Lemley DE, Ferrans VJ, Fox LM, et al. Cardiac manifestations of Weber-Christian disease: report and review of the literature. *J Rheumatol* 1991;18:756–760.
116. Smith KC, Su WPD, Pittelkow MR, et al. Clinical and pathologic correlations with 96 patients with panniculitis, including 15 patients with deficient levels of alpha-1-antitrypsin. *J Am Acad Dermatol* 1989;21;1192–1196.
117. O'Riordan K, Blei A, Rao MS, et al. Suppurative panniculitis associated with alpha 1-antitrypsin deficiency (PiSZ phenotype) treated with doxycycline. *Br J Dermatol* 2001;144:1282–1283.
118. Humbert P, Faivre B, Gibey R, et al. Use of anti-collagenase properties of doxycycline in treatment of α_1-antitrypsin deficiency panniculitis. *Acta Derm Venereol* 1992;71:189–194.
119. Chng WJ, Henderson CA. Suppurative panniculitis associated with alpha 1-antitrypsin deficiency (PiSZ phenotype) treated with doxycycline. *Br J Dermatol* 2001;144:1282–1283.
120. Zimmerman-Gorska I, Urbaniak M, Karwowski A. Co-existence of arthritis, subcutaneous fat necrosis, and pseudocyst of pancreas. *Rheumatol Int* 1986;6: 45–58.
121. Mourad FH, Hannoush HM, Bahlawan M, et al. Panniculitis and arthritis as the presenting manifestation of chronic pancreatitis. *J Clin Gastroenterol* 2001; 32:259–261.
122. Roenigk HH, Haserick JR, Arundell FD. Post steroid panniculitis: report of a case and review of the literature. *Arch Dermatol* 1964;90;387–391.
123. Winklemann RK, McEvoy MT, Peters MS. Lipophagic panniculitis of childhood. *J Am Acad Dermatol* 1989;21:971–978.
124. Crotty C, Winkelmann R. Cytophagic histiocytic panniculitis with fever, cytopenia, liver failure, and terminal hemorrhagic diathesis. *J Am Acad Dermatol* 1981;4:181–194.
125. Weenig RH, Ng CS, Perniciaro C. Subcutaneous panniculitis-like T-cell lymphoma: an elusive case presenting as lipomembranous panniculitis and a review of 72 cases in the literature. *Am J Dermatopathol* 2001;23:206–215.
126. Buss TJ, Fearneyhough P, Callen JP. Subcutaneous panniculitis-like T-cell lymphoma presenting as lupus erythematosus panniculitis (submitted).
127. Alegre VA, Winkelmann RK. Histiocytic cytophagic panniculitis. *J Am Acad Dermatol* 1989;20:177–185.
128. Pettersson T, Kariniemi AL, Teryonen S, et al. Cytophagic histiocytic panniculitis: a report of four cases. *Br J Dermatol* 1992;127:635–640.
129. Tuffanelli DL. Lupus erythematosus (panniculitis) profundus: a classic revisited commentary and report of 22 cases. *Hawaii Med J* 1982;41:394–397.
130. Izumi AK, Takiguchi P. Lupus erythematosus panniculitis. *Arch Dermatol* 1983;119:61–64.
131. Martens PB, Moder KB, Ahmed I. Lupus panniculitis: clinical perspectives from a case series. *J Rheumatol* 1999;26:68–72.
132. Day S, Klein BL. Popsicle panniculitis. *Pediatr Emerg Care* 1992;8:91–93.
133. Jorizzo JL, White WL, Zanolli MD, et al. Sclerosing panniculitis. *Arch Dermatol* 1991;127:554–558.
134. Herouy Y. Lipodermatosclerosis and compression stockings. *J Am Acad Dermatol* 2000;42:307–308.
135. Lugo-Somoliros A, Sanchez JL, Mendez-Coll J, et al. Calcifying panniculitis associated with polycystic kidney disease and chronic renal failure. *J Am Acad Dermatol* 1990;22:743–747.
136. Buchet S, Blanc D, Humbert P, et al. Panniculite calcifiante. *Ann Dermatol Venereol* 1992;119:659–660.
136a. Au S, Crawford RI. Three-dimensional analysis of a calciphylaxsis plaque. *J Am Acad Dermatol* 2002;47:53–57.
137. International Study Group for Behçet's Disease. Criteria for diagnosis of Behçet's disease. *Lancet* 1990;335:1078–1080.
138. Ohno S, Ohguchi M, Abanmi A, et al. Close association of HLA-Bw51 in Behçet's disease. *Arch Ophthalmol* 1982;100:1455–1458.
139. Jorizzo JL, Rogers RS III. Behçet's disease. *J Am Acad Dermatol* 1990;23: 738–741.
140. Lie JT. Vascular involvement in Behçet's disease: arterial and venous and vessels of all sizes. *J Rheumatol* 1992;19:341–343.
141. Jorizzo JR, Solomon AR, Zanolli MD, et al. Neutrophilic vascular reactions. *J Am Acad Dermatol* 1988;19:983–1005.
142. Chun ST, Su WPD, Lee S, et al. Erythema nodosum-like lesions in Behçet's syndrome: a histopathologic study of 30 cases. *J Cutan Pathol* 1989;16: 259–265.
143. Stratigos AJ, LasKaris G, Stratigos JD. Behçet's disease. *Semin Neurol* 1992;12: 346–357.
144. Colvard DM, Robertson DM, O'Duffy D. The ocular manifestations of Behçet's disease. *Arch Ophthalmol* 1977;95:1813–1817.
145. deBois MHW, Geelhoed-Duijvestijn PHLM, Westedt ML. Behçet's syndrome treated with colchicine. *Neth J Med* 1991;38:175–176.
146. Nishimura H, et al. Treatment of Behçet's disease with diamino-diphenyl sulfone (DDS). *J Dermatol Treat* 1993;4:77–79.
147. Hamuyrudan V, Mat C, Saip S, et al. Thalidomide in the treatment of the mucocutaneous lesions of the Behçet syndrome: a randomized, double-blind, placebo-controlled trial. *Ann Intern Med* 1998;128:443–450.
148. Kaklamani VG, Kaklamanis PG. Treatment of Behçet's disease-An update. *Semin Arthritis Rheum* 2001;30:299–312.
149. Jorizzo JL, White L, Wise CM, et al. Low-dose weekly methotrexate for unusual neutrophilic vascular reactions: cutaneous polyarteritis nodosa and Behçet's disease. *J Am Acad Dermatol* 1991;24:973–978.
150. Alpsoy E, Yilmaz E, Basaran E. Interferon therapy for Beçhet's disease. *J Am Dermatol* 1994 Oct;31(4):617–619.
151. Demiroglu H, Ozecebe OI, Barista I, et al. Interferon alfa-2a, colchicine, and benzathine penicillin versus colchicine and benzathine penicillin in Behçet's disease: a randomized trial. *Lancet* 2000; 355: 650–609.
152. O'Duffy JD. Vasculitis in Behçet's disease. *Rheum Dis Clin North Am* 1990;16: 423–431.
153. Tessler HH, Jennings T. High-dose, short-term chlorambucil for intractable sympathetic ophthalmioa and Behçet's disease. *Br J Ophthalmol* 1990;74: 353–357.
154. Huong DLT, et al. Interet des "bolus" de cyclophosphamide dans la maladie de Behçet: experience des 17 cas. *Presse Med* 1990;15:1335–1338.
155. Yazici H, Pazarli H, Barnes CG, et al. A controlled trial of azathioprine in Behçet's disease. *N Engl J Med* 1990;332:281–285.
156. Masada K, et al. Double-masked trial of cyclosporin versus colchicine and long-term open study of cyclosporin in Behçet's disease. *Lancet* 1989;1: 1093–1096.
157. Vansteenkiste JF, Penne P, Verschakelen JA, et al. Cyclosporin treatment in rapidly progressive pulmonary thromboembolic Behçet's disease. *Thorax* 1990;45:295–296.
158. Firestein GS, Gruber HE, Weisman MH, et al. Mouth and genital ulcers with inflamed cartilage: MAGIC syndrome. *Am J Med* 1985;79:65–72.
159. Gamboa F, Rivera JM, Mayoral L, et al. Behcet's disease and relapsing poly-

chondritis (MAGIC syndrome) associated with antiphospholipid syndrome. *Med Clin (Barc)* 1998;110:678–679.
160. Le Thi Huong D, Wechsler B, Piette JC, et al. Aortic insufficiency and recurrent valve prosthesis dehiscence in MAGIC syndrome. *J Rheumatol* 1993;20: 397–398.
161. Imai H, Motegi M, Mizuki N, et al. Mouth and genital ulcers with inflamed cartilage (MAGIC syndrome): a case report and literature review. *Am J Med Sci* 1997;314:330–332.
162. Katz SI, Gallin JI, Hertz KC, et al. Erythema elevatum diutinum: skin and systemic manifestations, immunologic studies and successful treatment with dapsone. *Medicine* 1977;56:443–455.
163. Yiannias JA, El-Azhary RA, Gibson LE. Erythema elevatum diutinum: a clinical and histopathologic study of 13 patients. *J Am Acad Dermatol* 1992;26: 38–44.
164. LeBoit P, Cockerell CJ. Nodular lesions of erythema elevatum diutinum in patients infected with the human immunodeficiency virus. *J Am Acad Dermatol* 1993;28:919–922.
165. Walker KD, Badame AJ. Erythema elevatum diutinum in a patient with Crohn's disease. *J Am Acad Dermatol* 1990;22:948–952.
166. Burns RE, Colville JM. Acne conglobata with septicemia. *Arch Dermatol* 1959;79:361–363.
167. Rosner IA, Burg A, Wisniewski JJ, et al. The clinical spectrum of the arthropathy associated with hidradenitis suppurativa and acne conglobata. *J Rheumatol* 1993;20:684–687.
168. Karvonen SL. Acne fulminans: report of clinical findings and treatment of twenty-four patients. *J Am Acad Dermatol* 1993;28:572–579.
169. Knitzer RH, Needleman BW. Musculoskeletal syndromes associated with acne. *Semin Arthritis Rheum* 1991;20:247–255.
170. Hellman DB. Spondyloarthropathy with hidradenitis suppurativa. *J Am Med Assoc* 1992;267;2363–2365.
171. Plewig G, Kligman AM. Acne fulminans. In: *Acne* Berlin: Springer-Verlag, 1975:196.
172. Seukeran DC, Cunliffe WJ. The treatment of acne fulminans: a review of 25 cases. *Br J Dermatol* 1999;141:307–309.
173. Hughes RA. Arthritis precipitated by isotretinoin treatment for acne vulgaris. *J Rheumatol* 1993;20:1241–1242.
174. McGee TC, Field RS, Loebl DH, et al. Pustulotic arthro-osteitis: a cause of atypical chest pain and a new arthritic syndrome. *South Med J* 1993;86: 469–472.
175. Kahn MF, Bouvier M, Palazzo E, et al. Sternoclavicular pustulotic osteitis (SAPHO): 20-year interval between skin and bone lesions. *J Rheumatol* 1991; 18:1104–1108.
176. Beretta-Piccoli BC, Sauvain MJ, Gal I, et al. Synovitis, acne, pustulosis, hyperostosis, osteitis (SAPHO) syndrome in childhood: a report of ten cases and review of the literature. *Eur J Pediatr* 2000;159:594–601.
177. Pras M, Zemer D, Langevitz P, et al. Familial Mediterranean fever. In: Maddison PJ, Isenberg DA, Woo PA, et al., eds. *Oxford textbook of rheumatology.* New York: Oxford University Press, 1993:913–917.
178. Majeed HA, Quabazard Z, Hijazi Z, et al. The cutaneous manifestation in children with familial Mediterranean fever (recurrent hereditary polyserositis): a six-year study. *Q J Med* 1990;75:607–616.
179. McDermott MF, Aksentijevich I, Galon J, et al. Germline mutations in the extracellular domains of the 55 kDa TNF receptor, TNFR1, define a family of dominantly inherited autoinflammatory syndromes. *Cell* 1999;97:133–144.
180. Goltz RW, Laymon CW. Multicentric reticulohistiocytosis of the skin and synovia. *Arch Dermatol* 1954;69:717–731.
181. Campbell DA, Edwards NL. Multicentric reticulohistiocytosis: systemic macrophage disorder. *Baillieres Clin Rheumatol* 1991;5:301–319.
182. Orkin M, Goltz RW, Good RA, et al. A study of multicentric reticulohistiocytosis. *Arch Dermatol* 1964;89:640–654.
183. Yee KC, Bowker CM, Tan CY, et al. Cardiac and systemic complications in multicentric reticulohistiocytosis. *Clin Exp Dermatol* 1993;18:555–558.
184. Maddison PJ. Multicentric reticulohistiocytosis. In: Maddison PJ, Isenberg, DA, Woo PA, et al., eds. *Oxford textbook of rheumatology.* New York: Oxford University Press, 1993:937–940.
185. Janssen BA, Kencian J, Brooks PM. Close temporal and anatomic relationship between multicentric reticulohistiocytosis and carcinoma of the breast. *J Rheumatol* 1992;19:322–324.
186. Lesher JL Jr, Allen BS. Multicentric reticulohistiocytosis. *J Am Acad Dermatol* 1984;11:713–723.
187. Ginsburg WW, O'Duffy JD, Morris JL, et al. Multicentric reticulo-histiocytosis: response to alkylating agents in six patients. *Ann Intern Med* 1989;111: 384–388.
188. Gourmelen O, Le Loet X, Fortier-Beaulieu M, et al. Methotrexate treatment of multicentric reticulo-histiocytosis. *J Rheumatol* 1991;18:627–628.
189. Cash JM, Tyree J, Recht M. Severe multicentric reticulohistiocytosis: disease stabilization achieved with methotrexate and hydroxychloroquine. *J Rheumatol* 1997;24:2250–2253.

CHAPTER 12

Infectious Diseases That Affect the Skin and Joint

Smeena Khan-Sabir and Victoria P. Werth

VIRAL INFECTIONS

Acute natural infection with many viruses can be associated with both skin and joint inflammation in humans. Viruses that affect joints include rubella, human Parvovirus, mumps, Epstein–Barr, hepatitis B and C, adenovirus, Coxsackie B, cytomegalovirus, varicella zoster, and several tropical arboviruses (1,2). Most of these viruses can also affect the skin. The arthritis induced by these viruses is usually self-limited, but a few can induce chronic or recurrent joint inflammation (3,4). The mechanisms of viral arthritis include immune complex formation, as in hepatitis B–associated arthritis (5), and direct viral invasion of synovial tissue, as seen in rubella-associated arthritis (6). *In vitro* joint tissue organ culture studies show that rubella, more than other arthritogenic viruses, replicates and penetrates deeply into the synovial membrane (7).

Parvovirus

HISTORY

Parvovirus B19 was discovered in 1974, while screening healthy blood donors for hepatitis B (8). In 1981, B19 was found in the serum of patients with aplastic crisis and sickle cell disease (9–11). Subsequently, B19 was found to play a role in aplastic anemias seen in those with other causes of chronic hemolytic anemias (12).

In 1983, erythema infectiosum, otherwise known as fifth disease, was found due to B19 (13,14). The association with hydrops fetalis and fetal death was made in 1984 (15); the association with arthropathy was made in 1985 (16,17).

EPIDEMIOLOGY

Asymptomatic infection may be diagnosed by finding elevated IgM antibodies to Parvovirus B19 and the seroprevalence of this in the adult population varies between 40% and 80% (18,19). These asymptomatic patients can be the source of outbreaks. The appearance of antibodies accelerates after 5 years of age suggesting that many individuals are infected after entering school and it appears that teachers, daycare center workers, and medical personnel are particularly at risk (20–22).

CUTANEOUS MANIFESTATIONS

The incubation period between infection and onset of symptoms may range from 6 to 18 days and has been reported to be as long as 28 days in some outbreaks. The disease begins with a prodrome, with onset of the rash within several days to a week (23). Erythema infectiosum is classically an erythematous, macular, or maculopapular eruption that gives a "slapped-cheek" appearance. The eruption, often pruritic, then spreads to the trunk and extremities, where it may develop a lacy or reticulated pattern. The lesions fade after several days. The viremia precedes the rash and the onset of the rash or polyarthralgias is associated with the development of the anti-B19 IgM antibody response that clears the viremia (19). Therefore, when patients present with cutaneous or joint symptoms, they are no longer infectious (2). Adults may have no eruption or only a lacelike erythema on the extremities and trunk, without the characteristic facial eruption (24) (Figs. 12.1 and 12.2).Unusual eruptions associated with Parvovirus B19 infection include purpura, petechiae, and vesiculopustules (25–28). One report described accentuation of petechiae on the wrists and ankles, in addition to the presence of Koplik spots (29).

RELATIONSHIP BETWEEN CUTANEOUS AND SYSTEMIC FEATURES

Most patients have pallor, fever, headache, lymphadenopathy, and malaise. Some have nonproductive cough, coryza, sore throat, vomiting, nausea, and abdominal pain. The course is typically more severe in adults than in children.

Up to 80% of adults, women more than men, develop joint pain. In adults, this is often an acute onset symmetric polyarthropathy most commonly involving the proximal interphalangeal and metacarpophalangeal joints. In children, the arthropathy can be asymmetric and pauciarticular most often affecting the knees (19). Arthropathy may occur with or without an exanthem. Joint complaints include severe pain, stiffness, and mild swelling (30). The joint pain lasts a median of five days, but has persisted for months to years, often with episodic flares. Many of these patients meet the American Rheumatism Association criteria for a diagnosis of rheumatoid arthritis (RA) (31). Associations have also been made with juvenile RA and adult Still disease associated with acute human Parvovirus B19 infection (32,33). Recently, there have been a number of reports of patients with chronic B19 associated arthritis developing systemic lupus erythematosus (34–36). Systemic vasculitis has been reported with B19 infection (37).

Complications of Parvovirus infection include encephalitis, meningitis, extremity numbness and tingling, and brachial

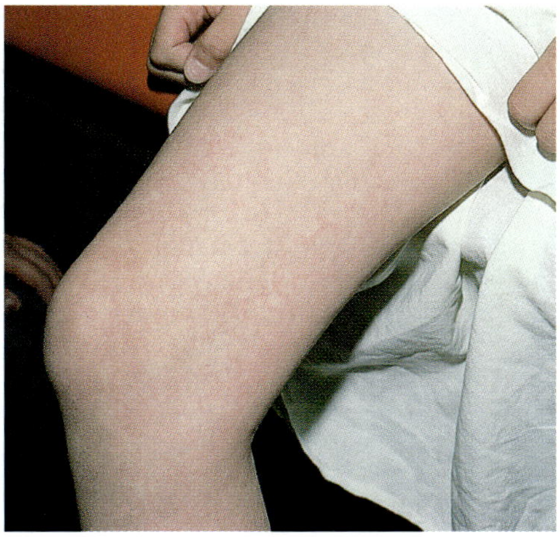

Figure 12.1. Parvovirus infection. Typical reticulated pattern on an extremity. (Courtesy of Paul Honig, M.D., Children's Hospital of Philadelphia, PA, with permission.)

plexus neuropathy (38,39). It is possible that a few cases of idiopathic thrombocytopenic purpura are related to B19 infection (37).

Transient aplastic crisis (TAC) occurs in a large number of patients with underlying hematologic disorders. Eighty percent to 93% of patients with TAC have evidence of recent B19 infection (31). In community outbreaks of infection, the incidence of TAC in patients with chronic hemolytic anemias has varied from 1.7% to 5% per year. Chronic B19 infection with anemia is seen with immunosuppressed hosts (40,41). Patients with acquired immunodeficiency syndrome (AIDS) and TAC have had a serum hemoglobin level less than 5 g/dL and absent reticulocytes. Chronic infection with B19 occurs with organ transplant recipients and has been associated with pancytopenia (42).

Infection of pregnant women is associated with an increased risk of fetal death and nonimmunologic hydrops (43,44). There does not appear to be an increase in birth defects. Approximately 50% of women are immune, but one study suggests that the annual incidence of infection in women of reproductive age was 1.5% (45,46). Two studies suggest that less than 10% of B19-infected pregnant women have adverse outcomes, with the greatest risk in the first 20 weeks of pregnancy (47,48). In one study, one third of the pregnant women with B19 infection were asymptomatic, and a recommendation was made to check B19 serologies in any pregnant woman exposed to erythema infectiosum (21).

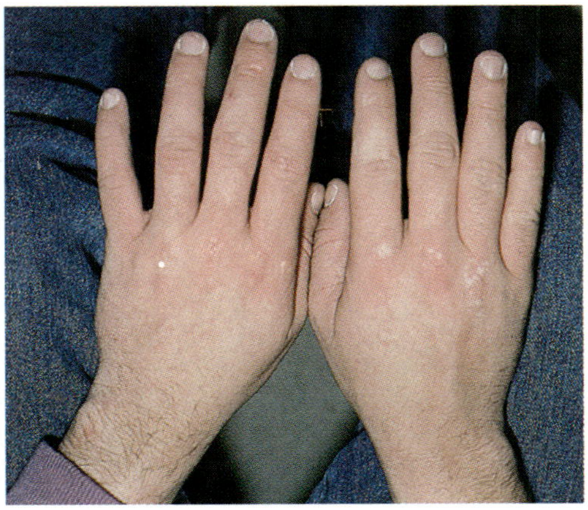

Figure 12.2. Parvovirus infection. Erythematous patches with fine desquamation localized in stocking-glove distribution.

PATHOLOGY AND IMMUNOPATHOLOGY

Histologic examination shows homogeneous, intranuclear inclusions with peripheral condensation of chromatin in erythroid precursor cells (15). Skin changes have not been well characterized and are not diagnostic.

LABORATORY FINDINGS

In the healthy host, an IgM antibody assay is optimal to detect recent B19 infection. The antibody test is usually positive by radioimmunoassay or enzyme immunoassay within 3 days of the development of symptoms and stays positive for 1 to 2 months (49). The test is usually positive at the time of the skin and arthritic manifestations. IgG becomes positive several days after IgM and lasts years.

Serologic results are less reliable in patients with hematologic disorders. They may present before the tests are positive and antibody levels can fluctuate in chronic infections. Tests for B19 DNA or viral antigens using hybridization assays or polymerase chain reaction (PCR) are best for these patients, and can be used in many different tissues and body fluids (31). There is no practical *in vitro* system for B19 isolation from clinical specimens.

Patients with hematologic diseases have severe anemia and a low reticulocyte count, with frequent transient thrombocytopenia and neutropenia. The bone marrow shows a near absence of red cell precursors. Bone marrow necrosis may be extensive. During recovery, 10 to 12 days after onset of symptoms, the peripheral smear shows reticulocytosis, leukocytosis, and thrombocytosis. The bone marrow is hypererythroblastic.

DIFFERENTIAL DIAGNOSIS

The differential diagnosis includes rubella, measles, scarlet fever, roseola, enteroviral infection, erysipelas, and drug hypersensitivity.

MANAGEMENT AND PROGNOSIS

Any patient with hereditary hemolytic anemias admitted to a hospital with a febrile illness should be evaluated for aplasia and, if an aplastic crisis is suspected, they should be placed in respiratory and contact isolation (20,43,50). Blood transfusion may be required for management of the anemia. Patients with AIDS or organ transplant recipients with B19 infection have responded to treatment with intravenous immunoglobulin (31). The management for B19-exposed pregnant women is unclear (31).

ETIOLOGIC FACTORS AND PATHOGENESIS

B19 is a small, nonenveloped single-stranded DNA virus belonging to the family Parvoviridae (51). One study showed human Parvovirus B19 DNA in the synovial tissue in 30 of 39 patients with joint fluid of two patients with arthritis, suggesting that direct invasion of the virus is responsible for the transient arthritis (52). Chronic B19 arthropathy is associated with persistence of either B19 virus or select B19 DNA sequences in the bone marrow and synovium (53,54).

Rubella

HISTORY

Before the live rubella vaccine, rubella was a common cause of a mild illness with exanthem. Since routine vaccination, the number of cases has dropped by 99% and it is now mainly seen in those over age 15 who have failed to be vaccinated (55).

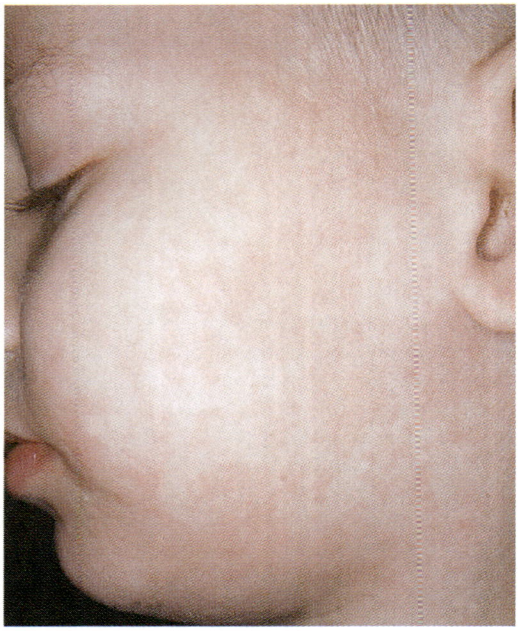

Figure 12.3. Rubella. Morbilliform eruption on face. (Courtesy of Bill Witmer, M.D., Department of Dermatology, University of Pennsylvania, with permission.)

EPIDEMIOLOGY

Rubella is most prevalent in the spring, is only moderately contagious, and is thus seen in group settings. The disease is spread via the respiratory route, and is contagious during the 5 days preceding and 7 days following the onset of the rash. It occurs most commonly in the spring.

CUTANEOUS MANIFESTATIONS

The rash is variable in extent and duration. Discrete pink macules and papules begin on the face and progress down to involve the trunk and extremities (Fig. 12.3). The rash may become confluent and at times may appear morbilliform or scarletiniform. An enathem (Forscheimer spots) consisting of pinpoint, rose-colored macules and petechiae on the soft palate occasionally occurs. The exanthem usually resolves in 2 or 3 days, clearing first on the face, and sometimes resolving with fine desquamation centrally.

RELATIONSHIP BETWEEN CUTANEOUS AND SYSTEMIC FEATURES

There is an incubation period of 14 to 21 days, followed by a prodrome of cough, fever, malaise, sore throat, loss of appetite, nausea, headache, lymphadenopathy, and eye pain. Tender enlargements of the suboccipital, postauricular, and anterior and posterior cervical nodes are most common, occurring just before or simultaneously with the rash. Prodromal symptoms occur mainly in older children and adults.

Rubella is one of the most arthritogenic viruses, and is associated with both acute and chronic joint inflammation, especially in adult women (7,56,57). In several outbreaks of natural rubella, more than 50% of adult women have developed joint inflammation and in 30%, the symptoms lasted over 6 months (58). Arthralgias and arthritis involve the fingers, wrists, and knees. Joint inflammation may precede the exanthem (59) or be the only manifestation of rubella, as seen in one case of rubella reinfection (60). There is evidence that rubella may play a role in both juvenile and adult RA: Rubella virus has been identified in the synovial fluid of patients with juvenile RA and RA (61–63). Rubella vaccination has also been associated with arthropathy and in a randomized placebo-controlled study of vaccination of nonimmune women with the live, attenuated rubella vaccine, acute arthropathy was significantly more frequent in the vaccinated women (64). However, chronic joint symptoms are not seen after rubella vaccination (65).

Acute encephalitis occurs 2 to 4 days after the rash in about one of 6,000 patients with rubella and may cause death in up to 20%. Ascending polyneuritis, thrombocytopenia, pericarditis, and myocarditis have been reported. The worst complication is the congenital rubella syndrome, with many specific organ defects and 20% to 30% mortality in the first year. First-trimester exposure causes infection in more than 90% of fetuses, with 50% having major organ damage in the first month.

PATHOLOGY AND IMMUNOPATHOLOGY

Skin biopsy shows a nondiagnostic, mild, superficial perivascular mononuclear cell infiltrate.

LABORATORY FINDINGS

Serologic testing by hemagglutination-inhibition, neutralization fluorescent complement fixation, immunodiffusion, or enzyme-linked immunosorbent assay (ELISA) confirms the diagnosis. The hemagglutination-inhibition antibodies are easily measured and a fourfold increase in titer in convalescence over acute titers is indicative of new infection. The hemagglutination-inhibition and neutralizing antibodies persist throughout life.

DIFFERENTIAL DIAGNOSIS

Other clinical considerations include other viral infections, such as rubeola, scarlet fever, or infectious mononucleosis.

MANAGEMENT AND PROGNOSIS

The prognosis is excellent, except for those with rare central nervous system (CNS) involvement. There are many risks to the fetus exposed to rubella in utero, and abortion is recommended in at least the first 18 weeks of gestation if the fetus is shown to be infected.

The arthritis can be either acute or chronic, and is treated symptomatically with aspirin or nonsteroidal antiinflammatory agents.

Prevention is the main goal, with immunization with live attenuated vaccine recommended since 1969 for all infants 15 months or older. The disease has rare sequelae, except for the effects on the fetus.

ETIOLOGIC FACTORS AND PATHOGENESIS

Rubella is caused by a togavirus, an RNA virus.

Varicella-Zoster Virus Infections

HISTORY

Varicella was confused with smallpox until 1767 (66). The name chickenpox is likely from the old English *gican*, "to itch" (67). The term shingles is from the Latin *cingulus*, meaning girdle (66).

EPIDEMIOLOGY

The United States adopted a universal vaccination against varicella in 1995 that has greatly reduced the frequency of this infection. However, varicella is highly contagious and children who are not vaccinated remain susceptible. Varicella usually occurs in the late winter and early spring in temperate climates. The distribution is worldwide, with no differing racial or sexual susceptibility. The prodromal and vesicular stages are highly infec-

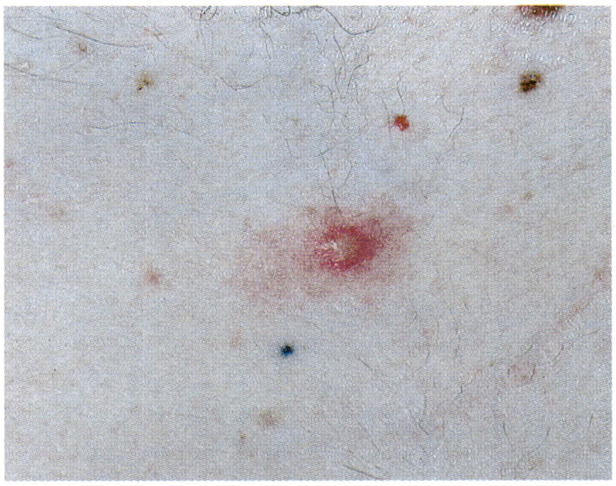

Figure 12.4. Varicella. Vesicle with surrounding erythema.

tious. Herpes zoster occurs at some point in 10% to 20% of all persons. The incidence and severity of herpes zoster increases with age.

CLASSIFICATION

Varicella is caused by primary infection with varicella-zoster virus, a member of the human herpesvirus family. Herpes zoster is due to reactivation of the latent virus in a host previously infected with the virus.

CUTANEOUS MANIFESTATIONS

Varicella spreads primarily by airborne respiratory droplets and has an incubation period that ranges from 10 to 21 days, with an average of 17 days. There is a 1- to 2-day prodrome with moderate fever, chills, myalgias, arthralgias, and malaise prior to or beginning with the skin lesions. The exanthem begins on the scalp or trunk, with subsequent spread to the extremities, as erythematous macules that develop into 2- to 4-mm vesicles surrounded by erythema (Fig. 12.4). New lesions develop over 3 to 4 days, and become pustular, umbilicated, and crusted. The vesicles characteristically appear in crops and are intensely pruritic. The hallmark of varicella infection is the simultaneous presence of different stages of the rash. A low-grade fever may accompany the eruption.

Herpes zoster begins as burning pain or pruritus in the affected dermatome for 4 to 5 days prior to the development of grouped vesicles on an erythematous base (Fig. 12.5). There can be associated symptoms of fever, malaise, and regional adenopathy. The lesions resolve over about 3 weeks. Dissemination occurs only in immunocompromised hosts.

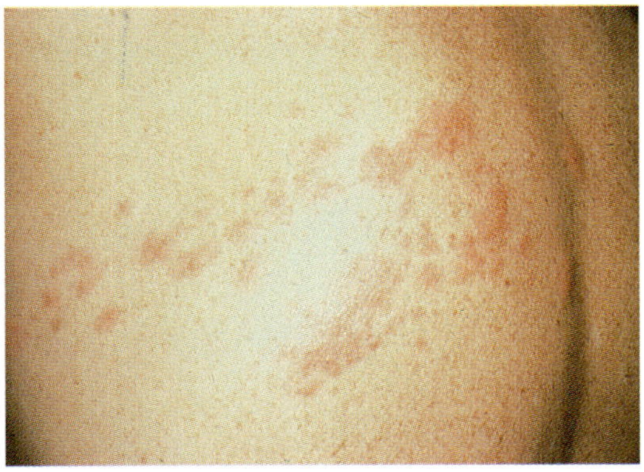

Figure 12.5. Herpes-zoster infection. Dermatomal vesicles on erythematous base.

RELATIONSHIP BETWEEN CUTANEOUS AND SYSTEMIC FEATURES

The most dreaded complications of varicella are pneumonia and encephalitis, seen more commonly in very young children, adults, and immunocompromised patients (68). Pneumonia is seen in 50% of adults with varicella and has a mortality rate of 10% to 30%. Symptoms of pneumonia include cough, dyspnea, and fever beginning 1 to 6 days after the rash. The mortality rate of varicella encephalitis in adults is about 35%. Other complications include bacterial superinfection, aseptic meningitis, Guillain–Barré syndrome, transverse myelitis, gastritis, appendicitis, glomerulonephritis, hepatitis, Reye syndrome, thrombocytopenia, conjunctivitis, carditis, orchitis, and syndrome of inappropriate secretion of antidiuretic hormone.

Neonatal varicella presents within 10 days of birth and is due to transmission of the virus late in pregnancy (69). Neonatal varicella can be severe, with a prolonged course, high fever, visceral complications, and a mortality rate of around 30% (70–72).

Congenital varicella syndrome is caused by maternal varicella infection between 8 and 20 weeks of gestation. The risk is less than 3%, but includes many neurologic and eye abnormalities, as well as skeletal, gastrointestinal, and genitourinary anomalies (70–72).

There are a number of reports on acute arthritis as a rare complication of varicella (73–75). It is usually a monoarthritis affecting large joints such as the knee most frequently, followed by the ankle, shoulder, hip, wrist, and small joints of the hands or feet. The arthritis typically begins 3.6 days after the rash, with only one report of arthritis occurring prior to the rash (76). Among 20 reported cases of varicella-associated arthritis, the average age was 6.1 years, with a range of 1.5 to 13 years. Varicella-associated arthritis in adults is exceedingly rare (77). Interestingly, there are reports of several cases of severe recalcitrant juvenile RA transiently developing remission during infection with varicella (78,79). Rarely the arthritis is due to bacterial pathogens, probably due to hematogenous spread to a joint from an infected varicella joint lesion (76). In herpes zoster, paresis and meningoencephalitis may be associated with involvement of motor neurons and the CNS, usually occurring 2 to 4 weeks after involvement of cranial nerve ganglia.

Arthritis associated with herpes zoster is rare, with four reports in the literature (80). Local joint pain with or without an effusion can precede the zoster.

PATHOLOGY AND IMMUNOPATHOLOGY

The pathology of skin lesions of varicella and zoster is identical. The characteristic changes in infected cells are enlarged cells with pale, vacuolated cytoplasm and formation of intranuclear inclusion bodies (81). Multinucleated giant cells are formed by the fusion of adjacent infected cells.

LABORATORY FINDINGS

Diagnosis of varicella or herpes zoster can be made by Tzanck smear or skin biopsy in 50% to 80% of patients. These show either balloon cells or multinucleated giant cells. Viral culture from vesicular fluid is most definitive, but takes at least 2 to 3 days. Rapid methods of identifying viral antigens in vesicular fluid include immunofluorescence, PCR, countercurrent immunoelectrophoresis, and gel diffusion. Serologic diagnosis of acute varicella infection depends on a fourfold rise in varicella-zoster antibody titer between an acute and convalescent sera.

In varicella arthritis, the white blood cell (WBC) count in the synovial fluid is usually quite low, but with a wide range up to 51,700/μL, with a predominance of mononuclear cells (74). Isolation of varicella virus from synovial fluid in nonbacterial cases is uncommon. It is important to aspirate joints to exclude treatable bacterial infection.

DIFFERENTIAL DIAGNOSIS

Varicella must be differentiated from disseminated herpes simplex, disseminated zoster, hand-foot-and-mouth disease, other vesicular enteroviral exanthems, and vesicular arthropod bites. Herpes simplex may present in a zosteriform distribution, and thus vesicle fluid culture can differentiate between simplex and zoster.

MANAGEMENT AND PROGNOSIS

Varicella in childhood should be treated with antipruritic lotion and oral antihistamines. Salicylates should not be used because of an association with Reye syndrome. Varicella and zoster are usually benign in healthy persons. Most complications occur in immunocompromised persons, neonates, adolescents, and adults. Intravenous acyclovir should be used in immunocompromised hosts. Vidarabine and parenteral human interferon-α have been also shown to be efficacious in the treatment of varicella in this population but significant side effects limit their use and acyclovir continues to be the drug of choice in treating varicella infections in the immunocompromised. Although varicella-zoster immunoglobulin (VZIG) is used in treating immunocompromised patients who have received a significant exposure to varicella, one third of these patients will still develop clinical infection. Vaccination remains an important modality in reducing infection in the immunocompromised as well as healthy individuals (82). Intravenous acyclovir therapy is used in patients with trigeminal zoster or in those at high risk of dissemination. High-dose oral acyclovir must be given within 3 days of onset of lesions to show any effect in terms of pain or decreased viral shedding (83). Adolescents or adults with respiratory symptoms should have a chest radiograph and arterial blood gas level, and be started on intravenous acyclovir if pneumonia is found. A pregnant woman exposed to varicella or zoster should have the ELISA test done for varicella-zoster virus. Immunoglobulin should be given to exposed seronegative pregnant women to prevent varicella complications.

ETIOLOGIC FACTORS AND PATHOGENESIS

The varicella-zoster virus is in the DNA herpesvirus group. The nasopharynx is the initial site of infection, followed by viremia, leading to spread to the skin and other organs. Infection of the sensory ganglia leads to latent infection of the ganglia. With increasing age or changes in immune status, possibly due to alterations in cellular immunity, replication of the latent virus resumes and the virus moves down the nerve toward the skin (84–86).

The etiology of the arthritis seen in varicella and herpes zoster is possibly due to the virus or to immune-complex deposition.

BACTERIAL, SPIROCHETAL, AND MYCOBACTERIAL INFECTIONS

Disseminated Gonorrhea Infection

HISTORY

Gonorrhea (GC) is derived from the Greek *gonos*, "seed," and *rhoea*, "flow," and was first used by Galen. GC has existed since ancient Egypt, and passages in the Old Testament and Talmud refer to genital exudates (87). Gonococcal urethritis was not differentiated from nongonococcal urethritis during the first half of the 20th century.

EPIDEMIOLOGY

Human beings are the only reservoir for the gonococcus. There has been a slow decrease overall in the incidence of GC in the past decade, with 150 cases per 100,000 Americans infected in 1995 (88). Approximately 0.5% to 3% of cases of GC disseminate (89–91). In the past decade, the strains of GC that cause disseminated gonorrhea infection (DGI) have become uncommon (92). Women are more commonly asymptomatic prior to DGI. However, asymptomatic male carriers are also an important part of the epidemiology of GC by virtue of their frequent asymptomatic infections of the pharynx and rectum (93). Antibiotic-resistant strains developed in the Far East and Africa and were imported to the United States.

CLASSIFICATION

Proven DIC requires a positive blood or synovial fluid culture. A diagnosis of probable DIC requires a positive primary mucosal site culture. The diagnosis of possible DIC is made if the symptoms respond to antibiotics.

CUTANEOUS MANIFESTATIONS

Fifty percent to 75% of patients with DGI develop skin lesions. The lesions, of which there may be from four to 50, are discrete erythematous papules or petechiae that rapidly evolve into pustules, often painful and necrotic, on an erythematous base (87,94). They are located on the extremities, usually acral and around joints, and only rarely on the trunk (Fig. 12.6). They may be macular, vesicular, bullous, or purpuric (95). New skin lesions may appear during the first 24 to 48 hours of treatment. The skin lesions are less common if arthritis is present (96).

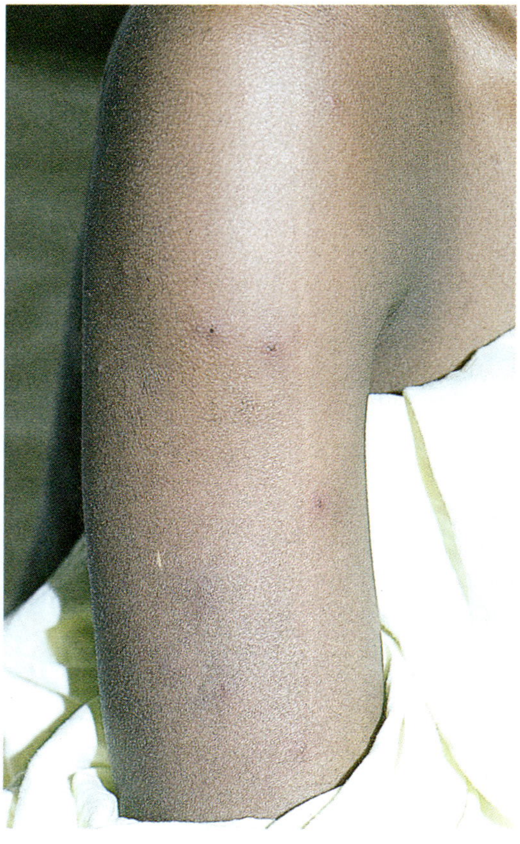

Figure 12.6. Disseminated gonorrhea. Erythematous papules on arm.

RELATIONSHIP BETWEEN CUTANEOUS AND SYSTEMIC FEATURES

Patients with DGI often lack local symptoms of gonococcal infection, but have positive cultures from urogenital, pharyngeal, or rectal sites. Dissemination in women often occurs several days after the start of the menstrual period (94,96,97). Pregnancy may be a risk factor for dissemination (94,96,97).

Patients with DGI typically develop either of two syndromes (97). In one, there is a triad of polyarthralgias (without purulent arthritis), tenosynovitis, and dermatitis. Involvement of the distal extremities is most common. 65% have tenosynovitis, often asymmetric, involving the dorsal tendons of the hand and wrist (97) Fever is usually present. Thirty percent to 40% of patients with dissemination develop a second syndrome, with development of a purulent arthritis later in the course, at times in an asymmetric pattern. The knee, ankle, elbow, wrist, and small joints of the hands and feet are frequently involved in a migratory pattern where one joint heals as the next become inflamed (98). The arthritis can lead to permanent joint damage.

Fifteen percent to 30% of women with urogenital GC develop salpingitis (99,100). Sterility and ectopic pregnancy are frequent problems (101). Ascending gonococcal infection during pregnancy may cause septic abortion before the twelvth week of gestation and chorioamnionitis after the 16th week. Chorioamnionitis can lead to premature rupture of membranes and premature labor (102).

Without treatment, patients can develop endocarditis, with rapid destruction of the aortic valve, meningitis, and perihepatitis.

PATHOLOGY AND IMMUNOPATHOLOGY

Pustular lesions are usually seen in an intraepidermal location with neutrophils both within them and in the dermis. The capillaries in the upper and mid dermis are surrounded by an infiltrate of neutrophils, often with nuclear dust, mononuclear cells, and red cells. Fibrinoid material may be seen in the walls of some vessels, and fibrin thrombi in some lumina (103). Cutaneous vasculitis has been reported as the sole manifestation of the disease (104). Bullae are subepidermal. Gram-negative diplococci in the walls of blood vessels are rarely seen in tissue sections (103). Immunoglobulin and complement have been detected in skin lesions (105). In one study, immunofluorescent staining techniques revealed gonococcal antigens in 14 of 16 sterile skin lesions (106).

LABORATORY FINDINGS

Diagnosis is made by culture of the blood, synovial fluid, endocervical canal, urethra, rectum, and pharynx. Culture of the columnar epithelium of the rectum and endocervix is better than culture of the vagina and anus. Specimens should be plated immediately on chocolate and Thayer-Martin agar and incubated at 37°C at a CO_2 concentration of 5% (87). Specimens for culture that must be transported to a central laboratory may be obtained using reduced, nonnutrient transport media containing activated charcoal to absorb inhibitors. These specimens are viable for up to 6 hours with minimal loss of viability (87). Sexual contacts should also be cultured.

The diagnosis of DGI can only be made if cultures are positive from blood, skin, or synovial tissue. Less than 50% of blood or synovial fluid cultures and less than 5% of vesicular skin lesions are culture-positive. Positive synovial cultures occur only in those with purulent joint effusions; GC is recovered from only 25% to 50% of these (107). PCR also allows identification of *Neisseria gonorrhoeae* in synovial fluid with a sensitivity of 78% (108). Eighty percent of mucosal cultures are positive (90). Immunofluorescence staining of skin lesions is more sensitive than PCR (98).

The synovial fluid leukocyte count has a mean of over 50,000 cells per cubic millimeter (98). Circulating immune complexes are common.

DIFFERENTIAL DIAGNOSIS

The differential includes meningococcemia, *Haemophilus influenzae,* and rare organisms such as *Streptobacillus moniliformis,* which can give similar skin lesions and arthritis (109).

MANAGEMENT AND PROGNOSIS

Hospitalization is recommended for patients with DGI to rule out serious complications, such as endocarditis and meningitis, and to evaluate the response to treatment. Hospitalization is especially important for noncompliant patients, those in whom diagnosis is uncertain, and those who have purulent synovial effusions or other complications (107).

There has been increased antibiotic resistance to GC since 1980 (110,111). The GC strains causing DGI are usually susceptible to penicillin, but a few cases of DGI due to β-lactamase–producing GC have been reported (112). Resistance to tetracyclines and fluoroquinolones has also been reported (111,113). The current recommendations by the Centers for Disease Control and Prevention (CDC) are shown in Table 12.1 (114).

More than 90% of patients improve within 48 hours after beginning antibiotic therapy (107). Failure to improve makes the diagnosis suspect; therefore, to assess clinical improvement, antipyretics or antiinflammatory medications should be avoided until the diagnosis is definitive.

It is important to test for coexisting *Chlamydia trachomatis* infection, which can be seen in up to 50% of those infected with GC (115,116). Patients treated for DGI should also be treated for concurrent *C. trachomatis* infection with oral doxycycline 100 mg twice daily or oral tetracycline 500 mg four times daily for 7 days. Approximately one in 2,500 females and one in 1,250 males with GC also have syphilis (117). Diagnosis of GC should prompt an evaluation for other sexually transmitted diseases, including human immunodeficiency virus (HIV).

Arthrocentesis is both diagnostic and therapeutic for the arthritis. Repeated arthrocentesis may be necessary for large effusions until the joint is no longer tense. Open drainage is rarely indicated, and instilling antibiotics in the joint is of no benefit (94).

TABLE 12.1. Centers for Disease Control and Prevention Recommendations

Recommended initial regimen
Ceftriaxone 1 g IM or IV every 24 h
Alternative initial regimens
Cefotaxime 1 g IV every 8 h
or
Ceftizoxime 1 g IV every 8 h
or
For persons allergic to β-lactam drugs:
Spectinomycin 2 g IM every 12 h
All regimens should be continued for 24–48 h after improvement begins, then therapy may be switched to one of the regimens that follow to complete a full week of antimicrobial therapy:
Cefixime 400 mg orally 2 times a day,
or
Ciprofloxacin 500 mg orally 2 times a day.
Ciprofloxacin is contraindicated for pregnant and lactating women, children, and adolescents ≤17 years of age.

IM, intramuscular; IV, intravenous.
From Centers for Disease Control and Prevention. 1998 Guidelines for treatment of sexually transmitted diseases. *MMWR Recomm Rep* 1998;217:1–111, with permission.

Barrier contraceptive methods are somewhat protective against GC and use of oral contraceptives is associated with a twofold increased relative risk of GC (118). Nonoxynol 9, found in vaginal spermicides, is bactericidal for GC (119).

Before antibiotics, gonococcal arthritis often resulted in residual inflammation in a single joint for several weeks, resulting in ankylosis of that joint.

ETIOLOGIC FACTORS AND PATHOGENESIS

Patients with deficiencies in the terminal components of the complement system are at increased risk of developing DGI (120). Two reports also suggest deficiency of the second component of complement can be associated with disseminated GC (121,122).

In addition, certain strains of GC are more likely to disseminate. It is known that strains of GC that disseminate are resistant to the complement-requiring bactericidal activity of normal human serum (123), share certain nutritional requirements (124), and may have defective complement-dependent chemotaxis of polymorphonuclear leukocytes (125). Certain proteins on the cell wall have been identified as important responsible factors participating in the extent and the severity of the infection (94,126,127). Strains of GC isolated from patients with septic arthritis tend to be less serum-resistant than strains isolated from patients with tenosynovitis and skin lesions (128).

Dissemination occurs several days after the start of menstruation because sloughing of the endometrium exposes the submucosal vessels to the bacteria (96,129). Alternatively, cervical mucus is a potential barrier to the passage of bacteria from the vagina to the uterus. Changes in the cervical mucus during menses may permit entrance of gonococci into the uterus (100). In addition, GC cells change their colony phenotype during menses, perhaps becoming more invasive (130). Changes in the endometrium or cervix seen in menses or pregnancy may select more virulent strains and account for the female prevalence of DGI (129).

The etiology of the skin lesions is due to the GC organism or to an immunologic reaction to the organism.

Antibiotic resistance is mediated by two different mechanisms. Plasmid-mediated production of penicillinase results in a high level of resistance to penicillin (131). A second mechanism is chromosomal resistance to the effects of penicillin (127,131).

Lyme Disease

HISTORY

Lyme disease was first described in the United States 17 years ago (132). The name is derived from Lyme, Connecticut, where the original cluster of Lyme arthritis was noted. Erythema chronica migrans (ECM) was first described in 1909 in Sweden (133). An association with lymphocytic meningitis, painful radiculitis, and cranial nerve palsy was subsequently noted (134, 135), as well as the association with ECM and tick bite (136). The CDC began surveillance for Lyme disease in 1982; it became a nationally reportable disease in 1990 (137).

EPIDEMIOLOGY

Lyme disease is now known to be the leading tickborne illness in the United States. There were 120 cases in 1980, 4,572 in 1988, 9,465 in 1991, and 12,952 cases reported to the CDC in 47 states in 1996 (138). The rise in incidence is due to increased recognition, reporting, transmission, and increased density of deer herds (139,140). Over 85% of cases are reported from Southern New England and the mid-Atlantic states (138). Children younger than 15 years and adults aged 25 to 44 years are at greatest risk because of greater outdoor exposures (139). The ECM lesions of Lyme disease have a seasonal distribution in most localities, with 80% of cases in Connecticut occurring in June and July. Lyme disease has been reported in western, middle, and Eastern Europe, trans-Ural areas, North America, England, China, Japan, Southeast Asia, Australia, and South Africa (141).

CLASSIFICATION

Like most spirochetal illnesses, the disease is divided into three stages, with only some patients having all three stages. Others present with stage II or III disease. Features of the individual stages may blend, so separation of stages may be difficult (142).

Stage I is early localized disease, where the skin lesions of ECM, often with minor constitutional symptoms, develop within 1 month of tick bite (range, 1 to 32 days; median, 7 days).

Stage II is early disseminated infection, with multiple ECM lesions, potential complications of carditis, neurologic disease, musculoskeletal symptoms, lymphocytoma, lymphadenopathy, ophthalmologic findings, and liver involvement. This is seen days to 10 months after the tick bite.

Stage 3 is chronic or persistent disease, with manifestations including musculoskeletal symptoms, fibromyalgia, neurologic disease, and skin lesions of acrodermatitis chronica atrophicans (ACA) and possibly morphea.

CUTANEOUS MANIFESTATIONS

ECM is the pathognomonic skin lesion of Lyme disease, is the first manifestation of Lyme disease in 60% to 80% of people, and occurs at the site of the tick bite (143). Only one third of the patients recall a bite (144). At the time of the skin lesion, which occurs within a few days to a month after the bite, the spirochetes enter the circulation and disseminate. The skin findings may be associated with fever, chills, fatigue, headache, neck stiffness, myalgias, arthralgias, conjunctivitis, erythematous throat, and regional or generalized lymphadenopathy. Rarely, hepatosplenomegaly and right upper quadrant tenderness occur.

The lesions of ECM begin as red macules that become papular and then expand into an erythematous, annular plaque. There are two forms of ECM. In one, there is an expanding red plaque with varying intensities of redness within the plaque. In the second, there is a target, with a central red plaque surrounded by normal-appearing skin, which in turn is surrounded by another band of erythema. As the lesion enlarges, the central erythema can fade. The central portion of the lesion may be edematous, vesicular, urticarial, or crusted. Triangular and elongated oval lesions have been described, but circular lesions are most frequent. The most common locations are the inguina, axillae, midriff or behind the knees (145). ECM lesions are usually asymptomatic, but can be pruritic or painful. They can enlarge very rapidly and multiple lesions due to hematogenous spread are seen 17% of the time (146) (Figs. 12.7 and 12.8). Untreated ECM lesions resolve in a median of 28 days (range, 1 day to 14 months) (143). Resolution is within a few days after treatment with antibiotics.

Borrelial lymphocytoma occurs a median of 30 to 45 days after a tick bite and is seen in 1% to 3% of patients with Lyme disease in Europe (147). There are no cases reported from the United States. Clinically, the lesion is a red–purple to bluish-red, sometimes-painful, nodule. The usual location is on the earlobe in children and nipple of the breast in adults (147), but cases have been seen on the nose, scrotum, upper arm, and shoulder. Spirochetal stains and cultures of biopsies of lymphocytoma lesions have revealed *Borrelia* species; patients have had positive Lyme antibody titers (147). Lymphocytoma can persist for months if untreated, but clears in 3 weeks with antibiotics (148).

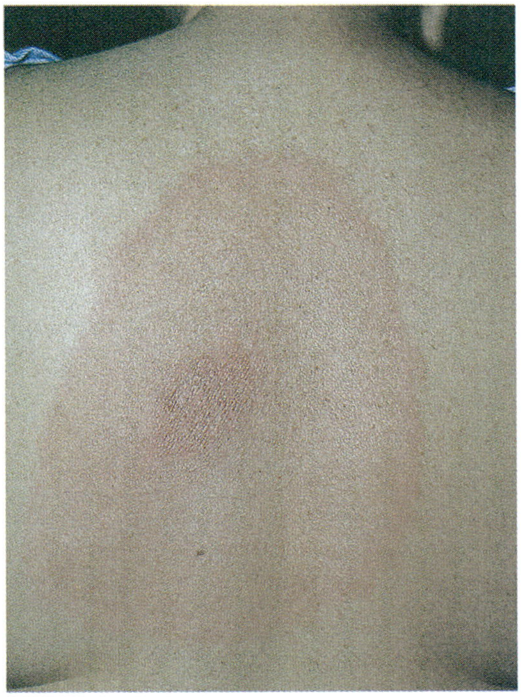

Figure 12.7. Erythema chronica migrans. Rapidly expanding target-appearing plaque on back.

ACA is associated with late Lyme disease. It occurs mainly in women between the ages of 40 and 70 years. The lesions begin on an extremity, usually the lower leg or foot, as a bluish-red edematous plaque. Fibrous bands may develop, especially on the ulnar and tibial regions, and fibrous nodules may form near joints. Regional lymphadenopathy is often present. Over many years, the skin becomes atrophic (149). *Borrelia burgdorferi* has been isolated from the skin of patients with ACA (150).

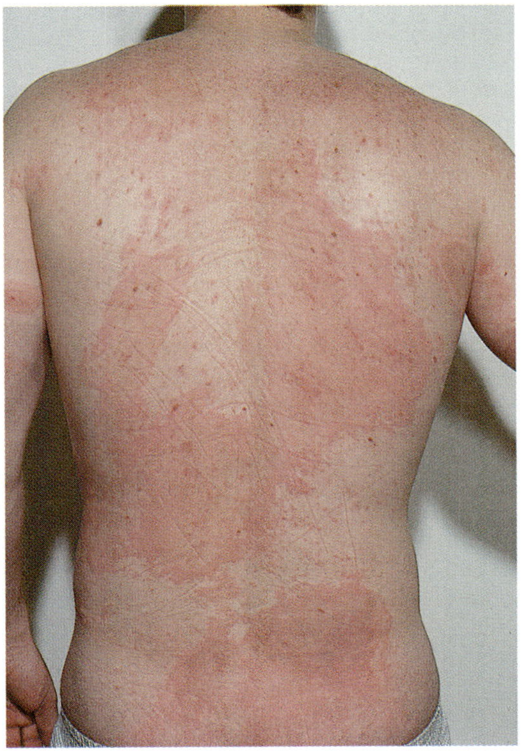

Figure 12.8. Erythema chronica migrans. Multiple, somewhat irregularly shaped erythematous plaques on back. (Courtesy of Bill Witmer, M.D., Department of Dermatology, University of Pennsylvania, with permission.)

Reports in Europe have suggested that some morphea lesions are also associated with Lyme disease (151). This issue has been controversial because morphea and lichen sclerosus et atrophicus–like lesions may develop in about 10% of patients with ACA and may represent sclerotic and atrophic changes of ACA (152). One recent German study used DNA amplification to show the presence of *B. burgdorferi* in lesions of morphea and lichen sclerosus et atrophicus in patients that were seronegative for *Borrelia* infection (153).

RELATIONSHIP BETWEEN CUTANEOUS AND SYSTEMIC FEATURES

With dissemination of the infection, usually several days to 10 months after the tick bite, prominent systemic symptoms of fever, myalgia, arthralgia, headache, regional or generalized lymphadenopathy, and stiff neck can be seen. Multiple, secondary skin lesions are occasionally seen. In this second stage of Lyme disease, other systemic findings may occur, including cardiac manifestations in 8% to 10% of untreated patients (myocarditis or conduction defects), neurologic abnormalities in 10% to 12% (cranial neuropathies especially facial, radiculopathies, meningitis, peripheral sensory and/or motor neuropathy, myelitis, chorea, ataxia, meningoencephalitis), musculoskeletal symptoms in 50% of untreated (migratory polyarthritis, polyarthralgias, fibromyalgia), ophthalmologic (conjunctivitis, iritis, choroiditis), hepatic (liver function test abnormalities, hepatitis), and renal (microscopic hematuria, proteinuria) (143). Approximately 20% with later manifestations of Lyme disease recall no history of tick bite or ECM (154).

In the third or chronic stage of Lyme disease, which occurs months to years after the tick bite, symptoms include musculoskeletal (migratory polyarthritis in 50% of untreated, chronic monoarthritis, usually of the knee, in about 10% of untreated, with erosion of cartilage and bone), fibromyalgia, neurologic (often subtle chronic encephalopathy or peripheral neuropathy, ataxia, dementia, and sleep disorder) (155). The joint symptoms in untreated Lyme disease include arthralgias, intermittent episodes of arthritis, usually monoarticular or asymmetric oligoarticular, and chronic arthritis, usually of the knees (156). Small joint inflammation is unusual. Episodes of Lyme arthritis may last several days to several months and typically remit after months to years but may become chronic (145).

Lyme encephalopathy and polyneuropathy are usually seen with subtle memory deficit, localized radicular pain, or distal paresthesias (155,157).

Prospective controlled studies in endemic areas showed no fetal abnormalities or deaths with Lyme disease, but infection during pregnancy is a concern and if there is an adverse effect, it is uncommon (142).

PATHOLOGY AND IMMUNOPATHOLOGY

Skin pathology is not diagnostic unless spirochetes are found (158). There is a superficial and deep perivascular and interstitial infiltrate composed mostly of lymphocytes with or without a mixture of plasma cells and/or eosinophils. The plasma cells are found mainly in biopsies from the periphery of lesions and eosinophils are seen in biopsies from the center of lesions. With Warthin-Starry or Dieterle silver staining, spirochetes can be identified in EM lesions, most commonly from the advancing border (158).

LABORATORY FINDINGS

In most cases of ECM, a carefully elicited history and a physical examination are all that is required and the CDC accepts physician-diagnosed ECM of greater than 5 cm in size as establishing the diagnosis (145). In cases where the diagnosis is uncertain, an elevated antibody response to *B. burgdorferi*, measured by a two-step procedure consisting of a screening ELISA test followed by a confirmatory Western immunoblot test, helps in making a diagnosis (159). Antibodies are commonly not detectable in the first few weeks of the illness. Occasionally patients inadequately treated with antibiotics early in the infection are seronegative later in the illness (160,161). Treated patients commonly maintain seropositivity after adequate treatment, so it is common to attribute new symptoms incorrectly to Lyme disease (162). False-positive results have been reported with other spirochetal diseases, varicella infections, infectious mononucleosis, RA, and systemic lupus erythematosus.

Culture of *B. burgdorferi* from the margin of untreated ECM skin lesions is commonly successful, with recent yields ranging from 72% to 86% (163,164). This provides a definitive diagnosis of Lyme disease.

CNS disease due to Lyme disease usually has cerebrospinal fluid (CSF) or electromyographic abnormalities that improve several months after intravenous antibiotics (155). There is a lymphocytic pleocytosis in the CSF. A comparison of levels of antibody in the CSF with the serum is probably a more sensitive and specific method of making an accurate diagnosis of CNS disease (142).

DIFFERENTIAL DIAGNOSIS

The differential diagnoses for ECM include granuloma annulare, erysipelas, tinea, fixed drug eruption, lupus erythematosus, dermatomyositis, erythema gyratum repens, and nonspecific tick or insect bite reaction. The differential diagnosis for multiple ECM lesions includes erythema multiforme and Sweet syndrome.

The differential for borrelial lymphocytoma includes granuloma faciale, granuloma annulare, sarcoidosis, lupus erythematosus, polymorphous light eruption, and arthropod bite granuloma. Breast lesions may be confused with a carcinoma.

The differential for ACA includes changes due to cold injury or poor circulation. The differential of erythematous ACA lesions includes dermatomyositis. The differential diagnosis for fibrotic nodules includes rheumatic nodules or gouty tophi.

MANAGEMENT AND PROGNOSIS

Current recommendations for the antibiotic treatment of Lyme disease are based on the stage of disease. For early localized infection, recommended regimens include 10- to 30-day courses of oral doxycycline 100 mg twice daily, tetracycline 250 to 500 mg four times daily, amoxicillin 500 mg three or four times daily, or amoxicillin plus probenecid 500 mg three times daily for early infections (142,165). A 30-day course of these antibiotics is required for Lyme arthritis (166).

Except for patients with facial palsy alone, patients with early disseminated disease or late Lyme disease with carditis or neurologic involvement require treatment with intravenous ceftriaxone sodium 1 g twice daily or 2 g daily, cefotaxime 3 g every 12 hours, or benzylpenicillin 14 g in divided doses for 2 to 4 weeks (142,167,168). Patients with carditis should be admitted for monitoring and intravenous antibiotics. In addition, some sources recommend corticosteroids if the heart block does not resolve by 1 to 2 days after treatment (169). The heart block is usually self-limited, but can be irreversible.

Patients with chronic arthritis of the knees, particularly those with the HLA-DR4 specificity and antibody reactivity to the outer-surface proteins A and B of the spirochete, may have immune-mediated processes that persist after treatment (170, 171). Lyme disease may also trigger fibromyalgia or chronic fatigue syndrome that does not respond to antibiotics (172,173). Symptoms include marked fatigue, severe headache, widespread musculoskeletal pain, multiple symmetric tender points, joint pain and stiffness, difficulty with concentration, and sleep disturbance (173).

Retreatment with antibiotics is seldom beneficial, and consideration should first be given as to whether the diagnosis is correct (154,162). Brief courses of antibiotics rapidly clear *B. burgdorferi* from the skin at ECM sites (163). Encephalopathy or polyneuropathy can respond to retreatment with intravenous antibiotics (162).

Prophylactic antibiotic treatment for tick bites is not routinely recommended (174). The risk from an asymptomatic tick bite is small and in many geographic areas would lead to almost continuous antibiotic use in the summer. Tick bite prevention is important. This includes use of repellents; wearing light-colored long-sleeved shirts and long pants, with the pants tucked into the socks; conducting periodic checks for ticks during outdoor exposure; avoiding tall grass and brush; removing and washing clothing suspected of exposure to ticks; and prompt removal of ticks with tweezers or forceps. The best overall repellent protection against ticks occurs with a combination of DEET (*N* ,*N*-diethyl-m-toluamide) as a skin repellent and a permethrin-containing clothing repellent (175).

There are reports of a recombinant vaccine that is well tolerated and effective at decreasing the incidence of ECM (176). Guidelines on who should be vaccinated and its long-term role in the overall disease prevention in populations have not been established (145).

Pregnant women with Lyme disease should be treated in a similar pattern to others infected with *Borrelia* organisms, and need not terminate the pregnancy (145).

Reinfection with Lyme is rare in chronic Lyme disease, and second episodes of Lyme disease are milder than the first episode (143,145).

ETIOLOGIC FACTORS AND PATHOGENESIS

The disease is caused by a bite from various species of ixodid tick, leading to transmission of *B. burgdorferi*, a spirochete (177, 178). *Ixodes dammini* is found in much of the northeastern United States and Michigan, Wisconsin, and Minnesota. *Ixodes pacificus* is primarily seen in the western United State and *Ixodes ricinus* and *Ixodes persulcatus* in Europe and Asia, respectively (175). Over a 2-year period, ixodid ticks undergo development from larva to nymph to adult. The ticks can become infected by ingesting blood from numerous bird and animal sources, especially the white-footed mouse preferred by nymphal ticks and the white-tailed deer preferred by adult ticks. Birds likely lead to geographic spread of the disease. Pets may become infected but do not serve as transmission hosts.

Larval, nymphal, and adult ticks can transmit the infection, although the nymphal stage, usually in May to early July, is the usual time of transmission. Most of the other cases are due to adult ticks feeding in the early spring or fall (179). The greatest risk of infection is after a tick has been attached to the skin for more than 24 hours (180). Spirochetes in *I. dammini* ticks are mostly in the midgut (181). The spirochetes likely disseminate from the midgut to the salivary glands when an infected tick starts to feed (181). Dissemination likely occurs prior to infectivity of the tick, and this may explain the approximate 2-day delay between attachment and transmission of the spirochete.

It is unclear if the late manifestations are due to persistent infection or to autoimmune disease. Recent *in vitro* experiments suggest that *B. burgdorferi* may be sequestered within fibroblasts and protected from extracellular microbial antibiotics (143,182).

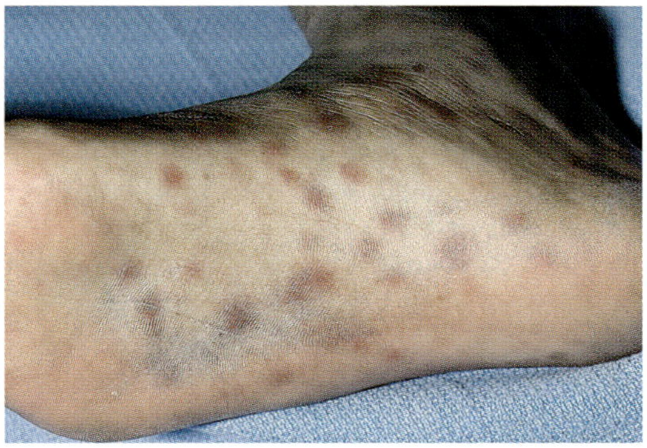

Figure 12.9. Secondary syphilis. Erythematous papules on plantar surface of fcot. (Courtesy of Bill Witmer, M.D., Department of Dermatology, Univers ty of Pennsylvania, with permission.)

Encephalopathy and polyneuropathy probably result from direct infection of the nervous system.

Syphilis

HISTORY

Osteoarticular syphilis was first recognized early in this century (183), although bone changes have been found in Australian, African, and Central American pre-Columbian fossils.

EPIDEMIOLOGY

The incidence of syphilis last peaked in 1989 with 20.3 cases per 100,000 persons, the greatest increase since 1949 (184). Since then, there has been a steady decline with 3.2 cases reported per 100,000 in 1998 (184). There is increased incidence in blacks, with the rate being 44 times that of white Americans (185).

CUTANEOUS MANIFESTATIONS

Congenital, secondary, and tertiary syphilis can be associated with musculoskeletal findings. In congenital syphilis, skin lesions include condyloma lata and mucous patches.

The variety of presentations that can occur with secondary syphilis has earned it a reputation as the "great imitator." The classic skin lesion seen with secondary syphilis is an erythematous copper-hued, maculopapular eruption, commonly involving the trunk, palms, and soles (Figs. 12.9 and 12.10). Occasionally, the lesions are pustular, nodular, ulcerative, or vasculitic (186–189). Annular plaques on the face are common (Fig. 12.11). These occur 6 to 12 weeks after the primary painless ulcer (chancre) and last 4 to 6 weeks. Condyloma lata are moist, smooth, verrucous plaques on the genitals. Mucous patches of the tongue and patchy alopecia on the scalp are also characteristic cutaneous features of secondary syphilis.

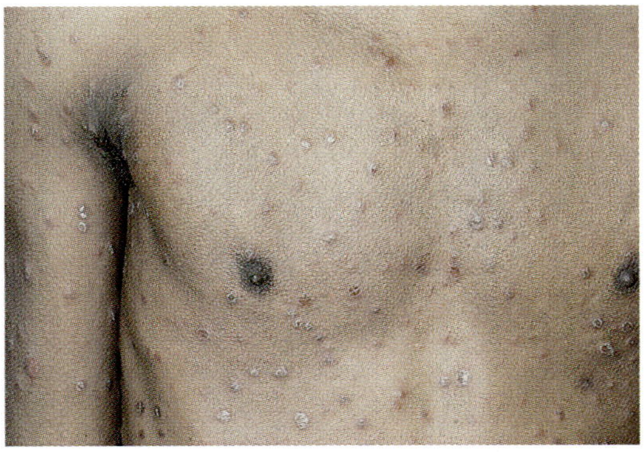

Figure 12.10. Secondary syphilis. Erythematous papules on trunk. (Courtesy of Bill Witmer, M.D., Department of Dermatology, University of Pennsylvania, with permission.)

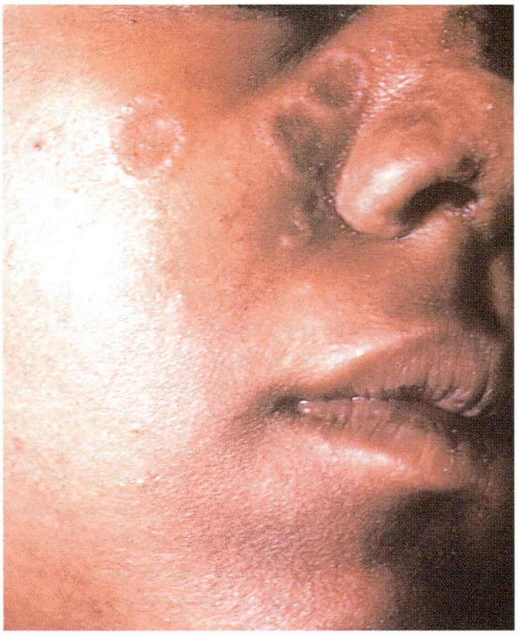

Figure 12.11. Secondary syphilis. Annular, erythematous plaques on face.

Even without treatment, only a third of patients progress to tertiary syphilis (190). Tertiary syphilis occurs with nodules and noduloulcerative lesions and gummas in the skin, usually 3 to 7 years, but as long as 60 years after the secondary stage resolves (191). The longer the interval from the secondary stage, the more solitary and damaging the lesions are. Gummas are painless pink to dusky red nodules of various sizes, often ulcerated, found on the scalp, forehead, buttocks, presternum, supraclavicular, and pretibial areas. There is a tendency to partial healing without treatment, but total healing is unusual (191).

RELATIONSHIP BETWEEN CUTANEOUS AND SYSTEMIC FEATURES

Syphilis, although a rare cause of joint symptoms, can cause musculoskeletal involvement during congenital, secondary, and tertiary syphilis (Table 12.2).

In congenital syphilis, the most common joint symptoms are periostitis and osteochondritis. Osteochondritis occurs in 70% of patients and can cause epiphyseal separation, where one sees periarticular swelling and immobility of the affected joint; this can resolve spontaneously. Clutton joints, with painless knee effusions, occur in children aged 8 to 16 years (192).

Four percent to 8% of patients with secondary syphilis have a symmetric nonmigratory polyarthritis that commonly affects the knees and ankles (192,193). Shoulders, proximal interphalangeal joints, and metacarpophalangeal joints are occasionally involved. The joints show mild tenderness, synovial effusion, and thickening, without redness or heat. Tenosynovitis of the wrists and ankles and osteitis of the tibia, ulna, clavicle, and skull may also occur. Five percent to 10% have arthralgias, usually worse at night and not worsened by exercise (192). Other features include generalized adenopathy, fever, malaise, and anorexia. A number of unusual clinical manifestations have been seen in secondary syphilis, including CNS involvement (meningitis, perceptive deafness, cranial nerve neuropathy), eye involvement (retinitis, optic neuritis, granulomatous con-

TABLE 12.2. Musculoskeletal Involvement of Syphilis

Congenital syphilis
- Osteochondritis (Parrot pseudoparalysis)
- Diaphyseal osteitis
- Periostitis
- Dactylitis
- Clutton joints
- Gummata of bones

Secondary syphilis
- Polyathralgias
- Polyarthritis
- Tenosynovitis
- Back pain
  - Normal radiographic findings
  - Unilateral sacroiliitis
  - Spondylitis
- Osteitis
- Periostitis

Tertiary syphilis
- Chronic syphilitic arthritis
- Gummatous arthritis
- Charcot joints

From Fish DG, Ampel NM, Galgiani JN, et al. Coccidioidomycosis during human immunodeficiency virus infection: a review of 77 patients. *Medecine (Baltimore)* 1990;69:384–391, with permission.

junctivitis), hepatitis, nephritis, parotid enlargement, enteritis, and gastritis.

PATHOLOGY AND IMMUNOPATHOLOGY

In secondary syphilis, there is epidermal hyperplasia; dilated, thickened, and increased large endothelial cells; and a superficial and deep perivascular and sometimes lichenoid infiltrate with plasma cells (194). In papulosquamous lesions, there can be spongiform pustules within the epidermis (194). Small, well-circumscribed epithelioid cell granulomas, some with giant cells, are present in the infiltrate (195). Pustular lesions show a subcorneal pustule. Warthin–Starry stain or silver stain shows spirochetes in the epidermis and in the dermis around the walls of capillaries in a third of cases of secondary syphilis. Condyloma lata show the same changes as other lesions of secondary syphilis, but usually has many more treponemes demonstrable on silver stain (196).

In nodular tertiary syphilis, there are small granulomas in the dermis amid a lymphoid and plasma cell infiltrate, blood vessels can show endothelial swelling, and there may be mild caseation necrosis. In gummas, there is an extensive granulomatous infiltrate involving the dermis and fat, involvement of vessels in the dermis and fat, and extensive caseation necrosis in the area of the granulomatous infiltrate (197).

LABORATORY FINDINGS

VDRL or rapid plasma reagin test is positive in most patients and needs to be confirmed by antitreponemal tests. Dark-field examination of skin lesions from skin, mucous patches, or condyloma lata lesions allows immediate diagnosis.

The CDC recommends that those infected with HIV due to sexual contact or intravenous drug abuse should be tested for syphilis (184). Patients with syphilis should be tested for HIV. HIV-infected patients with a positive serologic test for syphilis should probably undergo a lumbar puncture because asymptomatic neurosyphilis is commonly present, although this recommendation is controversial (192,198). The seronegativity seen in some cases of syphilis and HIV is usually due to a prozone phenomenon (193,198). It is thus important to dilute samples for RPR from patients with HIV to avoid a false-negative test.

Laboratory diagnosis of the etiology of the arthritis can be difficult. Radiographic findings are nonspecific. Serologic testing of the synovial fluid is rarely positive. Treponemes are rarely found in the synovial fluid or on synovial biopsy. Synovial fluid shows mild inflammation with cell counts ranging from 4,000 to 13,000 polymorphonuclear (PMN) cells/μL.

DIFFERENTIAL DIAGNOSIS

The skin lesions of secondary syphilis can resemble pityriasis rosea or a viral exanthem. The differential diagnosis of tertiary syphilis skin lesions includes bacterial or deep fungal infections. The musculoskeletal symptoms can mimic systemic lupus erythematosus, vasculitis, RA, Lyme disease, sarcoid, and lymphoma.

MANAGEMENT AND PROGNOSIS

Penicillin continues to be the mainstay of treatment. Early syphilis in non-HIV–infected patients is treated with 2.4 million IU of benzathine penicillin G intramuscularly per week, given in two doses, for 2 weeks. Treatment of HIV-infected early syphilis is unclear, but some recommend intravenous penicillin or two or three weekly doses of benzathine penicillin with 10 days of amoxicillin. For latent syphilis in the non-HIV–infected patient, treatment is three doses of 2.4 million IU of benzathine penicillin at weekly intervals. HIV-infected patients with neurosyphilis require treatment with intravenous penicillin G, 12 to 14 million IU per day, or ceftriaxone (198). Careful follow-up syphilis serologies should be monitored to assess the efficacy of treatment. In primary syphilis, the serologies will be negative in 1 year and in secondary syphilis, it takes 2 years (199).

The musculoskeletal manifestations usually resolve after antibiotic therapy (183).

ETIOLOGIC FACTORS AND PATHOGENESIS

Skin lesions show spirochetes with special stains. In secondary syphilis, high levels of circulating immune complexes have been found, and immune complexes with spirochete antigens have been found in the skin and kidney (200,201). The cause of the arthritis is unclear, but could include spirochetes, inflammation due to PMN cells, or immune-complex deposition.

Meningococcus

EPIDEMIOLOGY

Meningococcal disease occurs worldwide. Those at risk of infection include persons with no prior exposure, children younger than 5 years, new military recruits, and persons with terminal complement deficiencies.

DISEASE CLASSIFICATION

There are three clinical syndromes with cutaneous involvement in meningococcal disease. These are meningitis, acute meningococcemia, and chronic meningococcemia.

CUTANEOUS MANIFESTATIONS

Skin lesions are seen in half of those with meningitis and nearly all with acute meningococcemia. They begin as macules that blanch or have central petechiae or pustules. Over time, they become 1- to 15-mm petechial or purpuric macules to nodules or bullae, sometimes painful, occurring primarily on the trunk, lower extremities, and pressure areas. They can be angulated in contour, spread rapidly over hours, and generally spare the face, palms, and soles (Fig. 12.12).

In chronic meningococcemia, there are several different types of skin lesions. In 30% of the cases, the skin lesions are

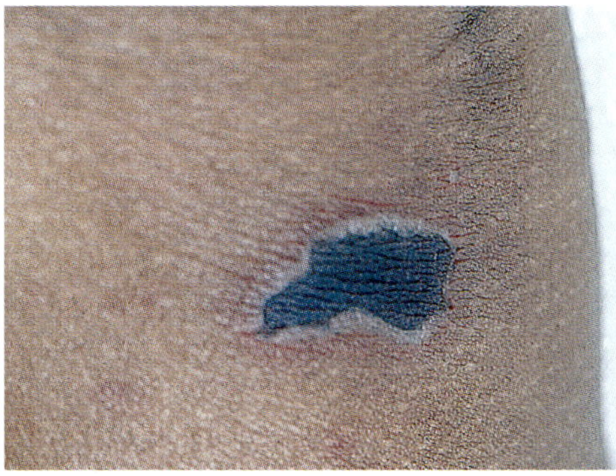

Figure 12.12. Meningococcemia. Purpuric, blue–gray macule. (Courtesy of Paul Honig, M.D., Children's Hospital of Philadelphia, PA, with permission.)

pale, erythematous 1- to 20-mm macules and papules. Skin lesions include erythema nodosum–like nodules, mainly on the legs, petechiae of variable size, some with vesicles or pustules in the center, hemorrhagic areas with blue–gray centers, and hemorrhagic tender nodules.

RELATIONSHIP BETWEEN CUTANEOUS AND SYSTEMIC FEATURES

Invasive disease occurs due to hematogenous spread from the upper respiratory tract, causing bacteremia or infection of other sites, including meningitis, pericarditis, or arthritis. Initial symptoms include mild upper respiratory complaints, headache, nausea, vomiting, malaise, and myalgias. Patients develop shock, cyanosis, and disseminated intravascular coagulopathy, and can die in less than a day.

In chronic meningococcemia, there may be an initial acute illness that culminates with vague intermittent complaints of myalgias, arthralgias, headaches, anorexia, and weight loss. The skin lesions occur with the fever and arthritis, and recurrences can occur for weeks to months.

Meningococcal arthritis is rare relative to DGI. The arthritis is clinically similar to DGI and thus is often misdiagnosed as DGI (202,203). There is occasional joint swelling and tenderness, but unlike DGI, there is no tenosynovitis. Most patients experience an inflammatory monoarthritis of a large joint, especially the knee (202–204). Cases of joint involvement mimicking acute rheumatic fever and chronic sacroiliitis have also been reported (205,206).

There have been a few reports of *Neisseria meningitidis* infection in HIV infection. In one report, the patient had group B arthritis–dermatitis syndrome, with acute pain and swelling of the knee from the meningococcus and multiple red, painful skin lesions on his chest and arms (207).

PATHOLOGY AND IMMUNOPATHOLOGY

In acute meningococcemia, skin biopsy shows dilated vessels, swollen endothelial cells, acute vasculitis, and vascular thrombi consisting of platelets, fibrin, and red cells. There is perivascular hemorrhage and inflammation. Organisms are often seen within the endothelium, neutrophils, and vascular thrombi (208).

In chronic meningococcemia, the skin lesions do not show bacteria. There is a mixed PMN and mononuclear cell infiltrate, without endothelial cell swelling or thrombi.

LABORATORY FINDINGS

Neutrophilic leukocytosis is common. Blood cultures are positive in most cases with acute meningococcemia without meningitis and in one third of those with meningitis. CSF should be obtained for Gram stain and cultures in those who have symptoms of meningitis. The most rapid diagnosis can be made by Gram stain of biopsy or needle aspirates from the petechial skin lesions (208). In chronic meningococcemia, blood cultures taken during fevers are often positive.

In patients with meningococcal arthritis, Gram stain of the synovial fluid usually reveals an intracellular gram-negative diplococcus and culture generally is positive for *N. meningitides* (203,204).

DIFFERENTIAL DIAGNOSIS

The differential diagnosis of acute meningococcemia includes acute septicemia with *Streptococcus pneumoniae*, *Streptococcus*, or *Staphylococcus aureus*, acute endocarditis, leukocytoclastic vasculitis, enteroviral infections, Rocky Mountain spotted fever, toxic shock syndrome, purpura fulminans, and leptospirosis. The differential of chronic meningococcemia, entities where there are fever, skin lesions, and joint involvement, includes subacute bacterial endocarditis, acute rheumatic fever, Henoch–Schönlein purpura, Rat-bite fever, erythema multiforme, and gonococcemia.

MANAGEMENT AND PROGNOSIS

Intravenous penicillin is the drug of choice. Chloramphenicol can be used in penicillin-allergic persons. The mortality rate for treated meningococcal meningitis is 5% and for acute meningococcemia is 20 to 30%. Those with larger purpuric lesions have a higher mortality (203). Untreated patients usually die.

In chronic meningococcemia, some recover spontaneously without treatment. Others develop acute meningococcemia. Nearly 100% are cured with antibiotic treatment.

Meningococcal arthritis generally responds to antibiotics. There is a report of a case of recurrent sterile arthritis following treated primary septic meningococcal arthritis (209).

ETIOLOGIC FACTORS AND PATHOGENESIS

Acute meningococcemia is caused by *N. meningitidis*. There are 13 serotypes, based on the type of capsular antigen. Groups A, B, C, Y, and W-135 are the major pathogens. It is an obligate, aerobic, gram-negative diplococci. Humans are the only reservoir, and *N. meningitides* is found in the upper respiratory tract of 2% to 10% of people. Colonization can occur for days to months and bacteria are spread through the air.

Mycobacterium Marinum

HISTORY

Mycobacterium marinum has been identified as the cause of a granulomatous eruption in swimmers since the 1950s (210).

EPIDEMIOLOGY

M. marinum is acquired through exposure to fresh water, salt water, fish tanks, swimming pools, fish or aquatic exposures, timber cuts, or splinters. The incubation period is usually about three weeks, although much longer periods are possible.

CLASSIFICATION

The disease can be solitary or sporotrichoid.

CUTANEOUS MANIFESTATIONS

The disease often occurs after inoculation into abrasions or after penetrating injuries to the fingers and hands. This is an indolent disease, with nodules or ulcerated plaques, occasionally with extension to deep tissue. Common areas of involvement are the fingers, dorsum of the hands, and knees (211,212). The lesions

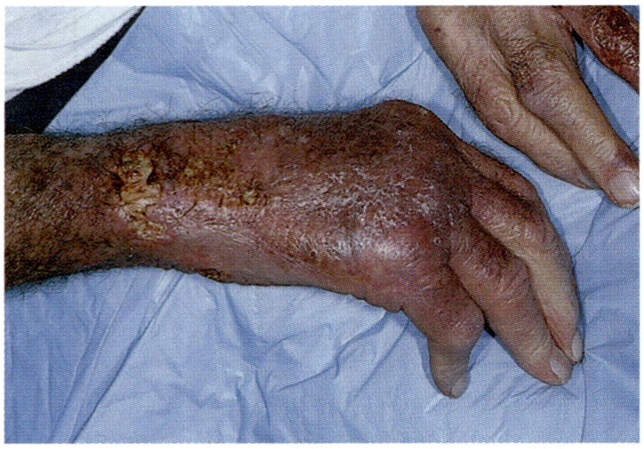

Figure 12.13. *Mycobacteria marinum.* Ulcerations on hands and wrist with underlying deformity of fingers in immunocompromised host bitten by a crab.

can be localized or sporotrichoid (25%), with dissemination 2% of the time (211,213,214) (Fig. 12.13).

RELATIONSHIP BETWEEN CUTANEOUS AND SYSTEMIC FEATURES

M. marinum can cause both tenosynovitis and rarely arthritis due to a direct extension of cutaneous infection or by direct inoculation (211,215). The arthritis generally presents with slow onset of a chronic monoarthritis, most commonly of the MCP and PIP joints (215,216). Although joint swelling may be marked, they are only mildly painful and systemic symptoms are usually absent (217). Diagnosis is generally delayed by many months (217).

PATHOLOGY AND IMMUNOPATHOLOGY

Noncaseating granulomas are commonly seen in the dermis, sometimes with abscess formation (210). Staining for acid–fast bacilli is positive in about 10% of cases (211).

LABORATORY FINDINGS

Diagnosis is best made by culture of a skin biopsy or joint fluid. Optimal growth of the organism from synovial specimens requires low temperatures (30°C to 32°C) and special culture medium (218). There is no standardized method for susceptibility testing for *M. marinum*.

DIFFERENTIAL DIAGNOSIS

Similar lesions are seen in sporotrichosis, other mycobacterial infections, blastomycosis, coccidioidomycosis, histoplasmosis, and nocardiosis, tertiary syphilis, yaws, verruca vulgaris, tuberculosis verrucosa cutis, and certain skin tumors.

MANAGEMENT AND PROGNOSIS

M. marinum can be treated with tetracyclines (tetracycline 2 g per day or minocycline 200 mg per day), but failures have been documented (219,220). Rifampin 600 mg per day and ethambutol 15 mg/kg/d can be used together, although there have been no documented episodes of resistance with single-drug treatment (211,219). Prolonged treatment, generally 3 to 6 months, is usually required (211). Joint involvement may require longer treatment. Spontaneous healing can occur.

Surgical debridement may be necessary for lesions with persistent pain or a discharging sinus, particularly with deep disease in the hand, although there is concern about extending the disease with surgical treatment (217).

ETIOLOGIC FACTORS AND PATHOGENESIS

M. marinum is a rapidly growing photochromogen. Cultures should be done at 30°C to 32°C, with about a 50% yield.

Mycobacterium Leprae

HISTORY

The first evidence of leprosy in skeletal remains was from the oasis of Dakhleh in Egypt, in four skulls buried in the second century BC. The number of cases in Europe was quite high in the thirteenth and fourteenth centuries, and the incidence in Europe has decreased since that time. However, the disease is endemic in many parts of the world today.

EPIDEMIOLOGY

The disease is most common in Latin America, Southeast Asia, Africa, and the Far East.

CLASSIFICATION

There are five clinical forms that cover a spectrum determined by the patient's cell-mediated immunity: tuberculoid (normal immunity), borderline tuberculoid, borderline, borderline lepromatous, and lepromatous (absent immunity).

CUTANEOUS MANIFESTATIONS

The incubation period is 2 to 6 years, and contagion is low. Tuberculoid leprosy has large, well-demarcated, xerotic, annular, asymmetric, anesthetic, erythematous, or hypopigmented plaques. Adjacent peripheral nerves are often enlarged. Paresthesias and anesthesias occur frequently, and ulcers and destruction of digits occur due to trauma secondary to the peripheral neuropathy (221).

In lepromatous leprosy, there are shiny brown or erythematous papules or plaques, often bilateral, symmetric, and not anesthetic, commonly on the face, nose, and ears. In borderline disease there are macules, papules, plaques, and nodules that are symmetric and hypoanesthetic (Fig. 12.14). Generalized neuropathy is common (221). Erythema nodosum leprosum is a reaction with painful, erythematous nodules (221).

RELATIONSHIP BETWEEN CUTANEOUS AND SYSTEMIC FEATURES

Leprosy commonly affects the ears and nose, with collapse of the nasal bridge not uncommon.

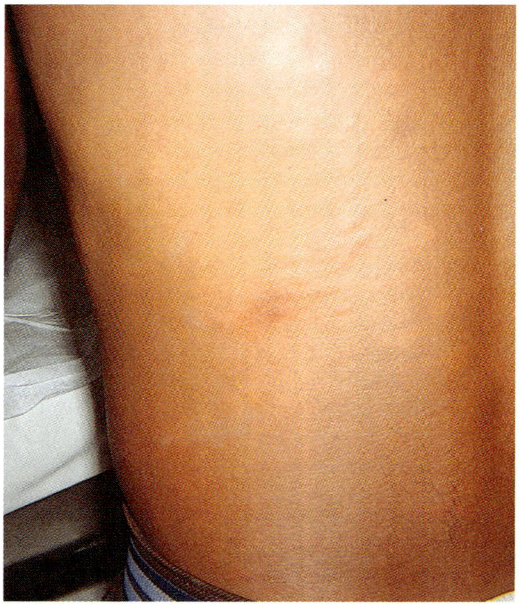

Figure 12.14. Hansen disease. Erythematous plaques on trunk.

Inflammatory changes include polyarthritis and swollen hands and feet. The polyarthritis typically involves the knees, wrists, metacarpophalangeal and interphalangeal joints, ankles, metatarsophalangeal joint, and elbows. Swan neck deformities, ulnar deviation, and atrophy of interosseal muscles of the hands, subcutaneous nodules, and radiographic evidence of juxtaarticular osteoporosis and erosions can be seen (222,223). Occasionally mono- or oligoarthritis is seen (223). Chronic sacroiliitis appears to be a common previously unrecognized manifestation of leprosy articular involvement (222). The arthritis usually occurs in type 1 and type 2 reactive states, particularly with erythema nodosum leprosum (ENL), and may occur before, during, or after ENL (221). ENL-associated arthritis has a sudden onset, is associated with morning stiffness, and is disabling. Other features of ENL include nephritis, neuritis, and hepatosplenomegaly.

PATHOLOGY AND IMMUNOPATHOLOGY

A deep biopsy to fat is important to evaluate nerves. Tuberculoid leprosy shows epithelioid cell granulomas with a mild to moderate mononuclear cell infiltrate and occasionally giant cells. The granulomas are often elongated along nerves. *Mycobacterium leprae* are rare, but are best visualized using the Fite stain on biopsies obtained from the edge of a lesion. *M. leprae* can sometimes be found in some synovial biopsies (223,224). Lepromatous leprosy shows an extensive cellular infiltrate separated from the epidermis by a grenz zone. There are foamy macrophages that resemble xanthoma cells and many acid–fast bacilli are seen on Fite stain.

LABORATORY FINDINGS

Diagnosis is made by skin biopsy or slit-skin smears. PCR will likely be helpful for paucibacillary disease in the future.

DIFFERENTIAL DIAGNOSIS

Skin lesions can resemble morphea, vitiligo, yaws, onchocerciasis, pityriasis alba, tinea versicolor, seborrheic dermatitis, tinea corporis, granuloma annulare, gyrate erythemas, syphilis, sarcoidosis, tuberculosis, lupus erythematosus, cutaneous leishmaniasis, and mycosis fungoides. The arthritis can resemble RA.

MANAGEMENT AND PROGNOSIS

Dapsone is the treatment of choice. Treatment continues 2 years after the skin clears in tuberculoid leprosy and for life in lepromatous leprosy. Table 12.3 shows the World Health Organization recommendations for the different types of leprosy.

ETIOLOGIC FACTORS AND PATHOGENESIS

The disease is caused by infection of the skin and peripheral nerves by *M. leprae,* a slow-growing acid–fast bacillus. The mode of transmission is uncertain, although the respiratory route is suspected. The arthritis is due to either a reactive process, especially since it is commonly associated with ENL or to bacilli in the joint (222,223). The ENL-related arthritis often resolves without sequelae, although prolonged episodes of inflammatory arthritis and joint disability can occur (222).

TABLE 12.3. Treatment of Leprosy

Lepromatous and borderline	
Rifampin	600 mg/mo for minimum 2 y
Dapsone	100 mg/d for life
Clofazimine	300 mg/mo supervised for minimum 2 y 50 mg/d unsupervised for minimum 2 y
Treat 2 y with minimum of 8 y of follow-up	
Indeterminate and tuberculoid	
Rifampin	600 mg/mo for 6 mo
Dapsone	100 mg/d for 2 y after lesions resolve
Minimum of 4 y of follow-up	

FUNGAL INFECTIONS

Like the mycobacteria, fungi are uncommon causes of infectious arthritis. Clinically, they resemble other inflammatory arthritides and synovial fluid leukocyte counts resemble noninfectious inflammatory arthritis. Routine cultures are often negative and delays in diagnosis leading to permanent joint deformity therefore often occur.

Sporotrichosis

HISTORY

Sporotrichosis was first reported by Shenck in 1898 (225). In 1909, DeBeurmann described gummatous intraosseus lesions (226).

EPIDEMIOLOGY

The distribution of sporadic infection is worldwide, with males predominating (75% to 95%) (227). Infection is usually due to cutaneous inoculation during outdoor work such as farming, gardening, or forestry. There have been 11 epidemics of cutaneous sporotrichosis reported in the U.S. literature since 1941. Eight were related to exposure to sphagnum moss, which is used to pack seedlings for shipping, and three to hay exposure. There was an outbreak due to sphagnum moss in 1988, in which there were 84 cases in 15 states (228). Endemic areas include the Mississippi and Missouri river valleys, Oklahoma, and Mexico (229).

CLASSIFICATION

There are cutaneous and extracutaneous forms of the disease. There are three cutaneous forms: typical lymphatic sporotrichosis, fixed cutaneous, and mucous membrane. Systemic forms, much more rare than cutaneous forms, include localized, multifocal, or disseminated forms.

CUTANEOUS MANIFESTATIONS

Cutaneous sporotrichosis typically appears as a succession of erythematous, often ulcerated nodules along the lymphatic drainage on an extremity (Fig. 12.15). Since the infection is usually acquired by traumatic inoculation, the fingers and hands are the most common sites. An indurated, freely movable, painless nodule develops at the site of inoculation after an incubation period of 1 week to 3 months. The nodule then can ulcerate. Spread to regional lymph nodes occurs in up to 75% of patients. Infection of the mucous membranes of the nose, mouth, and pharynx can occur (Fig. 12.16). Fevers and chills are uncommon.

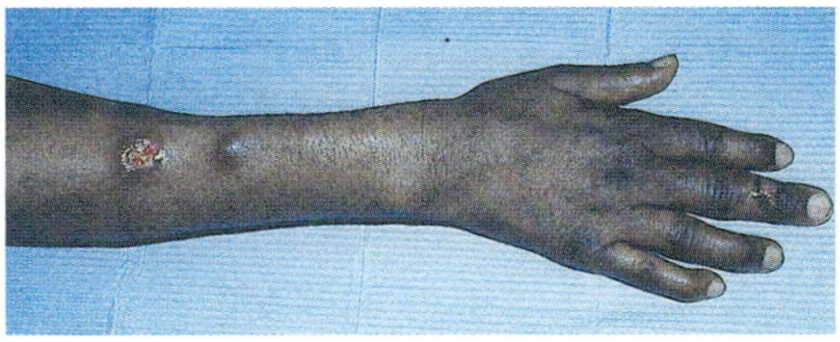

Figure 12.15. Lymphatic sporotrichosis. Multiple erythematous nodules on arms.

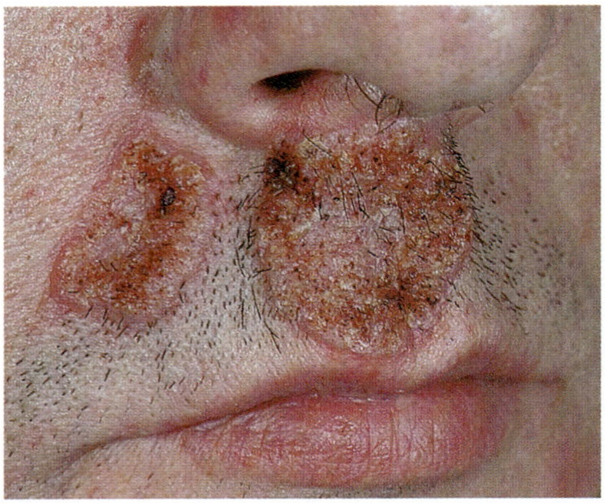

Figure 12.16. Sporotrichosis. Fixed cutaneous variant. Multiple erythematous plaques on face.

RELATIONSHIP BETWEEN CUTANEOUS AND SYSTEMIC FEATURES

Initial diagnosis is incorrect in many cases, leading to a delay in treatment. Cutaneous and systemic sporotrichosis can exist together, particularly in the multifocal systemic form of the disease (230). Sporotrichosis can disseminate to almost any organ, causing osteomyelitis, arthritis, granulomatous tenosynovitis, olecranon bursitis, myositis, pneumonia, genitourinary, eye, and CNS infection (227,231–234).

The arthritis is rare, with an incidence of 0.03% to 0.04%, and is usually chronic and indolent, mono- or polyarticular, and involving the knee, wrist, small joints of the hands and feet, and elbow. Half of patients have multiple joints involved, and half of patients with arthritis have a joint effusion (235). A delay in diagnosis of the arthritis (3 to 96 months) is related to the insidious onset, slowly progressive nature of the arthritis; the difficulty in visualizing the organism in synovial fluid or tissues; and the difficulty in culturing the fungus (227,236,237). Abscesses and fistulas are common due to invasion of parasynovial sites.

Cavitary upper lobe lesions are characteristic of unifocal systemic pulmonary sporotrichosis. In multifocal systemic disease, pulmonary involvement shows linear and nodular infiltrates (238).

PATHOLOGY AND IMMUNOPATHOLOGY

It is rare to see the organism on routine histology, although periodic acid–Schiff, methenamine silver, and Gridley stains can be helpful. *Sporothrix schenckii* occurs in tissue sections only as yeast cells. Cells are spherical, oval, or elongate (cigar shaped). The asteroid body is composed of a 5-μm-diameter budding yeast cell surrounded by a radiate eosinophilic substance. Immunostaining with anti-*S. schenckii* antibodies is far more sensitive than other routine histochemical methods (239). Synovial biopsy specimen will most commonly show a noncaseating granulomatous inflammation (235). A dense mononuclear infiltrate with coagulation necrosis and hypertrophic villi with pannus formation has also been described (240).

LABORATORY FINDINGS

Culture of the skin is the most productive way to make a diagnosis. An increased erythrocyte sedimentation rate is the most common abnormality found (227,233).

When the joint is affected, it may be difficult to diagnose. Synovial fluid may be serosanguinous and inflamed, with a moderate synovial fluid leukocytosis ranging from 8×10^6 to 2.36×10^8 WBCs per liter with low glucose levels (236). Synovial fluid or tissue cultures are required to diagnose the arthritis and often both and repeated specimens are necessary (235). Precipitins can be shown in 70% to 85% of infected subjects, and latex agglutination titers are elevated in a higher percentage. Higher agglutination titers are seen in patients with articular disease; titers decrease with treatment (227). Radiographic changes are usually present on initial evaluation, showing soft-tissue swelling and osteoporosis, juxtaarticular erosions, and intraosseous lytic lesions (231,241).

DIFFERENTIAL DIAGNOSIS

Hands and wrists are usually not involved in other fungal arthritides, such as with *Candida* species or coccidioidomycosis (Table 12.4).

MANAGEMENT AND PROGNOSIS

Early in the disease, heat alone may resolve the lesions. Oral potassium iodide [supersaturated potassium iodide (SSKI); 1 g KI per mL], 1 mL twice daily up to a maximum of 9 to 12 g daily for 4 weeks after symptoms have resolved, given orally in milk, remains highly effective in the treatment of cutaneous and lymphocutaneous forms of infection (242). Side effects of KI include acne, upset stomach, lacrimation, and salivation, sore throat, skin eruptions, menstrual irregularity, and lethargy. Itraconazole, 100 mg to 200 mg daily, is effective in cutaneous sporotrichosis (243,244), and recently has been shown effective in systemic forms of sporotrichosis (238,245). Main side effects include nausea, vomiting, hypertension, and elevated liver function tests. Less than 5% of patients develop hypokalemia, pedal edema, and hair loss. Cutaneous forms of the disease may resolve spontaneously (246). Surgical drainage is contraindicated and may slow healing.

Systemic sporotrichosis can be treated with intravenous amphotericin B, which is effective in 60% to 70% of patients at doses of more than 1 g over 12 weeks (231,239). Sometimes more than one course is necessary. Intraarticular amphotericin B and synovectomy are also helpful (236). Itraconazole appears to yield cure rates similar to those of amphotericin B (238,245, 247). In addition, 5-flurocytosis (100 mg/kg per day) may help when other treatments fail. Ketoconazole and potassium iodide are not effective treatments for the arthritis.

The arthritis can cause significant morbidity, with arthrodesis sometimes required.

TABLE 12.4. Organisms That Can Cause Nodular Lymphangitis

Common causes	Uncommon causes
Sporothrix schenckii	*Nocardia asteroides*
Mycobacterium marinum	*Mycobacterium chelonae*
Nocardia brasiliensis	*Leishmania major*
Leishmania braziliensis	*Mycobacterium kansasii*
Francisella tularensis	*Blastomyces dermatitidis*
	Coccidioides immitis
	Cryptococcus neoformans
	Histoplasma capsulatum
	Streptococcus pyogenes
	Staphylococcus aureus
	Pseudomonas pseudomallei
	Bacillus antracis
	Cowpox

From Winn RE, Anderson J, Piper J, et al. Systemic sporotrichosis treated with itraconazole. *Clin Infect Dis* 1993;17:210–217, with permission.

ETIOLOGIC FACTORS AND PATHOGENESIS

Sporotrichosis is caused by *S. schenckii*, a dimorphic fungus with low virulence that is saprophytic on a variety of vegetation and decomposing wood and in soil. The disease occurs by cutaneous inoculation or respiratory inhalation. Risk factors for dissemination include alcohol abuse, myeloproliferative disorders, malignancy, prolonged steroid use, diabetes, malnutrition, sarcoidosis, HIV infection, tuberculosis, chronic obstructive lung disease, and previous joint trauma (227,229,230,235,248). Spread to the joint is presumedly due to hematogenous spread, either from the skin or the lungs (238). Defects in cell-mediated immunity in patients with disseminated infection, as compared with lymphocutaneous sporotrichosis and healthy subjects, have been described (249).

Candida Species

HISTORY

Until 1980, infections caused by *Candida* species in drug addicts were infrequent (250). Osteoarticular infections (spondylitis and large-joint infections) were reported after 1971 and were due to *Candida* species other than *Candida albicans* (251). In 1981, there were several reports of *C. albicans* associated with infections of the skin, eye, and joints (251,252). This is now recognized as a new syndrome, seen particularly in drug addicts.

EPIDEMIOLOGY

Candida species are the most common fungi associated with opportunistic infections. The incidence of fungemias has increased with newer immunosuppressive therapies.

There have been 300 cases reported in the literature of a new candidal infection seen in drug addicts, and it is currently the most frequent fungal infection related to intravenous drug abuse (251). Epidemic outbreaks occurred in Europe and Australia during the 1980s (251,253,254), but only sporadic cases in the United States (255). The new candidal infection is associated with use of brown heroin, which, because of its poor water solubility, is dissolved in lemon juice or other acidic solvents (251). The candida presumably comes from the lemons or the plastic containers.

CLASSIFICATION

Disseminated candidiasis occurs in two clinically discrete settings. The first is with immunocompromised non–intravenous drug abusers. The second is with intravenous drug abusers. There are two clinical syndromes with candidal septic arthritis. The first is a monoarthritis caused by direct intraarticular inoculation of fungi that inhabit the skin. The second is the development of a mono- or polyarthritis due to hematogenous spread of candida (252,256).

CUTANEOUS MANIFESTATIONS

Patients with disseminated candidal infection, especially intravenous drug abusers, commonly develop skin lesions. Disseminated candidiasis in immunocompromised non–intravenous drug abusers develops skin lesions only 5% to 13% of the time. These are macular or nodular lesions found on the trunk and proximal extremities; they are not restricted to hair-bearing areas. Unilateral skin lesions in the same limb as candidal arthritis in a non–intravenous drug abuser were recently described (257).

The skin lesions in intravenous drug abusers with disseminated candidiasis, seen in about 75% of cases, are usually the first evidence of disseminated disease (251). There are painful nodules and pustules on the scalp and beard areas, with occasional involvement of other hair-bearing areas (258).

RELATIONSHIP BETWEEN CUTANEOUS AND SYSTEMIC FEATURES

Candidal arthritis due to joint injection is quite rare. It more commonly occurs in the immunocompromised or the elderly. In older individuals, often those with underlying osteoarthritis, it presents with an indolent, chronic course without fever or elevated WBC count. Patients with disseminated candidiasis, unlike those with the localized form, are immunocompromised and systemically ill; inflammation arises in normal joints through hematogenous dissemination.

In children, candidal arthritis is associated with metaphyseal osteomyelitis (252). The child usually has swollen, tender joints and a fever. Reduced joint function after treatment is rare.

Hematogenous dissemination after infancy occurs usually in persons with severe underlying condition or intravenous drug abusers. In non–intravenous drug abusers, clinical signs and symptoms include fever, pain, warmth, effusion, and restricted motion of the affected joint (254). Presentation can be either acute or indolent and osteomyelitis due to spread from the joint occurs in 70% to 85%. Bursitis can also occur.

One third of heroin addicts treated for systemic candidiasis have osteoarticular infection (253,259). Clinically, there is a short period of fever, followed in days to weeks by skin findings, eye involvement in 64% (chorioretinitis, endophthalmitis, panuveitis, episcleritis), and osteoarticular lesions in 20% (costochondral tumors, joints such as knee, hip, sacroiliac, vertebrae, and polyarticular, perichondritis, myositis) (251,260). The costochondral involvement involves a single, firm, slightly tender, often long-standing mass on the anterior region of the thorax (253). Eye symptoms include pain, photophobia, and blurred vision.

PATHOLOGY AND IMMUNOPATHOLOGY

Skin biopsies of disseminated *Candida* species in immunosuppressed patients show vascular involvement, a finding not usually seen with intravenous drug abusers. Cutaneous lesions in intravenous drug abusers with disseminated candidal infection show localized, limited abscesses with abundant PMN cells surrounded by foreign body reaction in the dermis. Periodic acid–Schiff and Grocott-Gomori methenamine-silver nitrate stains can show yeast and pseudomycelia in the hair shafts (252, 258).

LABORATORY FINDINGS

The diagnosis of candidal arthritis due to injections is made by a positive culture or biopsy. Synovial fluid shows leukocyte counts from 9,500 to 42,000/mm^3, with a predominance of PMN cells.

In disseminated candidal infection, *Candida* species can be cultured from the CSF. In disseminated infection, the synovial fluid shows 7,500 to 151,000 PMN cells per cubic millimeter (252,254). Diagnosis is made by culture of synovial fluid or tissue, urine (70% to 75%), blood (50%), or pharynx. Scanning with gallium and technetium should be done to localize the area for biopsy when there is bone or joint pain in a patient predisposed to candidal infections (252).

DIFFERENTIAL DIAGNOSIS

The differential diagnosis in the skin includes other fungal or bacterial sepsis. The arthritis can resemble infections from *S. aureus*, *Pseudomonas aeruginosa*, and tuberculosis.

MANAGEMENT AND PROGNOSIS

Ketoconazole has been the drug of choice for isolated cutaneous lesions, but fluconazole is replacing it (251). Amphotericin B (0.3 to 0.7 mg/kg body weight per day for a total of 1 to 3 g over

6 to 10 weeks), with or without flucytosine (150 mg/kg in four divided doses), or ketoconazole (400 to 800 mg orally per day), was used for treatment of the arthritis and disseminated candidiasis. The rapid development of resistant strains precludes the administration of flucytosine alone. Intraarticular amphotericin B can be helpful in localized disease or refractory disseminated joint disease (252). Fluconazole (200 to 400 mg per day for 30 to 45 days) has also been helpful in disseminated candidiasis (261). Surgical treatment, mainly joint drainage, is sometimes important. Deaths from disseminated candidiasis occur in approximately 25% of patients.

ETIOLOGIC FACTORS AND PATHOGENESIS

The direct intraarticular inoculation of fungi is usually seen in the setting of repeated aspiration and injection of corticosteroids to a joint. Corticosteroids may damage the local defense and clearance mechanisms of an already diseased joint (250). In patients with non–intravenous drug abuse disseminated candidiasis, 70% of cases are due to *C. albicans*. The other cases are usually caused by *Candida tropicalis*, *Candida parapsilosis*, *Candida guilliermondii* or *Candida glabrata* (250,262,263). In intravenous drug abusers with candidal arthritis, more than 90% of cases of osteoarticular infection are caused by *C. albicans*.

Histoplasmosis

HISTORY

The first report of histoplasmosis, which Darling thought was a protozoa, was in 1906 (264). In 1934, DeMonbreum (265) showed the agent to be a fungus.

EPIDEMIOLOGY

The disease is endemic in the Ohio and Mississippi river valleys and has been reported from 30 widely scattered countries, most commonly in temperate climates. In these areas, up to 80% of adults have skin test evidence of previous infection. The disease tends to occur in young children and adults over age 60, especially males. The largest epidemic was in Indianapolis and affected 100,000 people (266).

CLASSIFICATION

The primary infection is generally self-limited and asymptomatic. However, a flulike illness, pneumonia, and reticuloendothelial hyperplasia may occur, especially in those with heavy exposure or in young children. Reinfection can occur, leading to acute histoplasmosis or chronic pulmonary and disseminated disease, depending on the cell-mediated immunity.

CUTANEOUS MANIFESTATIONS

There are multiple, discrete papules on the extremities, trunk, and face, some in a follicular distribution (267) (Fig. 12.17). Erythema nodosum and/or erythema multiforme can occur during the primary infection. Disseminated disease is usually associated with underlying immunosuppression (227,267).

RELATIONSHIP BETWEEN CUTANEOUS AND SYSTEMIC FEATURES

The most frequent rheumatic manifestation occurs during primary infection, with 10% of patients having a migratory polyarthritic syndrome involving knees, ankles, wrists, and small joints of the hands. Pleuritis, pericarditis, and erythema nodosum can coexist (268). This is usually self-limited and resolves without sequelae.

Dissemination occurs in 0.1% of infections (236). Symptoms can include fever, weight loss, anemia, pulmonary micronodules, and hepatosplenomegaly. Arthritis and tenosynovitis,

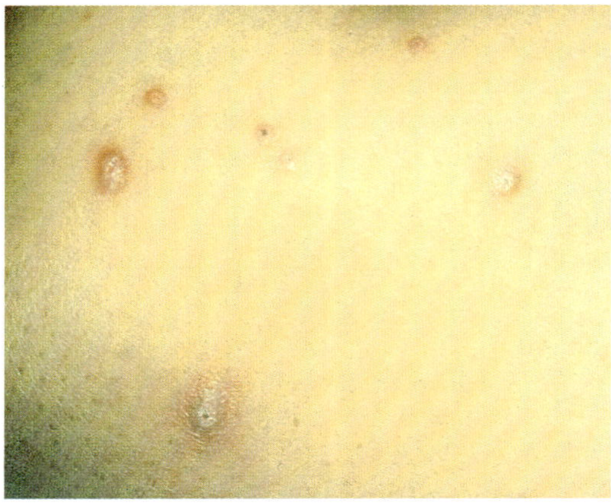

Figure 12.17. Histoplasmosis in a patient with human immunodeficiency virus. Multiple, erythematous papules on trunk.

sometimes complicated by carpal tunnel syndrome, are rare complications of disseminated histoplasmosis. The joint involvement is a monoarthritis affecting the knees most frequently. Focal bone lesions can be seen rarely. Radiographic changes include cortical subperiosteal thickening, widening of the medullary canal, osteopenia, and epiphyseal bone destruction (227,269). Histoplasma capsulatum reportedly causes prosthetic joint infection (270).

PATHOLOGY AND IMMUNOPATHOLOGY

The skin biopsy shows macrophages and histiocytes with intracellular yeast forms (271). There is often ulceration and foci of necrosis in a chronic inflammatory infiltrate, with at times a few giant cells. The spores can usually be seen with hematoxylin–eosin stain as round or oval 2- to 4-µm bodies surrounded by a clear space, but are accentuated with a silver stain (271). Synovial tissue biopsies may reveal granulomas (269).

LABORATORY FINDINGS

Diagnosis is based on detection of the organism in tissues or exudates. Complement fixation, immunodiffusion, and latex agglutination serology can detect infection. Complement fixation has 80% sensitivity, but cross-reaction with other mycoses may occur. *Histoplasma capsulatum* polysaccharide antigen can be detected rapidly and early in the urine and blood of those with disseminated disease (272). Rarely, the organism can be cultured from synovial fluid aspirates (269).

DIFFERENTIAL DIAGNOSIS

H. capsulatum must be differentiated from *Coccidioides immitis*, *C. neoformans*, *Blastomyces dermatitidis*, *Toxoplasma gondii*, *Leishmania donovani*, *Toluropsis glabrata*, *Pneumocystis carinii*, *Penicillium marneffei*, and other infectious diseases that occur in immunosuppressed hosts.

MANAGEMENT AND PROGNOSIS

The treatment of choice is itraconazole 400 mg daily for 6 months, although there are no reports of its use with musculoskeletal involvement. Amphotericin B is used if intravenous therapy is needed; disseminated disease with arthritic involvement has been treated with amphotericin B (227). Oral fluconazole has recently been reported to be effective (269). Surgical débridement has been performed in most reported cases, but recurrence has been reported with surgery alone and medical antifungal therapy, as monotherapy or as a surgical adjunct, is therefore regarded as necessary to exert a cure (269).

ETIOLOGIC FACTORS AND PATHOGENESIS

Histoplasmosis is caused by inhalation of spores of *H. capsulatum*, a worldwide dimorphic fungus. This fungus attacks cells of the reticuloendothelial system and spreads to the regional lymph nodes with granulomatous reaction, necrosis, followed by calcification.

Coccidioidomycosis

HISTORY

The first patient with coccidioidomycosis, thought to be a protozoan, was reported in 1891 in Argentina. In 1900, the etiology was found to be a fungus (273).

EPIDEMIOLOGY

There are over 50,000 cases of coccidioidomycosis per year, especially in immunocompromised persons (274). It is endemic in the Southwestern United States, Northern Mexico, and parts of Central and South America (272). Certain ethnic groups such as Filipinos and blacks experience disseminated disease more frequently (236).

CLASSIFICATION

The usual course is a self-limited or asymptomatic pulmonary infection. Sixty-six percent develop asymptomatic infection, which is identified by skin test only; 33% develop a primary pneumonia; and only 1% develop dissemination (275). Although uncommon, disseminated coccidioidomycosis often involves skin lesions when it does occur. The secondary forms include pulmonary disease (benign chronic and progressive types) and single or multisystem disseminated disease (chronic cutaneous, generalized, and meningeal types).

CUTANEOUS MANIFESTATIONS

Erythema nodosum, erythema multiforme, or urticaria can be early signs of the disease, and are seen in 25% of adult white women and 4% of white men. Primary cutaneous coccidioidomycosis is rare. Skin lesions are most common in the chronic cutaneous and generalized types of secondary disease. Disseminated disease involves granulomatous papules, pustules, and nodules that begin on the face, scalp, or neck. These evolve into confluent, sometimes verrucous plaques, and necrotic ulcers, sometimes resulting in a purulent exudate and scarring.

RELATIONSHIP BETWEEN CUTANEOUS AND SYSTEMIC FEATURES

Thirty-three percent have symptoms 2 to 3 weeks after exposure, with a primary lung infection and hilar adenopathy or pleural involvement, usually resolving completely. Migratory arthralgias may occur early in the infection. Eight to 15 days after the onset, one third develop musculoskeletal symptoms, including a migratory polyarticular arthritis that can affect any joint, without effusions; the joints are tender to pressure and painful to motion (275). The arthritis completely resolves with the acute episode in 2 to 3 weeks. Other symptoms include fever, pleuritic chest pain, cough, anorexia, and episcleritis.

Dissemination occurs after weeks, months, or years with extension to meninges, skin, lymph nodes, subcutaneous tissue, bones, and joints (275). In chronic coccidioidomycotic arthritis, the large weight-bearing joints are affected most frequently (276). The disease course is slow and insidious, with gradual onset of pain and loss of function. Eventually, the subchondral bone becomes involved in patients with a long duration of infection (276).

PATHOLOGY AND IMMUNOPATHOLOGY

Standard hematoxylin and eosin staining of skin biopsies shows the fungus well. There is a surrounding neutrophilic, granulomatous, or mixed infiltrate. Gomori methenamine-silver and period acid–Schiff also stain the endospores and spherules.

LABORATORY FINDINGS

The diagnosis is made by cultures and histopathologic studies demonstrating the spherule phase. Serologic testing is useful, but may be negative early on or in HIV-infected persons (277, 278).

DIFFERENTIAL DIAGNOSIS

The primary disease resembles influenza or a severe upper respiratory infection. Disseminated coccidioidomycosis must be distinguished from disseminated tuberculosis, blastomycosis, actinomycosis, or *S. aureus*.

MANAGEMENT AND PROGNOSIS

Therapies include itraconazole, fluconazole, amphotericin B, ketoconazole, open drainage, synovectomy, and arthrodesis (275,278). Amputation should be considered if therapies are ineffective. Untreated nonmeningeal disseminated coccidioidomycosis is fatal in 50% of cases and untreated meningeal disease is fatal in 100% of cases.

ETIOLOGIC FACTORS AND PATHOGENESIS

C. immitis is a dimorphic fungus. Infection begins after inhalation of the infectious arthroconidia in dust aerosols. Dissemination is more likely in Filipinos, blacks, pregnant women, and immunosuppressed hosts.

Cryptococcosis

HISTORY

Busse and Bushke first reported disease in humans due to cryptococci in 1895. *C. neoformans* was first isolated from soil in 1951 by Emmons.

EPIDEMIOLOGY

The disease occurs worldwide and affects twice as many men as women. *C. neoformans* is found in soil, particularly in areas where pigeons are located (280). After systemic candidiasis and aspergillosis, cryptococcosis is the next most frequent fungal pathogen (227).

CLASSIFICATION

Initial infection occurs in the lung, usually with rapid resolution. Primary cutaneous cryptococcosis is rare. Hematogenous dissemination can occur in immunosuppressed hosts, leading to skin lesions in 15% of cases.

CUTANEOUS MANIFESTATIONS

Skin lesions in disseminated cryptococcosis often show skin-colored or erythematous to purple papules or nodules with surrounding erythema (Fig. 12.18). Other presentations include acneiform pustules, subcutaneous abscesses, and ulcerations (Fig. 12.19).

RELATIONSHIP BETWEEN CUTANEOUS AND SYSTEMIC FEATURES

Disseminated disease can also involve the bones, viscera (myocarditis, pericarditis, pleuritis, prostatic infection), CNS (meningitis, meningoencephalitis, cryptococcemia), and lungs. Osteomyelitis occurs in 5% to 10% of cases with dissemination, is insidious in onset without fever or chills, and can occur con-

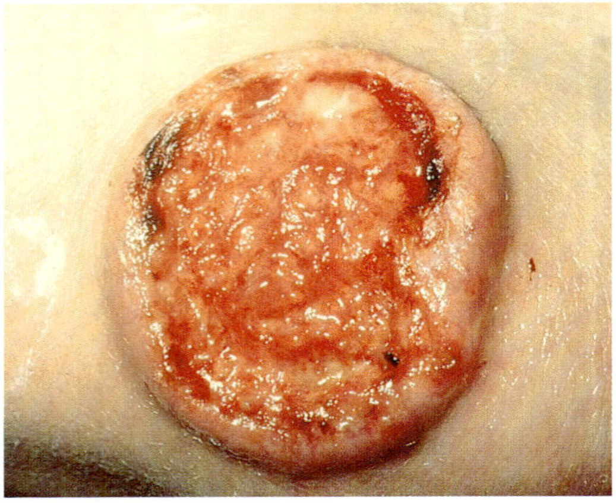

Figure 12.18. Cryptococcus.

tiguous to areas of skin infection. Arthritis is a rare manifestation of disseminated cryptococcosis and usually is due to extension from an osteomyelitis. The most common presentation is monoarthritis, most often of the knee, but oligoarthritis and polyarthritis can occur. Other joints involved include the elbow, sternoclavicular, sacroiliac, and ankle. Fever, malaise, and weight loss can occur. Synovial thickening and effusions can be seen. Synovial fluid is turbid and viscous, with leukocyte counts from 200 to 20,000 WBCs/μL, mostly mononuclear cells (227).

PATHOLOGY AND IMMUNOPATHOLOGY

The fungal organism can be seen best in skin biopsies using a periodic acid–Schiff or methenamine-silver stain.

LABORATORY FINDINGS

India ink preparations of skin aspirates or smears can show budding yeasts with a wide capsule. The organism can be cultured from tissue or spinal fluid. The latex agglutination test for capsular antigen can be used on serum or spinal fluid to aid in detection of infection, although false-negative results may occur. Serial titers can help evaluate the efficacy of therapy. Erythrocyte sedimentation rates are often elevated.

DIFFERENTIAL DIAGNOSIS

Disseminated cutaneous cryptococcosis can resemble molluscum contagiosum, pyoderma, and other fungal infections.

MANAGEMENT AND PROGNOSIS

Treatment has included combined therapy with amphotericin B (20 mg per day intravenously for 10 weeks) and 5-fluorocytosine (150 mg/kg per day orally in four divided doses). Patients with AIDS respond poorly and relapse frequently. Fluconazole or itraconazole is used for maintenance therapy in cases of AIDS to prevent relapse (281).

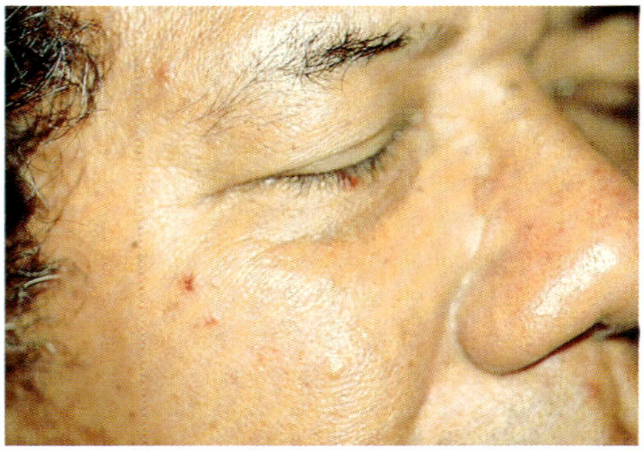

Figure 12.19. Cryptococcus.

ETIOLOGIC FACTORS AND PATHOGENESIS

The disease is caused by inhalation of dust containing *C. neoformans*, a dimorphic encapsulated yeastlike fungus. People with immunosuppression due to diabetes mellitus, cancers, sarcoidosis, AIDS, and medications are particularly at risk.

Other Fungal Infections

Immunocompromised patients get numerous other fungal infections involving skin and joints, including blastomycosis, aspergillosis, and *Trichosporon* species, and *Petriellidium boydii* (*Allescheria boydii*) infection (282–285).

PROTOZOA INFECTIONS

Entamoeba Histolytica

There has been one report in the literature describing a patient with cutaneous amoebiasis who developed an arthritic knee caused by ameba (284). The skin lesions are thought to be due to extension of underlying intestinal or hepatic lesions. Thus, most skin lesions occur in the abdominal, perianal, and perineal areas. Skin lesions grow very rapidly and are quite painful (286). Diagnosis is made by fresh preparations and iodine staining of synovial fluid and immunoperoxidase staining with antiameba monoclonal antibodies. Treatment is with metronidazole 750 mg per day for 3 days, with rapid resolution of symptoms.

PREVENTION OF INFECTIOUS ARTHRITIS FROM CUTANEOUS SOURCES

Patients with RA and joint replacements are particularly prone to bacterial joint infections, although any chronic arthritis may increase the likelihood of infection. Skin infections are the most common source of infection (287,288) (Fig. 12.20). Patients with RA may have an inherent phagocytic defect (289,290) or be predisposed to infection because of long-term oral or intraarticular corticosteroids or other immunosuppressives. The treatment of infected arthroplasties is difficult, with only 20% recovering with a functioning prosthesis and 2% culminating in death from the infection (287). Thus, good skin care and antibiotic prophy-

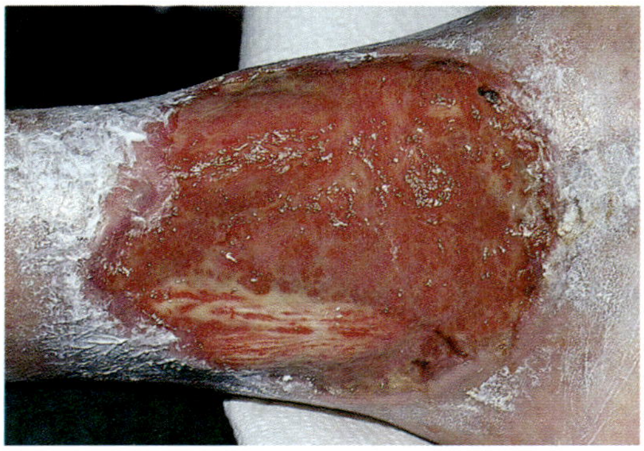

Figure 12.20. Pyoderma gangrenosum in patient with rheumatoid arthritis. (Courtesy of Bill Witmer, M.D., Department of Dermatology, University of Pennsylvania, with permission.)

laxis until healing of any skin ulcers is recommended, especially those distal to a joint with a prosthesis (291,292).

REFERENCES

1. Denman AM. Virus-host interaction and the connective-tissue diseases. In: Dick C, ed. *Immunological aspects of rheumatology.* North Holland: Elsevier, 1981.
2. Ytterberg SR. Viral arthritis. *Curr Opin Rheumatol* 1999;11:275–280.
3. The viral aetiology of rheumatoid arthritis [editorial]. *Lancet* 1984;1:772–774.
4. Phillips PE. Infections and chronic rheumatic disease in children. *Semin Arthritis Rheum* 1980;10:92–99.
5. Wands JR, Mann E, Alpert E, et al. The pathogenesis of arthritis associated with acute hepatitis-B surface antigen-positive hepatitis. *J Clin Invest* 1975;55: 930–936.
6. Horstmann DM, Liebhaber H, LeBouvier GL, et al. Rubella: reinfection of vaccinated and naturally immune persons exposed in an epidemic. *N Engl J Med* 1970;283:771–778.
7. Huppertz HI, Niki NPH, Chantler JK. Susceptibility of normal human joint tissue to viruses. *J Rheumatol* 1991;18:699–704.
8. Cossart YE, Field AM, Cant B, et al. Parvovirus-like particles in human sera. *Lancet* 1975;1:72–73.
9. Pattison JR, Jones SE, Hodson J, et al. Parvovirus infections and hypoplastic crisis in sickle-cell anaemia [letter]. *Lancet* 1981;1:664–665.
10. Serjeant GR, Topley JM, Mason K, et al. Outbreak of aplastic crises in sickle cell anaemia associated with Parvovirus-like agent. *Lancet* 1981;2:595–597.
11. Rao KRP, Patel AR, Anderson MJ, et al. Infection with Parvovirus-like virus and aplastic crisis in chronic hemolytic anemia. *Ann Intern Med* 1983;98: 930–932.
12. Young N. Hematologic and hematopoietic consequences of B19 Parvovirus infection. *Semin Hematol* 1988;25:159–172.
13. Anderson MJ, Jones SE, Fisher-Hoch SP, et al. Human Parvovirus, the cause of erythema infectiosum (fifth disease) [letter]? *Lancet* 1983;1:1378.
14. Plummer FA, Hammond GW, Forward K, et al. An erythema infectiosum-like illness caused by human Parvovirus infection. *N Engl J Med* 1985;313: 74–79.
15 Anand A, Gray ES, Brown T, et al. Human Parvovirus infection in pregnancy and hydrops fetalis. *N Engl J Med* 1987;316:183–186.
16 Reid DM, Reid TM, Brown T, et al. Human Parvovirus-associated with arthritis: a clinical and laboratory description. *Lancet* 1985;1:422–425.
17. White DG, Woolf AD, Mortimer PD, et al. Human Parvovirus arthropathy. *Lancet* 1985;1:419–421.
18. Naides SJ. Rheumatic manifestations of Parvovirus B19 infection. *Rheum Dis Clin North Am* 1998;24:375–401.
19. Nesher G, Moore TL. Human Parvovirus infection. *Infect Med* 1997;14: 638–642.
20. Bell LM, Naides SJ, Stoffman P, et al. Human Parvovirus B19 infection among hospital staff members after contact with infected patients. *N Engl J Med* 1989;321:485–491.
21. Schwarz TF, Roggendorf M, Hottentrager B, et al. Human Parvovirus B19 infection in pregnancy [letter]. *Lancet* 1988;2:566–567.
22. Gillespie SM, Cartter ML, Aech S, et al. Occupational risk of human Parvovirus B19 infection for school and day-care personnel during an outbreak of erythema infectiosum. *JAMA* 1990;263:2061–2065.
23. Anderson MJ, Higgins PG, Davis LR, et al. Experimental parvoviral infection in humans. *J Infect Dis* 1985;152:257–265.
24. Woolf AD, Campion GV, Chishick A, et al. Clinical manifestations of human Parvovirus B19 in adults. *Arch Intern Med* 1989;149:1153–1156.
25. Conway SP, Cohen BJ, Field AM, et al. A family outbreak of Parvovirus B19 infection with petechial rash in a 7-year-old boy. *J Infect* 1987;15:110–112.
26. LeFrere JJ, Meyer O, Menkes CJ, et al. Human Parvovirus and purpura [letter]. *Lancet* 1985;2:730–731.
27. Naides SJ, Piette W, Veach LA, et al. Human Parvovirus B19-induced vesiculopustular skin eruption. *Am J Med* 1988;84:968–972.
28. Loong TC, et al. Human serum Parvovirus associated vasculitis. *Postgrad Med J* 1986;62:493–494.
29. Evans LM, Grossman ME, Gregory N. Koplik spots and a purpuric eruption associated with Parvovirus B19 infection. *J Am Acad Dermatol* 1992;27:466–467.
30. Torok TJ. Parvovirus B19 and human disease. *Adv Intern Med* 1992;37: 431–455.
31. Naides SJ, Scharosch LL, Foto F, et al. Rheumatologic manifestations of human Parvovirus B19 infection in adults: initial two-year clinical experience. *Arthritis Rheum* 1990;33:1297–1309.
32. Kishore J, Misra R, Gupta D, et al. Raised IgM antibodies to Parvovirus B19 in juvenile rheumatoid arthritis. *Indian J Med Res* 1998;107:15–18.
33. Pouchot J, Ouakil H, Debin ML, et al. Adult Still's disease associated with acute human Parvovirus B19 infection. *Lancet* 1993;341:1280–1281.
34. Gran JT, Johnsen V, Myklebust G, et al. The variable clinical picture of arthritis induced by human Parvovirus B19. *Scand J Rheumatol* 1995;24:174–179.
35. Nesher ?, Osborn TG, Moore TL, et al. Parvovirus infection mimicking systemic lupus erythematosus. *Semin Arthritis Rheum* 1995;24:297–301.
36. Fawaz-Estrup F. Human Parvovirus infection: rheumatic manifestations, angioedema, C1 esterase inhibitor deficiency, ANA positivity, and possible onset of systemic lupus erythematosus. *J Rheumatol* 1996;23:1180–1185.
37. Finkel TH, Torok TJ, Ferguson A, et al. Chronic Parvovirus B19 infection and systemic necrotizing vasculitis: opportunistic infection or aetiological agent? *Lancet* 1994;343:1255–1258.
38. Walsh KJ, Armstrong RD, Turner AM. Brachial plexus neuropathy associated with human Parvovirus infection. *Br Med J (Clin Res Ed)* 1988;296:896.
39 Faden H, Gary GW, Korman M. Numbness and tingling of fingers associated with Parvovirus B19 infection [letter]. *J Infect Dis* 1990;161:354–355.
40. Kurtzman GJ, Ozawa K, Cohen B, et al. Chronic bone marrow failure due to persistent B19 Parvovirus infection. *N Engl J Med* 1987;317:287–294.
41. Kurtzman GJ, Cohen B, Meyers P, et al. Persistent B19 Parvovirus infection as a cause of severe chronic anaemia in children with acute lymphocytic leukaemia. *Lancet* 1988;2:1159–1162.
42. Marshall WF, Telenti A, Smith TF. Polymerase chain reaction detection of Parvovirus B19 viremia after organ transplantation. In: Program and Abstracts of the 30th Interscience Conference on Antimicrobial Agents and Chemotherapy; MONTH DATE, 1990; Atlanta, Georgia.
43. Evans JPM, Rossiter MA, Kumaran TO, et al. Human Parvovirus aplasia: case due to cross infection in a ward. *Br Med J (Clin Res Ed)* 1984;288:681.
44. Anderson LJ, Hurwitz ES. Human Parvovirus B19 and pregnancy. *Clin Perinatol* 1988;15:273–286.
45. Cartter ML, Farley TA, Rosengren S, et al. Occupational risk factors for infection with Parvovirus B19 among pregnant women. *J Infect Dis* 1991;163: 282–285.
46. Koch WC, Adler SP. Human Parvovirus B19 infections in women of childbearing age and within families. *Pediatr Infect Dis J* 1989;8:83–87.
47. Public Health Laboratory Service Working Party on Fifth Disease. Prospective study of human Parvovirus (B19) infection in pregnancy. *Br Med J* 1990; 300:1166–1170.
48. Rodis JF, Quinn DL, Cary GW Jr, et al. Management and outcomes of pregnancies complicated by human B19 Parvovirus infection: a prospective study. *Am J Obstet Gynecol* 1990;163:1168–1171.
49. Kurtzman GJ, Cohen B, Field AM, et al. Immune response to B19 Parvovirus and an antibody defect in persistent viral infection. *J Clin Invest* 1989;84: 1114–1123.
50. Centers for Disease Control. Risks associated with human Parvovirus B19 infection. *MMWR Recomm Rep* 1989;38:81–88.
51. Young NS, Mortimer PP, Moore JG, et al. Characterization of a virus that causes transient aplastic crisis. *J Clin Invest* 1984;73:224–230.
52. Cassinotti P, Siegl G, Michel BA, et al. Presence and significance of human Parvovirus B19 in synovial membranes and bone marrow from patients with arthritis of unknown origin. *J Med Virol* 1998;56:199–204.
53. Foto F, Saag KG, Scharosch LC, et al. Parvovirus B19 -specific DNA in bone marrow from B19 arthropathy patients: evidence for B19 virus persistence. *J Infect Dis* 1993;167:744–748.
54. Soderlund M, von Essen R, Haapasaari J, et al. Persistence of Parvovirus B19 DNA in synovial membranes of young patients with and without chronic arthropathy. *Lancet* 1997;349:1063–1065.
55. Rubella and congenital rubella syndrome—United States, 1994–1997. *MMWR Morb Mortal Wkly Rep* 1997;46:350–354.
56. Chantler JK, Ford DK, Tingle AJ. Persistent rubella infection and rubella-associated arthritis. *Lancet* 1982;1:1323–1325.
57. Ford DK, Tingle AJ, Chantler JK. Rubella arthritis. In: Espinoza L, ed. *Infections in the rheumatic diseases.* Orlando: Grune & Stratton, 1988:103–106.
58. Ytterberb SR. Viral arthritis. In: Koopman WJ, ed. *Arthritis and allied conditions,* 13th ed. Baltimore: Lippincott Williams & Wilkins, 1997;2341–2360.
59. Chambers RJ, Bywaters EGL. Rubella synovitis. *Ann Rheum Dis* 1963;2: 263–267.
60. Kudesia G, McKendrick M, Morgan-Capner P, et al. Clinical rubella reinfection: a case of arthropathy. *J Infection* 1991;23:81–83.
61. Chantler JK, Tingle AJ, Petty RE. Persistent rubella virus infection associated with chronic arthritis in children. *N Engl J Med* 1985;313:1117–1123.
62. Ogra PL, Chiba Y, Ogra SS, et al. Rubella-virus infection in juvenile rheumatoid arthritis. *Lancet* 1975;1:1157–1161.
63. Chantler JK, da Roza DM, Bonnie ME, et al. Sequential studies on synovial lymphocyte stimulation by rubella antigen and rubella virus isolation in an adult with persistent arthritis. *Ann Rheum Dis* 1985;44:564–568.
64. Tingle AJ, Mitchell LA, Grace M, et al. Randomised double-blind placebo-controlled study on adverse effects of rubella immunization in seronegative women. *Lancet* 1997;349:1277–1281.
65. Ray P, Black S, Shinefield H, et al. Risk of chronic arthropathy among women after rubella vaccination: vaccine Safety Datalink Team. *JAMA* 1997;278: 551–556.
66. Zaia JA. Clinical spectrum of varicella-zoster virus infections. In: Nahmias A, Dowdle W, Schinazi R, eds. *The human herpesviruses, an interdisciplinary approach.* New York: Elsevier, 1981:10–19.
67. Schott-Wilson J. Why "chicken" pox [letter]? *Lancet* 1978;1:1152.
68. Law B, MacDonald N, Halpern S, et al. The Immunization Monitoring Program Active (IMPACT) prospective five year study of Canadian children hospitalized for chickenpox or an associated complication. *Pediatr Infect Dis J* 2000;19:1053–1059.
69. Derrick CW, Lord L. In utero varicella-zoster infections. *South Med J* 1998;91: 1064–1066.
70. Tseng HW, Liu CC, Wang SM, et al. Complications of varicella in children: emphasis on skin and central nervous system disorders. *J Microbiol Immunol Infect* 2000;33:248–252.
71. Sauerbrei A. Varicella-zoster virus infections in pregnancy. *Intervirology* 1998; 41:191–196.

72. Issacs D. Neonatal chickenpox. *J Pediatr Child Health* 2000;36:76–77.
73. De Juan Martin F. Artritis varicelosa en la infancia. *Anales Espanoles de Pediatria* 1986;24:323–324.
74. Priest JR, Urick JJ, Grothp KE, et al. Varicella arthritis documented by isolation of virus from joint fluid. *J Paediatr* 1978;93:990–992.
75. Stebbings S, Highton J, Croxson MC, et al. Chickenpox monoarthritis: demonstration of varicella-zoster virus in joint fluid by polymerase chain reaction. *Br J Rheumatol* 1998;37:311–313.
76. Fierman AH. Varicella-associated arthritis occurring before the exanthem: case report and literature review. *Clin Pediatr* 1990;29:188–190.
77. Evans E, Sofat N, Turner J, et al. An unusual case of adult varicella-associated arthritis. *Rheumatology* 2000;39:806–808.
78. Aihara Y, Katakura S, Imagawa T, et al. Transient remission of intractable systemic-type of juvenile rheumatoid arthritis after chickenpox in a 2-year-old boy. *Ped Internat* 2001;43:95–97.
79. Saulsbury FT. Remission of juvenile rheumatoid arthritis with varicella infection. *J Rheumatol* 1999;26:1606–1608.
80. Aarons EJ, Beeching NJ. Aseptic arthritis associated with herpes zoster. *J Infect* 1993;26:87–88.
81. Penneys N. Diseases caused by viruses. In: Elder D, et al., eds. *Lever's histopathology of the skin,* 8th ed. Philadelphia: Lippincott-Raven, 1997.
82. McCrary ML, Severson J, Tyring SK, et al. Varicella zoster virus. *J Am Acad Dermatol* 1999;41:1–14.
83. Whitley RJ. Therapeutic approaches to varicella-zoster virus infections. *J Infect Dis* 1992;166[Suppl 1]:551–557.
84. Miller A. Selective decline in cellular immune response to varicella-zoster in the elderly. *Neurology (Minneap)* 1980;30:582–587.
85. Berger R, Florent G, Just M. Decrease of the lymphoproliferative response to varicella-zoster antigen in the aged. *Infect Immunol* 1982;32:24–27.
86. Burke B, Steele R, Beard O, et al. Immune responses to varicella-zoster in the aged. *Arch Intern Med* 1982;142:291–293.
87. Hook EW, Holmes KK. Gonococcal infections. *Ann Intern Med* 1985;102: 229–243.
88. Sexually transmitted disease surveillance. Atlanta, GA: Centers for Disease Control and Prevention, 1995: Title 3600.
89. Hook EW, Handsfield HH. Gonococcal infections in the adult. In: Holmes KK, ed. *Sexually transmitted diseases,* 2nd ed. New York: McGraw-Hill, 1990: 149–158.
90. Handsfield HH. *Neisseria gonorrhoeae*. In: Mandell GL, Douglas RG Jr, Bennett JE, eds. *Principles and practice of infectious diseases,* 3rd ed. New York: Churchill Livingston, 1990:1622–1623.
91. Barr J, Danielsson D. Septic gonococcal dermatitis. *Br Med J* 1971;1:482–485.
92. Levine B. Sexually transmitted diseases: treatment guidelines. *MMWR* 1993; 42:56–67.
93. Handsfield HH. Asymptomatic gonorrhea in men: diagnosis, natural course, prevalence and significance. *N Engl J Med* 1974;290:117–123.
94. Cucurull E, Espinoza LR. Gonococcal arthritis. *Rheum Dis Clin North Am* 1998;24:305–322.
95. Manicourt DH, Orloff S. Gonococcal arthritis-dermatitis syndrome: study of serum and synovial fluid immune complex levels. *Arthritis Rheum* 1982;25: 574–578.
96. Britigan BE, Cohen MS, Sparling PF. Gonococcal infection: a model of molecular pathogenesis. *N Engl J Med* 1985;312:1683–1694.
97. Wise CM, Morris CR, Wasilauskas BL, et al. Gonococcal arthritis in an era of increasing penicillin resistance. *Arch Intern Med* 1994;154:2690.
98. O'Brien JP, Goldenberg DL, Rice PA. Disseminated gonococcal infection: a prospective analysis of 49 patients and a review of pathophysiology and immune mechanisms. *Medicine* 1983;62 :395–406.
99. Platt R, Rice PA, McCormack WM. Risk of acquiring gonorrhea and prevalence of abnormal adnexal findings among women recently exposed to gonorrhea. *JAMA* 1983;250:3205–3209.
100. Ross JDC. Systemic gonococcal infection. *Genitourin Med* 1996;72:404.
101. Westrom L. Incidence, prevalence, and trends of acute pelvic inflammatory disease and its consequences in industrialized countries. *Am J Obstet Gynecol* 1980;138:880–892.
102. Brunham RC, Holmes KK, Eschenbach D. Sexually transmitted diseases in pregnancy. In: Holmes LKK, Mardh PA, Sparling PF, et al., eds. *Sexually transmitted diseases.* New York: McGraw-Hill, 1984:782–711.
103. Masi AT, Eisenstein BI. Disseminated gonococcal infection (DGI) and gonococcal arthritis (GCA), II: clinical manifestations, diagnosis, complications, treatment , and prevention. *Semin Arthritis Rheum* 1981;10:173–197.
104. Mastrolonardo M, et al. Cutaneous vasculitis as the sole manifestation of disseminated gonococcal infection: case report. *Genitourin Med* 1970;70:130–131.
105. Shapiro L, Teisch JA, Brownstein MH. Dermatohistopathology of chronic gonococcal sepsis. *Arch Dermatol* 1973;107:403–406.
106. Bayer AS. Gonococcal arthritis syndromes: an update on diagnosis and management. *Postgrad Med* 1980;67:200.
107. Angulo JM, et al. Gonococcal arthritis. *Comp Ther* 1999;25:155–162.
108. Liebling MR, Arkfeld DG, Michelini GA, et al. Identification of *Neisseria gonorrhoeae* in synovial fluid using the polymerase chain reaction. *Arthritis Rheum* 1994;37:702–709.
109. Krauss DS, Aronson MD, Gump DW, et al. *Hemophilus influenzae* septic arthritis: a mimicker of gonococcal arthritis. *Arthritis Rheum* 1974;17:267.
110. Rinadi RZ, Harrison WO, Fan PT. Penicillin-resistant gonococcal arthritis: a report of four cases. *Ann Intern Med* 1982;97:43–45.
111. Gorwitz RJ, Nakashima AK, Moran JS, et al. Sentinel surveillance for antimicrobial resistance in *Neisseria gonorrhoeae,* United States, 1998–1991: the Gonococcal Isolate Surveillance Project Study Group. *MMWR CDC Surveill Summ* 1993;42:29.
112. Stewart K, Carlson M, Segal AM, et al. Gonococcal arthritis caused by penicillinase producing strains of *Neisseria gonorrhoeae. Arthritis Rheum* 1991;34: 245.
113. Fox KK, Knapp JS, Holmes KK, et al. Antimicrobial resistance in *Neisseria gonorrhoeae* in the United States, 1988–1994: the emergence of decreased susceptibility to the fluoroquinolones. *J Infect Dis* 1997;175:1396.
114. Centers for Disease Control and Prevention. 1998 Guidelines for treatment of sexually transmitted diseases. *MMWR Recomm Rep* 1998;47:1–111.
115. Gang-related outbreak of penicillinase-producing *Neisseria gonorrhoeae* and other sexually transmitted diseases, Colorado Springs, Colorado. *MMWR Recomm Rep* 1993;42:25–28.
116. Tapsall JW, et al. The frequency of co-infection with *Neisseria gonorrhoeae* and *Chlamydia trachomatis* in men and women in eastern Sydney. *Pathology* 1996; 28:84.
117. LeSaux N, Ronald AR. Role of ceftriaxone in sexually transmitted diseases. *Rev Infect Dis* 1982;11:299–309.
118. Gardner JAS. The role of oral contraceptives in cervical infection with sexually transmitted diseases. Seattle, Washington: University of Washington; 1980. Dissertation.
119. Singh B, Cutler JC, Utidjian HM. Studies on the development of a vaginal preparation providing both prophylaxis against venereal disease and other genital infections and contraception, II: effect *in vitro* of vaginal contraception and noncontraception preparations on *Treponema pallidum* and *Neisseria gonorrhoeae. Br J Vener Dis* 1972;48:57–64.
120. Ross SC, et al. Complement deficiency states and infection. *Medicine* 1984;63: 243.
121. Kelly WN, Harris ED, Ruddy S, et al., eds. *Textbook of rheumatology,* 3rd ed. Philadelphia: WB Saunders, 1989.
122. McWhinney PH, Langhorne P, Love WC, et al. Disseminated gonococcal infection associated with deficiency of the second component of complement. *Postgrad Med J* 1991;67:297–298.
123. Rice PA, McCormack WM, Kasper DL. Natural serum bactericidal activity against *Neisseria gonorrhoeae* isolates from disseminated, locally invasive, and uncomplicated disease. *J Immunol* 1980;124:2105–2109.
124. Knapp JS, Holmes KK. Disseminated gonococcal infections caused by *Neisseria gonorrhoeae* with unique nutritional requirement. *J Infect Dis* 1975;132: 204–208.
125. Densen P, MacKeen LA, Clark RA. Dissemination of gonococcal infection is associated with delayed stimulation of complement-dependent neutrophil chemotaxis *in vitro*. *Infect Immun* 1982;38:563–572.
126. Gregg CR, et al. Toxic activity of purified lipopolysaccharide of *Neisseria gonorrhoeae* for human fallopian tube mucosa. *J Infect Dis* 1985;143:432.
127. Dallabeta G, et al. Gonococcal infections. *Infect Dis Clin North Am* 1987;1:25.
128. Rice PFA, Goldenberg DL. Clinical manifestations of disseminated infection caused by *Neisseria gonorrhoeae* are linked to differences in bactericidal reactivity of infecting strains. *Ann Intern Med* 1981;95:175–178.
129. Britigan BE, et al. Gonococcal infections: a model of molecular pathogenesis. *N Engl J Med* 1985;312:1683.
130. Draper DL, James JF, Brooks GF, et al. Comparison of virulence markers of peritoneal and fallopian tube isolates with endocervical *Neisseria gonorrhoeae* isolates from women with acute salpingitis. *Infect Immun* 1980;27:882.
131. Lind I. Antimicrobial resistance in *Neisseria gonorrhoeae. Clin Infect Dis* 1997; 24[Suppl]:93.
132. Steere AC, Malawista SE, Snydman DR et al. Lyme arthritis: an epidemic of oligoarticular arthritis in children and adults in three Connecticut communities. *Arthritis Rheum* 1977;20:7–17.
133. Afzelius A. Erythema chronicum migrans. *Acta Derm Venereol* 1921;2:120–125.
134. Garin-Bujadoux C. Paralysie par les tiques. *J Med Lyons* 1922;3:765–767.
135. Bannwarth A. Chronische Lymphocytare Meningitis, entzuundliche Polyneuritis and Rheumatismus, Ein Beitrag zum Problem Allergie und Nervensystem. *Archiv fur Psychiatric und Nervenkrankheiten* 1941;113:284–376.
136. Hellerstrom S. Erythema chronica migrans afzelius with meningitis. *Acta Dermato-Venereologica* 1951;31:227–234, 1951.
137. Lyme disease: United States, 1991–1992. *MMWR* 1993;42:345–378.
138. Centers for Disease Control and Prevention: Lyme disease—United States, 1996. *MMWR* 1997;46:531–535.
139. Centers for Disease Control. Lyme disease—United States, 1987 and 1988. *JAMA* 1989;262:2209–2210.
140. Tsai TF, Bailey RE, Moore PS. National surveillance of Lyme disease, 1987–1988. *Conn Med* 1989;53:324–326.
141. Sigal LH. Lyme disease: a worldwide borreliosis. *Clin Exp Rheum* 1988;6: 411–421.
142. Sigal LH. Current recommendations for the treatment of Lyme disease. *Drugs* 1992;43:683–699.
143. Steere A. Lyme disease. *N Engl J Med* 2001;345:115–125.
144. Asbrink E, Hovmark A. Early and late cutaneous manifestations in Ixodes-borne borreliosis (erythema migrans borreliosis, Lyme borreliosis). *Ann N Y Acad Sci* 1988;539:4–15.
145. Sigal LH. Musculoskeletal manifestations of Lyme arthritis. *Rheum Dis Clin North Am* 1998;24:323–351.
146. Berger BW, Lesser RL. Lyme disease. *Dermatol Clin* 1992;4:763–775.
147. Strle F, et al. Solitary borrelial lymphocytoma: report of 36 cases. *Infection* 1992;20:201–206.

148. Strle F, et al. Treatment of borrelial lymphocytoma. *Infection* 1996;24:80–84.
149. Aberer E, et al. Success and failure in the treatment of acrodermatitis chronica atrophicans. *Infection* 1996;24:85–87.
150. Asbrink E, Hovmark A. Successful cultivation of spirochetes from skin lesions of patients with erythema chronicum migrans Afzelius and acrodermatitis chronica atrophicans. *Acta Pathol Mirobiol Immunol Scand* 1985;93: 161–163.
151. Buechner SA, et al. Localized scleroderma associated with *Borrelia burgdorferi* infection. Clinical, histologic, and immunohistochemical observations. *J Am Acad Dermatol* 29:190–196, 1993.
152. Olsson I, Hovmark A, Asbrink E, et al. Sclerotic skin lesions as manifestations of Ixodes-borne borreliosis. *Ann N Y Acad Med* 539:480–482, 1988.
153. Schempp C, et al. Further evidence for *Borrelia burgdorferi* infection in morphea and lichen sclerosus et atrophicus confirmed by DNA amplification. *J Invest Dermatol* 100:717–720, 1993.
154. Sigal LH, Patella SJ. Lyme arthritis as the incorrect diagnosis in pediatric and adolescent fibromyalgia. *Pediatics* 90:523–528, 1992.
155. Logigian EL, Kaplan RF, Steere AC. Chronic neurologic manifestations of Lyme disease. *N Engl J Med* 323:1438–1444, 1990.
156. Steere AC, et al: The clinical evolution of Lyme arthritis. *Ann Intern Med* 107:725–731, 1987.
157. Halprin JJ, et al. Lyme neuroborreliosis: central nervous system manifestations. *Neurology* 39:753–549, 1989.
158. Berger BW, Clemmensen OJ, Ackerman AB. Lyme disease is a spirochetosis. *Am J Dermatopathol* 5:111–124, 1983.
159. Nadelman RB, et al: Lyme Borreliosis. *Lancet* 352:557–565, 1998.
160 Dattwyler RJ, et al. Seronegative Lyme disease: dissociation of the specific T- and B-lymphocyte responses to Borrelia burgdorferi. *N Engl J Med* 319: 1441–1446, 1988.
161. Dressler F, Yoshinari NH, Steere AC. The T-cell proliferative assay in the diagnosis of Lyme disease. *Ann Intern Med* 115:533–539, 1991.
162. Steere AC, Taylor E, McHugh GL, et al. The overdiagnosis of lyme disease. *JAMA* 1993;269:1812–1816.
163. Nadelman RB, et al. Failure to isolate *Borrelia burgdorferi* after antimicrobial therapy in culture-documented lyme borreliosis associated with erythema migrans: report of a prospective study. *Am J Med* 1993;94:583–588.
164. Berger BW, Johnson RC, Kodner C, et al. Cultivation of *Borrelia burgdorferi* from erythema migrans lesions and perilesional skin. *J Clin Microbiol* 1992;30: 359–361.
165. Massarotti EM, et al. Treatment of early lyme disease. *Am J Med* 1992;92: 396–403.
166. Liu NY, et al. Randomized trial of doxycycline vs amoxicillin/probenecid for the treatment of Lyme arthritis: treatment of non-responders with intravenous penicillin or ceftriaxone. *Arthr Rheum* 1989;32:S46.
167. Steere AC, Pachner A, Malawista SE. Neurologic abnormalities of Lyme disease: successful treatment with high-dose intravenous penicillin. *Ann Intern Med* 1983;99:767–772.
168. Dattwyler RJ, Halperin JJ, Volkman DJ, et al. Treatment of late Lyme borreliosis-randomized comparison of ceftriaxone and penicillin. *Lancet* 1988;1: 1191–1194.
169. McAlister HF, et al. Lyme carditis: an important cause of reversible heart block. *Ann Intern Med* 110:339–345, 1989.
170. Steere AC, Dwyer E, Winchester R. Association of chronic Lyme arthritis with HLA-DR4 and HLA-DR2 alleles. *N Engl J Med* 1990;323:219–223.
171. Kalish RA, Leong JM, Steere AC. Association of treatment-resistant chronic Lyme arthritis with HLA-DR4 and antibody reactivity to OspA and OspB of Borrelia burgdorferi. *Infect Immun* 1993;61:2774–2779.
172. Dinerman H, Steere AC. Lyme disease associated with fibromyalgia. *Ann Intern Med* 1992;117:281–285.
173. Hsu V, et al."Chronic Lyme disease" as the incorrect diagnosis in patients with fibromyalgia. *Arthritis Rheum* 1993;3:1493–1500.
174. Agre F, Schwartz R. The value of early treatment of deer tick bites for the prevention of Lyme disease. *Am J Dis Child* 1993;147:945–947.
175. Couch P, Johnson CE. Prevention of Lyme disease. *Am J Hosp Pharm* 1992;49: 1164–1173.
176. Sigal LH, et al. Multicenter efficacy trial of a prophylactic recombinant Borrelia burgdorferi outer surface protein (OspA) vaccine for Lyme disease. *Arthritis Rheum* 1997;40[Suppl]:142.
177. Steere AC, Malawista SE. Cases of Lyme disease in the United States: location correlated with distribution of *Ixodes dammini*. *Ann Intern Med* 1979;91: 730–735.
178. Burgdorfer W, et al. Lyme disease: a tick-borne spirochetosis? *Science* 1982; 1317–1320.
179. Anderson JF. Ecology of Lyme disease. *Conn Med* 1989;53:343–346.
180. Sood SK, et al. Duration of tick attachment as a predictor of the risk of Lyme disease in an area in which Lyme disease is endemic. *J Infect Dis* 1997;175: 996–999.
181. Ribeiro JM, Mather TN, Piesman J, et al. Dissemination and salivary delivery of Lyme disease spirochetes in vector ticks (acari: ixodidae). *J Med Entomol* 1987;24:201–205.
182. Klempner MS, Noring R, Rogers RA. Invasion of human skin fibroblasts by the Lyme disease spirochete, *Borrelia burgdorferi*. *J Infect Dis* 1993;167: 1074–1081.
183. Wile UJ. Arthropathy in secondary syphilis. *J Cutan Dis Incl Syph* 1914;32: 20–23.
184. Division of STD Prevention. Sexually Transmitted Disease Surveillance, 1997. US Department of Health and Human Services, Public Health Service. Atlanta: Centers for Disease Control (CDC), September 1998.
185. Centers for Disease Control: Primary and Secondary Syphilis—United States, 1997. *MMWR Recomm Rep* 1998;47:493–497.
186. Cohen PR, Hymes SR. Secondary syphilis presenting as cutaneous nodules in a patient previously treated for laryngeal carcinoma. *Cutis* 1992;49:51–54.
187. Noppakun N, Dinehart SM, Solomon AR. Pustular secondary syphilis. *Int J Dermatol* 1987;26:112–114.
188. Pavithran K. Nodular secondary syphilis. *Int J Dermatol* 1991;30:799–800.
189. Sharma VK, Sharma R, Kumar B, et al. Ulcerative secondary syphilis. *Int J Dermatol* 1990;29:585–586.
190. Goens JL, et al. Dermatologic and systemic manifestation s of syphilis. *Am Fam Physician* 1994;50:1013–1020.
191. Sanchez M, Luger AFH. Syphilis. In: Fitzpatrick TB, Eisen AZ, Wolff K, et al., eds. *Dermatology in general medicine*. 1993:2699–2743.
192. Reginato AJ. Syphilitic arthritis and osteitis. *Rheum Dis Clin N Am* 1993;19: 379–398.
193. Burgoyne M, Agudelo C, Pisko E. Chronic syphilitic polyarthritis mimicking systemic lupus erythematosus/rheumatoid arthritis as the initial presentation of human immunodeficiency virus infection. *J Rheumatol* 1992;19: 313–315.
194. Abell E, Marks R, Wilson JE. Secondary syphilis: a clinicopathological review. *Br J Dermatol* 1975;93:53–61.
195. Kahn LB, Gordon W. Sarcoid-like granulomas in secondary syphilis. *Arch Pathol* 1971;92:334–337.
196. Poulsen A, Kobayasi T, Secher L, et al. *Treponema pallidum* in macular and papular secondary syphilis skin eruptions. *Acta Derm Venereol (Stockh)* 1986; 66:251–258.
197. Crowson AN, et al. Treponemal diseases. In: Elder D, et al., eds. *Lever's histopathology of the skin*, 8th ed. Philadelphia: Lippincott-Raven, 1997:503–508.
198. Dowell ME, et al. Response of latent syphilis or neurosyphilis to ceftriaxone therapy in persons infected with human immunodeficiency virus. *Am J Med* 1992;93:481–488.
199. Brown TJ, et al. An overview of sexually transmitted diseases, I. *J Am Acad Dermatol* 1999;41:511–529.
200. McNeely MC, et al. Cutaneous secondary syphilis: Preliminary immunohistopathologic support for a role for immune complexes in lesion pathogenesis. *J Am Acad Dermatol* 1986;14:564–571.
201. Bhorade MS, Carag HB, Lee HJ, et al. Nephropathy of secondary syphilis: a clinical and pathological spectrum. *JAMA* 1986;261:1159–1166.
202. Laurenson I, et al. Meningococcal disease. *N Engl J Med* 2001;345:699.
203. Rosenstein NE, at al. Meningococcal disease. *N Engl J Med* 2001;344: 1378–1388.
204. Damany DS, et al. Primary meningococcal pyoarthrosis of the knee. *J Infection* 1997; 35:320–321.
205. Person DA, et al. Chronic meningococcemia mimicking acute rheumatic fever. *Hawaii Med J* 1998;57:583–584.
206. Austin TW, et al. Chronic meningococcal sacroiliitis: case report. *Clin Infect Dis* 1995;20:473.
207. Nitta AT, Douglas JM, Arakere G, et al. Disseminated meningococcal infection in HIV-seropositive patients. *AIDS* 1993;7:87–90.
208. Van Deuren M, et al. Rapid diagnosis of acute meningococcal infections by needle aspiration or biopsy of skin lesions. *BMJ* 1996;306:1229–1232.
209. Mader R, et al. Recurrent sterile arthritis following primary septic meningococcal arthritis. *Clin Exp Rheumatol* 1994;12:531–533.
210. Linell F, Norden A. *Mycobacterium balnei*. A new acid-fast bacillus occurring in swimming pools and capable of producing skin lesions in humans. *Acta Tuberc Scand* 1954;33[Suppl]:1.
211. Iredell J, Whitby M, Blacklock Z. Mycobacterium marinum infection: epidemiology and presentation in Queensland 1971–1990. *Med J Austr* 1992;157: 596–598.
212. Johnston JM, Izumi AL. Cutaneous *Mycobacterium marinum* infection ("swimming pool granuloma"). *Clin Dermatol* 1987;5:68–75.
213. Williams CS, Riordan DC. *Mycobacterium marinum* (atypical acid-fast bacillus) infections of the hand. *J Bone Joint Surg Am* 1973;55:1042–1050.
214. King AJ, et al. Disseminated cutaneous *Mycobacterium marinum* infection. *Arch Dermatol* 1983;119:268.
215. Harth M, et al. Septic arthritis due to *Mycobacterium marinum*. *J Rheumatol* 1994;21:95.
216. Barton A, et al. *Mycobacterium marinum* infection causing septic arthritis and osteomyelitis. *Br J Rheum* 1997;36:1207–1209.
217. Alloway JA, et al. *Mycobacterium marinum* arthritis. *Semin Arthritis Rheum* 1985;24:382.
218. Pioro MH, et al. Septic arthritis. *Rheum Dis Clin North Am* 1997;23:239–258.
219. Forsgren A. Antibiotic susceptibility of *Mycobacterium marinum*. *Scand J Infect Dis* 1993;25:779–782.
220. Ljungberg B, Christensson B, Grubb R. Failure of doxycycline treatment in aquarium-associated *Mycobacterium marinum* infections. *Scand J Infect Dis* 1987;19:539–543.
221. Gibson T, et al. Arthritis of leprosy. *Br J Rheumatol* 1994;33:963–966.
222. Cossermelli-Messina W, et al. Articular inflammatory manifestations in patients with different forms of leprosy. *J Rheumatol* 1998;25:111–119.
223. Pernambuco C, Cossermelli-Messina W. Rheumatic manifestations of leprosy: clinical aspects. *J Rheumatol* 1993;20:897–899.
224. Holla VV, Kenetkar MV, Kolhatkar MK, et al. Leprous synovitis: a study of fifty cases. *Int J Leprosy* 1983;51:29–32.

225. Shenck BR . On refractory subcutaneous abscesses caused by a fungus possibly related to the sporotricha. *Bull Hopkins Hosp* 1898;9:286.
226. Altner PC, Turner RR. Sporotrichosis of bones and joints: review of the literature and report of six cases. *Clin Orthop Rel Res* 1970;68:138–148.
227. Cuellar ML, et al. Other fungal arthritides. *Rheum Dis Clin North Am* 1993;19: 439–455.
228. Coles FB, et al. A multistate outbreak of sporotrichosis associated with sphagnum moss. *Am J Epidemiology* 1992;136:475–487.
229. Winn RE. Systemic fungal infections—diagnosis and treatment, I: sporotrichosis. *Infect Dis Clin North Am* 1988;2:899–911.
230. Lynch PJ, Voorhees JJ, Harrell EJ. Systemic sporotrichosis. *Ann Intern Med* 1970;73:23–30.
231. Chowdhary G, Weinstein A, Klein R, et al. Sporotrichal arthritis. *Ann Rheum Dis* 1991;50:112–114.
232. Gullberg RM, et al. Sporotrichosis: recurrent cutaneous, articular, and central nervous system infection in a renal transplant recipient. *Rev Infect Dis* 1987;9: 369–376.
233. Fitzpatrick JE, Eubanks S. Acquired immunodeficiency syndrome presenting as disseminated cutaneous sporotrichosis. *Int J Dermatol* 1988;27:406–407.
234. Lipstein-Kresch E, et al. Disseminated *Sporothrix schenckii* infection with arthritis in a patient with acquired immunodeficiency syndrome. *J Rheumatol* 1985;12:805–808.
235. Purvis RS, et al. Sporotrichosis presenting as arthritis and subcutaneous nodules. *J Am Acad Dermatol* 1993;28:879–884.
236. Cuellar ML, et al. Fungal arthritis. *Ann Rheum Dis* 1992;51:690–697.
237. Yacobucci GN, Santilli MD. Sporotrichosis of the knee: a case report. *Orthopedics* 1986;9:387–390.
238. Sharkey-Mathis PK, et al. Treatment of sporotrichosis with itraconazole. *Am J Med* 1993;95:279–285.
239. Marques ME, Coelho KIR, Sotto MN, et al. Comparison between histochemical and immunohistochemical methods for diagnosis of sporotrichosis. *J Clin Pathol* 1992;45:1089–1093.
240. Bayer AS, Scott VJ, Guze LB. Fungal arthritis, III: sporotrichal arthritis. *Semin Arthritis Rheum* 1979;9:66–74.
241. Ortiz O, Lefkowitz Z. Case report 678. *Skeletal Radiol* 1991;20:376–378.
242. Graybill JR. Future directions of antifungal chemotherapy. *Clin Infect Dis* 1992;14[Suppl 1]:S1700–1781.
243. Viviani MA, Tortorano AM, Pagano A, et al. European experience with itraconazole in systemic mycoses. *J Am Acad Dermatol* 1990;23:587–593.
244. Oscherwitz SL, et al. Disseminated sporotrichosis in a patient infected with human immunodeficiency virus. *Clin Infect Dis* 1992;15:568–569.
245. Winn RE, et al. Systemic sporotrichosis treated with itraconazole. *Clin Infect Dis* 1993;17:210–217.
246. Iwatsu T, Nishimura K, Miyaji M. Spontaneous disappearance of cutaneous sporotrichosis: report of two cases. *Dermatology* 1985;24:524–525.
247. Baker JH, Goodpasture HC, Kuhns HR, et al. Fungemia caused by an amphotericin B-resistant isolate of *Sporothrix schenkii*: successful treatment with itraconazole. *Arch Pathol Lab Med* 1989;113:1279–1281.
248. Heller HM, Fuhrer J. Disseminated sporotrichosis in patients with AIDS: case report and review of the literature. *AIDS* 1991;5:1243–1246.
249. Plouffe JF, et al. Cell mediated immune responses to sporotrichosis. *J Infect Dis* 1246;139:152–157.
250. Katzenstein D. Isolated *Candida* arthritis: report of a case and definition of a distinct clinical syndrome. *Arthritis Rheum* 1985;28:1421.
251. Bisbe J, et al. Disseminated candidiasis in addicts who use brown heroin: report of 83 cases and review. *Clin Infect Dis* 1992;15:910–923.
252. Silveira LH, et al. *Candida* arthritis. *Rheum Dis Clin North Am* 1993;19:427–437.
253. Miro JM, et al. Costochondral involvement in systemic candidiasis in heroin addicts: clinical, scintigraphic, and histologic features in 26 patients. *Arthritis Rheum* 1988;31:793–797.
254. Bayer AS, Guze LB. Fungal arthritis, I: *Candida* arthritis—diagnostic and prognostic implications and therapeutic considerations. *Semin Arthritis Rheum* 1978;89:142.
255. Grubb BP, Manders MM, Haile CA. Candidal costochondritis responsive to ketoconazole in an iv drug abuser. *Postgrad Med* 1986;79:57–60.
256. Cuende E, et al. *Candida* arthritis in adult patients who are not intravenous drug addicts: report of three cases and review of the literature. *Semin Arthritis Rheum* 1993;22:224–241.
257. Marcus J, Grossman ME, Yunakov MJ, et al. Disseminated candidiasis, *Candida* arthritis and unilateral skin lesions. *J Am Acad Dermatol* 1992;26:295–297.
258. Bielsa I, et al. Systemic candidiasis in heroin abusers: cutaneous findings. *Int J Dermatol* 1987;26:314–319.
259. Dupont B, Drouhet E. Cutaneous, ocular, and osteoarticular candidiasis in heroin addicts: new clinical and therapeutic aspects in 38 patients. *J Infect Dis* 1985;152:577–591.
260. Collignon P, Sorrell TC. Disseminated candidiasis: evidence of distinctive syndrome in heroin abusers. *Br Med J* 1983;287:861.
261. Anaissie E. Opportunistic mycoses in the immunocompromised host: experience at a cancer center and review. *Clin Infect Dis* 1992;14[Suppl 1]:S43–S53.
262. Weems JJ. *Candida parapsilosis*: epidemiology, pathogenicity, clinical manifestations, and antimicrobial susceptibility. *Clin Infect Dis* 1992;14:756–766.
263. Zmierczak H, et al: *Candida glabrata* arthritis: case report and review of the literature. *Clin Rheumatol* 1999;18:406–409.
264. Darling ST. A protozoon general infection producing pseudotubercles in the lungs and focal necrosis in the liver, spleen, and lymph nodes. *JAMA* 1906;46: 1283.
265. DeMonbreun WA. The cultivation and cultural characteristics of Darling's *Histoplasma capsulatum*. *Am J Trop Med* 1934;14:93.
266. Wheat LJ, et al. A large urban outbreak of histoplasmosis: clinical features. *Ann Intern Med* 1982;94:331.
267. Eidbo J, Sanchez RL, Tschen JA, et al. Cutaneous manifestations of histoplasmosis in acquired-immune-deficiency-syndrome. *Am J Surg Pathol* 1993;17: 110–116.
268. Bridgeford PH. Histoplasmosis arthritis. In: Espinoza LR, ed. *Infections in the rheumatic diseases.* Orlando: Grune & Stratton, 1988:173–180.
269. Darouiche RO, et al. Articular histoplasmosis. *J Rheumatol* 1992;19:1991–1993.
270. Fowler VG. Prosthetic joint infection due to *Histoplasma capsulatum*: case report and review. *Clin Infect Dis* 1998;26:1017.
271. Longley BJ. Fungal diseases. In: Elder D, et al., eds. *Lever's histopathology of the skin,* 8th ed. Philadelphia: Lippincott-Raven, 1997:517–551.
272. Kaufman L. Laboratory methods for the diagnosis and confirmation of systemic mycoses. *Clin Infect Dis* 1992;14[Suppl 1]:S23–S29.
273. Ophuls W, Moffitt HC. A new pathogenic mould (formerly described as a protozoan): *Coccidioides immitis*: preliminary report. *Phila Med J* 1900;5:1471.
274. Galgiani JN. Coccidioidomycosis: changes in clinical expression, serological diagnosis, and therapeutic options. *Clin Infect Dis* 1992;14[Suppl 1]:S100–S105.
275. Kushwaha VP, et al. Musculoskeletal coccidioidomycosis: a review of 25 cases. *Clin Orthop* 1996;332:190–199.
276. Lund PJ, et al. Magnetic resonance imaging in coccidioidal arthritis. *Skeletal Radiol* 1996;25:661–665.
277. Fish DG, et al. Coccidioidomycosis during human immunodeficiency virus infection. A review of 77 patients. *Medicine (Baltmore)* 1990;69:384–391.
278. Pappagianis D, Zimmer BL. Serology of coccidioidomycosis. *Clin Microbiol Rev* 1990;3:247–268.
279. Graybill JR, Stevens DA, Galgiani JN, et al. Itraconazole treatment of coccidioidomycosis. *Am J Med* 1990;84:282–290.
280. Patterson TF, Andriole VT. Current concepts in cryptococcosis. *Eur J Clin Microbiol Infect Dis* 1989;8:457–469.
281. Graybill JR. Future directions of antifungal chemotherapy. *Clin Infect Dis* 1992;14[Suppl 1]:S170–S181.
282. Abril A, et al. Polyarticular blastomycotic arthritis. *J Rheumatol* 1998;25: 1019–1021.
283. Alvarez L, et al. Articular aspergillosis: case report. *Clin Infect Dis* 1995;20: 457–460.
284. Garcia-Porrua C, et al. Septic arthritis by *Aspergillus fumigatus*: a complication of corticosteroid infiltration. *Br J Rheumatol* 1997;36:610–611.
285. McWhinney PHM, et al. Successful surgical management of septic arthritis due to trichosporon beigelii in a patient with acute myeloid leukaemia. *Scan J Infect Dis* 1992;24:245–247.
286. Than-Saw, Mar-Mar-Nyein, Oo MM. Isolation of *Entamoeba histolytica* from arthritic knee joint. *Trop Geogr Fed* 1992;44:355–358.
287. Benstson S, Knutson K. The infected knee arthroplasty. *Acta Ortop Scand* 1991; 62:301–311.
288. Golz R, Kuschner SH, Gellman H. Sequential infection of silicone metacarpophalangeal joint arthroplasties resulting from skin breakdown. *J Hand Surg Am* 1992;17:150–152.
289. Mowat AG, Baum J. Chemotaxis of polymorphonuclear leukocytes from patients with rheumatoid arthritis. *J Clin Invest* 1971;50:2541–2549.
290. Turner RA, Schumacher HR, Myers AR. Phagocytic function of polymorphonuclear leukocytes in rheumatic diseases. *J Clin Invest* 1973;52:1632–1635.
291. Thomas BJ, Moreland JR, Amstutz HC. Infection after total joint arthroplasty from distal extremity sepsis. *Clin Orthop* 1983;181:121–125.
292. Bengtson S, Borgquist L, Lidgren L. Cost analysis of prophylaxis with antibiotics to prevent infected knee arthroplasty. *BMJ* 1989;299:710–720.

CHAPTER 13

Special Considerations Concerning the Cutaneous Manifestations of Rheumatic Diseases in Children

Lela A. Lee and William L. Weston

This chapter focuses on cutaneous manifestations of rheumatic diseases in children. Many of the diseases covered in this chapter have been discussed in preceding chapters. Consequently, the discussion will be limited to those aspects of disease unique to the pediatric population.

NEONATAL LUPUS ERYTHEMATOSUS

Neonatal lupus erythematosus (NLE) is a uniquely pediatric disease. It is not systemic lupus erythematosus that happens to occur in a newborn; rather it is a disease with a distinctive constellation of organ pathophysiology. It is an experiment of nature demonstrating a probable pathogenic role of autoantibodies produced in the mother and passed across the placenta to the unborn fetus. It also constitutes the best evidence suggesting a role of antibodies in the pathogenesis of a specific lupus cutaneous lesion. NLE is characterized primarily by congenital heart block or subacute cutaneous lupus lesions. Hepatobiliary disease and thrombocytopenia may also occur. Almost all babies with NLE have maternal anti-Ro (also known as SS-A) autoantibodies.

Historical Perspective

In 1954, McCuistion and Schoch (1) reported a case of cutaneous lupus lesions occurring transiently in a newborn whose mother subsequently developed systemic lupus erythematosus (SLE). It was their hypothesis that a factor transferred from mother to child during gestation caused the transient lupus skin lesions. In 1957, Hogg (2) reported a case of congenital heart block with subendocardial fibroelastosis in a newborn whose mother had SLE. She proposed that the pathology in the baby represented a congenital form of lupus erythematosus (LE).

The relationship between connective tissue disease in the mother and congenital heart block or lupus skin lesions in her offspring became clearer as more reports were added to the literature in the following decades. In 1980, Franco et al. (3) and Weston et al. (4) reported that anti-Ro autoantibodies are associated with NLE and may serve as a serologic marker for the disease. Since that time, many more cases of NLE have been recognized and reported, with a few hundred cases in the literature (5,6).

Although most cases have been reported relatively recently, NLE clearly existed, but was unrecognized, prior to the reports of McCuistion and Schoch and Hogg. For example, in 1928, Aylward (7) reported siblings with congenital heart block, born to a mother with Sjögren syndrome, but made no association between the Sjögren syndrome in the mother and the congenital heart block in the babies.

Epidemiology

The incidence of NLE is not known with certainty. However, information is available about the incidence of congenital heart block, which has been estimated to occur in one of 20,000 live births (8). NLE is the most common cause of congenital heart block (9,10), accounting for perhaps 50% to 75% of cases (11). Heart block is present in about half of NLE cases. Taken together, this information indicates that the incidence of NLE is likely to be at least one in 20,000 live births.

NLE probably occurs in all ethnic groups. In our series, the ethnic composition of the group reflects that of the general population of the region. In a large series from a national registry for NLE, females outnumber males two to one among children with skin lesions, whereas the ratio of females to males is about one to one among children with cardiac disease (12,13).

Although almost all children with NLE have maternal anti-Ro autoantibodies, the likelihood that a given woman with anti-Ro autoantibodies will have a baby with NLE is low. In a survey of sera from 800 pregnant women, we found four (0.5%) with anti-Ro precipitins (14). If the estimated incidence of NLE at one in 20,000 births is correct, then the risk for an anti-Ro–positive mother is about 1%. It should be emphasized that these are estimates only, but they do provide some perspective about the risk for NLE.

It is possible that some subgroups of anti-Ro–positive mothers have a higher risk. Women who have previously had a child with NLE may have as much as a 25% risk of having an affected child in a subsequent pregnancy (15). In addition, women with

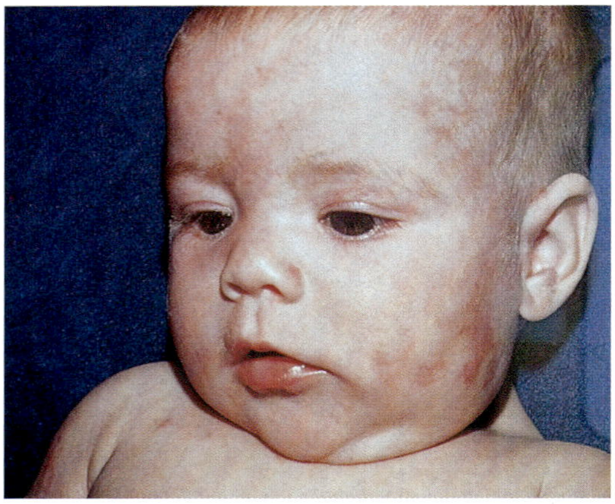

Figure 13.1. Neonatal lupus erythematosus. The eruption consists of confluent erythematous macules and plaques and is most prominent on the face.

anti-Ro who have SLE have been reported to have a 6% (16) to 13% (17) risk of having a baby with NLE in a given pregnancy.

Cutaneous Manifestations

Cutaneous disease is present in about one half of cases of NLE. Skin lesions of NLE are usually annular erythematous plaques, sometimes with fine scale (Figs. 13.1 and 13.2) (5,18). Hypopigmentation is common and may be the most cosmetically significant feature, particularly in babies with dark skin (Fig. 13.3). Fine wrinkling indicative of epidermal atrophy is not unusual, and telangiectasias may occur, but follicular plugging, dermal atrophy, and scarring rarely occur. Occasionally, cutis marmorata congenita–type lesions occur. We have observed a child with blistering lesions on the head and more typical NLE lesions elsewhere. The blisters presumably occurred in some of the lesions because of intense basal cell destruction.

Lesions of NLE occur most frequently on the face and scalp, although any area of the skin may be affected. Lesions may be concentrated in the periorbital or malar areas, giving an "owl-eye" appearance (19) (Fig 13.4). On unusual occasions, targetoid-like lesions have been detected (Fig 13.5). In some cases, the eruption is initiated or exacerbated by exposure of the skin to sunlight. However, sunlight is not a prerequisite for lesion formation, as NLE lesions have been observed at birth and may develop in the relatively sun-protected diaper area.

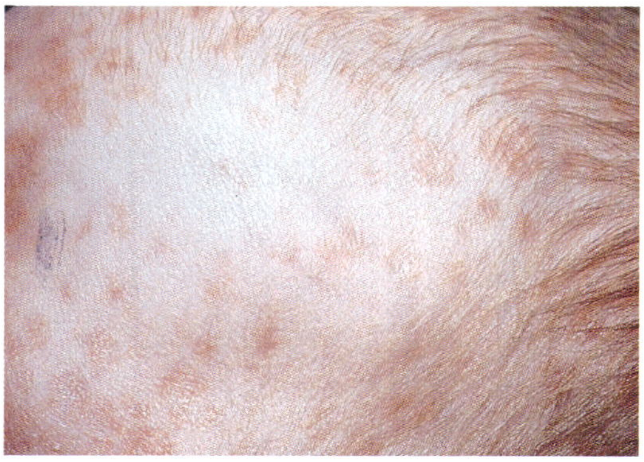

Figure 13.2. Neonatal lupus erythematosus. The lesions are smaller and more discrete than those shown in Fig. 13.1. This is the sister of the child in Fig. 13.1. (From Lee LA, Weston WL. New findings in neonatal lupus syndrome. *Am J Dis Child* 1984;138:233–236, with permission.)

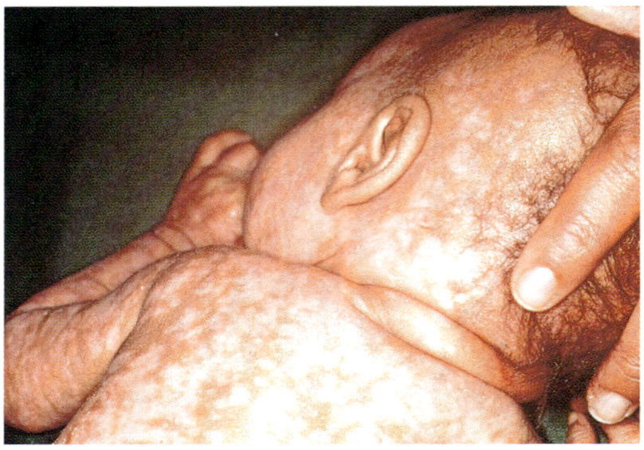

Figure 13.3. Neonatal lupus erythematosus. The eruption has resulted in extensive hypopigmentation in this infant whose normal skin color is black. The hypopigmentation later resolved. (From Lee LA, Weston, WL. Lupus erythematosus in childhood. *Dermatol Clin* 1986;4:151–160, with permission.)

Cutaneous lesions appear at birth or, more commonly, during the first weeks of life. Lesions last for a few weeks or months and then resolve spontaneously. Hypopigmentation may take several months to resolve (Fig. 13.3). In a few cases, there may be permanent telangiectasias or pigmentary abnormalities (Fig 13.6).

The cutaneous lesions of NLE surely represent subacute cutaneous lupus erythematosus (SCLE) of the newborn. They are associated with anti-Ro autoantibodies, may be brought on by sun exposure, and generally have relatively superficial inflammation without adnexal involvement, dermal atrophy, or scarring. These characteristics are more typical of SCLE than of discoid lupus erythematosus (DLE) (20,21). There are some differences between NLE lesions and those of SCLE in adults, however. The occurrence of lesions in the mid-facial region, including the periorbital and malar areas, is quite common in NLE but not typical of SCLE of adults. Lesions of NLE sometimes occur in areas of skin that are sun-protected, whereas SCLE lesions in adults are typically confined to sun-exposed skin. Nevertheless, the morphology of individual lesions, the pathology, the immunopathology, and the circulating autoantibodies are shared by NLE and SCLE of adults.

Cutaneous findings may occur in NLE as a result of extracutaneous disease. In some babies, petechiae or purpura due to thrombocytopenia are a presenting sign of NLE. Jaundice may be present in babies with hepatobiliary disease.

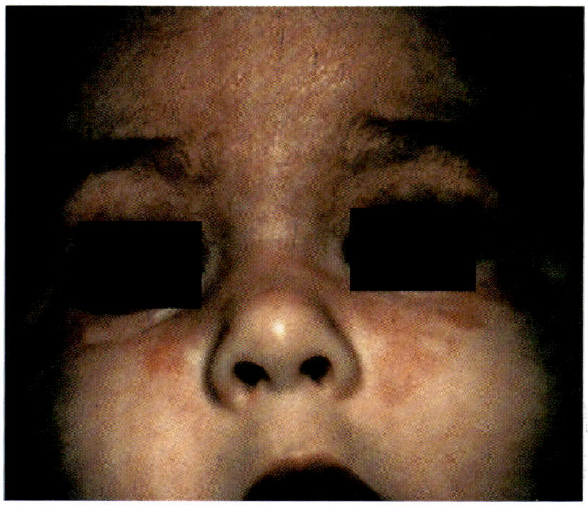

Figure 13.4. Periorbital involvement in patient with neonatal lupus erythematosus.

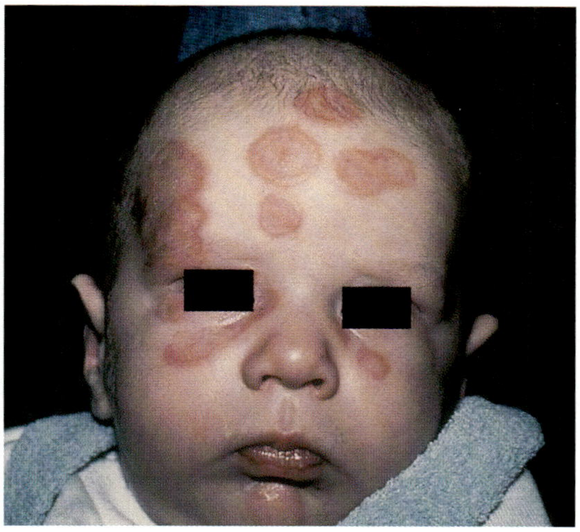

Figure 13.5. Targetoid lesions in infant with neonatal lupus erythematosus.

Extracutaneous Features

Congenital heart block occurs in perhaps one half or more of the cases of NLE. The heart block is usually complete heart block, although other conduction abnormalities such as bundle branch block and even asymptomatic prolonged QT interval have been observed (12,22,23). In most cases, heart block develops during gestation, often during the second trimester. However, complete heart block may develop during the third trimester or even shortly after birth (24). It is possible, but quite unusual, for heart block to resolve spontaneously (25), and indeed, autopsy examination has shown replacement of atrioventricular nodal tissue with fibrosis (26,27).

Most babies with NLE heart block require permanent pacemaker implantation during the newborn period or early childhood (12). In 10% to 20% of cases, heart failure persists despite a normal heart rate, and it is presumed that these babies have cardiac muscle involvement as well (5,12,28). The mortality rate for babies with persistent heart failure is very high. Although heart failure is usually evident during the neonatal period, there have been a few cases of children with congenital heart block who developed dilated cardiomyopathy noted months later (29).

Hepatobiliary disease may occur in as many as 10% of cases of NLE (5,30–32). In a review of cases from a national registry (32), three variants of hepatobiliary disease were noted: (a) liver failure present in utero or shortly after birth, often with a phenotype of neonatal iron storage disease or neonatal "hemochromatosis"; (b) transient conjugated hyperbilirubinemia noted during the first few weeks of life; and (c) transient aminotransferase elevations occurring at a few months of age. The prognoses for the latter two variants are excellent, with no apparent lasting hepatobiliary damage.

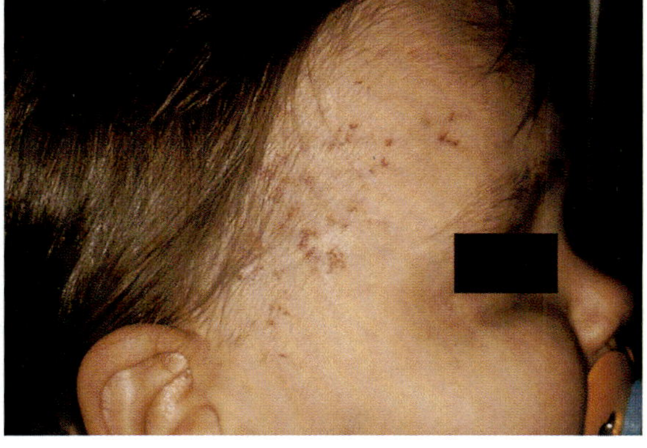

Figure 13.6. Neonatal lupus erythematosus. Residual telangiectasia in an infant with neonatal lupus erythematosus born of a mother with anti U_1 ribonucleic protein antibodies.

Thrombocytopenia occurs in about 10% of cases and is typically transient, but may be severe (33). In one of our cases, the baby had gastrointestinal bleeding thought to be due to thrombocytopenia.

Other extracutaneous findings reported in one or a few cases include hemolytic anemia, leukopenia, splenomegaly, pneumonitis, hypocalcemia, and myelopathy (18). The true relationship of these findings to NLE is not known.

Relationship Between Cutaneous and Systemic Features of the Disease

Cutaneous NLE may coexist with any of the extracutaneous features, but often occurs as an isolated finding. In a review of 18 cases of cutaneous NLE from a single institution, four children had thrombocytopenia, and three each had cardiac disease and hepatobiliary disease (19).

Pathology and Immunopathology

The histology of the cutaneous lesions of NLE is the same as that of SCLE of adults, with basal cell damage and a relatively sparse, superficial mononuclear cell infiltrate, and little adnexal involvement or deep infiltrate (21,34).

We have observed particulate deposits of IgG in the epidermis of NLE skin lesions and in the skin of adult patients with SCLE (21). The pattern of deposition is distinct from what is typically described in SLE and DLE, where immunoglobulin deposits are present at the dermal–epidermal junction. The particulate epidermal deposits can be reproduced in human skin grafted onto severe combined immunodeficient or nude mice by injecting affinity-purified anti-Ro antibodies (35).

Laboratory Manifestations

NLE is characteristically associated with maternal autoantibodies to Ro. The originally described Ro protein is a 60-kDa protein that binds any of four small RNAs called hY RNAs (36). In sera containing antibodies to 60-kDa Ro, it is common to find other autoantibodies concurrently, and perhaps consequently, there have been several different autoantibodies associated with NLE. These include antibodies to 52-kDa Ro (37), a protein whose sequence is not homologous to 60-kDa Ro; La (SS-B), an RNA-binding protein that can bind the Ro hY RNAs (38); calreticulin (39); a 57-kDa protein (40); a 75-kDa phosphoprotein (41); α-fodrin (42); and, occasionally, U_1RNP (43).

A variety of autoantibody assays may be available to the practitioner, including screening antinuclear antibody (ANA), immunodiffusion (Ouchterlony test), immunoblotting, and enzyme-linked immunosorbent assay (ELISA). Although the screening ANA should be positive in maternal sera, it is a nonspecific test and therefore of limited use. In the experience of the authors, immunodiffusion is the most useful assay, as virtually all maternal NLE sera have precipitin lines to Ro and/or La (44). Immunoblotting, which is generally performed as a research tool rather than a commercial test, is reasonably reliable for detection of antibodies to 52-kDa Ro and to La, but is insufficiently sensitive for detection of antibodies to 60-kDa Ro. ELISAs are not currently highly standardized, and the clinical relevance of detection of low levels of autoantibodies in ELISA is not known. In summary, many autoantibodies have been associated with NLE, but the diagnostic standard remains the presence of high titers of antibodies to Ro and/or La, detectable by immunodiffusion.

Children with the skin findings of NLE should be evaluated for other signs of NLE. Laboratory testing may include liver function tests (e.g., bilirubin and aminotransferase levels), complete blood count (including platelet count), and electrocardiogram.

Differential Diagnosis

Differential diagnosis of skin lesions of NLE is usually not difficult because the skin lesions are quite distinctive. On occasion, the lesions may appear similar to those of papulosquamous eruptions such as tinea, atopic dermatitis, or seborrheic dermatitis.

Management of Skin Lesions and Prognosis

Skin lesions should generally be managed conservatively, with much attention to sun protection. Topical steroids may be used on active lesions. Antimalarials would be expected to be of no benefit as the skin lesions would likely be resolving before the antimalarials would take effect. In addition, administration of antimalarials in an appropriate dose may be difficult in babies, and accidental overdosage has resulted in cardiac toxicity and death. It is possible that systemic steroids would be helpful, but we do not recommend their use for skin disease unless there is some indication that significant permanent deformity, such as scarring, is likely to occur. The telangiectasias that may result from NLE have been, in our experience, small lesions that should be amenable to treatment with a modality such as a pulsed dye laser if treatment is desired.

The prognosis for skin lesions is excellent, as discussed before, with few children having residua. The overall prognosis for the health of the child is not entirely known. Children who have had NLE are usually healthy in childhood, although many of those with heart block do require permanent pacemaker implantation (12). It is likely that there is some increased risk for the development of autoimmune disease later in life, and cases have been reported of such in individuals who had NLE (18). In a review of cases of cutaneous NLE from a national registry, it is noteworthy that three of 57 children developed an autoimmune disease during childhood (one with Hashimoto thyroiditis and two with juvenile rheumatoid arthritis) (13).

The prognosis for mothers of babies with NLE is also not fully known. In our experience, it is common for mothers to have no symptoms suggestive of autoimmune disease at the time that they have the babies with NLE. In another 5 years or so, most of these mothers develop symptoms (15). In our group, the symptoms consist largely of dry eyes, dry mouth, and arthralgias—symptoms more suggestive of Sjögren syndrome than systemic lupus. In other series, maternal symptoms of systemic lupus or undifferentiated connective tissue disease occur more frequently (45,46). One group proposed that mothers of babies with skin disease are more likely to have significant symptoms than are mothers of babies with cardiac disease (47).

A woman who has had one baby with NLE may or may not have other children affected in subsequent pregnancies. The risk for having another affected baby is probably in the range of 15% to 25% (12,15,45,48). Mothers do not appear to have an increased risk for spontaneous abortion, although it would be expected that there is a significant risk for fetal loss later in pregnancy due to hydrops fetalis.

Etiologic Factors and Pathogenesis

The etiology of NLE is not known, but circumstantial evidence points very strongly to autoantibodies. Autoantibodies are universally present in NLE sera and disease activity resolves as maternal antibody titers lower in the baby circulation. Deposits of IgG are present in the heart (49) and skin (50) of affected babies. There is strong evidence in an animal model that the antibody deposits seen are specific deposits of anti-Ro rather than a nonspecific antibody deposition (35).

Autoantibodies of the anti-Ro family have been shown to have an adverse effect on the heart. Alexander et al. (51) reported that anti-Ro–containing serum inhibited repolarization of isolated perfused neonatal rabbit cardiac tissue. Garcia et al. (52) reproduced heart block with anti-Ro–containing IgG and affinity-purified anti–52-kDa Ro (53) in isolated perfused rabbit hearts. Kalush et al. (54) immunized mice with anti-DNA 16/6 idiotype. Some of the immunized mice developed antibodies to Ro and had offspring with congenital heart block. Mazel et al. (55) reported the induction of bradycardia and prolonged PR interval (although not complete heart block) in newborn mice whose mothers received anti-Ro/La–containing IgG during pregnancy. A cross-reactivity between 52-kDa Ro and the serotoninergic 5-HT4 receptor has been identified, and antibodies to this cross-reactive epitope antagonize the serotonin-induced L-type calcium channel activation on human atrial cells (56). Miranda-Carus et al. (57) have proposed that anti-Ro/La autoantibodies binding apoptotic cells in the heart trigger an inflammatory reaction mediated in part by tumor necrosis factor-α (TNF-α).

It is noteworthy that most babies exposed to anti-Ro in utero do not develop disease. The most likely explanation is that autoantibodies, particularly anti-Ro, are necessary but not sufficient for disease to occur. Other factors, whether random events or whether genetically or environmentally determined, must also be involved in disease production.

The reasons for the organ specificity of NLE are not known. When guinea pigs were injected with anti-Ro–containing serum, antibody deposits were found in all organs, including organs that are apparently never involved in NLE (50). In a study of 20 sera, we found that mothers of babies with skin disease had significantly lower titers of anti–60-kDa Ro than did mothers of babies with heart disease (44). A potential explanation for this finding is that the lower titers of anti–60-kDa Ro in the skin disease sera may be the greater affinity of those antibodies for the skin, leading to a substantial deposition of antibodies in the skin. Since the skin is an extremely large organ, autoantibody deposits in the skin could then lower the circulating titers of autoantibodies. However, differences among anti-Ro autoantibodies in affinity for different organs have not been conclusively demonstrated. Possibly, cross-reactivities with antigens such as the 5-HT4 receptor explain the organ specificity of NLE.

The reason that mothers of babies with NLE do not have the same symptoms as their babies is not known. It is relatively uncommon for NLE mothers to have SCLE lesions, and heart block has never been reported in an NLE mother. A study of isolated perfused rabbit cardiac muscle showed effects on repolarization when neonatal, but not adult, cardiac muscle was bathed in anti-Ro–containing serum (51), raising the possibility that Ro or a cross-reacting antigen is highly expressed on the surface of cells in the conduction system early in development, but not later in life. Other studies indicate that 52-kDa Ro isoforms are expressed differently during different stages of gestation (58) and that the Ro hY RNAs are expressed differently at different stages of gestation (59).

Genetic factors that may contribute to NLE have been examined. HLA serologic typing shows an association with DR3 and DQw2 in NLE mothers and no HLA associations apparent in infants (60). Watson et al. (61) found an association with abnormal C4 genes, with 15 of 18 NLE mothers having C4-null allotypes. Since these genetic associations are present in NLE mothers, they may be related more to a predisposition to produce anti-Ro autoantibodies than to other events in the pathogenesis of NLE. Genetic factors in babies associated with increased risk for disease have not been determined.

LUPUS ERYTHEMATOSUS OF CHILDHOOD

The preceding section described a transient disease of newborns that has been called neonatal lupus. Whether this is the most accurate name is debatable, as the disease is not the same as that of LE of adults. This section discusses true LE of childhood, a disease in which the child produces his or her own lupus autoantibodies, in which the disease is not necessarily transient, and in which the clinical features are similar to those of adult LE. Because LE has been covered comprehensively in a preceding chapter in this book, this section will focus on characteristics of childhood LE that are unique to children.

It should be noted that some of the literature concerning childhood LE does not carefully distinguish LE developing after puberty from LE developing before puberty. It is probable that LE developing in a 13-year-old girl has much more in common with lupus developing in a 20-year-old woman than it has with lupus in a 6-year-old child.

Epidemiology

Few data are available concerning the incidence of LE in childhood, with one estimate of an incidence of 0.6 per 100,000 per year (62). Although the effect of female sex may not be as strong in prepubertal children as it is in adults (63), the effect of race is striking, with prevalences of LE in black, Asian, and Hispanic children more than three times that of white children in one study (64).

Cutaneous Manifestations

Children with SLE may develop the same cutaneous lesions as those seen in adults with SLE. Malar rash has been noted in about one third to one half of children with SLE (Fig. 13.7) (62, 63,65). Lesions on the hands are commonly observed (Fig. 13.8).

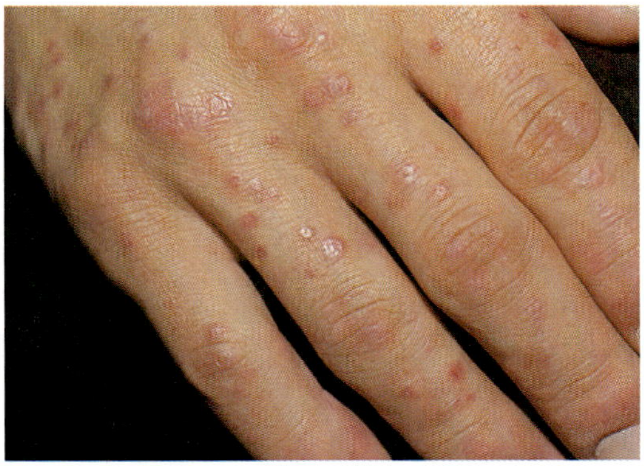

Figure 13.8. Systemic lupus erythematosus. Typical involvement of the dorsum of the hand with lesions between the knuckles of a 12-year-old girl (note contrast with hand of child with dermatomyositis shown in Fig. 13.14).

Discoid lupus lesions in the absence of systemic disease have been noted infrequently in children (Fig. 13.9) (66,67). A review of 16 cases of childhood discoid LE occurring before age 10 notes a lack of female predominance (10 boys, six girls) and a high rate of progression to systemic disease (five cases) (66). If one considered only those cases in which follow-up was available through adulthood, five of 10 patients developed SLE.

SCLE lesions also occur infrequently in children (68). Individuals with C4 or C2 deficiency may be predisposed to have anti-Ro autoantibodies and SCLE lesions (69), and individuals with genetic deficiencies of complement may develop disease at a very early age (70).

Lupus panniculitis may occur in children and has been reported in a case of partial deficiency of C2 and C4 (71). A case has been reported of bullous LE occurring as the presenting sign of childhood SLE (72).

Relationship Between Cutaneous and Systemic Features of the Disease

Cutaneous findings have similar implications in children as they do in adults. However, as stated before, discoid lesions may carry a more ominous prognosis in children, as it appears that a much higher percentage develops systemic disease.

The internal manifestations of lupus in children have been described in several reviews (62,63,73,74).

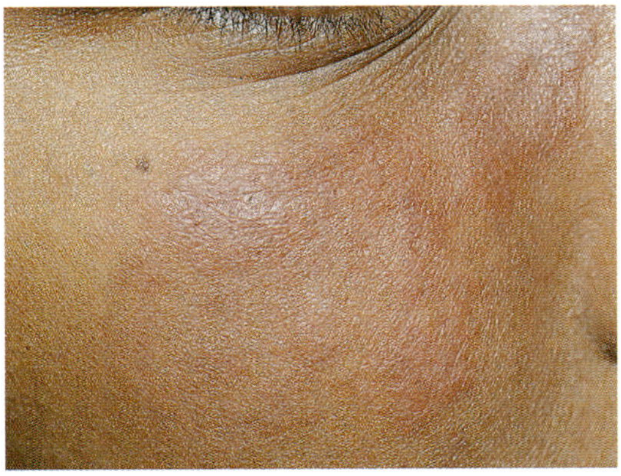

Figure 13.7. Systemic lupus erythematosus. Shown is the eruption of acute cutaneous lupus erythematosus on the face of an 8-year-old child with systemic disease.

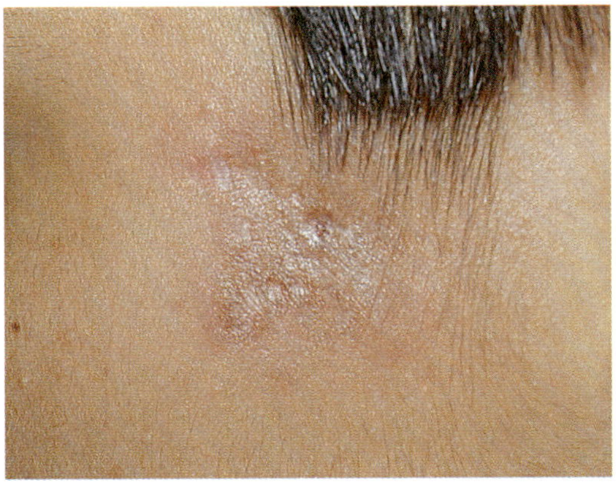

Figure 13.9. Discoid lupus erythematosus. Scarring lesions are present on the preauricular skin of a 10-year-old child.

Laboratory Manifestations

Laboratory manifestations are similar to those of adults with SLE. Anti-Ro autoantibodies have been associated with early-onset LE (before age 10) (75). In addition, genetic deficiencies of complement may be detected in a relatively higher percentage of children with LE than adults with LE.

Management of Skin Lesions and Prognosis

First-line treatment of cutaneous LE in children consists of sun-protective measures and topical or intralesional corticosteroids. If these measures fail, antimalarial therapy may be used. In general, high-dose systemic corticosteroids and immunosuppressive agents are not indicated for the treatment of cutaneous LE in children because of their risks. However, these agents have been used successfully for severe systemic disease in children. If antimalarial agents fail, and if the skin disease is debilitating and/or scarring, one might consider the use of a short-acting systemic retinoid such as 13-*cis*-retinoic acid, which has been reported to be helpful in adults with cutaneous lupus (76). However, neither of the authors has direct experience with the use of retinoids to treat cutaneous LE in children.

Etiologic Factors and Pathogenesis

The etiology of lupus is not known, although genetic factors clearly play a role. In addition, sex steroids have a profound effect on the development of disease, with young postpubertal females being disproportionately affected with SLE. Genetic factors may be particularly important in individuals who develop LE at an early age. Possibly, the occurrence of multiple genes predisposing an individual to LE overrides the usual requirement for postpubertal sex steroid levels.

It has been noted that early-onset childhood LE and childhood LE in males has a correlation with the presence of anti-Ro antibodies in the mother's serum (77). Thus, the genotype that is associated with anti-Ro may be important in the pathogenesis of some cases of childhood LE. In addition, the association of childhood LE with genetic deficiencies of complement components has been discussed. There are case reports of cutaneous and systemic lupus occurring in association with chronic granulomatous disease (78).

JUVENILE DERMATOMYOSITIS

Dermatomyositis (DM) in children tends to be of a somewhat different character than DM in adults, and so merits a separate discussion. Notably, in contrast to DM in adults, childhood DM is frequently associated with significant calcinosis and with infarctive skin lesions. Contractures and muscle atrophy can result in lifelong disability.

Epidemiology

The incidence of juvenile DM is estimated to be more than three per million per year (79). A greater prevalence in females has been noted by some authors (80–82), whereas others have not noted a definite gender predominance (83,84). The average age of onset is approximately 9 years, but it is not unusual for very young children to be affected (80,83). The incidence drops off in the teenage years. On occasion, an adult will present with features more consistent with childhood DM than with adult DM.

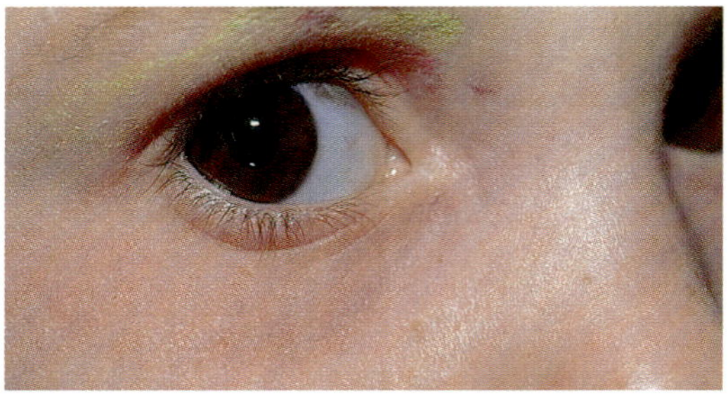

Figure 13.10. Dermatomyositis. The eyelids have a light purplish-red erythema in 3-year-old.

Disease Classification

The classification scheme of Bohan and Peter (85) has been discussed in a previous chapter. It is not always clear in an individual child whether his or her disease is best classified as type IV (juvenile DM with vasculitis) or type II (primary idiopathic DM). It is quite unusual for DM in childhood to be type III (DM with neoplasia).

Cutaneous Manifestations

Children with DM have cutaneous findings similar to those of adults with DM, with a photosensitive facial heliotrope rash (Figs. 13.10–13.12), Gottron papules (Figs. 13.13 and 13.14), psoriasiform lesions (Fig. 13.15), and periungual telangiectasias. Gingival telangiectasias have been noted as a helpful diagnostic finding (86). The cutaneous manifestations of DM have been discussed in a previous chapter. Two cutaneous features of

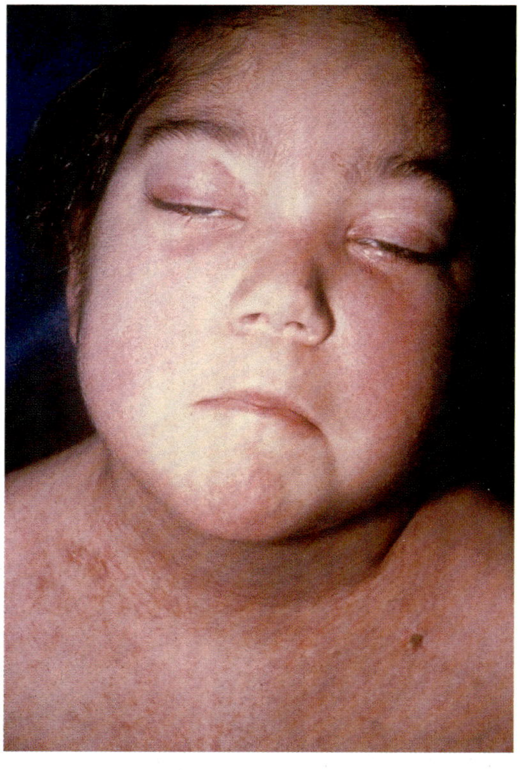

Figure 13.11. Dermatomyositis. Diffuse erythema and edema in a patient with dermatomyositis.

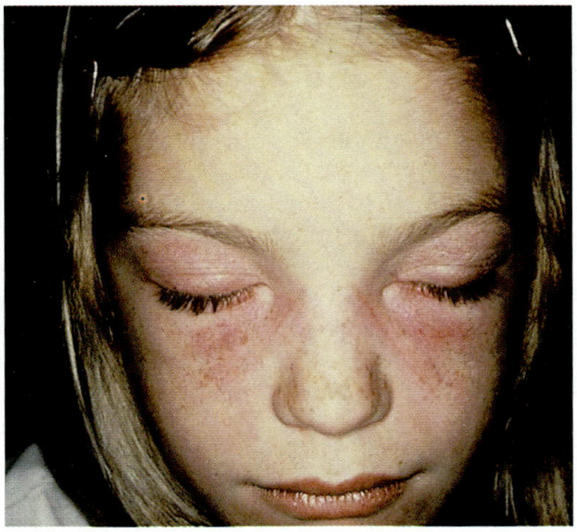

Figure 13.12. Dermatomyositis. Periorbital dermatitis in a child with dermatomyositis.

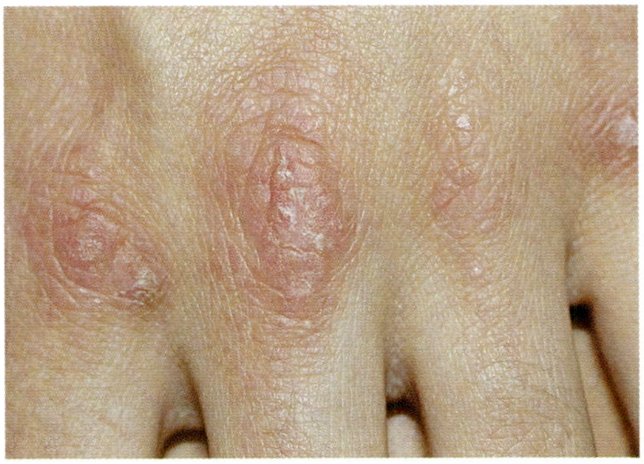

Figure 13.13. Dermatomyositis. Typical Gottron papules involving the knuckles of a 10-year-old.

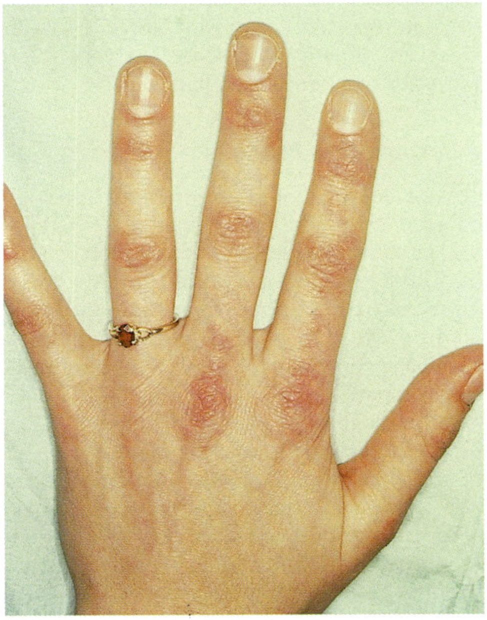

Figure 13.14. Dermatomyositis. Gottron sign in a teenager with dermatomyositis.

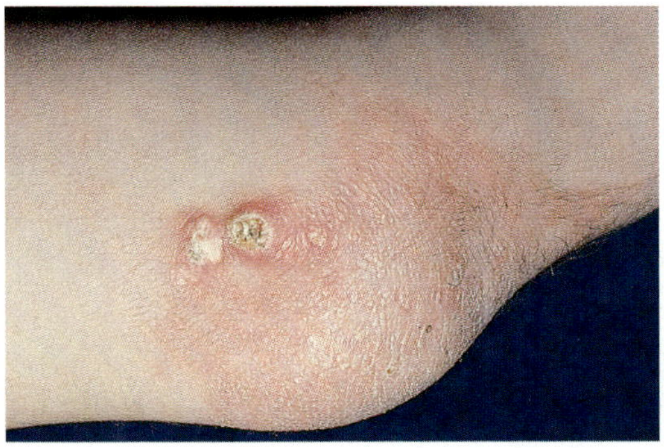

Figure 13.15. Dermatomyositis. Erythema and scaling of the knee plus hard white papules of cutaneous calcinosis in a 7-year-old boy.

childhood DM deserve special mention, as they are more characteristic of childhood than adult DM. These are calcinosis and infarctive skin lesions.

Calcinosis, seen in 30% or more of children with DM (82), appears in the skin as dermal or subcutaneous nodules (see Fig. 13.15). The nodules may ulcerate, in which case the calcium is visible as a hard white substance in the center of the ulceration. The calcium can eventually be extruded from the skin, although the process is usually very slow, and significant scarring may result. The lesions may be quite symptomatic when they occur over areas of trauma or weight bearing such as the elbows or the buttocks. Calcinosis is more common in children with long-standing disease, but may occur within a few months of onset (87) or even many months prior to other findings (88).

Ulcerative skin lesions may occur independently of the process of calcinosis, due to a vasculopathy in the cutaneous blood vessels (89,90). The lesions may initially appear as dusky erythematous papules, similar to those of leukocytoclastic vasculitis. Mucous membranes may be affected. It has been noted that children with DM may develop vitiliginous-appearing patches due to locally decreased blood flow (80). Whether these white patches are related to the same process that causes the infarctive lesions is not clear.

In patients with long-standing disease, permanent contractures may occur. Muscle atrophy may be a prominent, very debilitating long-term sequela of juvenile DM. There are reports of lipodystrophy occurring in association with juvenile DM (89, 91) as well as panniculitis (92) and palmar–plantar hyperkeratosis (93).

Relationship Between Cutaneous and Systemic Features of the Disease

The onset of DM may be gradual or abrupt. Cutaneous lesions may precede or follow extracutaneous features of the disease. In unusual cases, clinically apparent muscle disease never develops (94,95).

The calcinosis that occurs in the skin may be accompanied by calcinosis in muscles, where it may compromise muscle function. The infarctive skin lesions are often accompanied by infarctive lesions in internal organs. Of particular note are lesions in the gastrointestinal tract, which may cause perforation and may be a presenting sign of childhood DM (89). While adults with DM commonly have gastrointestinal involvement with weak musculature, infarctive lesions of the gastrointestinal tract are not a typical feature of adult DM.

Pathology and Immunopathology

The pathology and immunopathology of DM have been discussed in a preceding chapter. Vascular abnormalities in skin biopsies include endothelial cell swelling (which may be so pronounced that occlusion of the vessel results), capillary basement membrane thickening, endothelial cell proliferation, and perivascular fibrosis (90).

Laboratory Manifestations

Muscle enzyme and electromyelographic abnormalities, and detection of circulating autoantibodies have been discussed in a previous chapter. An autoantibody specificity uniquely associated with childhood DM has not been identified. In contrast to adult myositis, childhood DM has a lower prevalence of autoantibodies of a defined specificity, a lower prevalence of myositis-specific autoantibodies, and a much lower prevalence of antibodies to Jo-1 (96,97). Antibodies to Mi-2 do occur in childhood DM sera. Screening ANA is positive in most cases (79,98).

Differential Diagnosis

The diagnosis of childhood DM is not usually difficult when the typical cutaneous findings are accompanied by clinically evident muscle involvement. The diagnosis may be difficult in cases in which muscle involvement is not evident and characteristic cutaneous findings such as Gottron papules are absent. In situations where there is an erythematous eruption on the face, but other specific signs of DM are absent, the differential diagnosis of sun-sensitive rashes must be entertained. Occasionally, the facial eruption of DM is indistinguishable from childhood SLE. The papulosquamous lesions of DM may mimic those of psoriasis. Lesions on the dorsa of the hands may look like eczema.

Management of Skin Lesions and Prognosis

Management of skin lesions in childhood DM is similar to that for adult DM. Sun protection must be stressed as an essential component in the management of the photosensitive lesions. Systemic treatments such as high-dose corticosteroids are given primarily for life-threatening or highly debilitating features of the disease such as vasculopathy and skeletal muscle involvement. Antimalarials have been used for cutaneous lesions (81), although the authors generally do not use them. Intravenous γ-globulin (IVGG) has been reported to have a salutary effect on both muscle disease and skin lesions of childhood DM (99). Antihistamines may be useful for pruritus management.

Calcinosis may be a difficult problem. In general, lesions of calcinosis are managed with attention to wound care and to protection from trauma, such as providing extra cushions for chairs or padding for elbows. It may be worthwhile to surgically remove the calcinosis in a few selected lesions that are particularly symptomatic, but that is not practical or desirable for most lesions. There have been reports of benefit with aluminum hydroxide (100); early, aggressive systemic steroid therapy (101); diltiazem (102); alendronate (103); and probenecid (104).

The course of childhood DM is variable. Some children experience an explosive onset of disease and some develop the disease very gradually. Different courses have been described as being monocyclic, recurrent, or continuous. Monocyclic disease, in which remission occurs within 2 years or less, occurs in perhaps 25% to 40% of cases (82,105). The remainder of children has a more prolonged course, with remissions and relapses occurring over several years, or with persistent disease requiring continuous therapy. In some cases, the disease may persist into adulthood.

It is estimated that about 7% of children with DM die as a result of the disease (82,106). Causes of death include gastrointestinal perforation, myocardial disease, and complications from systemic therapy. Children with vasculopathy have a worse prognosis than those without vascular involvement (101, 107). Most children who have DM have reasonable functional outcomes, although sequelae of some type are common (82, 108). In about 15%, there is major disability (80), much of it occurring as a result of muscle atrophy and contractures.

Etiologic Factors and Pathogenesis

Although it would be expected that the etiology of juvenile DM would be similar to that of adult DM, the targeting of the endothelium in juvenile DM and the prominence of calcinosis in the clinical picture indicate that there may be some differences in etiology between juvenile and adult DM. The vascular involvement, calcinosis, and fibrosis that may be present in biopsies led some investigators to postulate that juvenile DM is similar to scleroderma and may share etiologic factors (90).

As is the case for many autoimmune diseases, infections have been postulated to initiate the disease process (109–112). Genetic determinants are important, with the HLA-DQA1*0501 allele conferring susceptibility (113), and the TNF-α-308A allele associated with a longer disease course and increased risk of calcifications (114). In some children, there is evidence for maternal chimerism (115).

THE PERIARTERITIS NODOSA SYNDROMES

There are three distinct syndromes in infancy and childhood in which periarteritis nodosa is a major feature: (a) infantile periarteritis nodosa, (b) Kawasaki disease, and (c) chronic primarily cutaneous periarteritis nodosa. There are overlapping features of the three. Kawasaki disease is by far the most prevalent, with over 5,000 cases reported each year (116,117). Infantile periarteritis nodosa and Kawasaki disease are very different from forms of periarteritis nodosa seen in adults.

Infantile Periarteritis Nodosa

Since 1870, a severe form of periarteritis nodosa in infants has been recognized (118,119). These infants all had in common periarteritis of coronary arteries that evolved to coronary aneurysms. The infants were reported to have fever and irritability, but usually did not have skin findings. In the few that did have skin findings, they were described as transient exanthems without a specific morphology (120). Diagnosis was usually made at autopsy.

Some authors have suggested that such infants may represent "atypical" examples of Kawasaki disease (120). Despite the absence of the skin signs typical of Kawasaki disease, these infants had coronary artery aneurysms, prolonged fever, increased erythrocyte sedimentation rates (ESRs), and thrombocytosis—all prominent findings in Kawasaki disease.

The mortality rate in infantile periarteritis nodosa is quite high. This diagnosis is infrequently made as a high index of clinical suspicion is required and the major signs of fever and irritability are nonspecific in infants. Most infants with periarteritis nodosa die of myocardial infarction or rupture of the coronary aneurysms. Many of the cases are still diagnosed at autopsy, although cardiac ultrasound studies may be quite useful in early diagnosis.

Kawasaki Disease

HISTORICAL PERSPECTIVE

In 1967, a Japanese pediatrician, Tomisaku Kawasaki, reported a unique and prolonged mucocutaneous illness characterized by persistent fever, lymphadenopathy, conjunctivitis, red and cracked lips, a strawberry tongue, and red palms and soles (120). Peeling of the fingertips, distally to proximally, developed in almost all of the 50 cases initially reported. All of the children had an elevated sedimentation rate and leukocytosis.

After the initial report, it became evident that during the recovery phase about 1% to 2% of the children suddenly died (116). It was later learned that coronary aneurysms were the cause of death. It has been estimated that about 20% of untreated children will develop coronary artery disease (116, 117). Since 1970, there have been criteria for the diagnosis developed by the U.S. Centers for Disease Control and Prevention (CDC), and evaluation of cardiac status has become a routine in affected children (117). In the absence of a diagnostic test for Kawasaki disease, the CDC clinical and laboratory criteria remain the standard for diagnosis.

CLINICAL FEATURES

Three stages of the disease are recognized (116,117). In the acute febrile stage, prolonged fever of 40°C is accompanied by bilateral conjunctival injection, red oropharynx, strawberry tongue, red lips, red palms and soles, and edema of the hands and feet (Figs. 13.16 and 13.17). Although cervical lymphadenopathy was a major feature of the earliest described cases, it has subsequently been found in 50% to 75% of cases (116,117). Lymphadenopathy may be so severe that it mimics bacterial cervical adenitis, although it may also be absent (116). Erythema of the perineal region is observed in half the affected infants (116). The acute febrile stage lasts at least 5 days and often up to 14 days.

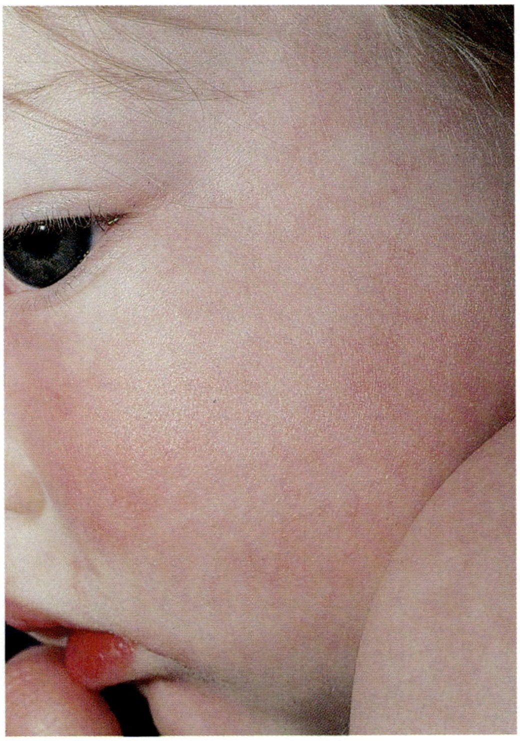

Figure 13.16. Kawasaki disease. Erythema of cheeks and bright red lips characteristic of the illness in this toddler.

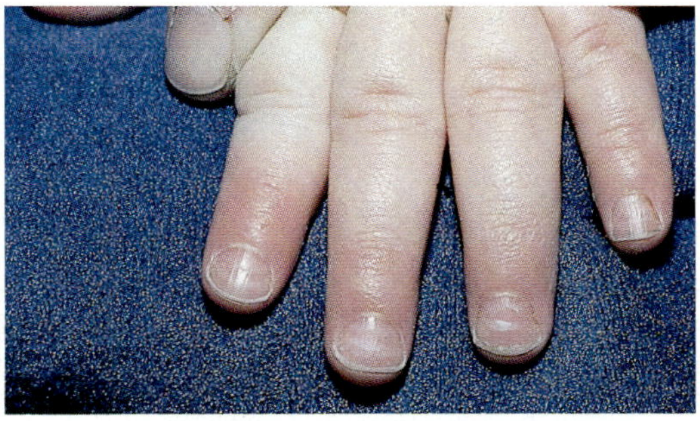

Figure 13.17. Kawasaki disease. Erythema and edema of the toddler's fingers plus Beau lines in the fingernails.

In the next phase, called the subacute phase, the fever, lymphadenopathy, and skin lesions resolve, but irritability, anorexia, and the conjunctival injection persist (117). Desquamation of the fingers and toes is observed in 29% of patients during the subacute phase (116) (Fig. 13.18). At the time of desquamation, a few children have demonstrated red transverse lines across their fingernail beds (117) (see Fig. 13.17). The transverse lines last up to 2 weeks and disappear at the time the desquamation of the fingertips resolves. Arthritis (9%) or arthralgias (23%), thrombocytosis (95%), and myocardial dysfunction (20%) also first appear during the subacute stage (117). Hepatomegaly is found in 15% of children and splenomegaly in 3% during the subacute stage (117). The subacute stage lasts until day 25 of the illness.

The convalescent stage lasts 6 to 8 weeks, until all the signs and symptoms have resolved. Recurrent skin peeling has been noted to occur for several years after apparent recovery from Kawasaki disease (122). This recurrent skin peeling has been associated with nasal colonization with *Staphylococcus aureus* (122). Most fatalities have occurred from 2 to 12 weeks after the onset of symptoms, when the child is apparently recovering (117). Throughout the illness, the ESR is quite elevated, and its return to normal signifies the end of the illness to some authorities (117). Recently, discrepancies in the ESR and C-reactive protein (CRP) levels (high ESR and normal CRP or normal CRP and high ESR) correlated with the presence of cardiac disease (123). Conspicuously absent are the cutaneous findings usually associated with periarteritis nodosa, including livedo reticularis and palpable tender nodose lesions in the skin.

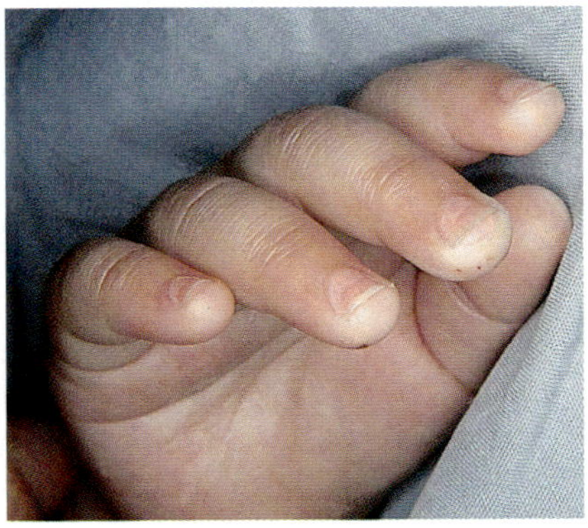

Figure 13.18. Kawasaki disease. Peeling of the fingertips from distal to proximal.

There are a great number of associated features that emphasize the systemic and multiorgan nature of Kawasaki disease. Hydrops of the gallbladder is an unique symptom of Kawasaki disease and may be observed in 10% of children (117). Diarrhea and vomiting (25%) is sometimes observed, as is aseptic meningitis (9%) (117). Pyuria is found in 25% of children and pneumonia in 2% (117). Despite the dramatic cardiovascular findings, hypertension is rarely observed (117). A rare but serious complication, observed in eight children to date, is gangrene of the digits (117). It is always seen in association with severe coronary artery aneurysms. Acute encephalopathy is also recognized in Kawasaki disease (124).

EPIDEMIOLOGY

Kawasaki disease is virtually limited to toddlers and young children, with more than 80% of the reported cases occurring in children younger than 4 years of age (117). Asians appear to have the highest risk of acquiring the disease, and whites the lowest (116,117,121). There is a 1.5:1 ratio of males to females, and most cases occur in the late winter and spring (117,123). Although many authorities believe Kawasaki disease is the result of an infection, there is little evidence of child-to-child spread. Residence near a body of water may be a predisposing factor (117).

ETIOLOGIC FACTORS AND PATHOGENESIS

The etiology of Kawasaki disease is unknown and many infectious pathogens have been implicated. The sore throat and high fever may mimic streptococcal infections, although the bacteria is only occasionally isolated from affected children (117,125). There are isolated reports of seroconversion to, or recovery of Epstein–Barr virus, human herpesvirus 6, rubeola, adenovirus, coxsackievirus B4, influenza, group A streptococci, *Staphylococcus aureus*, Parvovirus B19 and *Leptospira* organisms (117). Recent reports of a Kawasaki-like syndrome occurring in adults with human immunodeficiency virus infection are intriguing (126). Prior shampooing of rugs also has been implicated with perhaps some pathogen or antigen liberated during the process (117). There are a few instances thought to be drug-related. In a few cases, the disease may have preceded juvenile rheumatoid arthritis or leukemia (117).

Recently, adhesion molecules (endothelin, intercellular adhesion molecule-1) and cytokines (TNF-α, interleukin-1, and interferon-γ) have been detected in elevated levels in the blood (117). Whether these substances participate in the vascular injury or represent nonspecific acute-phase reactants in the blood is unclear.

PATHOLOGY

Periarteritis nodosa lesions in the heart are the hallmark of the disease and are found primarily during the acute febrile phase (116,117,121). Aneurysms of coronary arteries are observed in the last two phases and are felt to be a major pathologic association with Kawasaki disease. A panarteritis may ensue and endothelial injury may predispose the patient to thrombosis and occlusion of coronary vessels. Pericarditis and myocarditis may also be observed.

LABORATORY MANIFESTATIONS

An elevated ESR occurs in all cases with the mean in one study at 73 mm per hour (117). Leukocytosis (mean white blood cell count, 19,400/mm^3) and thrombocytosis (mean platelet count, 793,000/mm^3) are usually found (117). C-reactive protein, antistreptolysin O titers, anti-DNAse B titers, and immunoglobulins may also be elevated (117,122). Because of cardiac prognosis, it is recommended that both ESR and C-reactive protein tests be obtained in children with Kawasaki disease (122). ANAs are usually not detected (127).

COURSE AND PROGNOSIS

Mortality in untreated Kawasaki disease is 1% (117). Cardiovascular sequelae, however, may be seen in as many as 20% of cases, with evidence of coronary aneurysms, abnormal left ventricular function, or pericardial effusions lasting several months (116,117). About 1% of children will have coronary aneurysms that persist for several years.

A peculiarity is the development of a recurrence of Kawasaki disease (117). During subsequent infectious diseases, a reappearance of at least some of the Kawasaki disease findings has been observed in about 10% of cases. Several instances have been described where a child had no evidence of coronary artery disease during a first episode of Kawasaki disease only to develop the typical findings during a second episode (117).

In addition to residual cardiovascular findings, sensorineural hearing loss was observed in seven of 40 children who recovered from Kawasaki disease (117). Whether this is due to the disease itself or to aspirin therapy is not certain.

MANAGEMENT

The consensus among authorities who treat Kawasaki disease is that the treatment of choice is IVGG and oral aspirin (116,117, 128). The recommended doses are 2 g/kg per day of IVGG and 30 mg/kg per day of aspirin. The IVGG is administered on a single day as a 10- to 12-hour infusion (117,121,128). Rapid regression of coronary artery dilatation has been reported following IVGG infusion (117,128). The combination of IVGG and aspirin has been demonstrated to greatly reduce the cardiovascular complications (116,117). In one study, 6.5% of children were resistant to this therapy (129). Retreatment with either intravenous immunoglobulin or pulse intravenous steroids did not improve outcomes (129). In contrast, systemic steroid therapy actually increases the likelihood of coronary aneurysms and is contraindicated in Kawasaki disease (117). Giant coronary artery aneurysms and severe myocardial disease may require coronary artery bypass surgery (129). The long-term prognosis is good if bilateral internal mammary artery grafts are used (130).

Chronic Relapsing Primarily Cutaneous Periarteritis Nodosa in Children

Characteristic cutaneous findings of livedo reticularis plus palpable, linear, often tender, nodules (nodose lesions) are found in 80% of children with periarteritis nodosa (118,131–134) (Fig. 13.19). Typically, children (rather than infants or toddlers) are

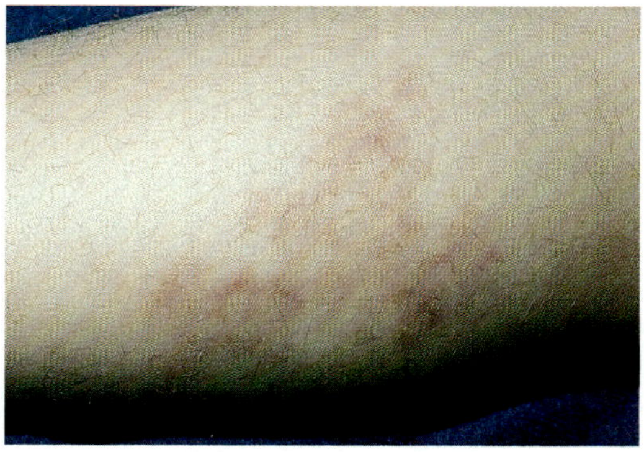

Figure 13.19. Cutaneous periarteritis nodosa. Livedo reticularis pattern and oval nodules on the leg of a 5-year-old child.

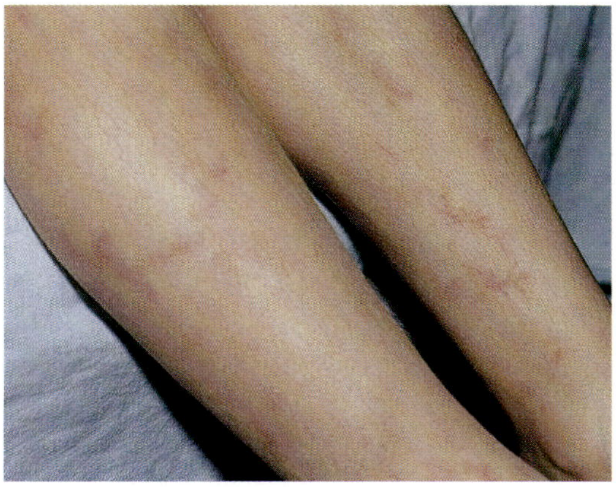

Figure 13.20. Cutaneous periarteritis nodosa. Typical "adult" pattern of livedo reticularis of the legs in an adolescent.

affected and they develop other signs and symptoms of the systemic disease along with the cutaneous lesions. Fever, myalgias, arthralgias, and gastrointestinal symptoms are observed in 70% of children (118). Hypertension, renal disease, pulmonary involvement, and neuropathy (mononeuritis multiplex) are also noted (118,131–134). The lesions tend to persist for weeks, with crops of new nodules appearing (Fig. 13.20).

The course tends to be chronic and relapsing in children, with the disease persisting for months to years (118,131–134). Distinct from the adult form is the frequent association with preceding streptococcal infections and the presence of anti-streptococcal antibodies (133). Newborns of mothers affected with periarteritis nodosa have also developed typical cutaneous disease with livedo reticularis and nodose lesions; in these cases, the disease was transient, lasting up to 3 months of age (118).

The high prevalence of periarteritis nodosa in familial Mediterranean fever provides clues to the pathogenesis. Pyrin, an abnormal neutrophil protein encoded by *MEFV*, the gene mutated in familial Mediterranean fever, makes children susceptible to develop periarteritis nodosa with streptococcal infection (134).

Biopsies of the nodular lesions demonstrated the typical pathology of periarteritis nodosa. In addition to oral steroids, low-dose methotrexate has been successful in steroid-resistant children with cutaneous periarteritis nodosa (118).

CUTANEOUS FINDINGS IN ACUTE RHEUMATIC FEVER

Erythema marginatum, one of the Jones criteria for the diagnosis of acute rheumatic fever, is present in less than 10% of affected children (135,136). Although it is one of the Jones criteria for diagnosis, it is often not present (137). Erythema marginatum is characterized by slightly elevated red, annular areas that rapidly move from site to site over hours (135,136). Half-circle and quarter-circle arrangements may also be observed. It is more frequently observed during periods of high fever, and is seen on the trunk and proximal extremities.

Subcutaneous nodules are rarely seen in children with acute rheumatic fever. When present, these mobile subcutaneous nodules are seen on the scalp, over the spine, and over the joints (135,138). The subcutaneous nodules of acute rheumatic fever in childhood are often confused with granuloma annulare (139). Neither erythema marginatum nor subcutaneous nodules have any prognostic significance in acute rheumatic fever (138,140).

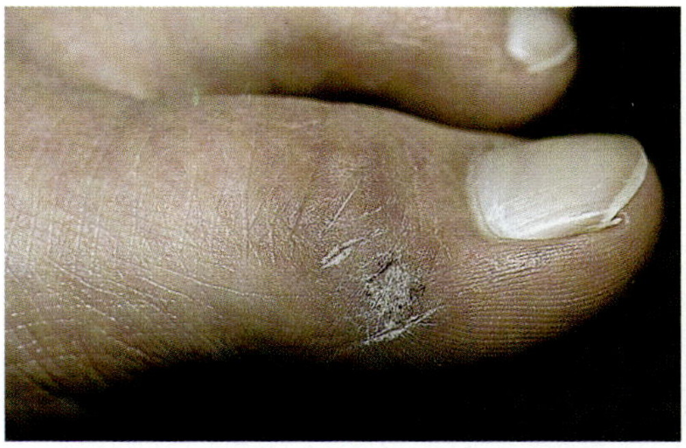

Figure 13.21. Perniosis. Figure shows ulcerated purple nodule of toe (kibes) in a 12-year-old girl.

CUTANEOUS FINDINGS IN JUVENILE RHEUMATOID ARTHRITIS

The only form of juvenile rheumatoid arthritis regularly associated with cutaneous findings is the classic Still disease. In this form, high fever without obvious cause is the presenting symptom. During the fever spikes, an evanescent pink macular eruption on the trunk may be seen (140,141). The macules are 2 to 6 mm, and are often paler in the center. The skin eruption is quite evanescent and may recur with the next febrile episode (140–142). Intermittent episodes are characteristic of young children with juvenile rheumatoid arthritis (140). Hepatosplenomegaly, arthritis, and polyserositis often accompany the skin eruption. The other forms of juvenile rheumatoid arthritis are usually without a rash.

PERNIOSIS IN CHILDREN

Perniosis, or chilblain, is seen as persistent purple–red nodules on the digits. When it ulcerates, it is called kibes (143) (Fig. 13.21). Exposure to cold, wet conditions precipitates the lesions. The nodules are slow in onset and may last 4 to 8 weeks once established. Radiographic evidence of speckled bodies resembling geodes may been seen in the digits and this finding is termed "microgeodic disease." Recently, childhood perniosis has been associated with a family history of rheumatoid arthritis and the presence of cryoglobulins (143). Keeping the extremities warm and dry and use of nifedipine may help (143).

CHRONIC, INFANTILE, NEUROLOGIC, CUTANEOUS, AND ARTICULAR SYNDROME

Chronic, infantile, neurologic, cutaneous, and articular syndrome (CINCA) presents in early infancy with an urticarial eruption (144). It characteristically varies from day to day and flares with the many febrile episodes of the syndrome. It has been described as nonpruritic, but that is difficult to determine in infants. The articular eruption follows with recurrent episodes of redness and tenderness of large joints. Seizures and spasticity of the legs are major neurologic findings and older children complain of headaches (144). Most infants develop cerebral atrophy with mental retardation, deafness, and visual impairment (145,146).

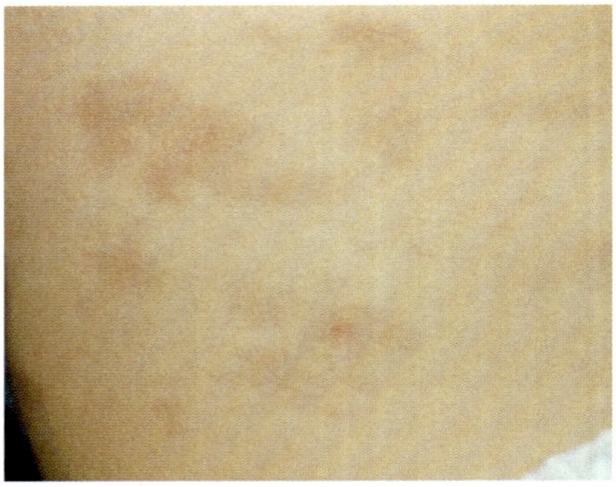

Figure 13.22. Guttate morphea. Multiple early lesions represented by dusky slightly depressed areas of skin in a teenager.

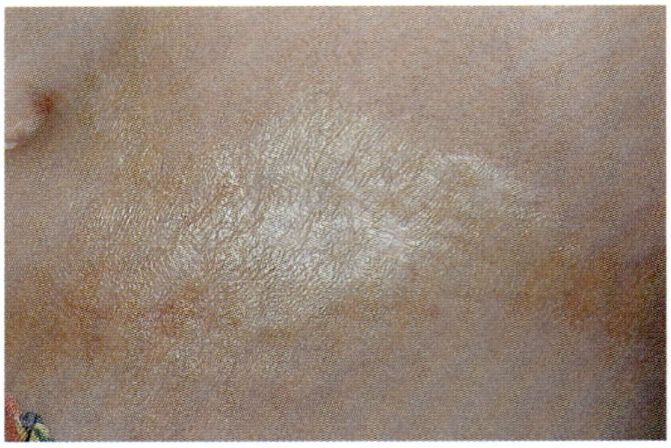

Figure 13.24. Guttate morphea. White, immobile plaque on a child's abdomen.

SCLERODERMA IN CHILDREN

Generalized scleroderma in the form of progressive systemic sclerosis is exceedingly rare in childhood (147–149). More often, the clinician will see children with localized forms of scleroderma called morphea. It is always preferable to use the term "morphea" rather than scleroderma when speaking to parents to avoid the fear produced when information on scleroderma is found. In childhood morphea, both oval circumscribed plaques (the so-called "guttate" morphea), and linear plaques may be seen. As in adults, lesions usually begin with a dusky discoloration to the skin associated with a slight depression in the skin surface. The lesions then evolve to hypopigmentation within the dusky area, and finally to skin immobility. In children, lesions will frequently remain in the dusky early phase for months to years, which makes the clinical diagnosis quite difficult (Fig. 13.22). With progression of the lesions, the center may become totally white with a lilac-colored border (Fig. 13.23). Children may have some lesions that remain in the dusky discoloration stage with normal skin mobility, and some lesions which become immobile (Fig. 13.24).

Guttate morphea lesions may be solitary or may involve multiple areas of the trunk. Both guttate and linear lesions may be present on the same child (148,149) (Fig. 13.25). Unique to childhood are the consequences of having a linear, immobile morphea lesion extend over a growing bone. This may result in shortening of that bone and resultant body asymmetry (134). On a leg, it may result in one leg longer than the other, on the face, facial hemiatrophy (Parry–Romberg syndrome) (Fig. 13.26), or on the scalp, failure of frontal bone growth, leading to a deep linear depression (en coup de sabre).

In a few children, guttate or linear morphea lesions may precede other collagen vascular diseases such as fasciitis or SLE by months to years. Such cases are exceptional, and most children with morphea have a benign course. About 5% of children with morphea will have a positive ANA and antibodies to anticentromere, SCL-70, and anti–microfillin I are found in less than half the children (150). There is no evidence that *Borrelia* infections are associated with childhood morphea in North America (151).

Overall, the prognosis for children with morphea is quite good, although the skin changes persist for years. There are some children with onset before adolescence in whom there is significant tissue remodeling and clearing of the morphea lesions. There are no good predictors of spontaneous clearing and the frequency of clearing is not well documented.

There are no double-blind studies on any therapeutic approach to childhood morphea (148). Treatment should be considered for linear morphea that crosses joints. Most pediatric dermatologists suggest physical therapy as a cornerstone of therapy. One open trial of intravenous immunoglobulin was effective in severe childhood morphea (152). There are recent studies that narrow-band UV-A1 phototherapy (153) or calcipitriol ointment plus UV-A1 is efficacious in childhood morphea (154).

Figure 13.23. Guttate morphea. Solitary slightly immobile plaque with "lilac" colored borders in a 7-year-old.

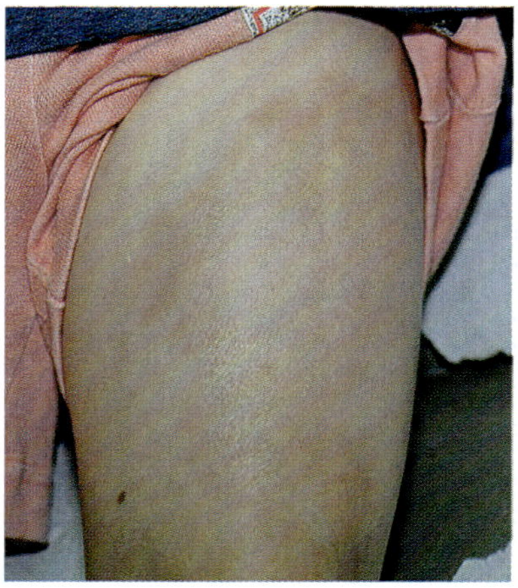

Figure 13.25. Linear morphea. Dusky, dyspigmented plaque over thigh of preadolescent.

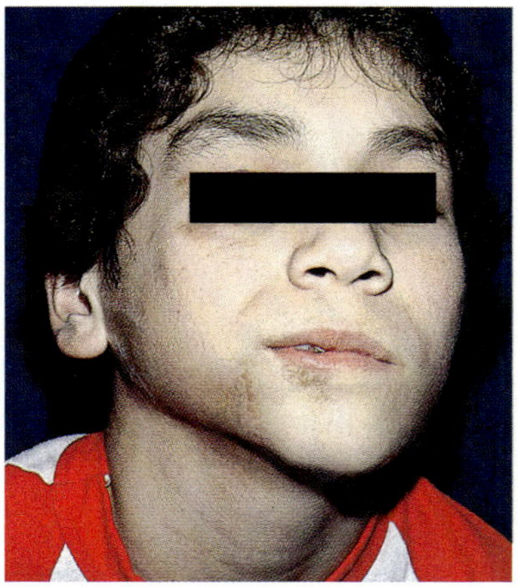

Figure 13.26. Linear morphea. Immobility of skin of right mandible led to failure of growth of mandibular bone, facial asymmetry, and atrophy (Romberg syndrome).

REFERENCES

1. McCuistion CH, Schoch EP Jr. Possible discoid lupus erythematosus in newborn infant: Report of a case with subsequent development of acute systemic lupus erythematosus in mother. *Arch Dermatol* 1954;70:782–785.
2. Hogg GR. Congenital, acute lupus erythematosus associated with subendocardial fibroelastosis: report of a case. *Am J Clin Path* 1957;28:648–654.
3. Franco HL, Weston WL, Tan EM, et al. Association of antibodies to sicca syndrome antigens in newborns with lupus erythematosus and their mothers. *Clin Res* 1980;28:134A(abst).
4. Weston WL, Harmon C, Peebles C, et al. A serological marker for neonatal lupus erythematosus. *Br J Dermatol* 1982;107:377–382.
5. Lee LA. Neonatal lupus erythematosus. *J Invest Dermatol* 1993;100:9S–13S.
6. Buyon JP. Neonatal lupus. *Curr Opin Rheumatol* 1996;8:485–490.
7. Aylward RD. Congenital heart-block. *Br Med J* 1928;1:943.
8. Michaëlsson M, Engle MA. Congenital complete heart block: an international study of the natural history. In: Brest AN, ed. *Cardiovascular clinics.* Philadelphia: FA Davis Co., 1972:85–101.
9. Reed BR, Lee LA, Harmon C, et al. Autoantibodies to SS-A/Ro in infants with congenital heart block. *J Pediatr* 1983;103:889–891.
10. Scott JS, Maddison PJ, Taylor PV, et al. Connective-tissue disease, antibodies to ribonucleoprotein, and congenital heart block. *N Engl J Med* 1983;309:209–212.
11. Esscher E, Scott JS. Congenital heart block and maternal systemic lupus erythematosus. *Br Med J* 1979;1:1235–1238.
12. Buyon JP, Hiebert R, Copel J, et al. Autoimmune-associated congenital heart block: demographics, mortality, morbidity and recurrence rates obtained from a national neonatal lupus registry. *J Am Coll Cardiol* 1998;31:1658–1666.
13. Neiman AR, Lee LA, Weston WL, et al. Cutaneous manifestations of neonatal lupus without heart block: characteristics of mothers and children enrolled in a national registry. *J Pediatr* 2000;137:674–680.
14. Harmon CE, Lee LA, Huff JC, et al. The frequency of antibodies to the SSA/Ro antigen in pregnancy sera. *Arthritis Rheum* 1984;28:S20(abst).
15. McCune AB, Weston WL, Lee LA. Maternal and fetal outcome in neonatal lupus erythematosus. *Ann Intern Med* 1987;106:518–523.
16. Ramsey-Goldman R, Hom D, Deng J-S, et al. Anti-SS-A antibodies and fetal outcome in maternal systemic lupus erythematosus. *Arthritis Rheum* 1986;29: 1269–1273.
17. Lockshin MD, Bonfa E, Elkon K, et al. Neonatal lupus risk to newborns of mothers with systemic lupus erythematosus (published erratum appears in *Arthritis Rheum* 1988;31:1203). *Arthritis Rheum* 1988;31:697–701.
18. Lee LA. Maternal autoantibodies and pregnancy, II: the neonatal lupus syndrome [review]. *Baillieres Clin Rheumatol* 1990;4:69–84.
19. Weston WL, Morelli JG, Lee LA. The clinical spectrum of anti-Ro-positive cutaneous neonatal lupus erythematosus. *J Am Acad Dermatol* 1999;40[5 Pt 1]: 675–681.
20. Sontheimer RD. Subacute cutaneous lupus erythematosus: a decade's perspective. *Med Clin North Am* 1989;73:1073–1090.
21. David-Bajar KM, Bennion SD, DeSpain JD, et al. Clinical, histologic, and immunofluorescent distinctions between subacute cutaneous lupus erythematosus and discoid lupus erythematosus. *J Invest Dermatol* 1992;99:251–257.
22. Stephensen O, Cleland WP, Hallidie-Smith K. Congenital complete heart block and persistent ductus arteriosus associated with maternal systemic lupus erythematosus. *Br Heart J* 1981;46:104–106.
23. Cimaz R, Stramba-Badiale M, Brucato A, et al. QT interval prolongation in asymptomatic anti-SSA/Ro-positive infants without congenital heart block. *Arthritis Rheum* 2000;43:1049–1053.
24. Geggel RL, Tucker L, Szer I. Postnatal progression from second- to third-degree heart block in neonatal lupus syndrome. *J Pediatr* 1988;113:1049–1052.
25. McCue CM, Mantakas ME, Tingelstad JB, et al. Congenital heart block in newborns of mothers with connective tissue disease. *Circulation* 1977;56: 82–90.
26. Lev M, Silverman J, Fitzmaurice FM, et al. Lack of connection between the atria and the more peripheral conduction system in congenital atrioventricular block. *Am J Cardiol* 1971;27:481–488.
27. Ho SY, Esscher E, Anderson RH, et al. Anatomy of congenital complete heart block and relation to maternal anti-Ro antibodies. *Am J Cardiol* 1986;58: 291–294.
28. Eronen M, Siren MK, Ekblad H, et al. Short- and long-term outcome of children with congenital complete heart block diagnosed in utero or as a newborn. *Pediatrics* 2000;106[1 Pt 1]:86–91.
29. Taylor-Albert E, Reichlin M, Toews WH, et al. Delayed dilated cardiomyopathy as a manifestation of neonatal lupus: case reports, autoantibody analysis, and management. *Pediatrics* 1997;99:733–735.
30. Laxer RM, Roberts EA, Gross KR, et al. Liver disease in neonatal lupus erythematosus. *J Pediatr* 1990;116:238–242.
31. Lee LA, Reichlin M, Ruyle SZ, et al. Neonatal lupus liver disease. *Lupus* 1993;2:333–338.
32. Lee LA, Sokol RJ, Buyon JP. Hepatobiliary disease in neonatal lupus: prevalence and clinical characteristics in cases enrolled in a national registry. *Pediatrics* 2002;109:E11.
33. Watson R, Kang JE, May M, et al. Thrombocytopenia in the neonatal lupus syndrome. *Arch Dermatol* 1988;124:560–563.
34. Bangert JL, Freeman RG, Sontheimer RD, et al. Subacute cutaneous lupus erythematosus and discoid lupus erythematosus: comparative histopathologic findings. *Arch Dermatol* 1984;120:332–337.
35. Lee LA, Gaither KK, Coulter SN, et al. Pattern of cutaneous immunoglobulin G deposition in subacute cutaneous lupus erythematosus is reproduced by infusing purified anti-Ro (SSA) autoantibodies into human skin-grafted mice. *J Clin Invest* 1989;83:1556–1562.
36. Farris AD, Puvion-Dutilleul F, Puvion E, et al. The ultrastructural localization of 60-kDa Ro protein and human cytoplasmic RNAs: association with novel electron-dense bodies. *Proc Natl Acad Sci U S A* 1997;94:3040–3045.
37. Ben-Chetrit E, Chan EKL, Sullivan KF, et al. A 52-kD protein is a novel component of the SS-A/Ro antigenic particle. *J Exp Med* 1988;167:1560–1571.
38. Gottlieb E, Steitz JA. Function of the mammalian La protein: evidence for its action in transcription termination by RNA polymerase III. *EMBO J* 1989;8: 851–861.
39. McCauliffe DP, Zappi E, Lieu T-S, et al. A human Ro/SS-A autoantigen is the homologue of calreticulin and is highly homologous with onchocercal RAL-1 antigen and an Aplysia "memory molecule." *J Clin Invest* 1990;86:332–335.
40. Maddison PJ, Lee L, Reichlin M, et al. Anti-p57: a novel association with neonatal lupus. *Clin Exp Immunol* 1995;99:42–48.
41. Wang D, Buyon JP, Zhu W, et al. Defining a novel 75-kDa phosphoprotein associated with SS-A/Ro and identification of distinct human autoantibodies. *J Clin Invest* 1999;104:1265–1275.
42. Miyagawa S, Yanagi K, Yoshioka A, et al. Neonatal lupus erythematosus: maternal IgG antibodies bind to a recombinant NH2-terminal fusion protein encoded by human alpha-fodrin cDNA. *J Invest Dermatol* 1998;111:1189–1192.
43. Provost TT, Watson R, Gammon WR, et al. The neonatal lupus syndrome associated with U1RNP (nRNP) antibodies. *N Engl J Med* 1987;316:1135–1138.
44. Lee LA, Frank MB, McCubbin VR, et al. The autoantibodies of neonatal lupus erythematosus. *J Invest Dermatol* 1994;102:963–966.
45. Waltuck J, Buyon JP. Autoantibody-associated congenital heart block: outcome in mothers and children. *Ann Intern Med* 1994;120:544–551.
46. Press J, Uziel Y, Laxer RM, et al. Long-term outcome of mothers of children with complete congenital heart block. *Am J Med* 1996;100:328–332.
47. Lawrence S, Luy L, Laxer R, et al. The health of mothers of children with cutaneous neonatal lupus erythematosus differs from that of mothers of children with congenital heart block (see comments). *Am J Med* 2000;108:705–709.
48. Julkunen H, Kaaja R, Wallgren E, et al. Isolated congenital heart block: fetal and infant outcome and familial incidence of heart block. *Obstet Gynecol* 1993; 82:11–16.
49. Lee LA, Coulter S, Erner S, et al. Cardiac immunoglobulin deposition in congenital heart block associated with maternal anti-Ro autoantibodies. *Am J Med* 1987;83:793–796.
50. Lee LA, Weston WL, Krueger GG, et al. An animal model of antibody binding in cutaneous lupus. *Arthritis Rheum* 1986;29:782–788.
51. Alexander E, Buyon JP, Provost TT, et al. Anti-Ro/SS-A antibodies in the pathophysiology of congenital heart block in neonatal lupus syndrome, an experimental model: *in vitro* electrophysiologic and immunocytochemical studies. *Arthritis Rheum* 1992;35:176–189.
52. Garcia S, Nascimento JHM, Bonfa E, et al. Cellular mechanism of the conduction abnormalities induced by serum from anti-Ro/SSA-positive patients in rabbit hearts. *J Clin Invest* 1994;93:718–724.
53. Viana VST, Garcia S, Nascimento JHM, et al. Affinity purified anti-52 kD Ro/SSA antibody induces A-V heart block "*in vitro.*" *Arthritis Rheum* 1995;38: S306(abst).
54. Kalush F, Rimon E, Mozes E. Neonatal lupus erythematosus in offspring of mothers with experimental systemic lupus erythematosus. *Am J Reprod Immunol* 1992;28:264–268.
55. Mazel JA, El-Sherif N, Buyon J, et al. Electrocardiographic abnormalities in a murine model injected with IgG from mothers of children with congenital heart block. *Circulation* 1999;99:1914–1918.
56. Eftekhari P, Salle L, Lezoualc'h F, et al. Anti-SSA/Ro52 autoantibodies block-

ing the cardiac 5-HT4 serotoninergic receptor could explain neonatal lupus congenital heart block (In Process Citation). *Eur J Immunol* 2000;30:2782–2790.
57. Miranda-Carus ME, Askanase AD, Clancy RM, et al. Anti-SSA/Ro and anti-SSB/La autoantibodies bind the surface of apoptotic fetal cardiocytes and promote secretion of TNF-alpha by macrophages. *J Immunol* 2000;165: 5345–5351.
58. Buyon JP, Tseng C-E, Di Donato F, et al. Cardiac expression of 52β: an alternative transcript of the congenital heart block-associated 52-kd SS-A/Ro autoantigen, is maximal during fetal development. *Arthritis Rheum* 1997;40: 655–660.
59. Fraire-Velazquez S, Herrera-Esparza R, Villalobos-Hurtado R, et al. Ontogeny of Ro hY RNAs in human heart. *Scand J Rheumatol* 1999;28:100–105.
60. Lee LA, Bias WB, Arnett FJ, et al. Immunogenetics of the neonatal lupus syndrome. *Ann Intern Med* 1983;99:592–596.
61. Watson RM, Scheel JN, Petri M, et al. Neonatal lupus erythematosus syndrome: analysis of C4 allotypes and C4 genes in 18 families. *Medicine* 1992;71: 84–95.
62. Lehman TJA. Systemic lupus erythematosus in childhood and adolescence. In: Wallace DJ, Hahn BH, eds. *Dubois' lupus erythematosus.* Philadelphia: Lea & Febiger, 1993:431–441.
63. Schaller J. Lupus in childhood. *Clin Rheumat Dis* 1982;8:219–228.
64. Siegel M, Lee SL. The epidemiology of systemic lupus erythematosus. *Semin Arthritis Rheum* 1973;3:1–54.
65. Wananukul S, Watana D, Pongprasit P. Cutaneous manifestations of childhood systemic lupus erythematosus. *Pediatr Dermatol* 1998;15:342–346.
66. George PM, Tunnessen WW Jr. Childhood discoid lupus erythematosus. *Arch Dermatol* 1993;129:613–617.
67. Winklemann RK. Chronic discoid lupus erythematosus in children. *JAMA* 1968;205:675–678.
68. Siamopoulou MA, Stefanou D, Drosos AA. Subacute cutaneous lupus-erythematosus in childhood. *Clin Rheumatol* 1989;8:533–537.
69. Provost TT, Arnett FC, Reichlin M. Homozygous C2 deficiency, lupus erythematosus and anti-Ro (SSA) antibodies. *Arthritis Rheum* 1983;26:1279–1282.
70. Meyer O, Hauptmann G, Tappeiner G, et al. Genetic deficiency of C4, C2 or C1q and lupus syndromes: association with anti-Ro (SS-A) antibodies. *Clin Exp Immunol* 1985;62:678–684.
71. Taieb A, Hehunstre J-P, Goetz J, et al. Lupus erythematosus panniculitis with partial genetic deficiency of C2 and C4 in a child. *Arch Dermatol* 1986;122: 576–582.
72. Kettler AH, Bean SF, Duffy JO, et al. Systemic lupus erythematosus presenting as a bullous eruption in a child. *Arch Dermatol* 1988;124:1083–1087.
73. Fish AJ, Blau EB, Westberg NG, et al. Systemic lupus erythematosus within the first two decades of life. *Am J Med* 1977;62:99–117.
74. Walravens PA, Chase HP. The prognosis of childhood systemic lupus erythematosus. *Am J Dis Child* 1976;130:929–933.
75. Lehman TJA, McCurdy D, Spencer C, et al. Prognostic value of antibodies to SSA/Ro, SSB/La, and RNP in children with systemic lupus erythematosus. *Arthritis Rheum* 1990;33[suppl]:S145(abst).
76. Newton RC, Jorizzo JL, Solomon AJ, et al. Mechanism-oriented assessment of isotretinoin in chronic or subacute cutaneous lupus erythematosus. *Arch Dermatol* 1986;122:170–176.
77. Lehman TJA, Reichlin M, Santner TJ, et al. Maternal antibodies to Ro (SS-A) are associated with both early onset of disease and male sex among children with systemic lupus erythematosus. *Arthritis Rheum* 1989;32:1414–1420.
78. Manzi S, Urbach AH, McCune AB, et al. Systemic lupus erythematosus in a boy with chronic granulomatous disease: case report and review of the literature. *Arthritis Rheum* 1991;34:101–105.
79. Pachman LM. An update on juvenile dermatomyositis. *Curr Opin Rheumatol* 1995;7:437–441.
80. Norins AL. Juvenile dermatomyositis. *Med Clin North Am* 1989;73:1193–1209.
81. Pachman LM. Juvenile dermatomyositis: a clinical overview. *Pediatr Rev* 1990;12:117–125.
82. Huber AM, Lang B, LeBlanc CM, et al. Medium- and long-term functional outcomes in a multicenter cohort of children with juvenile dermatomyositis. *Arthritis Rheum* 2000;43:541–549.
83. Hiketa T, Matsumoto Y, Ohashi M, et al. Juvenile dermatomyositis: a statistical study of 114 patients with dermatomyositis. *J Dermatol* 1992;19: 470–476.
84. Miller LC, Michael AF, Kim Y. Childhood dermatomyositis: clinical course and long-term follow-up. *Clin Pediatr* 1987;26:561–566.
85. Bohan A, Peter JB. Polymyositis and dermatomyositis. *N Engl J Med* 1975;292: 344–347, 403–407.
86. Ghali FE, Stein LD, Fine JD, et al. Gingival telangiectases: an underappreciated physical sign of juvenile dermatomyositis. *Arch Dermatol* 1999;135: 370–374.
87. Pachman LM, Hayford JR, Chung A, et al. Juvenile dermatomyositis at diagnosis: clinical characteristics of 79 children. *J Rheumatol* 1998;25:1198–1204.
88. Wananukul S, Pongprasit P, Wattanakrai P. Calcinosis cutis presenting years before other clinical manifestations of juvenile dermatomyositis: report of two cases. *Australas J Dermatol* 1997;38:202–205.
89. Ansell BM. Juvenile dermatomyositis. *J Rheumatol* 1992;19[Suppl 33]:60–62.
90. Bowyer SL, Clark RAF, Ragsdale CG, et al. Juvenile dermatomyositis: histological findings and pathogenetic hypothesis for the associated skin changes. *J Rheumatol* 1986;13:753–759.
91. Huemer C, Kitson H, Malleson PN, et al. Lipodystrophy in patients with juvenile dermatomyositis—evaluation of clinical and metabolic abnormalities. *J Rheumatol* 2001;28:610–615.
92. Ghali FE, Reed AM, Groben PA, et al. Panniculitis in juvenile dermatomyositis. *Pediatr Dermatol* 1999;16:270–272.
93. See Y, Rooney M, Woo P. Palmer plantar hyperkeratosis—a previously undescribed skin manifestation of juvenile dermatomyositis. *Br J Rheumatol* 1997; 36:917–919.
94. Euwer RL, Sontheimer RD. Amyopathic dermatomyositis: a review. *J Invest Dermatol* 1993;100:124S–127S.
95. Peloro TM, Miller OF III, Hahn TF, et al. Juvenile dermatomyositis: a retrospective review of a 30-year experience. *J Am Acad Dermatol* 2001;45:28–34.
96. Targoff IN. Humoral immunity in polymyositis/dermatomyositis. *J Invest Dermatol* 1993;100:116S–123S.
97. Feldman BM, Reichlin M, Laxer RM, et al. Clinical significance of specific autoantibodies in juvenile dermatomyositis. *J Rheumatol* 1996;23:1794–1797.
98. Montecucco C, Ravelli A, Caporali R, et al. Autoantibodies in juvenile dermatomyositis. *Clin Exp Rheumatol* 1990;8:193–196.
99. Lang BA, Laxer RM, Murphy G, et al. Treatment of dermatomyositis with intravenous gammaglobulin. *Am J Med* 1991;91:169–172.
100. Wang WJ. Calcinosis cutis in juvenile dermatomyositis: remarkable response to aluminum hydroxide therapy. *Arch Dermatol* 1988;124:1721–1722.
101. Bowyer SL, Blane CE, Sullivan DB, et al. Childhood dermatomyositis: factors predicting functional outcome and development of dystrophic calcification. *J Pediatr* 1983;103:882–888.
102. Ichiki Y, Akiyama T, Shimozawa N, et al. An extremely severe case of cutaneous calcinosis with juvenile dermatomyositis, and successful treatment with diltiazem. *Br J Dermatol* 2001;144:894–897.
103. Mukamel M, Horev G, Mimouni M. New insight into calcinosis of juvenile dermatomyositis: a study of composition and treatment. *J Pediatr* 2001;138: 763–766.
104. Harel L, Harel G, Korenreich L, et al. Treatment of calcinosis in juvenile dermatomyositis with probenecid: the role of phosphorus metabolism in the development of calcifications. *J Rheumatol* 2001;28:1129–1132.
105. Spencer CH, Hanson V, Singsen BH, et al. Course of treated juvenile dermatomyositis. *J Pediatr* 1984;105:399–408.
106. Pachman LM, Maryjowski MC. Juvenile dermatomyositis and polymyositis. *Clin Rheumat Dis* 1984;10:95–115.
107. Crowe WE, Bove KE, Levinson JE, et al. Clinical and pathogenetic implications of histopathology in childhood polydermatomyositis. *Arthritis Rheum* 1982;25:126–139.
108. Collison CH, Sinal SH, Jorizzo JL, et al. Juvenile dermatomyositis and polymyositis: a follow-up study of long- term sequelae. *South Med J* 1998;91: 17–22.
109. Christensen ML, Pachman LM, Schneiderman R, et al. Prevalence of Coxsackie B virus antibodies in patients with juvenile dermatomyositis. *Arthritis Rheum* 1986;29:1365–1370.
110. Bowles NE, Sewry CA, Dubowitz V, et al. Dermatomyositis, polymyositis, and coxsackie-B virus infection. *Lancet* 1987;1:1004–1007.
111. Martini A, Ravelli A, Albani S, et al. Recurrent juvenile dermatomyositis and cutaneous necrotizing arteritis with molecular mimicry between streptococcal type 5 M protein and human skeletal myosin. *J Pediatr* 1992;121:739–742.
112. Moore EC, Cohen F, Douglas SD, et al. Staphylococcal infections in childhood dermatomyositis: association with the development of calcinosis, raised IgE concentrations and granulocyte chemotactic defect. *Ann Rheum Dis* 1992;51: 378–383.
113. Reed AM, Pachman LM, Hayford J, et al. Immunogenetic studies in families of children with juvenile dermatomyositis. *J Rheumatol* 1998;25:1000–1002.
114. Pachman LM, Liotta-Davis MR, Hong DK, et al. TNFalpha-308A allele in juvenile dermatomyositis: association with increased production of tumor necrosis factor alpha, disease duration, and pathologic calcifications. *Arthritis Rheum* 2000;43:2368–2377.
115. Reed AM, Picornell YJ, Harwood A, et al. Chimerism in children with juvenile dermatomyositis. *Lancet* 2000;356:2156–2157.
116. Burns JC, Kushner HI, Bastian JF, et al. Kawasaki disease: a brief history. *Pediatrics* 2000;106:E27.
117. Burns JC. Kawasaki disease. *Adv Pediatr* 2001;48:157–77.
118. Yalcindag A, Sundel R. Vasculitis in childhood. *Curr Opin Rheumatol* 2001:13; 422–427.
119. Corbeel L, Gewillig M, Baeton E, et al. Carotid and coronary artery involvement in infantile periarteritis nodosa possible induced by Coxsackie B4 infection. *Eur J Pediatr* 1987;146:441–442.
120. Boven K, DeGraeff-Meeder ER, Spliet W, et al. Atypical Kawasaki disease: an often missed diagnosis. *Eur J Pediatr* 1992;151:577–580.
121. Kawasaki T, Kosaki F, Okawa S, et al. A new infantile mucocutaneous acute febrile mucocutaneous lymph node syndrome (MLNS) prevailing in Japan. *Pediatrics* 1974;54:271–276.
122. Michie C, Kinsler V, Tulloh R, et al. Recurrent skin peeling following Kawasaki disease. *Arch Dis Child* 2000;83:353–355.
123. Anderson MS, Burns J, Treadwell TA, et al. Erythrocyte sedimentation rate and C-reactive protein discrepancy and high prevalence of coronary artery abnormalities in Kawasaki disease. *Pediatr Infect Dis J* 2001;20:698–702.
124. Tabarki B, Mahdhaoui A, Selmi H, et al. Kawasaki disease with predominant central nervous system involvement. *Pediatr Neurol* 2001;25:239–241.
125. Cox F, Foshee W, Miller J Jr, et al. Simultaneous Kawasaki disease and group A streptococcal pharyngitis. *Clin Pediatr* 1993;32:48–52.

126. Johnson RM, Little JR, Storch GA. Kawasaki-like syndromes associated with human immunodeficiency virus infection. *Clin Infect Dis* 2001;32:1628–1634.
127. Lee LA, Burns J, Glode M, et al. No autoantibodies to nuclear antigens in the Kawasaki syndrome. *N Engl J Med* 1983;308:1034.
128. Saalouke MG, Venglarcik JS, Baker DR, et al. Rapid regression of coronary dilatation in Kawasaki disease with intravenous gamma globulin. *Am Heart J* 1991;121:905–909.
129. Hashino K, Ishii M, Iemura M, et al. Re-treatment for immune globulin-resistant Kawasaki disease: a comparative study of additional immune globulin and steroid pulse therapy. *Pediatr Int* 2001;43:211–217.
130. Inoue T, Otaki M, Oku H, et al. Follow-up study of coronary artery bypass grafting in patients with Kawasaki disease. *Am Heart J* 2001;142:740–744.
131. Ozen S, Besbas N, Saatci U, et al. Diagnostic criteria for polyarteritis nodosa in childhood. *J Pediatr* 1992;12:206–209.
132. Jones SK, Lane AL, Golitz LE, et al. Cutaneous periarteritis nodosa in childhood. *Am J Dis Child* 1985;139:920–922.
133. Tonnelier JM, Ansart S, Tilly-Gentric A, et al. Juvenile relapsing periarteritis nodosa and streptococcal infection. *Joint Bone Spine* 2000;67:356–358.
134. Ozen S, Ben-Chetrit F, Bakkaloglu A, et al. Polyarteritis nodosa in patients with familial Mediterranean fever (FMF): a concomitant disease or feature of FMF? *Semin Arthritis Rheum* 2001;30:281–287.
135 Burke JB. Erythema marginatum. *Arch Dis Child* 1955;30:359–365.
136 Secord S, Emre U, Shah BR, et al. Erythema marginatum in acute rheumatic fever. *Am J Dis Child* 1992;146:637–638.
137 Jones TD. The diagnosis of rheumatic fever. *JAMA* 1944;126:481–484.
138. Yavuz H, Ozel A, Yilmaz O, et al. Benign rheumatoid nodules. *Am J Dis Child* 1993;147:1011–1012.
139. Cunnigham MW. Pathogenesis of group A streptococcal infections. *Clin Microbiol Rev* 2000;13:470–511.
140. Bont L, Brus F, Dijkman-Neerincx RH, et al. The clinical spectrum of post-streptococcal syndromes with arthritis in children. *Clin Exp Rheumatol* 1998; 16:750–752.
141. Calabro JJ, Marchesano JM . Rash associated with juvenile rheumatoid arthritis. *J Pediatr* 1968;72:611–619.
142. Cate RH, de Vries van der Vlugt NBCM, van Suijlekom-Smit LWA, et al. Disease patterns in early onset pauciarticular juvenile chronic arthritis. *Eur J Pediatr* 1992;151:339–341.
143. Weston WL, Morelli JG. Childhood pernio and cryoproteins. *Pediatr Dermatol* 2000;17:97–99.
144. Prieur AM, Griscelli C, Lampert F, et al. A chronic, infantile, neurological, cutaneous and articular (CINCA) syndrome: a specific entity analyzed in 30 patients. *Scand J Rheumatol* 1987;66:57–68.
145. Prieur AM. A recently recognized chronic inflammatory disease of early onset characterized by a triad of rash, central nervous system involvement and arthropathy. *Clin Exp Rheumatol* 2001;19:103–106.
146. Dollfus H, Hafner R, Hofmann HM, et al. Chronic infantile neurological cutaneous and articular/neonatal onset multisystem inflammatory disease syndrome: ocular manifestations in a recently recognized chronic inflammatory disease of childhood. *Arch Ophthalmol* 2000;18:1386–1392.
147. Martini A. Juvenile systemic scleroderma. *Curr Rheumatol Rep* 2001;3: 387–3890.
148. Hawk A, English JC Jr. Localized and systemic scleroderma. *Semin Cutan Med Surg* 2001;20:27.
149. Miller JJ III. The fasciitis-morphea complex in children. *Am J Dis Child* 1992; 146:733–736.
150. Arnett FC, Tan FK, Uziel Y, et al. Autoantibodies to the extracellular matrix microfibrillar protein, fibrillin I, in patients with localized scleroderma. *Arthritis Rheum* 1999;42:2656–2659.
151. Weide B, Schittek B, Klyscz T, et al. Morphoea is neither associated with the features of *Borelli burgdorferi* infection, nor is this agent detectable in lesional skin by polymerase chain reaction. *Br J Dermatol* 2000;143:780–785.
152. Wollins U, Looks A, Schneider R, et al. Disabling morphea of childhood: beneficial effects of intravenous immunoglobulin therapy. *Clin Exp Dermatol* 1998;23:292–293.
153. Gruss CJ, von Kobyletzki G, Behrens-Williams SC, et al. Effects of low dose ultraviolet A1 phototherapy on morphea. *Photodermatol Photoimmunol Photomed* 2001;17:149–155.
154. Kreuter A, Gambicher T, Avermaete A, et al. Combined treatment with calcipotriol ointment and low-dose ultraviolet A1 phototherapy in childhood morphea. *Pediatr Dermatol* 2001;18:241–245.

CHAPTER 14

Immunosuppressive Therapies

Adrienne Rencic, Daniel Mimouni and Carlos H. Nousari

Cutaneous manifestations of rheumatic disease are treated with a variety of topical and systemic immunosuppressive agents. Some of these agents have been approved by the U.S. Food and Drug Administration (FDA). Other agents, because of their anti-inflammatory and immunosuppressive effects in other diseases, have been adapted to the treatment of rheumatic diseases. This chapter will provide a brief overview of the most commonly prescribed agents.

TOPICAL THERAPY

Corticosteroids

Topical corticosteroids (CSs) are commonly prescribed to ameliorate cutaneous lesions in rheumatic disease. They may be divided into fluorinated and nonfluorinated. Fluorinated compounds are more potent due to increased efficacy within the cell and decreased breakdown into metabolites. The mineralocorticoid side-effect profile of the fluorinated compounds, however, is increased as well. Methylation or hydroxylation increases efficacy without a corresponding increase in mineralocorticoid side effects.

The potency of topical CSs is determined by the vasoconstriction effects on the skin. However, vehicle can increase potency of a topical steroid. For example, the more occlusive vehicles such as ointments are more potent. Occlusion with various agents including tape impregnated with CS also increases potency. Pretreatment of the skin by tape stripping or acetone may also result in increased permeability of the CSs.

Clinical Use

High-potency topical CSs are most commonly used in the treatment of discoid lupus erythematosus (DLE). These are commonly used in conjunction with antimalarials and sun-protective measures. Topical steroids may also be used in subacute cutaneous lupus, systemic lupus, and dermatomyositis for symptomatic relief of skin discomfort due to active disease. Topical CSs in these patients should always be combined with thorough sun protection and systemic drugs including antimalarials for optimal treatment. High-potency topical CSs may also be useful in localized morphea, the treatment of cutaneous lesions in Reiter syndrome, or for symptomatic relief in Still disease.

Side Effects

Side effects of topical CSs are primarily limited to cutaneous problems, including telangiectasia, striae, atrophy, steroid acne, perioral or periorbital dermatitis, folliculitis, and exacerbation of rosacea. Additionally, miliaria and hypopigmentation may be seen. Preservatives and fragrances in topical CSs may cause contact or irritant dermatitis. If ultrapotent steroids are used on a large body surface area, particularly in conditions in which the barrier function is impaired, systemic absorption and side effects occur similar to those seen with systemic administration of glucocorticosteroids, such as adrenal suppression or iatrogenic Cushing syndrome. Clobetasol propionate used at a dosage of 50 g per week has resulted in adrenal suppression (1). However, there are many reports of adrenal failure in patients using lower doses over a long period (2). New topical steroids with potent local activity and little systemic effect are being developed. This class of CS is effective at its application site, but is rapidly transformed to inactive metabolites, thus decreasing systemic absorption and side effects (3).

SUN PROTECTION

Sun protection is an essential part of treatment of connective tissue diseases. Adequate sun protection should be considered a steroid-sparing adjuvant therapy, particularly in conditions such as cutaneous lupus erythematosus and dermatomyositis. Studies have shown induction of cutaneous lesions upon photo-provocation in 25% of patients with systemic lupus erythematosus (SLE), 64% of patients with subacute cutaneous lupus erythematosus (SCLE), and 42% of patients with DLE, and *in vitro* experiments have shown increased susceptibility of cultured cells from patients with lupus to UV-A, but particularly to UV-B irradiation (4–6). Patients with dermatomyositis have also been shown to have increased photosensitivity, however, the mechanism is unclear (6,7). One study demonstrated a clear benefit of sunscreen in prevention of lesions with photo-provocation (8).

Sunscreens are either physical blockers or chemical blockers. Physical blockers do not allow UV light to penetrate them, whereas chemical blockers absorb particular wavelengths of light.

Chemical blockers may be divided into UV-A blocking agent and UV-B blocking agents. The sun-protection factor of a sunscreen is based solely on its ability to block UV-B, the wavelengths causing erythema of the skin, and the primary wavelength responsible for triggering lupus flares (4,5). There is no corresponding factor that indicates the ability of a sunscreen to protect against UV-A radiation. However, secondarily, the wavelengths may contribute to disease flare in some connective tissue diseases. It is therefore essential to recommend sunscreens that contain either physical blockers or broad-spectrum UV-A and UV-B coverage. The most common physical blockers include zinc oxide and titanium dioxide. These now come in a micronized form, which is invisible when applied. Specific UV-A blocking agents include avobenzone (Parsol 1789) and both the physical blockers, zinc oxide and titanium dioxide. UV-B blocking agents include aminobenzoates, salicylates, cinnamates, PABA, and PABA derivatives (padimate A and O).

Additional sun protection may be achieved using sun-protective clothing (Solumbra; Sun Solutions, Falmouth, MA) and by application of UV-A protective film on car windows (Llumar, Martinsville, VA; and Vista UV Shield, Vista, Cary, NC).

Side Effects

Side effects to sunscreens include primarily nonspecific irritant dermatitis and less commonly, allergic contact dermatitis and photoallergic contact dermatitis. Photocontact dermatitis has been reported in decreasing order of frequency with oxybenzone, avobenzone, methoxycinnamate, and benzophenone. Reportedly, 19 individuals were allergic over the course of 8 years in a long-term study conducted in Australia (9). Lenique et al. (10) reported that 13% of 54 patients had allergic reactions to oxybenzone, two with allergic contact dermatitis, three with photoallergic contact dermatitis, and two with both.

In patients with known allergy to sunscreens, it is safest to use physical blockers, since these are inert and have not been reported to cause any allergic reactions.

MACROLACTAM IMMUNOMODULATORS

Tacrolimus

Topical tacrolimus is a new topical macrolide immunomodulator. It will be only briefly mentioned, because it has not been used widely in the treatment of rheumatic disease. Its mechanism of action involves inhibition of the phosphatase, calcineurin, blocking the activity of the transcription factor NF-AT (nuclear factor of activated T cells) and, consequently, the transcription of a variety of cytokines, including interleukin-2 (IL-2). Without these cytokines, early stages of T-cell activation are prevented (11).

CLINICAL USE

There is a single published report describing successful treatment of facial erythema in six of 11 patients with lupus and dermatomyositis (12). All three patients with SLE responded and a fourth of the patients with DLE and half the patients with dermatomyositis responded well to treatment. Fully evolved lesions of DLE did not respond in any of the patients (12). Tacrolimus may be useful in symptomatic relief of skin discomfort in some rheumatic conditions, without the undesired cutaneous atrophy and telangiectasia formation of topical steroids, but this requires further investigation.

Approximately half the patients experienced skin burning and pruritus with application of tacrolimus. This improved with continued use. This was the primary adverse effect. There is little systemic absorption of topical tacrolimus in most patients treated. However, three patients with Netherton syndrome developed blood levels equivalent to that seen in transplant recipients (13). Care must be taken in these patients to avoid systemic toxicity, although none was seen in the three patients described.

Pimecrolimus

This macrolactam, also known as ASM 981, is a derivative from the parent compound ascomycin. Pimecrolimus is a cell-selective inhibitor of inflammatory cytokines specifically developed for the treatment of inflammatory dermatoses. Pimecrolimus has a mechanism of action similar to that of other calcineurin inhibitors. It forms a complex with macrophilin-12, which will inhibit calcineurin. Calcineurin inhibition leads to inhibition of synthesis of proinflammatory T helper cells type 1 (T_H1) and type 2 (T_H2) cytokines. Other immunomodulatory effects, including stabilization of mast cells and inhibition of tumor necrosis factor-α (TNF-α) and other late-phase cytokines have also been observed with the use of pimecrolimus.

CLINICAL INDICATIONS

Pimecrolimus is formulated in vehicle cream at concentrations of 0.2 %, 0.6 %, and 1%. Pimecrolimus has not been reported to cause atrophy, and the systemic absorption rate appears to be clinically insignificant. Topical pimecrolimus appears to be associated with less burning sensation in comparison with tacrolimus. There are no reported uses of pimecrolimus in the treatment of rheumatic disorders. Although preliminary studies have not shown that pimecrolimus is superior to topical tacrolimus, this ascomycin derivative has a role in the topical therapeutic armamentarium of T-cell–mediated skin disorders (11).

SYSTEMIC THERAPY

The most common agents used in treatment of cutaneous rheumatic diseases are systemic CSs, alone or in combination with a steroid-sparing agent: antimalarials, thalidomide, antimetabolites, or cytotoxic drugs. Other less commonly used agents include thalidomide, intravenous immunoglobulin (IVIG), methotrexate, and dapsone. The backbone of CSs consists of a four-ring compound called the cyclopentenoperhydrophenanthrene nucleus. Each carbon is designated with a number. There are 21 carbons. Hydrocortisone (cortisol) has a hydroxyl group at C-11. Fluorination of the 9α position produces fludrocortisone, a more potent glucocorticoid, but increases mineralocorticoid activity as well. By adding a double bond at the 1,2 position and hydroxylation or methylation of the 16-carbon, triamcinolone, dexamethasone, and betamethasone result. These compounds are potent glucocorticoids, but have less mineralocorticoid effect than the parent compound, fludrocortisone.

Drug Metabolism

CSs are absorbed in the jejunum. Peak serum levels occur between 30 and 100 minutes. Food does not decrease absorption. Exogenous CSs do not bind well to plasma proteins and achieve a higher free fraction in the plasma than endogenous CSs. All CSs require reduction of the 4,5 double bond (intra- and extrahepatic) to be inactivated; inactive metabolites are excreted by the kidneys.

MECHANISM OF ACTION

CSs exert their physiologic effects via binding to the glucocorticoid receptor (GR). Once the CS binds to its receptor, it is translocated into the nucleus and binds glucocorticoid-responsive elements (GRE) in the promoters of a variety of genes. Transcription may be activated or suppressed by its action.

There are two isoforms, alternatively spliced variants of the GR, GRα and GRβ. GRβ differs from GRα only in its C-terminal domain. The terminal 50 amino acids of GRα are replaced by 15 unique amino acids in GRβ. GRβ does not bind CS. *In vitro* experiments have shown that GRβ inhibits GRα-mediated transcriptional activity. Unfortunately, physiologic experiments have not confirmed these data (14). Although this remains a potential target to increase therapeutic specificity of CS, more research is required to elucidate the precise function of the GRβ isoform.

Two important genes involved in inflammatory response, which CS is known to inhibit, are *NFkB* and *AP1*. *NFkB* inhibitor production is increased by CS, which can also bind directly to *NFkB*. Via inhibition of *NFkB* and *AP1*, CSs can block production of a variety of inflammatory mediators including cytokines, growth factors and adhesion molecules. Furthermore, CSs induce apoptosis of lymphocytes and eosinophils, inhibit phospholipase A2, and as a direct result, decrease production of the downstream inflammatory mediators of the arachidonic acid cascade (15).

CSs decrease the effector function of a variety of inflammatory cells including T cells, B cells, natural killer cells, polymorphonuclear leukocytes, mast cells, monocytes, macrophages, Langerhans cells, eosinophils, basophils, and fibroblasts. The net effect is decreased cell-mediated and humoral immunity, via impaired cytokine release; decreased chemotaxis; reduced recruitment to sites of inflammation; defective antigen presentation; and decreased production of extracellular matrix and angiogenesis (15).

Clinical Use and Dosage

Daily oral CS use should not exceed the equivalent of 1 mg/kg (ideal body mass) of prednisone. This should be tapered as quickly as possible with early introduction of CS-sparing agents as necessary to control disease activity (16). Having stated this, care should be taken not to taper too quickly as frequent raising and lowering of CS may prolong the disease course rather than hasten it (17). The initial portion of the taper from 60 mg to 30 mg may be done over the course of 3 months; however, the taper from this point should be much more gradual.

Conditions in which CS are used include SLE, dermatomyositis; scleroderma; rheumatoid arthritis; Still disease; relapsing polychondritis; Sjögren syndrome; cutaneous and systemic vasculitides including polyarteritis nodosa, Churg–Strauss syndrome, Wegener granulomatosis, and hypocomplementemic urticarial vasculitis syndrome; as well as neutrophilic dermatoses [pyoderma gangrenosum (PG), Behçet disease, Sweet syndrome, bowel-related dermatosis–arthritis syndrome]. Essentially, CSs are the cornerstone of immunosuppressive therapy in virtually all rheumatic diseases.

Side Effects

Acute adverse effects with systemic CSs include hypertension, hyperglycemia, agitation, insomnia, and precipitation of psychosis. Longer term use may result in osteoporosis, osteonecrosis, adrenal insufficiency, cataracts, opportunistic infections, impaired growth, proximal myopathy, weight gain, and cushingoid habitus.

TABLE 14.1. Osteoporosis Prophylaxis with Long-Term Corticosteroid Use

Baseline bone densitometry scan, repeat each year
Calcium 1,500 mg elemental per day
Vitamin D 800 IU per day
Alendronate once weekly at 40 mg for prophylaxis
Risedronate at 5 mg daily
Women
Hormone replacement controversial, should be discussed with physician
Men
Check serum testosterone and prostate-specific antigen × 3 measurements (consecutive months), then yearly
If testosterone is low (in the absence of prostate cancer), testosterone replacement should be administered
If there is greater than 5% loss on annual dual-energy x-ray absorptiometry scan, begin alendronate 70 mg weekly
If hypercalciuria is present, consider addition of hydrochlorothiazide

One of the most concerning, yet preventable side effects mentioned before is osteoporosis. Steroid-induced osteoporosis occurs most rapidly during the first 3 to 6 months of treatment (18). Appropriate prophylaxis at the initiation of therapy can prevent a significant amount of bone loss. All patients should receive prescriptions for calcium, vitamin D, and alendronate 40 mg weekly with their first prescription for CS. Additional preventive measures should be guided by patient history and individual risk factors. Postmenopausal women should discuss hormone replacement therapy or selective estrogen receptor modulators with their physician due to the recent controversy associated with this issue (19,20). Men with low levels of testosterone should also receive replacement therapy if they do not have prostate cancer. Patients with baseline osteoporosis should receive a therapeutic dosage of a bisphosphonate (i.e., alendronate 70 mg weekly). Any patient with hypercalciuria should receive hydrochlorothiazide. The roles of fluoride and miacalcin are controversial in the treatment of osteoporosis, but some physicians use these agents as well in severely osteoporotic patients (21).

Another important, yet frequently overlooked method of preventing osteoporosis is rational use of immunosuppressants with initial CS treatment with addition of CS-sparing agents and tapering of CS as quickly as possible.

Patients with hepatic failure should receive prednisolone or hydrocortisone rather than their precursors because 11β-hydroxydehydrogenase is required to convert prednisone or cortisol into prednisolone and hydrocortisone, their respective active metabolites. This enzyme is only present in the liver.

Monitoring Guidelines and Prophylaxis

See Tables 14.1 and 14.2.

TABLE 14.2. Infection Prophylaxis with Long-Term Corticosteroid

Check purified protein derivative and human immunodeficiency status
Pneumococcal vaccine
Influenza vaccine
If long-term use necessary or with antimetabolites, consider *Pneumocystis carinii* pneumonia prophylaxis.
Repeat diphtheria and tetanus if antibody titers are low.

ANTIMALARIALS

Antimalarials are effective drugs for maintenance therapy in connective tissue diseases including chronic cutaneous lupus erythematosus, DLE, tumid LE, lupus panniculitis, SCLE, Sjögren syndrome, and dermatomyositis. Hydroxychloroquine (HCQ) and chloroquine (CQ) are 4-aminoquinolones, which are the most commonly used drugs in this class.

Drug Metabolism

HCQ is very well absorbed in the gastrointestinal (GI) tract (75% to 100%). In the serum, 50% is protein-bound. Consequently, it can take 2 to 3 months to achieve a therapeutic dose and 6 to 12 months to see maximal therapeutic effect. Forty-five percent is renally excreted, 20% is excreted through the bowel, and 3% is excreted by the skin. Epidermal levels are 100 to 200 times that seen in plasma.

CQ is typically administered at 250 to 500 mg daily and is 100% absorbed in the GI tract. Peak plasma concentrations are reached within 8 hours and steady-state concentrations are reached in 4 to 6 weeks. Consequently, therapeutic drug levels are achieved more quickly than with HCQ. CQ too has a predilection for the skin and has been detected in the skin as long as 7 months after cessation of treatment. Fifty percent of CQ is renally excreted. Ninety percent of patients on standard therapeutic doses of CQ have corneal deposits. Acidification of the urine increases excretion of both CQ and HCQ. Hemodialysis is ineffective in removal of CQ and HCQ.

MECHANISM OF ACTION

The exact mechanism of action by which antimalarials exert their therapeutic effect is unclear. Both CQ and HCQ in the epidermis can absorb UV light in a dose-dependent fashion. HCQ and CQ concentrate within intracellular acidic cytoplasmic vesicles, such as lysosomes. The accumulation of HCQ or CQ in lysosomal vesicles decreases phagocytosis, chemotaxis, and delays recycling of enzymes and cell surface receptors. Additionally, HCQ and CQ can inhibit natural killer cell activity and IL-2 production.

Drug Interactions and Side Effects

HCQ should be avoided with concomitant use of anticonvulsants, digoxin, cimetidine, and amiodarone. CQ should be avoided with anticonvulsants, D-penicillamine, cimetidine, and cyclosporine. Smoking may decrease the efficacy of antimalarials.

Side effects of HCQ and CQ include hemolysis in patients with glucose-6-phosphate dehydrogenase (G6PDH) deficiency, nausea and vomiting, blue–black hyperpigmentation, bleaching of hair, and exacerbation of psoriasis. The most concerning side effects are ocular. Corneal deposits present as bright halos around objects. This is reversible and is more prominent in CQ treatment, but is not an indication to discontinue therapy. Retinopathy is dose-related. The earliest sign is premaculopathy with retinal pigment deposition and pericentral and paracentral scotoma and decreased visual acuity may signal irreversible retinopathy. Ocular problems occur less frequently because the therapeutic dosing is lower than that used in the past.

Clinical Indications and Dosage

Antimalarials are most frequently used in lupus erythematosus (LE), particularly DLE, dermatomyositis, and Sjögren syndrome to treat sicca symptoms. Dosage for HCQ is typically 200 mg twice daily. Alternatively, dosing may be calculated by ideal body mass at 6.5 mg/kg daily. CQ dosage is 250 to 500 mg daily or 3.5 to 4 mg/kg per day.

Monitoring Guidelines

Baseline ophthalmologic examination should be performed with slit lamp, visual acuity, and visual field testing with a red object. The patient should use an Amsler grid monthly to evaluate visual fields. If the patient notices fading of the squares, visual field testing should be repeated immediately. Slit lamp and visual acuity examinations should be repeated every 6 months. Bilateral visual field defects should prompt immediate discontinuation of the antimalarial drug.

In patients who may be predisposed, a G6PDH level should be checked because G6PDH-deficient patients may develop severe hemolysis and agranulocytosis.

Liver function tests, chemistry profile, and complete blood count (CBC) should be checked at baseline and monthly for the first 3 months. Subsequently they may be monitored every 4 to 6 months (22).

THALIDOMIDE

Thalidomide has gained notoriety due to its teratogenic effects and has fallen out of favor with many dermatologists; however, it is an extremely useful agent in the treatment of inflammatory dermatoses, specifically DLE, Behçet disease, and PG, when in combination with other immunosuppressive agents.

Drug Metabolism

Thalidomide is a synthetic analog of glutamic acid. It is composed of two rings, a phthalimide ring and glutarimide ring. It is lipid soluble, and readily crosses the placenta. Peak plasma concentration is reached within 3 to 6 hours after ingestion, but may be delayed by ingestion with fatty foods. Primary metabolism is by nonenzymatic hydrolytic cleavage of its four amide bonds, which occurs above pH 6. Excretion is primarily nonrenal, with less than 1% of the original present in the urine 24 hours after administration.

MECHANISM OF ACTION

Although thalidomide's many clinical effects have been well characterized, there is little known regarding the molecular or biochemical pathways by which it acts to exert these effects. Table 14.3 summarizes its physiologic effects.

Clinical Indications and Dosage

Dosing varies with the disease being treated and its severity. The typical range is 50 to 200 mg per day. DLE responds well to

TABLE 14.3. Mechanisms of Action of Thalidomide

Inhibition tumor necrosis factor-α
Decreased interleukin-12 production
Inhibition of interferon-γ
Inhibition of histamine, prostaglandins, serotonin
Decreased monocyte phagocytosis
Decreased neutrophil chemotaxis and phagocytosis
Inhibition of angiogenesis
Activation of sleep center

smaller initial doses and often responds within the first month of treatment. Cutaneous lesions in SCLE and SLE and lupus profundus may also respond well to thalidomide treatment. Higher initial doses are used with tapering to a lower maintenance dosage (i.e., 25 to 50 mg per day).

PG, particularly atypical PG associated with an underlying hematologic malignancy, such as multiple myeloma or myelodysplastic syndrome, may respond well to treatment with high-dose thalidomide, since it will also be treating the underlying disorder. Thalidomide in these cases is not used as a sole agent but in conjunction with CS as a steroid-sparing agent.

Behçet syndrome has been reported to respond to 100 to 300 mg of thalidomide daily. Mucocutaneous lesions respond well; however, ocular lesions may be recalcitrant to treatment. Recurrence on withdrawal of thalidomide is common (23).

Side Effects and Drug Interactions

The most feared adverse effect is teratogenicity. The only means to prevent this is through strict adherence to effective contraceptive methods for men and women and their respective partners. Teratogenic effects include limb malformations, ocular and external ear deformities, facial palsies, congenital heart disease, and GI tract and genitourinary anomalies. There is a reported increased mortality rate of occurring perinatally.

Peripheral neuropathy is of significant concern in patients using thalidomide. This primarily affects the sensory nerves, presenting as painful paresthesias in the hands and feet and loss of sensation in the distal limbs. It is not clearly related to daily dose or cumulative dose of the drug, but may be related to slow acetylation in some individuals (24). Motor signs such as muscle weakness may be present. It is either slow to resolve or irreversible.

Sedation is one of the most common side effects, but does improve with time.

Concurrent administration of thalidomide and barbiturates, chlorpromazine, reserpine, and alcohol will increase the activity of the latter drugs. Acetaminophen toxicity may be potentiated by coadministration with thalidomide.

Prudence should be exercised in administration of thalidomide with agents that could cause neuropathy, decrease the effectiveness of oral contraceptives, or cause somnolence.

Monitoring Guidelines

Celgene (Warren, NJ), the primary manufacturer of thalidomide in the United States, has a System for Thalidomide Education and Prescribing Safety (STEPS) program designed to monitor the use of thalidomide. This program requires extensive patient counseling regarding the risks and benefits of thalidomide and requires written informed consent signed by the patient and submitted to a national registry prior to the initiation of therapy. Women of childbearing age are required to have pregnancy tests before and during (every 2 weeks) therapy, until 4 weeks after discontinuation of thalidomide use. They are also required to use effective contraceptive measures. Only 28 days may be prescribed at a time. No refills are permitted and an authorization number may be obtained after both the physician and the patient have completed a monthly telephone survey.

Laboratory monitoring includes serum human chorionic gonadotropin as described previously, electrophysiological nerve studies at baseline and every 6 months, or more frequently if symptoms or with a greater than 30% decrease in sensory nerve action potential amplitude. Human immunodeficiency virus (HIV) RNA should be monitored at baseline, 1 month, 3 months, and every 3 months subsequently. In HIV-positive or neutropenic patients. Thalidomide should not be initiated or should be discontinued if the absolute neutrophil count (ANC) drops below 750/mm^3.

AZATHIOPRINE

Azathioprine, a purine analog, was first synthesized in 1959 by attaching an imidazole group to 6-mercaptopurine, which is an analog of hypoxanthine. *In vivo*, azathioprine is rapidly converted to its active metabolite, 6-mercaptopurine.

Drug Metabolism

Azathioprine is usually given orally. It is very well absorbed into the GI system, with more than 88% bioavailability (25). Nevertheless, a negligible quantity is excreted in urine, mandating dosage adjustments in patients with renal failure. Peak plasma level is reached after 2 hours, and the half-life elimination rate is 5 hours. Maximal immunosuppression is achieved after 8 to 12 weeks of intake. Azathioprine and 6-mercaptopurine are only partially bound to plasma proteins and are moderately dialyzable. Azathioprine can cross the placenta and is therefore contraindicated in pregnancy.

The active drug, 6-mercaptopurine, is further metabolized in three pathways (26) (Fig. 14.1). A good understanding of all three is of utmost importance, because impairment of one will affect the activity of the others. Only the first enzymatic pathway, which is catalyzed by hypoxanthine-guanine phosphoribosyltransferase (HGPRT), produces the active metabolite, a purine analog. Genetic absence of HGPRT causes Lesch–Nyhan syndrome, and patients with this syndrome are not susceptible to immunosuppression after exposure to azathioprine. The second pathway is mediated by xanthine oxidase and produces an inactive metabolite. Xanthine oxidase can be inhibited by allo-

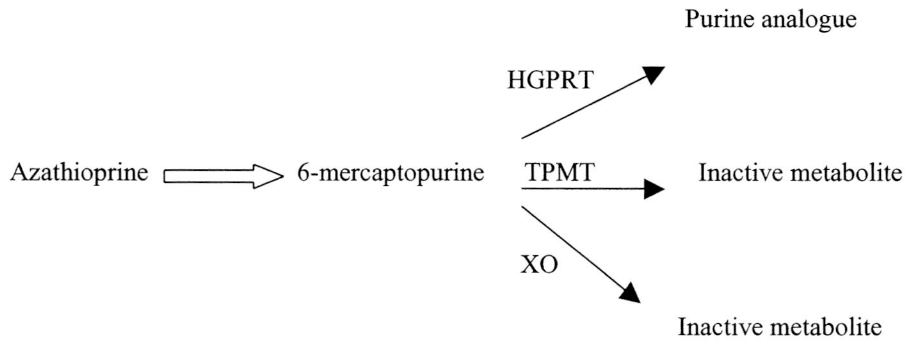

Figure 14.1. Azathioprine metabolism.

purinol. Patients treated with allopurinol may have increased immunosuppression following intake of azathioprine owing to diversion of the metabolite to the first pathway, thereby creating more active metabolite. The third pathway is mediated by thiopurine methyltransferase (TPMT) and also produces an inactive metabolite. Three mutations in the gene encoding for TPMT have been identified. Studies in white populations have shown that TPMT activity is high in 89%, moderate in 11%, and very low or absent in 0.3% (27). Patients in the latter group who take azathioprine will have extremely high levels of the active metabolite, which can lead to severe, life-threatening myelosuppression.

MECHANISM OF ACTION

The mechanism of action of azathioprine is not fully understood. Its active metabolite, 6-thioguanine, which is formed by the HGPRT pathway, is a purine analog that inhibits the synthesis and repair mechanism of DNA and RNA. It contains a thiol group that is attached to guanine. The similarity of 6-thioguanine to guanine allows for the incorporation of 6-thioguanine in DNA and RNA and prevents cell division. The reason for its particular affinity for B- and T-lymphocytes, which is responsible for the drug's immunosuppressive ability, remains obscure.

Clinical Indications and Dosage

The FDA approved the use of azathioprine for organ transplantation and severe rheumatoid arthritis. The dermatologic uses of azathioprine are all off-label. Dermatologic diseases that reportedly benefit from azathioprine include vasculitis, connective tissue diseases, and Behçet disease. CBC and liver function tests must be performed at baseline, before therapy, to detect cytopenias during therapy. The recommended initial dosage is 1 to 2 mg/kg daily, which can be increased to a maximum of 5 mg/kg daily. The narrow therapeutic window of all immunosuppressive agents necessitates dosage adjustment according to ideal body weight and not the patient's actual weight.

Side Effects and Drug Interactions

The major and most worrisome side effect of azathioprine is myelosuppression, which usually manifests as leukopenia, although thrombocytopenia and anemia have been reported. This adverse reaction is relatively rare, occurring mainly in patients very low or absent TPMT activity. Cessation of the drug on findings of cytopenias may prevent life-threatening events. A recent pharmaco-economic analysis based on a target case has suggested that pretreatment screening for *TPMT* mutations will reduce the risk of myelosuppression and may be cost effective (28). Other possible side effects of azathioprine are toxic hepatitis, pancreatitis, hypersensitivity syndrome (azathioprine-induced shock), and drug fever (29–31). Many patients suffer from mild GI distress. Patients taking azathioprine are at increased risk of opportunistic infections as well as future malignancy. The most important drug interaction is with allopurinol, as explained in the drug metabolism section. In addition, patients taking concurrent azathioprine and warfarin may need an increased dosage of warfarin. The combination of azathioprine and captopril may induce severe anemia or pancytopenia and should be avoided.

Monitoring Guidelines

CBC and liver and kidney function tests should be performed at baseline, before treatment. Screening for *TPMT* mutation is advisable where possible. During treatment, CBC and liver function tests should be performed weekly for the first month, bimonthly to monthly for the next 3 months, and every 2 months thereafter.

MYCOPHENOLATE MOFETIL

Mycophenolate mofetil (MMF), the 2-morpholinoethyl ester of mycophenolic acid (MPA), which is the active compound. MMF was originally isolated from a fermentation product of *Penicillium* species. It was used in the 1970s to successfully treat severe psoriasis, but concerns regarding a possible carcinogenetic effect and an increased incidence of herpes zoster led to its discontinuation (32). Today, the esterified reformulated product is widely used as an immunosuppressive agent in patients after kidney transplantation. Its use in dermatology is becoming more prevalent.

Drug Metabolism

MMF is rapidly absorbed and completely hydrolyzed to form its active ingredient, MPA. As opposed to MPA, the drug has an excellent bioavailability. In the liver, it is inactivated by the hepatic enzyme glucuronyl transferase and subsequently reactivated within the epidermis and GI tract by β-glucuronidase. Peak plasma level is reached after less than an hour, with a half-life elimination rate of 18 hours. Another reactivation pathway in the liver itself causes secondary plasma peaks 6 to 12 hours after administration (32). Optimal immunosuppression is achieved after 8 to 12 weeks of intake. Most of the drug (87%) is excreted in the urine as the inactive phenolic glucuronide of MPA.

MECHANISM OF ACTION

MPA is a selective and noncompetitive inhibitor of inosine monophosphate dehydrogenase (IMPDH), a key enzyme in the *de novo* synthesis of purine. It blocks the conversion of inosine-5-phosphate and xanthine-5-phosphate to guanosine-5-phosphate. This inhibits the proliferation of B- and T-lymphocytes, which relies more on the *de novo* than the salvage pathway for synthesis of purine, and antibody synthesis (32). In addition, MMF blocks the glycosylation of adhesion molecules, thereby inhibiting leukocyte recruitment and adhesion to endothelial cells (33).

Clinical Indications and Dosage

The FDA has approved MMF for the immunosuppression of patients after organ transplantation. All dermatologic uses of MMF are off-label. It is prescribed for DLE; particular success may be seen in palmoplantar and lupus pernio variants. Dermatomyositis sine myositis responds very well to MMF (34). There may an allergic reaction; thus, MMF is contraindicated in patients with known hypersensitivity to the drug or one of its compounds. MMF has been shown to have teratogenic effects in animals and should not be used in pregnancy unless the benefits clearly outweigh the possible risks. Severe neutropenia has been reported in 2% to 4% of patients after organ transplantation, but this is a rare complication in dermatology patients.

Although the recommended dosage of MMF for renal transplant recipients is 30 mg/kg daily, 35 to 45 mg/kg daily may be necessary to achieve remission in dermatologic diseases. This is likely due to concomitant treatment of transplant recipients with multiple immunosuppressive agents such as cyclosporine or tacrolimus, which act synergistically with

MMF, but also increases the incidence of significant side effects. MMF in dermatologic disorders is typically used in combination only with CS, a combination that is additive, but not synergistic. The dosage should also be adjusted in patients with renal impairment.

It is important to emphasize to both patients and physicians that the drug has a delayed onset of action, and clinical improvement becomes apparent only after 2 to 3 months of use.

Side Effects and Drug Interactions

The most common side effects of MMF are GI disturbances. Patients may complain of abdominal cramping, nausea, and less frequently, diarrhea and vomiting, although significant GI distress is uncommon. Being an immunosuppressive agent, MMF may induce a greater susceptibility to infections and may increase the lifetime risk of lymphoma. The risk of lymphoproliferative disease with MMF treatment is unknown, but is likely low. Other, less common, side effects are genitourinary disturbances, such as burning sensation, urgency, frequency, and sterile pyuria (but not nephrotoxicity), and neurologic symptoms, such as fatigue, weakness, headache, tinnitus, and insomnia. In summary, the safety profile of MMF is high, with clinically insignificant side effects. Most of the side effects are dose-dependent and, the most common GI disturbances tend to subside with time. No idiosyncratic reactions are documented.

MMF has reduced absorption when administered with antacids containing magnesium and aluminum hydroxide; their simultaneous administration should therefore be avoided if possible. Live vaccines should be avoided during drug intake as well.

Monitoring Guidelines

The recommended baseline laboratory tests include CBC and liver and kidney function tests. During treatment, CBC should be done weekly for the first month, twice monthly for the second and third months, and then monthly throughout the first year.

CYCLOPHOSPHAMIDE

Cyclophosphamide is an alkylating agent derived from nitrogen mustard.

Drug Metabolism

Cyclophosphamide is metabolized into phosphoramide mustard and acrolein by hepatic enzymes. Oxidative enzymes are required to detoxify phosphoramide mustard, which is the more toxic compound.

MECHANISM OF ACTION

Cyclophosphamide inhibits DNA replication and therefore acts preferentially in cells that are rapidly dividing. B cells are preferentially affected over T cells. Tumor cells contain lower levels of the oxidative enzymes that are needed to detoxify phosphoramide mustard than normal cells, making this an effective chemotherapeutic agent.

Clinical Indications and Dosage

Cyclophosphamide may be administered either as a pulsed intravenous monthly dosage (0.5 to 1.5 g/m^2) or oral low dosage daily (2 to 3 mg/kg) when used as a standard immunosuppressive agent. The typical treatment course lasts 18 to 24 months (35).

There are certain protocols in which bone marrow ablation is achieved by high-dose intravenous cyclophosphamide administration (36). The principle behind this treatment is that stem cells are refractory to cell death by cyclophosphamide due to high levels of aldehyde dehydrogenase, but other bone marrow–derived cells are not. Consequently, after death of the other cells, the stem cells can repopulate the marrow.

The most common uses for daily or pulse cyclophosphamide are in the treatment of severe SLE and in medium-sized vessel vasculitis, such as polyarteritis nodosa, rheumatoid vasculitis, Wegner granulomatosis, and Churg–Strauss syndrome, which is refractory to treatment with azathioprine in combination with oral CSs. Cyclophosphamide treatment of scleroderma with pulmonary inflammation has been shown to have a beneficial effect on pulmonary function and overall survival of patients (37).

Side Effects and Drug Interactions

The most concerning acute side effects include hemorrhagic cystitis and leukopenia. The risk of hemorrhagic cystitis may be reduced by administration of intravenous mesna, which binds acrolein, the substance responsible for the cystitis (38). Additionally, patients should be advised to take the full dose of cyclophosphamide in the morning with at least 48 oz of water. The nadir of leukopenia following pulse-dose cyclophosphamide occurs 10 to 12 days after administration.

Long-term adverse effects include increased risk of bladder cancer with oral cyclophosphamide administration and increased risk of lymphoma with daily oral cyclophosphamide use. Bladder cancer may occur several decades after cyclophosphamide administration. Premature ovarian failure, azospermia, and teratogenic effects are well recognized. Less severe side effects include nausea and vomiting, alopecia (anagen effluvium), and photo-induced hyperpigmentation of skin and nails.

Cyclophosphamide should not be administered with other bone marrow suppressants such as allopurinol or zidovudine. Coadministration with doxorubicin increases chances of hemorrhagic cystitis. Administration of succinylcholine and cytoxan may lead to prolonged neuromuscular blockade.

Monitoring Guidelines

Baseline CBC, urinalysis, blood urea nitrogen level, creatinine level, and liver function tests should precede administration of daily oral cyclophosphamide. Urinalysis and CBC should be checked weekly for the first month and biweekly for the next 2 months. If the laboratory results remain normal, they may be monitored on a monthly basis thereafter. Women of childbearing age require monthly human chorionic gonadotropin levels. With pulse-dose cyclophosphamide administration, CBC should be monitored 10 days after the administration of the medication. ANC below 1,500 should prompt temporary discontinuation of the medication with weekly monitoring of the CBC. Once the ANC is greater than 3,000 the medication may be reinitiated at a lower dosage with weekly monitoring of the CBC. In cases of severe leukopenia or thrombocytopenia, filgrastim or pegfilgrastim may be administered. Even after discontinuation of cyclophosphamide, urinalysis must be monitored approximately every 3 months for life (38).

Prophylaxis for patients on cyclophosphamide includes trimethoprim–sulfamethoxazole double strength three times weekly for *Pneumocystis carinii* pneumonia prophylaxis, pneumonia vaccination, influenza vaccination, and revaccination with diphtheria and tetanus vaccines if titers are low.

INTRAVENOUS IMMUNOGLOBULIN

IVIG is pooled from plasma of healthy donors, as many as 3,000 to 10,000 donors. Commercially obtained immunoglobulins consist primarily of IgG, but have trace amounts of IgA, cytokines, and soluble CD4, CD8, and HLA. IVIG has been used in many inflammatory diseases that are mediated by autoantibodies or immune complexes. Anecdotal successes have been reported; however, conclusive data from controlled clinical trials are lacking for many conditions (39).

Drug Metabolism/Mechanism of Action

The mechanism of action of IVIG is controversial, but there are several proposed mechanisms. Fc receptor blockade, the presence of antiidiotype antibodies, and effects on cytokines, cytokine receptors, and complement. A relatively new theory proposes that an intracellular receptor FcRn (Fc receptor of the neonate), of which α_2-microglobulin is an essential component, is essential in immunoglobulin metabolism. Normally the FcRn binds to immunoglobulin, which has been pinocytosed. This is then recycled and released at the cell surface. If IgG is unbound, it is degraded within the lysosomes of the cell. When the system is flooded with immunoglobulin and all receptors are saturated, there will be a dose-dependent degradation of immunoglobulin. This information has been discovered using mouse models; however, a homologous protein to the mouse FcRn is present in humans (40). The half-life of IVIG is approximately 3 to 5 weeks.

Clinical Indications and Dosage

IVIG may be administered at different dosages: 0.4 g/kg per day for 4 days or 1 g/kg per day over 2 days. Treatments are usually monthly. CS-resistant dermatomyositis has been treated successfully with IVIG infusions (41). This is a fairly safe and effective treatment for those patients who have failed adequate trials of standard immunosuppressants, such as CSs, MMF, or azathioprine, with broad-spectrum sun protection and antimalarial treatment. Disadvantages of the treatment are restricted availability, hospital admission required for infusion, and great expense.

Side Effects and Drug Interactions

Fevers, chills, nausea, vomiting, and malaise are the most common responses to IVIG infusion. These symptoms occur most frequently in people with severe hypogammaglobulinemia or agammaglobulinemia who have not received IVIG previously. These reactions may be improved by decreasing the rate of infusion.

Acute renal failure may occur in patients who have preexisting renal dysfunction, patients with diabetes mellitus, or in anyone over the age of 65. This has been disproportionately associated with IVIG preparations containing sucrose. In these patients, one should be sure to assess for adequate hydration before infusion and infusion should be slow, at a rate of less than 3 mg/kg per minute. Periodic monitoring of renal function and patient education regarding signs and symptoms of renal dysfunction are essential.

Serum sickness–like reaction may occur in patients receiving IVIG. This is characterized by fever arthralgia; urticarial skin lesions, which may be purpuric; leukocytoclastic vasculitis; angioedema; lymphadenopathy; and hypocomplementemia. Hypocomplementemia is a result of activation of the complement cascade by immune complex deposition. This is thought to occur in many cases as a result of IgG antibodies directed against IgA. This situation is most common in patients with IgA deficiency, but may occur in patients who have had multiple transfusions and even in a small percentage of otherwise healthy individuals. Patients with IgA deficiency or albumin allergy may develop anaphylaxis in response to IVIG infusion.

Aseptic meningitis is a possible adverse effect seen with human IVIG infusion. It most commonly occurs with high dosage, 2 g/kg per month. It resolves within several days after discontinuation of IVIG. One study of 54 patients treated with IVIG showed that 11% developed aseptic meningitis. Of the patients with a history of migraines, 50% developed aseptic meningitis, whereas only 4% of patients without a history of migraines developed aseptic meningitis (42).

Decreased response to live attenuated vaccines has been noted in patients receiving IVIG (43).

LEFLUNOMIDE

Leflunomide is a new immunomodulatory agent that inhibits the proliferation of B- and T-lymphocytes. This drug has a special importance due to its unique mechanism of both inhibition of the biosynthesis of the pyrimidines as well as cytokines.

Drug Metabolism

Leflunomide is metabolized to its major active form, A77 1726 (M1), and other minor active metabolites. The exact location of its metabolism is not clear. The M1 metabolite has a bioavailability of 80%. The time to peak plasma concentration is 6 to 12 hours, and the half-life is 14 days. Forty-three percent of the drug is eliminated in the urine and 48% in the feces.

MECHANISM OF ACTION

Leflunomide acts primarily via two pathways. The first involves the noncompetitive and reversible inhibition of dihydroorotate dehydrogenase (DHODH), a key enzyme in the *de novo* biosynthesis of the pyrimidines. As a result, p53 is translocated to the cell nucleus, arresting the cells in the G_1 phase. B- and T-lymphocytes, which rely mostly on the *de novo* synthesis of pyrimidines, are especially affected. In the second pathway, the tyrosine kinases involved in signal transduction pathways are inhibited by higher dosages of the drug (44). The inhibition of JAK3 tyrosine phosphorylation and STAT6 tyrosine phosphorylation reduces the production of IL-4 and thus inhibiting complex mechanisms induced by this cytokine including the production of IgG1 (45).

Other possible actions of leflunomide seem to be less important. It increases the messenger RNA level of IL-10 receptor, decreases IL-8 messenger RNA concentrations, and blocks the activation of TNF-dependent nuclear factors (46).

Clinical Indications and Dosage

Leflunomide has been used successfully in the treatment of rheumatoid arthritis. The recommended dosage is 20 mg per day. Some researchers propose starting with a loading dosage of 1.4 mg/kg daily for 3 days, followed by 0.3 mg/kg daily (>20 mg daily) (44), although higher doses may be necessary in T_H2-mediated diseases. The drug has been found to be teratogenic in laboratory animals and is contraindicated in pregnancy. The long half-life of the drug (14 days) in this context is very important and in young women who wish to conceive, cholestyramine is needed for complete washout. Drug interactions exist with methotrexate (induces hepatotoxicity), rifampin (increases the plasma level of leflunomide), and cholestyramine (inhibits leflunomide absorption).

Side Effects and Drug Interactions

Common side effects of leflunomide include elevation of liver enzymes, anemia, GI symptoms with transient diarrhea, morbilliform drug eruption, and alopecia (47). The liver enzyme levels usually increase less than twofold and normalize with dose reduction. If they are elevated more than threefold, the drug should be discontinued and replaced with cholestyramine.

Monitoring Guidelines

The recommended baseline laboratory tests include CBC and liver function tests. During treatment, CBCs and liver function tests should be done monthly, as well as regular monitoring of blood pressure.

METHOTREXATE

Methotrexate is an irreversible dihydrofolate reductase inhibitor. Methotrexate is commonly used in the treatment of psoriasis, psoriatic arthritis, rheumatoid arthritis, and Reiter syndrome and has more recently been found to be a steroid-sparing agent in dermatomyositis.

Drug Metabolism

Methotrexate is generally well absorbed with a mean bioavailability of 67%. Fifty percent to 60% binds to plasma proteins. It is metabolized to a weakly active compound in the liver and is renally excreted. Its serum half-life is 6 to 7 hours, but it may act longer because it is retained in the tissue.

MECHANISM OF ACTION

Methotrexate inhibits the enzyme dihydrofolate reductase. It is a competitive inhibitor of dihydrofolate. Methotrexate most effectively blocks the synthesis of thymidylate, which is the rate-limiting step in DNA synthesis. Glutamylation of methotrexate enhances the efficacy by allowing more avid binding to dihydrofolate reductase and by allowing retention of methotrexate within cells, increasing the concentration at its target. Methotrexate decreases epidermal and mononuclear cell proliferation, inhibits response to IL-2, decreases chemotaxis by both monocytes and neutrophils, and impairs Langerhans cell activity. It is now thought that many of methotrexate's antiinflammatory effects may be mediated by adenosine (48).

Clinical Indications and Dosage

Methotrexate is most often used in psoriatic arthritis (49), rheumatoid arthritis (50), and dermatomyositis (51) as a steroid-sparing agent. Dosages range from 7.5 mg to 30 mg per week. Methotrexate may be administered in one dose either orally, intramuscularly, intravenously, or subcutaneously or may be given in three divided doses 12 hours apart orally. All patients receiving methotrexate should also receive daily folic acid, 1 mg. Daily dosing causes a higher rate of side effects and is therefore no longer used.

Side Effects and Drug Interactions

Methotrexate has two concerning adverse reactions. The first is an idiosyncratic reaction causing bone marrow suppression, leading to primarily neutropenia, but can result in pancytopenia. To prevent this reaction, patients should be given a test dosage of 2.5 mg initially. A CBC should be checked at baseline and 3 days later. If significant drop in white blood cell count is noted, the patient should be closely monitored because the maximal suppression occurs at 7 to 10 days after the dose is given. Leukovorin may be administered orally or parenterally to counteract the effects of myelosuppression. In cases of renal insufficiency or overdose by the patient with resulting toxic serum levels of methotrexate, leukovorin should be administered every 6 hours until the methotrexate level is below 1×10^{-8} mol/L. If methotrexate toxicity is suspected, it is wise to administer an oral dose of leukovorin immediately, even before admission to a hospital for parenteral administration.

Drugs decreasing renal clearance of methotrexate should be avoided. These include: nonsteroidal antiinflammatory drugs, colchicine, sulfonamides, penicillins, and any potentially nephrotoxic drug (i.e., cyclosporine or aminoglycosides). Drugs that displace methotrexate from proteins in the serum include phenytoin, barbiturates, sulfonamides, sulfonylureas, tetracyclines, sulfonylureas, retinoids, salicylates, and others. Drugs causing hepatotoxicity should be avoided as well (e.g., ethanol, retinoids). Trimethoprim–sulfamethoxazole is absolutely contraindicated while taking methotrexate due to synergistic toxicity: Both drugs target the same biochemical pathway.

Hepatotoxicity is a well-known and concerning side effect of methotrexate treatment. Certain patients are at higher risk for hepatotoxicity. The following risk factors are listed in order of importance: history of excessive alcohol consumption, persistently elevated liver function tests, hepatitis, cirrhosis, family history of genetic hepatic disease, diabetes mellitus, obesity, and exposure to hepatotoxic drugs.

Pulmonary fibrosis has been reported in patients treated with methotrexate, particularly in those with rheumatoid arthritis. It has not been seen in patients treated for psoriasis (52) and has not been reported in patients with dermatomyositis treated with methotrexate.

Other reactions include nausea, vomiting, ulcerative stomatitis, megaloblastic anemia, alopecia, drug eruptions, reactivation of phototoxicity, impaired fertility, and teratogenicity.

Monitoring Guidelines

Baseline evaluation includes CBC, liver function tests, renal function tests with urinalysis, blood urea nitrogen, creatinine, creatinine clearance, folate level, and pregnancy test in women, and hepatitis A, B, C, and HIV serologies. Purified protein derivative testing may be considered as well. Patients with impaired hepatic or renal function, pregnant or nursing mothers, and patients with hepatitis or HIV or other active infectious process should not be started on methotrexate.

CBC should be repeated 3 days and 1 week after the test dose is administered and biweekly for the first 3 months. Thereafter, it may be checked monthly along with liver function tests and renal function tests.

The consensus conference for methotrexate in psoriasis established a set of recommendations to guide decisions regarding appropriate timing for liver biopsy. In patients without risk factors, the first liver biopsy may be done after a total dosage of 1.0 to 1.5 g. In patients with risk factors, biopsy should be done early in the treatment course and repeated at 1- to 1.5-g intervals. The biopsy may be postponed for several months, until the determination is made whether the patient will commit to long-term therapy with methotrexate, but it should be performed within the first 4 months (49).

DAPSONE

Dapsone is a sulfone that is frequently used in the treatment of neutrophilic dermatoses, and less frequently as a steroid-sparing agent in conditions, such as dermatomyositis or less often, SLE.

Drug Metabolism

Dapsone is well, but slowly absorbed. It is largely protein bound. Its half-life may range from 14 to 83 hours. Dapsone is acetylated in the liver and within erythrocytes. It is further hydroxylated and conjugated with glucuronic acid and 90% is renally excreted. The remaining 10% may persist in the body for up to 35 days as a result of extensive protein binding and enterohepatic circulation.

MECHANISM OF ACTION

Antiinflammatory activity of dapsone is particularly effective against diseases mediated by neutrophils. Dapsone is effective in scavenging reactive oxygen species, which are frequently generated following neutrophil activation. Dapsone also inhibits the myeloperoxidase–peroxide–halide system of neutrophils. Dapsone inhibits prostaglandin D_2 production and glutathione reduction. It also inhibits neutrophil chemotaxis.

Clinical Indications and Dosage

The best evidence for use of dapsone is in neutrophil-mediated dermatoses including PG, erythema elevatum diutinum, vasculitis, and Sweet syndrome. It has also been used with some success as a steroid-sparing agent in autoimmune diseases such as relapsing polychondritis and dermatomyositis.

Typical dosage of dapsone is 50 to 200 mg per day. However, some conditions, such as PG, may require higher doses of up to 300 mg daily to adequately control the disease.

Side Effects and Drug Interactions

Dapsone has several major side effects: hemolytic anemia, methemoglobinemia, agranulocytosis, and dapsone hypersensitivity syndrome. Virtually all patients develop a dose-dependent hemolytic anemia and mild methemoglobinemia as a result of a hydroxylamine metabolite of dapsone. Patients who are G6PDH-deficient, often either of Mediterranean or African heritage, may develop severe hemolysis. Dosages of dapsone should not exceed 1.5 mg/kg daily or 100 mg in healthy individuals and 50 mg in patients with G6PDH deficiency to avoid excessive hemolysis. Patients with a deficiency of methemoglobin reductase or a hemoglobinopathy may develop severe methemoglobinemia even on low-dose dapsone, otherwise methemoglobinemia becomes significant only at dosages greater than 200 mg per day. Agranulocytosis is also caused by the hydroxylamine metabolite of dapsone as a result of direct bone marrow toxicity. In general, individuals who are slow acetylators are at particular risk for toxicity to dapsone.

Dapsone hypersensitivity syndrome consists of an erythematosus pruritic skin eruption comprising papules, pustules, plaques or eczematous areas, lymphadenopathy, fever, hepatosplenomegaly, and lymphocyte pleocytosis. Laboratory findings include elevated erythrocyte sedimentation rate, elevated liver function tests, and eosinophilia. This may occur from 1 to 6 weeks after initiation of dapsone therapy (53).

Neurotoxicity manifests as a sensory and motor peripheral neuropathy, which is reversible with early discontinuation of dapsone. Patients receiving high dosages of dapsone (i.e., 200 to 400 mg per day) seem to be more predisposed to neuropathy.

Clinically relevant drug interactions include trimethoprim, rifampin, pyrimethamine, cimetidine, and omeprazole.

Monitoring

Baseline testing includes a CBC with differential, reticulocyte count, liver function tests, renal function test, urinalysis, and G6PDH level. CBC with differential and reticulocyte count should be monitored every 2 weeks for 3 months, then monthly. Renal and liver function tests may be monitored every 3 to 6 months and methemoglobinemia should be checked if patient becomes symptomatic (53).

CYCLOSPORINE

Cyclosporine is a calcineurin inhibitor that prevents activation of T cells. There is little evidence supporting its use in the treatment of rheumatic diseases. It is used as a second-line therapeutic agent in relapsing polychondritis and dermatomyositis. Its most frequent use in rheumatic disease is PG, which may be associated with a variety of connective tissue diseases. It will be discussed only briefly (54).

Drug Metabolism

Cyclosporine is variably absorbed. It is excreted primarily through the biliary system, with only 6% of the dosage present in the urine. The half-life of the drug is approximately 8 hours. It is metabolized by cytochrome P450 IIIA. Consequently, there are many potential drug interactions (Table 14.4).

MECHANISM OF ACTION

The high-affinity receptor for cyclosporine is a 17-kDa immunophilin called cyclophilin A. The drug–immunophilin complex binds to calcineurin. Calcineurin is a serine/threonine protease. Calcineurin activity directly correlates with IL-2 production. Calcineurin is also involved in the induction of apoptosis and degranulation of cytotoxic T-lymphocytes. It is well established that calcineurin activation is not only a rate-limiting step but also a crucial propagating factor in calcium-dependent T-cell signaling pathways. Subsequently, calcineurin regulates the transcription factor NF-AT, which is implicated in the regulation of the cytokine-encoding genes, including the gene regulating IL-2 production. Once NF-ATc is dephosphorylated by calcineurin, the protein translocates into the nucleus where it binds NF-ATn, a nuclear AP-1 family member whose synthesis is induced by protein kinase C–dependent signals. Experimental data have shown that the cyclosporine, tacrolimus, and pimecrolimus–calcineurin complex inhibits the nuclear translocation of the NF-ATc by blocking its dephosphorylation (11).

Side Effects and Drug Interactions

Cyclosporine has many significant adverse effects. The most dangerous of these is nephrotoxicity. Care must be taken in administering cyclosporine to patients with preexisting renal dysfunction, and renal function must be closely monitored during therapy. Proper hydration status of the patient is important,

TABLE 14.4. Drug Interactions with Cyclosporine

Potentiate Renal Dysfunction	Increase Cyclosporine (Inhibit P450)	Decrease Cyclosporine (Induce P450)
Aminoglycosides	Calcium channel blockers	Nafcillin
Trimethoprim–sulfmethoxazole	Azole antifungals	Rifampin
Melphalan	Macrolide antibiotics	Phenytoin, phenobarbitol, carbamazepine
Amphotericin	Glucocorticoids	Octreotide
Azole antifungals	Allopurinol	Ticlopidine
Diclofenac, naproxen, suldinac	Bromocriptine	
Cimetidine, ranitidine	Danazol	
Tacrolimus	Metoclopramide	
	Grapefruit juice	

and care must be taken in administering medications that could potentiate renal toxicity (see Table 14.4). Other risks include hypertension, malignancy risk including increased number of cutaneous malignancies and lymphomas, hepatotoxicity, and hyperkalemia. Hirsutism and gum hyperplasia, particularly with coadministration with calcium channel blockers or anticonvulsants, are quite disturbing to the patient. Patients should not receive cyclosporine, while receiving psoralen plus UV-A therapy, UV-B therapy, or radiation, because this significantly increases the risk for cutaneous malignancies.

In addition to the drug interactions outlined in Table 14.4, cyclosporine can increase methotrexate levels by up to 30%. Cyclosporine may potentiate digitalis toxicity and myositis with concomitant lovastatin use. Additionally, seizures have been noted in patients receiving cyclosporine and high-dose methylprednisolone. Vaccines may be less effective if administered while using cyclosporine, and live vaccines should be avoided.

Monitoring Guidelines

Baseline blood pressure, potassium level, uric acid level, and magnesium level, lipid profile, and renal function tests, including creatinine, blood urea nitrogen, and urinalysis should be obtained. These should be repeated every 2 weeks for the first 3 months, and then may be reevaluated on a monthly basis. Additionally, the cyclosporine level should be monitored on a weekly basis until a stable therapeutic level is reached, then may be monitored monthly. Weekly monitoring of trough level is prudent with dosage changes or when initiating medications known to interact with cyclosporine.

If patients develop hypertension or a rise in creatinine level 25% above baseline, cyclosporine dose should be reduced 25% to 50%. These parameters should be reevaluated every 2 weeks until they normalize. If the creatinine level does not return to within 25% of the patient's baseline creatinine level after two dose adjustments, cyclosporine should be discontinued. If hypertension cannot be controlled with antihypertensive medications, cyclosporine should be discontinued.

TUMOR NECROSIS FACTOR INHIBITORS

TNF inhibitors are exciting new agents that specifically target one cytokine within the inflammatory cascade. Currently there are two FDA-approved agents, infliximab and etanercept (55). These have been used in the treatment of rheumatoid arthritis and psoriatic arthritis. Case reports regarding their use in inflammatory skin disease abound, but there are no reliable clinical trials as of yet. Nonetheless, these are exciting biologic agents that may prove to be invaluable tools in the dermatologist's armamentarium in the future.

Drug Metabolism

Infliximab is a chimeric antibody engineered against the TNF-α receptor, both soluble and membrane-bound forms. It can also bind to a receptor already bound to a TNF molecule. It contains a human constant region and a mouse variable region. This is a recombinant protein produced by a cell line. Its half-life is 8 to 10 days. Maximal effect was seen between weeks two and four (55).

Etanercept is a fusion protein of the extracellular ligand-binding portion of the p75 TNF receptor and the constant domain of IgG1. Etanercept binds to only soluble TNF-α, preventing its binding to and activation of TNF receptors.

Clinical Indications and Dosage

Infliximab is administered intravenously. Dosage is 3 to 5 mg/kg. Typically, after the first dose, subsequent doses are administered at 2 weeks, 6 weeks, and every 8 weeks thereafter. In patients with rheumatoid arthritis, it is usually administered with methotrexate (56).

Etanercept is administered 25 mg subcutaneously twice weekly. It is currently approved for the treatment of rheumatoid arthritis. Nonsteroidal antiinflammatory drugs and methotrexate may be continued while receiving etanercept.

Side Effects and Drug Interactions

The most prominent side effects of infliximab are infusion reactions including fever, chills, pruritus, and urticaria; cardiopulmonary symptoms develop in 1% of patients. Only 2% discontinued infliximab due to adverse reactions. There are rare reports of fatal infections, including one case (57) of disseminated tuberculosis and one case of disseminated coccidioidomycosis. Both these patients were receiving concurrent immunosuppression with other drugs. Three of 428 patients developed a lupus-like syndrome, which resolved with discontinuation of therapy.

The most common side effects seen with etanercept include fever, chills, skin eruption, and cough, and an injection-site reaction (37%). More serious side effects include infection, most commonly upper respiratory; however, there have been reported cases of sepsis and death, primarily in patients with comorbid conditions other than rheumatoid arthritis, making them more susceptible to infection.

REFERENCES

1. Allenby CF, Main RA, Marsden RA, et al. Effect on adrenal function of topically applied clobetasol propionate (Dermovate). *Br Med J* 1975;4:619–621.
2. Ohman EM, Rogers S, Meenan FO, et al. Adrenal suppression following low-dose topical clobetasol propionate. *J R Soc Med* 1987;80:422–424.
3. Ko DH, Heiman AS, Hudson CE, et al. New steroidal anti-inflammatory

antedrugs: methyl 3,20-dioxo-9α-fluoro-11β, 17a,21-trihydroxy-1,4-pregnadiene-16α-carboxylate and its 21-O-acyl derivatives. *Steroids* 2002;67: 211–219.
4. Golan TD, Foltyn V, Roueff A. Increased susceptibility to *in vitro* ultraviolet B radiation in fibroblasts and lymphocytes cultured from systemic lupus erythematosus patients. *Clin Immunol Immunopathol* 1991;58:289–304.
5. Lehmann P, Holzle E, Kind P, et al. Experimental reproduction of skin lesions in lupus erythematosus by UVA and UVB radiation. *J Am Acad Dermatol* 1990; 22:181–187.
6. Cheong Wk, Hughes GR, Norris PG, et al. Cutaneous photosensitivity in dermatomyositis. *Br J Dermatol* 1994;131:205–208.
7. Sontheimer RD. Photoimmunology of lupus erythematosus and dermatomyositis: a speculative review. *Photochem Photobiol* 1996;63:583–594.
8. Stege H, Budde MA, Grether-Beck S, et al. Evaluation of the capacity of sunscreens to photoprotect lupus erythematosus patients by employing the photoprovocation test. *Photodermatol Photoimmunol Photomed* 2000;16:256–259.
9. Cook N, Freeman S. Report of 19 cases of photoallergic contact dermatitis to sunscreens seen at the Skin and Cancer Foundation. *Australas J Dermatol* 2001; 42:257–259.
10. Lenique P, Machet L, Vaillant L, et al. Contact and photocontact allergy to oxybenzone. *Contact Dermatitis* 1992;26:177–181.
11. Nghiem P, Pearson G, Langley RG. Tacrolimus and pimecrolimus: from clever prokaryotes to inhibiting calcineurin and treating atopic dermatitis. *J Am Acad Dermatol* 2002;46:228–241.
12. Yoshimasu T, Ohtani T, Sakamoto, T, et al. Topical FK506 (tacrolimus) therapy for facial erythematous lesions of cutaneous lupus erythematosus and dermatomyositis. *Eur J Dermatol* 2002;12:50–52.
13. Allen A, Siegfried E, Silverman R, et al. Significant absorption of topical tacrolimus in 3 patients with Netherton syndrome. *Arch Dermatol* 2001;137: 747–750.
14. Brogan IJ, Murray IA, Cerillo G, et al. Interaction of glucocorticoids receptor isoforms with transcription factors AP-1 and NFκB: lack of effect of glucocorticoid receptor β. *Molec Cell Endocrinol* 1999;157:95–104.
15. Baraniuk JN. Molecular actions of glucocorticoids: an introduction. *J Allergy Clin Immunol* 1996;97(1 Pt 2):141–142.
16. Fauci A, Wolff S. Wegener's granulomatosis: studies in 18 patients and a review of the literature. *Medicine* 1973;52:535–561.
17. Hricik DE. Steroid withdrawal in renal transplant recipients: pro point of view. *Transplant Proc* 1998;30:1380–1382.
18. Clowes JA, Peel N, Eastell R. Glucocorticoid-induced osteoporosis. *Curr Opin Rheumatol* 2001;13:326–332.
19. Hulley S, Furberg C, Barrett-Connor E, et al. HERS Research Group. Noncardiovascular disease outcomes during 6.8 years of hormone therapy: Heart and Estrogen/progestin Replacement Study follow-up (HERS II). *JAMA* 2002;3; 288:58–66.
20. Grady D, Herrington D, Bittner V, et al. Cardiovascular disease outcomes during 6.8 years of hormone therapy: Heart and estrogen/progestin replacement study follow-up (HERS II). *JAMA* 2002;288:49–57.
21. Recommendations for the prevention and treatment of glucocorticoid-induced osteoporosis: 2001 update: American College of Rheumatology Ad Hoc Committee on Glucocorticoid-Induced Osteoporosis. *Arthritis Rheum* 2001;44: 1496–1503.
22 Callen JP, Camisa C. Antimalarial agents. In: Wolverton SE, ed. *Comprehensive dermatologic drug therapy*, 1st ed. Philadelphia: WB Saunders, 2001:251–268.
23 Radomsky CL, Levine N. Thalidomide. *Dermatol Clin* 2001;19:87–103.
24. Hess CW, Hunzicker T, Kupfer A, et al. Thalidomide induced peripheral neuropathy: a prospective clinical neurophysiological and pharmacogenetic evaluation. *J Neurol* 1986;233:88–89.
25. Chan GL, Canafax DM, Johnson CA. The therapeutic use of azathioprine in renal transplantation. *Pharmacotherapy* 1987;7:165–177.
26. Lennard L. The clinical pharmacology of 6-mercaptopurine. *Eur J Clin Pharmacol* 1992;43:329–339.
27. Snow JL, Gibson LE. The role of genetic variation in thiopurine methyltransferase activity and the efficacy and/or side effects of azathioprine therapy in dermatologic patients. *Arch Dermatol* 1995;131:193–197.
28. Tavadia SM, Mydlarski PR, Reis MD, et al. Screening for azathioprine toxicity: a pharmacoeconomic analysis based on a target case. *J Am Acad Dermatol* 2000; 42:628–632.
29. Gross R. Hepatotoxicity of 6-mercaptopurine and azathioprine. *Mayo Clin Proc* 1994; 69:498.
30. Kawanishi H, Rudolph E, Bull FE. Azathioprine-induced acute pancreatitis. *N Engl J Med* 1973;289:357.
31. Pozniak AL, Ahern M, Blake DR. Azathioprine-induced shock. *Br Med J (Clin Res Ed)* 1981;283:1548.
32. Kitchin JE, Pomeranz MK, Pak G, et al. Rediscovering mycophenolic acid: a review of its mechanism, side effects, and potential uses. *J Am Acad Dermatol* 1997;37:445–449.
33. Nousari HC, Anhalt GJ. Immunosuppressive and immunomodulatory drugs. In: Freedberg IM, Eisen AZ, Wolff K, et al., eds. *Fitzpatrick's dermatology in general medicine*, 5th ed. New York: McGraw-Hill, 1999:2853–2868.
34. Nousari HC, Sragovich A, Kimyai-Asadi A, et al. Mycophenolate mofetil in autoimmune and inflammatory skin disorders. *J Am Acad Dermatol* 1999;40:265–268.
35. Guillevin L, Cordier JF, Lhote F, et al. A prospective, multicenter, randomized trial comparing steroids and pulse cyclophosphamide versus steroids and oral cyclophosphamide in the treatment of generalized Wegeners granulomatosis. *Arthritis Rheum* 1997;40:2187–2198.
36. Brodsky RA, Petri M, Smith BD, et al. Immunoablative high-dose cyclophosphamide without stem cell rescue for refractory severe autoimmune disease. *Ann Intern Med* 1998;129:1031–1035.
37. White B, Moore WC, Wigley FM, et al. Cyclophosphamide is associated with pulmonary function and survival benefit in patients with scleroderma and alveolitis. *Ann Intern Med* 2000;132:947–954.
38. Drake MJ, Nixon PM, Crew JP. Drug-induced bladder disorders: incidence, prevention, and management. *Drug Saf* 1998;19:45–55.
39. Ratko TA, Burnett DA, Foulke GE, et al. Recommendations for off-label use of intravenously administered immunoglobulin preparations: University Hospital Consortium Expert Panel for Off-Label Use of Polyvalent Intravenously Administered Immunoglobulin Preparations. *JAMA* 1995;273:1865–1870.
40. Yu Z, Lennon V. Mechanism of intravenous immune globulin therapy in antibody mediated autoimmune diseases. *N Engl J Med* 1999;340:227–228.
41. Dalakas MC, Illa I, Dambrosia JM, et al. A controlled trial of high dose intravenous immunoglobulin infusions as treatment for dermatomyositis. *N Engl J Med* 1993;329:1993–2000.
42. Sekul EA, Cupler EJ, Dalakas MC. Aseptic meningitis associated with high-dose intravenous immunoglobulin therapy: frequency and risk factors. *Ann Intern Med* 1994;121:259–262.
43. US Department of Health and Human Services, Public Health Service, Centers for Disease Control and Prevention. Guide to contraindications to childhood vaccinations. 2000.
44. Laan RF, van Riel PL, van de Putte LB. Leflunomide and methotrexate. *Curr Opin Rheumatol* 2001;13:159–163.
45. Siemasko K, Chong AS, Jack HM, et al. Inhibition of JAK3 and STAT6 tyrosine phosphorylation by the immunosuppressive drug leflunomide leads to a block in IgG1 production. *J Immunol* 1998;160:1581–1588.
46. Alldred A, Emery P. Leflunomide: a novel DMARD for the treatment of rheumatoid arthritis. *Exp Opin Pharmacother* 2001;2:125–137.
47. Nousari HC, Anhalt GJ. Immunosuppressive and immunomodulatory drugs. In: Freedberg IM, Eisen AZ, Wolff K, et al., eds. *Fitzpatrick's dermatology in general medicine*, 5th ed. New York: McGraw-Hill, 1999:2853–2868.
48. Seitz M. Molecular and cellular effects of methotrexate. *Curr Opin Rheumatol* 1999;11:226–232.
49. Roenigk HH, Auerbach R, Maibach H, et al. Methotrexate in psoriasis: consensus conference. *J Am Acad Dermatol* 1998;38:478–485.
50. Pisetsky DS, St Clair EW. Progress in the treatment of rheumatoid arthritis. *JAMA* 2001;286:2787–2790.
51. Zieglschmid-Adams ME, Pandya A, Cohen SB, et al. Treatment of dermatomyositis with methotrexate. *J Am Acad Dermatol* 1995;32:754–757.
52. Belzunegui J, Intxausti JJ, De Dios JR, et al. Absence of pulmonary fibrosis in patients with psoriatic arthritis treated with weekly low-dose methotrexate. *Clin Exp Rheumatol* 2001;19:727–730.
53. Zhu YI. Stiller MJ. Dapsone and sulfones in dermatology: overview and update. *J Am Acad Dermatol* 2001;45:420–433.
54. Capella GL, Casa-Alberighi OD, Finzi AF. Therapeutic concepts in clinical dermatology: cyclosporine A in immunomediated and other dermatoses. *Int J Dermatol* 2001;40:551–561.
55. Kalden JR. Emerging role of anti-tumor necrosis factor therapy in rheumatic diseases. *Arthritis Res* 2002;4:S34–S40.
56. Blumenauer B, Judd M, Wells G, et al. Infliximab for the treatment of rheumatoid arthritis [review]. *Cochrane Database Syst Rev* 2002;3:CD003785.
57. Maini R, St. Clair EW, Breedveld F, et al. Infliximab (chimeric anti-tumor necrosis factor alpha monoclonal antibody) versus placebo in rheumatoid arthritis patients. ATTRACT Study Group. Lancet. 1999 Dec 4;354(9194): 1932–1939.

Subject Index

NOTE: A *t* following a page number indicates tabular material and an *f* following a page number indicates a figure. Drugs are listed under their generic names. When a drug trade name is listed, the reader is referred to the generic name.

B

I

N

Q

R

T